Intravenous Medications
A Guide to Preparation,
Administration and
Nursing Management

Diane Proctor Sager, R.N., M.S.N.

*Formerly Clinical Specialist in Medical Nursing
at the District of Columbia General Hospital,
Washington, D.C. Presently in private practice*

Suzanne Kovarovic Bomar, R.N., M.S.N.

*Formerly Clinical Specialist in Medical Nursing
and Critical Care at the District of Columbia General
Hospital, Washington, D.C.*

SPECIAL CONSULTANT:

Joseph G. Barbaccia, Pharm.D.

*Clinical Pharmacist,
Washington Hospital Center,
Washington, D.C.*

PHOTOGRAPHY BY
Michael A. Stein

Intravenous Medications

A guide to preparation, administration and nursing management

J. B. Lippincott Company   Philadelphia • Toronto

ISBN 0-397-54325-5

Library of Congress Catalog Card Number 79-28541
Printed in the United States of America
9 8 7 6 5 4 3 2 1

Library of Congress Cataloging in Publication Data

Sager, Diane Proctor.
    Intravenous medications.

    Includes bibliographical references and index.
    1. Intravenous therapy. 2. Injections, Intravenous. 3.
Nursing. I. Bomar, Suzanne Kovarovic, joint author. II.
Title. [DNLM: 1. Infusions, Parenteral. 2. Parenteral
feeding. WB354 S129i]
RM170.S23   615.8'55   79-28541
ISBN 0-397-54325-5

Note to the Reader

Dosages of the drugs included in this text are the manufacturer's suggestions, except where indicated, and are up to date to the time of printing. As with other aspects of the practice of medicine and nursing, the dosages of drugs are constantly subject to change. Therefore the reader is advised to consult the package insert of all drugs administered for the latest information.

Dedication

In memory of my beloved sister Elaine,
To David for his limitless patience, support and love,
And
To my parents who were always there.

D.P.S.

To Lamar, without whose untiring patience and steadfast encouragement this book could never have been written.

S.K.B.

Preface

In recent years, the number of drugs that are intended for intravenous use has been growing at an ever-increasing rate. More and more responsibility for the administration of these drugs has been delegated to the nurse, making it mandatory for her to increase her skills and knowledge in order to safeguard the patient and to fulfill legal requirements. Three years ago it became apparent to us that there was a need for a reference on intravenous medications that would contain all information needed to correctly prepare and administer these drugs. Until this time, information was scattered in various references, and was difficult to obtain and use, especially by the nurse practicing on a busy hospital unit. A colleague, Judith Beasley, a clinical supervisor on the surgical division of our hospital, began developing such a composite reference for use on our nursing units. With her permission, ideas and encouragement, we took this concept, expanded it and developed it into what we consider to be the most complete reference on intravenous equipment, techniques, management, and the drugs themselves.

During the development of this reference, we have kept in mind the student and the experienced nurse clinician who insert and maintain intravenous lines and who prepare and administer medications. The drugs were our primary focus in the early stages. However, since drug administration is dependent upon an access to the venous system, we felt that the inclusion of material on insertion techniques and maintenance of the intravenous line would make the reference more useful. This text should not be considered as an intravenous therapy text, however. Detailed material on phlebotomy, total parenteral nutrition, fluid and electrolyte balance and other specific topics was not included, except where it related to more general topics such as infection control. Despite this format, intravenous therapists and other medical and paramedical practitioners such as medical students, pharmacists, and physicians should certainly find this material useful.

The book is divided into two parts. Part One describes the theories and techniques of the intravenous administration of drugs. It is essential for the nurse to have a clear understanding of the legal basis of practice. Chapter 1 places emphasis on general legal aspects of nursing practice as well as specific implications surrounding the administration of medications.

Intravenous therapy in itself can be a source of stress to the patient, and coupled with the stress of illness and hospitalization, can generate much anxiety. These and related psychological considerations are included in the text to assist the nurse in identifying problems and helping the patient cope with the stress.

Knowledge of the correct technique for the insertion of an intravenous cannula is essential not only for those responsible for performing the venipuncture, but for those involved in preparing the equipment and assisting with the insertion. Serial photographs have been included to provide a clear understanding for those who are exposed to these techniques for the first time.

Maintaining a patent intravenous line and regulating the flow rate of fluids and drugs is a major responsibility for the nurse. Because of the potential hazards, this area has been given considerable emphasis. The emergence of specific devices such as intravenous infusion pumps to insure increased accuracy in flow rate regulation, has prompted an extensive discussion on the use of such devices.

Information throughout this text is geared toward all patients, young and old. However, since there are numerous considerations which are applicable to the pediatric population, a separate chapter has been devoted to the needs of this age group.

The administration of intravenous drugs can be associated with numerous complications, some relatively minor, but others potentially lethal. The nurse, by virtue of her role in the administration of drugs, is responsible for the prevention of complications to the fullest extent possible. When unavoidable complications arise, the nurse must be able to recognize them and immediately institute remedial action. The major complications of intravenous drug therapy are discussed in depth.

To administer intravenous drugs safely and effectively, the nurse must have a solid foundation in general pharmacologic principles, as well as in aspects specific to intravenously administered drugs. Monitoring for adverse effects, including allergic reactions, is another major nursing responsibility. Measures required to insure sterility, compatibility and dosage accuracy are included. Finally, the three modes of intravenous administration are discussed with emphasis on the appropriate techniques for each.

Part Two, the Drug Information Section, presents detailed information in column form on all drugs currently approved for intravenous use. This material includes drug actions, indications, dosage (pediatric and adult), preparation and storage in-

structions, guidelines on the appropriate modes of administration, incompatibilities, contraindications, warnings, precautions to observe, adverse reactions and how to manage them, treatment of overdosage, nursing implications and suggested readings. An Introduction to Part Two gives detailed information on the use of this section.

This text represents current concepts and practices of the nursing, medical and pharmacy professions. Such concepts are supported throughout by reference to the literature of these professions. The techniques presented represent our philosophy but do not exclude the possibility of other correct approaches. It is hoped that our material has been organized and presented in a meaningful, logical and therefore useful manner, to facilitate its application in day-to-day nursing practice. We feel that this reference will be most useful when used on the nursing unit, in the medication and intravenous preparation areas.

Due to the lack of a neutral personal pronoun, the authors have arbitrarily used the pronoun "he" throughout, except in regard to the nursing profession, in which "she" is used because of the predominance of women in that population.

D.P.S.
S.K.B.

Acknowledgments

A work such as this becomes a reality only because of the support and guidance given by friends, colleagues and family. The authors gratefully acknowledge them.

W. LAMAR BOMAR, JR., M.D.

For the countless hours of medical advice; and for technical assistance with the photography for this book.

MARJORIE S. CLARK, R.N., M.S.N.

For her friendship, encouragement and suggestions.

MARILYN CRAWFORD, R.N.

For references on renal failure and anticoagulation.

BONNIE DULEY

For typing the endless pages of manuscript for this book in a superior manner.

The late LOIS A. FEDERICO, R.N., M.S.N.

For reading the materials from the drug information section, and for her valuable suggestions.

LYNN D. GORDON, R.N., M.S.N.

For her assistance in the development of materials on renal disease.

PEARLINE HANSEN, R.N.

For evaluating materials on critical care medications from the viewpoint of the experienced bedside practitioner.

GAIL LINDENBARGER, C.R.N.A.

For references on medications used in anesthesia, and for invaluable suggestions on the care of the patient receiving a neuromuscular blocking agent.

LEILANI B. McCONNELL, R.N., B.S.N.

For valued suggestions used in the early development of this book.

MAUREEN C. MAGUIRE, R.N., M.S.N., P.N.P.

For reading the pediatric portion of this book.

JUDITH R. McPHERSON, R.N., M.S.N., N.P. 'C'

For her friendship, unending moral support, and guidance throughout the writing of the work.

CASSANDRA J. MORGAN, R.N., M.S.N.

For time spent reading information on medications, and for excellent ideas on nursing care.

ALONA J. MYERS, R.N., M.A.

For her encouragement and support during the initial phases in the development of this book.

KATHLEEN A. RESCH, R.N., M.S.N., C.C.R.N.

For reading and evaluating materials on medications used in critical care, and for her beneficial recommendations and references on nursing care.

ROSALIE STARCHOK, R.N.

For her enthusiastic promotion of the ideas upon which this work is based.

MICHAEL A. STEIN

For his fine photographic work used throughout this book.

TALMAGE G. WILSON, B.S.Ph.

For assisting with references on medications during the early development of the work.

The authors also wish to extend their thanks to the many manufacturers of intravenous drugs and products, who supplied information and sample products shown in this book.

Special appreciation is expressed by the authors to Mr. David T. Miller, Managing Editor of the Nursing Department, J. B. Lippincott Company, for his invaluable advice, guidance and confidence given during the writing of this book.

Contents

Appendix

Index

Part One

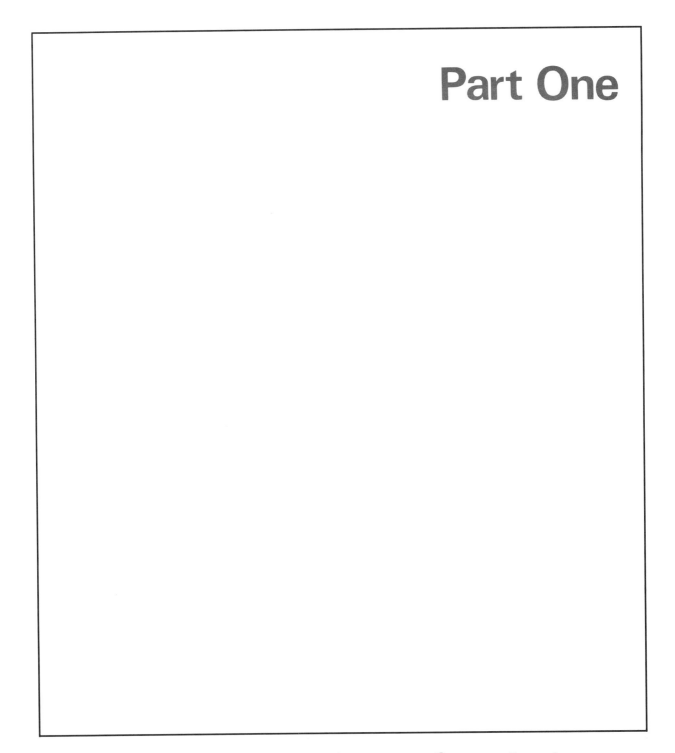

Theories and Techniques

1 The History of Intravenous Drug Therapy and Its Current Legal Implications

Intravenous drug therapy was first used in humans over three hundred years ago when, in 1662, the first successful intravenous injection was administered by J. D. Major (27). Experiments with blood transfusions were attempted a few years later, but since animal blood was used, death was a common outcome. Further experimentation stopped until the early nineteenth century when attempts were made to transfuse human blood. Because it was unmatched and unsterile, results were frequently fatal (27). Around the same time, large volumes of saline solution were infused intravenously to cholera victims by Dr. Thomas Latta (28). Although his efforts met with some success, complications including infections and death remained serious problems.

A major advance occurred near the end of the nineteenth century, when the germ theory was advanced by such individuals as Pasteur, Koch (10), and Lister. But technical limitations in the manufacture of products, along with resistance to acceptance of this principle, prevented its immediate application. Since 1923, when pyrogens were discovered and measures to eliminate them from intravenous drugs and fluids were applied, a significant reduction in complications has been seen (28).

Another twenty years passed before any major improvements were made in delivery apparatus. Prior to 1945, the only type of cannula in use was the metal needle, which was uncomfortable for the patient, was prone to infiltration, and, being nondisposable, offered a great risk of cross-contamination. In 1945, the plastic intravenous catheter was introduced (14), and since that time great improvements have been made in every aspect of intravenous equipment—from cannulae, tubing, and containers to specialized devices such as micropore filters and infusion pumps.

During most of the three hundred years of its existence, intravenous therapy, including intravenous administration of drugs, has been solely a medical function and responsibility, since until recently it was regarded as an extreme measure reserved for the most seriously ill patients. In the early 1900s, some responsibility was delegated to the nurse, but prior to World War II, the role of the nurse was confined to assisting the physician with the venipuncture and administration of fluids. As intravenous therapy became more commonplace and less hazardous, hospitals recognized the value of teaching selected nurses to perform venipuncture and related functions, such as changing fluid containers and tubing and caring for the insertion site. A pioneer in this role at Massachusetts General Hospital, Ada Lawrence Plumer, began as the sole intravenous therapist in 1940 and developed a departmental program which today has more than thirty-five intravenous therapists (17).

The concept of the intravenous therapy team has now become widely accepted, and hospitals are increasingly recognizing the merits of such a team. The primary advantage is a significant decrease in the incidence of infections and other complications associated with the procedure (3, 8). Such a reduction is due to several factors:

1. A small select group of individuals is responsible for insertion and maintenance of intravenous cannulae. This helps to insure uniformity regarding the techniques utilized. When problems arise, identifying the cause of the problem and the individual responsible is easier.
2. All members of the team are specially trained. Since they specialize in intravenous-related functions, their level of knowledge and skill pertaining to insertion and management of intravenous lines exceeds that of most other nurses and many physicians.
3. Daily inspection and care of the insertion site, changing of tubing and other equipment, and replacing the cannula at specified times (every 48 to 72 hours) are done consistently. These measures contribute significantly to the decrease in intravenous-associated infections. Early recognition of minor local problems can prevent development of systemic complications.

There is, however, one drawback inherent in the concept of the intravenous therapy team: the introduction of yet another specialist into the patient's overall care. This may be viewed by some as a throwback to the earlier functional nursing approach where different nurses were delegated the responsibilities for various aspects of care. This approach is in contrast to the more recent idea of having a primary nurse responsible for almost all an individual patient's nursing care (11).

While this concern is a valid one, it would seem to be considerably outweighed by the advantages offered by the intravenous team approach.

The responsibility for administering medications via the intravenous route has gradually become an accepted nursing function as nursing education has evolved and the scope of nursing practice has expanded. The administration of drugs in large-volume solutions via continuous infusion was the first mode of administration to be accepted as a nursing responsibility. In recent years the intermittent administration of a drug in a relatively small volume of fluid has also become a standard nursing function. The third mode of administration, that of giving the drug virtually undiluted by injection (sometimes also referred to as "IV push") has still not gained widespread acceptance as a legitimate nursing responsibility because of the added risks involved. However, exceptions are often made in specialized areas such as intensive care units and emergency departments where life-threatening situations are commonplace. In these instances nurses are generally required to have special training and to demonstrate their skill before being authorized to administer intravenous injections. (Methods, advantages and hazards of each mode are discussed in Chapter 8.)

The legal basis for all nursing duties, including intravenous therapy, is determined by several kinds of statutes and policies. These include:

1. Nursing practice acts
2. Joint policy statements
3. Specific hospital or institutional policies

These policies and acts provide legal protection for the nurse *as long as she acts correctly and within the framework they provide;* however, should the nurse fail to perform a function that is legitimately expected, perform it in an incorrect manner, or perform it outside the legal scope of nursing practice, she is liable to charges of negligence or malpractice. Although negligence and malpractice are considered synonymous by many, they are technically different, even though the line differentiating them is often hazy.

Negligence is the failure to do something which would normally be expected in a given situation. An example is the failure to monitor the infusion of a drug, such as Levophed, resulting in infiltration and subsequent extensive tissue necrosis.

Negligence also implies doing something normally performed, but in such a manner that is not generally accepted practice. An example would be giving an intramuscular injection in the wrong site, resulting in paralysis. In general, negligence usually results from *failure to use one's knowledge and skills properly* (14).

Malpractice refers to the performance of acts which are beyond the scope of accepted nursing practice. In some hospitals, for example, a nurse is not allowed to perform venipunctures. If a nurse at such an institution does draw blood or insert an intravenous cannula, she is technically guilty of malpractice should any ill effects result.

NURSING PRACTICE ACTS

Each state has a nursing practice act. While some of these do not in fact define nursing practice, most of them do, stating in broad terms those acts a nurse may and may not perform (15). Among those acts a nurse can perform is the administration of medications prescribed by a licensed physician. It may also specify as a responsibility the observation for symptoms and reactions related to such administration (24). By being rather broad, the nursing practice acts allow flexibility, yet cannot deal with specific therapeutic measures. By establishing boundaries within which the nurse may function, they distinguish nursing from the practice of medicine or pharmacy—a nurse is legally restricted to administering medications, while their preparation, compounding and dispensing is within the realm of the pharmacist. Physicians in rendering care to patients may also compound, dispense or administer medications and may direct medication to be administered by a nurse (9).

Many functions traditionally within the realm of medicine have gradually been delegated to nursing, but most of these are not specifically dealt with in nursing practice acts (15). Among these are many activities associated with intravenous drug therapy. Since they are in a "gray zone," they need amplification and clarification for legal purposes.

JOINT POLICY STATEMENTS

One means of meeting such a need is through the issuance of policy statements by state nurses' associations. Focusing on specific therapeutic measures which have traditionally belonged in the realm of medical practice such as intravenous drug therapy, the statements are authoritative documents or position papers (2). They are issued in conjunction with at least two other organizations, including state medical societies, state hospital associations or other significant health organizations (4). Such joint issuance signifies their official endorsement. These statements, which represent a professional standard of practice rather than a law, generally include the following elements (1):

1. Definition of the therapeutic measures
2. Limitations or directions under which a nurse may act
3. Special training or preparation required
4. Need for the institution to develop a specific policy which is within the framework of the joint statement

In a survey done by Plumer in 1972, thirty-three states and the District of Columbia had issued joint policy statements pertaining to intravenous therapy, most focusing on administration of intravenous fluids and/or performance of venipuncture (17). Some also deal with intravenous administration of medications. Of the states having no such policy statement at that time, nursing responsibility regarding intravenous therapy in six states was dealt with by rulings of the state nursing association or attorney general. Rulings by an attorney general are legal *opinions* which may be tested in court. An additional four states relied on the nursing practice act as a guide. The remaining seven states had no statements or rulings. Since that time, however, additional policy statements may have been issued or revisions made in existing statements; thus it behooves each nurse to be familiar with any joint policy statement issued by the state in which she is employed. Any such statement can be obtained from the state nurses' association.

HOSPITAL OR INSTITUTIONAL POLICY

Both the nursing practice acts and joint policy statements serve only as general guides and set limits on the nurse's responsibility in the area of intravenous therapy. The final determinant of a nurse's role is the policy of the hospital or institution. While it cannot exceed the limits set by the nursing practice act or joint policy statement, a hospital can choose to clarify or place further restrictions on a nurse's actions by establishing guidelines or criteria for performance of specific functions such as intravenous therapy.

The three aspects of intravenous therapy for which guidelines or criteria for performance are essential for nursing personnel include: insertion of the intravenous line (venipuncture); preparation of admixtures; and administration of intravenous medications.

Insertion of the intravenous line

1. Individuals who may perform venipuncture must be designated. Rather than allow all members of the nursing staff to perform such functions, it is not uncommon to specify clinical areas in which nursing staff are permitted to perform venipunctures, such as critical care units and emergency departments, or to limit venipuncture to members of the intravenous therapy team.
2. Staff members who are permitted to perform venipuncture are generally required to have had specialized training and supervised practice to insure their competence.
3. A structured and comprehensive in-service training program is essential to insure standardized performance.
4. A current roster should be maintained of nurses who have completed the training and are certified to perform venipuncture and related tasks.
5. Hospitals utilizing an intravenous therapy department or team must formulate specific objectives, policies and procedures for the administration and functioning of such a service. Kimmell points out some of the considerations in the development of an intravenous therapy team (12).

Preparation of admixtures

Hospital policy should specify which department is responsible for admixture preparation. (An admixture is the addition of a drug, drugs, or a different fluid to a given fluid [see Chapter 8].) Admixture preparation is regarded by some as "compounding" and as such would fall under the scope of the pharmacist rather than the nurse (6,

9). However, the addition of drugs to intravenous fluids has evolved to become an accepted nursing role from the time of nursing's first involvement in intravenous therapy. Although a pharmacy-based admixture program is preferable (see Chapter 8), the staffing patterns of many hospital and other health care institutions do not currently allow a pharmacy-based program. Nursing involvement, therefore, is mandatory to guarantee that the patients receive the needed therapy (4). When nurses are responsible for admixture preparation, it should be governed by a specific policy and detailed procedures emphasizing adherence to aseptic technique, avoidance of incompatibilities and correct preparation of drugs.

Even in institutions where the nursing staff is responsible for adding drugs to intravenous fluids, complex admixtures such as total parenteral nutrition (TPN) solutions are often prepared by the pharmacy. TPN solution preparation tends to be a compounding function because of the *number* and *volume* of additives involved.

Intravenous administration of drugs

Regardless of the system utilized for insertion of the intravenous line and preparation of admixtures, in most institutions the administration of some medications via the intravenous route has become an accepted nursing role. However, because of the hazards associated with specific drugs and the increased risk attendant upon certain modes of administration (injection versus continuous or intermittent infusion), a policy formulated by the hospital administration and nursing service must delineate all limitations and exceptions.

It is essential that the policy list all categories of drugs or specific drugs which are limited to administration by physicians. Certain antineoplastic agents, particularly those given intra-arterially, and experimental drugs might well be included among these. Nurses working on an oncology unit or clinic might be exempted from this restriction if they have been given specialized training and have demonstrated their knowledge and skill.

The modes of intravenous administration allowed and those restricted must also be specified. Nurses are generally permitted to administer drugs by infusion since this involves addition of the drug to a certain volume of solution. The resulting dilution of the drug and relatively slow rate of administration (usually over 30 minutes to several hours) decrease the likelihood of complications. Should any adverse reaction be noted, the infusion can be interrupted immediately before the remainder of the drug has been infused, and more serious reactions can be prevented. However, an intravenous injection which involves administering the drug in a virtually undiluted form directly into the vein is potentially more hazardous. Since the total dose is injected over a short period of time (ranging from instantaneously to over several minutes), adverse reactions may occur with equal rapidity. Once the drug has been administered it obviously cannot be recalled. For this reason, this mode of administration has usually been reserved for the physician.

In recent years exceptions have been made for specific drugs or clinical situations. Heparin, for example, is now routinely injected by nurses. In critical care units, drugs such as lidocaine and atropine are commonly administered by nurses when immediate treatment is required for cardiac arrhythmias and blocks. As with venipunctures, when selected nurses are granted the responsibility for administering specific intravenous drugs or giving drugs via intravenous injection, the institution must insure that such nurses have received the required instruction and have demonstrated their knowledge and skill and that a roster of nurses authorized to perform these functions is maintained.

To legally administer a medication prescribed by the physician, three conditions must be met: the order must be valid; the physician must be licensed; and the nurse must have an understanding of both the reason for and effect of the medication order (6). Many situations which the nurse might encounter in the intravenous administration of drugs fail to satisfy these conditions; thus these shortcomings will have legal implications.

VALIDITY OF AN ORDER

A valid medication order is one in which the drug, dose, and mode of administration are correct and appropriate for a given patient. Before carrying it out, the nurse must interpret it to insure that it is correct and that it contains precise instructions which the nurse understands. Potential problems are:

Illegible or Unclear Orders. Although a medication order may be validly written, if the nurse is unable to read and interpret it, it cannot be carried out. A nurse must never attempt to "guess" the meaning of an order. If unclear, the order should always be reconfirmed with the physician who wrote it (19).

Verbal and Telephone Orders. Most institutions have a specific policy regarding verbal and telephone orders; often they are not allowed except in emergency situations. Verbal communication, particularly via telephone, is subject to error and leaves no permanent record to check. In an emergency, when time is critical, a medication may be prescribed verbally, even by telephone (25). However, it is very important that the order be written in the patient's record as soon as time permits.

Incomplete Orders. An order may contain the drug and dose but omit the route, or in the case of intravenous medication, it might fail to specify the mode or rate of administration. Although a nurse must use her knowledge, this does not include assuming what was intended. Obtaining clarification is essential, for both safety of the patient and legal protection of the nurse.

Incorrect Orders. This problem is one of great concern to nurses who wonder whether they have the right to question a physician's order. Although in dependent functions such as intravenous drug administration the nurse is acting under the orders of a physician, she is nonetheless responsible for her own actions. Some nurses (and some physicians as well) erroneously believe that because a nurse is carrying out a treatment prescribed by a physician, the nurse is absolved from any legal responsibility if an incorrect order is carried out (15). On the contrary, the physician cannot relieve the nurse of responsibility for her actions; to carry out an order which the nurse knows to be incorrect would constitute negligence on her part (7). It is likewise illegal for the nurse to independently modify the order; even to substitute the correct dose or route. To do so would be to cross the line from nursing practice into medical practice, and should any harm result to the patient, the nurse would be guilty of malpractice. Whenever a nurse encounters an order which she believes to be wrong, the following steps should be taken:

1. Check an appropriate resource to ascertain whether the order is in fact in error. Recommendations and instructions provided by the drug manufacturer are becoming a widely accepted legal standard for drug information (26). (The drug information section in this book conforms with drug manufacturers' recommendations.) Information not only about dose range, method of preparation and mode

of administration, but also any other precautions or explicit instructions regarding use of the drug represent professional standards of care which should be followed. Failure to heed manufacturer's recommendations with resultant injury is evidence of negligence (26).

2. If the manufacturer's information confirms that the order is in error, the nurse must inform the physician. Because such a situation can create conflict between the physician and nurse, it is one which requires good nursing judgment and diplomacy. Avoid a tone of criticism or condescension; rather, provide documentation.

3. If, after reviewing the order, the physician wants it to stand as written, can the nurse give it and be freed of liability because she is under the physician's order? As mentioned above, any person (including a nurse) is responsible for the acts he or she performs and cannot be absolved by another person. To carry out an improper medication order which would be reasonably expected to result in injury is to be liable for negligence (7). The nurse must inform the physician that she cannot legally carry it out since it conflicts with the information available and thus could potentially be detrimental to the patient.

If the physician still insists that the drug be given, he may choose to prepare and administer it himself, thereby relieving the nurse of the responsibility. However, since this action may potentially harm the patient, the nurse should report the situation to the nursing supervisor for appropriate action.

LICENSED PHYSICIAN

While the nurse is obliged to carry out the valid orders of a licensed physician, what about instances in which a medication or other order is given by a nonlicensed intern or resident, medical student, or physician's assistant? Opinions differ as to whether a nurse may act under the orders of nonlicensed interns. Since their legal status varies according to the jurisdiction and institution, the nurse must be familiar with the laws that apply in the area in which she works. It is generally accepted that the nurse may not carry out orders prescribed by medical students and physician's assistants (4). And only the countersignature of a physician, denoting confirmation of the order, can authorize the nurse to carry it out.

NURSE'S UNDERSTANDING OF THE CAUSE AND EFFECT OF THE ORDER

With medication, especially one given by the intravenous route, it is of utmost importance that the nurse be familiar with the drug's actions, intended use for a particular patient, anticipated therapeutic response and potential adverse reactions (15). To administer an unfamiliar drug without obtaining information from an appropriate source would be considered negligent on the part of the nurse if administration resulted in harm to the patient. General information about the use of the drug, dosage range, mode of administration, precautions, etc., can be found in the drug literature supplied by the manufacturer or in the drug information section of this book. If, after consulting such a reference, the nurse has doubts as to the intent of the order, she is legally required to verify the order with the prescribing physician (7). The necessity for such verification is illustrated by the case of *Norton* v. *Argonaut Insurance Co.,* in which a nurse who was unfamiliar with pediatric drug preparations administered 3 cc. of *injectable* Lanoxin to a three-month-old infant, instead of using the pediatric *elixir*. The child died, and in the resultant suit the nurse was found to be negligent (4).

Another case demonstrating a nurse's negligence involved a patient receiving intravenous Levophed who was not monitored properly. The drug infiltrated, undetected, for an estimated 2 hours. This resulted in a permanent injury to the patient (*North Shore Hosp* v. *Luzi*—194 So. 2d 63) (21). In every instance in which a nurse administers medications (especially via the intravenous route), she must be able to recognize adverse reactions and know what remedial measures to take if they occur (18). Insofar as is possible, the nurse should keep abreast of new intravenous drugs by reading current nursing, medical, and pharmaceutical literature. Since the current proliferation of new drugs prevents a thorough acquaintance with all such drugs, the nurse must rely on authoritative resources which can supply essential information in a readily accessible form. Furthermore, institutions should include in their routine inservice programs a refresher course focusing on new drugs. In some institutions, the pharmacy department issues periodic newsletters with essential information about current drugs.

Not only is the nurse legally bound to be familiar with drugs which she administers, but she is likewise obligated to be skilled in the operation of any adjunctive devices required for their administration. One such device is the intravenous infusion pump, which is now in use in many hospitals. Each nurse responsible for operating such pumps must be skilled in their use and in detection of malfunction. Details regarding the use of infusion pumps are included in Chapter 5.

Although a nurse may possess the skill and knowledge needed to administer intravenous drugs safely, failure to apply such knowledge can result in harm to the patient and constitutes negligence.

Failure to Exercise Good Judgment in Administration of Intravenous Drugs or Fluids. If a nurse observes an adverse reaction to a drug, the infusion should be terminated. If infiltration or signs of phlebitis are noted, the cannula should be removed and the physician notified. Although administration of a medication represents a dependent function, the nurse is obliged to exercise independent judgment when carrying it out (23).

Administering a Drug to Which a Patient States He is Allergic. A patient may state he is allergic to a drug which has been ordered for him. If, acting on the assumption that the physician must know what the patient can safely take, the nurse proceeds to administer it, she risks both harm to the patient and legal liability. Court action was brought against a nurse who failed to heed the patient's warning of an aspirin allergy. Administration of that drug resulted in an anaphylactic reaction, but fortunately was not fatal (16). Suspicion of an allergy must *never* be disregarded, particularly with drugs given intravenously, because of the speed and severity of any reactions that occur. (A detailed discussion of drug allergies is presented in Chapter 8.)

Intravenous-Associated Infections Due to Lack of Adherence to Aseptic Practices. Not all instances of phlebitis or infections at the insertion site are preventable. Contamination can sometimes occur at the time of insertion or subsequently in spite of following correct procedures (22). However, when such infections result from a lack of reasonable care during the venipuncture or failure to inspect and clean the insertion site, the nurse can be held liable (4).

Use of Equipment Known to be Defective. While the institution is ultimately responsible for properly maintaining all equipment, especially that involved in direct patient care, each employee using the equipment shares in the responsibility. A nurse is responsible for noting any defects in equipment and reporting them to the appropriate hospital authorities. This responsibility is derived from her employment contract with the hospital (5). Single-use supplies and equipment such as intravenous cannulae, fluids, and adjunctive devices are rarely defective, but should a problem be detected, the item should not be used but rather returned to the appropriate hospital department so that it can be reported to the manufacturer, and so that it may be determined whether other items from the same lot need to be inspected.

Specialized electronic equipment which is used repeatedly, such as intravenous infusion pumps, must have preventive maintenance to insure correct functioning. The nurse must be alert to any defects, remove such equipment from use, and report it to the proper authorities. By continuing to use an infusion pump or other equipment which is known to be defective, the nurse is negligent in that she is failing to meet a legal standard of nursing care (5).

Inadequate Documentation of Intravenous Drug Therapy. Accurate written records are mandatory not only to insure continuity of care but also to provide legal evidence of all care that has been given. In documenting intravenous drug therapy it is essential to include both a record of the drugs administered (including dosage, times, rates, mode of administration, etc.) and of the infusion itself, such as type of cannula, date and location of insertion, all fluids given, daily observation and care of the site, including changing of the dressing and administration set (13). Thorough documentation provides evidence that the expected care has been given, and, in the event of unavoidable complications such as an adverse drug reaction or phlebitis, the record provides a legal defense for the nurse in case a lawsuit is brought against her. Without thorough documentation, even when the proper care has been given, the nurse's position is significantly weakened by absence of a written record of the care she provided (4).

AVOIDANCE OF LEGAL ACTIONS

In today's consumer-conscious age, in which lawsuits against professionals are increasingly frequent occurrences, the nurse is understandably concerned about the risk of involvement in a malpractice suit. This concern is intensified by the expanding scope of nursing practice, particularly in the area of intravenous drug therapy where the nurse now is expected to perform tasks which until recently were clearly within the realm of medicine.

In spite of one's best efforts, an adverse outcome will sometimes occur. In such a situation, how can the nurse be free of liability? To avoid suits claiming negligence or malpractice it is very important that the nurse adhere to three basic principles (20):

1. Always stay within the bounds of statutory legal requirements. Never perform an action which is not sanctioned by hospital policy, joint policy statement and nursing practice act. For all nursing functions, and especially those related to intravenous drug administration, know the laws of the state and the policies of the institution.
2. Avoid performing any function for which the required degree of knowledge and skill is lacking. When assigned a task which a nurse realizes she is not competent to perform, she must inform her appropriate superior. A nurse must never carry out such a responsibility simply because she has been told that there is no one else to do it. In the event of harm to the patient, she would have no legal protection.
3. Should an adverse reaction occur in spite of skillful care, provide the appropriate remedial measures, report the situation to the physician and *document it in the patient's record.* If a reaction to an intravenous drug is observed, the remainder of the dose should be discontinued immediately; if phlebitis or an infiltration is noted, the cannula should be removed without delay.

In addition to following these principles, the nurse can further help to avoid involvement in a legal action by maintaining good rapport with the patient and family. Suits sometimes arise out of a general dissatisfaction with care given, generated by a poor relationship between the patient and doctor or nurse (17). Nurses may be tempted to avoid patients who exhibit negative behavior such as lack of cooperation or hostility. However, it must be remembered that such behavior is often a manifestation of the patient's apprehensions and lack of knowledge. These and related psychological aspects will be discussed in greater detail in the next chapter.

REFERENCES

1. American Nurses' Association (Nursing Practice Department): *The Fundamentals of Joint Statements on Nursing Practice,* Kansas City, 1968.
2. Bullough, Bonnie: *The Law and the Expanding Nursing Role,* New York: Appleton-Century-Crofts, 1975.
3. Corso, J. A., Agostinelli, R., Brandriss, M. W.: Maintenance of Venous Polyethylene Catheters to Reduce Risk of Infection. *Journal of the American Medical Association,* 210:2075-2077, 1969.
4. Creighton, Helen: *Law Every Nurse Should Know* (3rd ed.), Philadelphia: W. B. Saunders Company, 1975.
5. Creighton, Helen: Liability for Defective Equipment. *Supervisor Nurse,* 5(1):45-46, January 1974.
6. Creighton, Helen: Nurses' Adding of Drugs to IV's. *Supervisor Nurse,* 4:62-64, March 1973.
7. Creighton, Helen: The Nurse's "Right" to Question a Physician's Order. *Supervisor Nurse,* 2:12-13, September 1971.
8. Fuchs, Peter C.: Indwelling Intravenous Polyethylene Catheters—Factors Influencing the Risk of Microbial Colonization and Sepsis. *Journal of the American Medical Association,* 216(9):1447-1450, May 31, 1971.
9. The Health Law Center and Streiff, Charles J. (editors): *Nursing and The Law,* Rockville, Maryland: Aspen Systems Corporation, 1975.
10. Hook, Ingrid L.: New Problems Replace Old in IV Fluid Administration. *Hospital Formulary,* 10:340-347, June 1975.
11. Jenner, Elizabeth A.: Intravenous Infusion—a Cause for Concern? *Nursing Times,* 73(5):156-158, February 3, 1977.
12. Kimmell, Rosemary A.: Dream to Working Reality: How to Start an IV Team. *American Journal of I.V. Therapy,* 4:38-45, February/March 1977.
13. Lind, Mildred D.: Documenting Intravenous Treatment. *American Journal of I.V. Therapy,* 4:54-56, 59, February/March 1977.
14. Meyers, Lawrence: Intravenous Catheterization. *American Journal of Nursing,* 45(11):930-931, November 1945.
15. Murchison, Irene A., and Nichols, Thomas S.: *Legal Foundations of Nursing Practice,* New York: The Macmillan Company, 1970.
16. Murchison, Irene, Nichols, Thomas S., and Hanson, Rachel: *Legal Accountability in The Nursing Process,* Saint Louis: The C.V. Mosby Company, 1978.
17. Plumer, Ada Lawrence: *Principles and Practice of Intravenous Therapy* (2nd ed.). Boston: Little, Brown and Company, 1975.
18. Regan, William Andrew (editor): Drug Reactions and Nursing Liability. *The Regan Report on Nursing Law,* 10(12):1, May 1970.

19. Regan, William Andrew (editor): Illegible Orders. *The Regan Report on Nursing Law,* 11(4):4, September 1970.
20. Regan, William Andrew (editor): Intravenous Medication—Liability for Accidents. *The Regan Report on Nursing Law,* 11(2):1, July 1970.
21. Regan, William Andrew (editor): Levophed Infiltration Due to RN Negligence. *The Regan Report on Nursing Law,* 7(11):3, April 1967.
22. Regan, William Andrew (editor): Needle Infection and Nursing Liability. *The Regan Report on Nursing Law,* 18(1):2, June 1977.
23. Regan, William Andrew (editor): Nursing Judgment vs. Medical Judgment. *The Regan Report on Nursing Law,* 9(4):1, September 1968.
24. Regan, William Andrew (editor): Nursing Practice and Intravenous Medication. *The Regan Report on Nursing Law,* 1(11):1, April 1961.
25. Regan, William Andrew (editor): Telephone Orders and Legal Risks. *The Regan Report on Nursing Law,* 8(1):1, June 1967.
26. Reimer, Douglas M.: Are a Drug Manufacturer's Instructions Standards of Care? *American Association of Nurse Anesthetists Journal,* 42:152-154, April 1974.
27. Williams, Jon T., and Moravec, Daniel F.: *Intravenous Therapy,* Hammond, Indiana: Clissold Publishing, 1967.
28. Wilson, Jacqueline A.: Infection Control in Intravenous Therapy. *Heart and Lung,* 5(3):430-436, May/June 1976.

2 Psychological Considerations

While the technical details of intravenous drug therapy (venipuncture, administration of the drugs, and monitoring of specialized equipment such as infusion pumps) are attended to, the special psychological needs of the patient are often minimized or disregarded. At best, the patient is receiving therapy which is uncomfortable and potentially hazardous; in addition, the drug therapy is often given for a serious, if not life-threatening, condition. With many medications, the untoward effects of the therapy may prove worse than the condition for which they are given. And, as with all types of therapy, the individual's response can be influenced by psychological factors.

To many patients an intravenous line may represent little more than an annoyance or uncomfortable procedure. Such patients may not exhibit overt anxiety and may demonstrate a willingness to cooperate. Yet, many harbor some fears about the prospect of intravenous drug therapy. Television and the news media have increased public awareness of advances in medical care both through factual accounts and fictionalized reports. Though some of these presentations focus on positive aspects of health care, others tend to emphasize complications associated with current medical therapy. Often exaggerated and misleading, such information can generate skepticism and apprehension among health-care consumers. Such feelings of apprehension are present in most patients to some degree and can intensify the discomfort associated with intravenous therapy as well as interfere with its effectiveness.

The anxiety experienced by patients receiving intravenous drug therapy is due in part to the therapy itself, which is often painful, particularly if the cannula must be reinserted frequently. More often though, the anxiety is associated both with the hospitalization, which to most patients is a stressful situation, and with the underlying illness, which can invoke considerable fear and anxiety.

Illness and hospitalization represent a situational crisis for the patient, which necessitates the utilization of psychological coping mechanisms. Terminal illness represents the most extreme type of crisis that one can experience. The stages of anticipatory grieving that dying patients and their families go through have been extensively studied

12

and described by Kübler-Ross (5). The same grieving process is experienced by individuals who have experienced the loss of a significant body structure or function and, to a lesser extent, by any individual facing acute illness and hospitalization. Regardless of the magnitude of the crisis, the individual will pass through the same stages, though the time required to achieve a resolution will vary considerably.

A person's anxiety level can vary considerably according to which stage he is in at that time. For example, in the initial stage of shock and disbelief in which denial predominates, a person may refuse intravenous drug therapy or other treatments if he will not admit their necessity. Essentially he is saying, "I am not really that sick; therefore, I do not need the treatment." On the other hand, some critically ill or dying patients may view this therapy as a certain cure for their condition and thus may accept it readily. Fortunately, except for severe and terminal illnesses, the denial phase is usually brief.

The feelings of anger which evolve next are also likely to be transient in less severe conditions. In the presence of marked disability or impending death, however, this stage can present a challenge for anyone providing care. Since the patient's anger is displaced onto everyone around, complaints about all aspects of care are commonplace. Thus, the intravenous line can become an object of the displaced anger and there may be a lack of cooperation with its insertion, attempts to remove it, or multiple complaints about it while it is in place.

Resistance toward personnel diminishes during the phases of bargaining and depression which follow. In the former, the patient is likely to exhibit his best behavior in order to obtain what has been "bargained for"—usually a reprieve from the illness. Later as depression emerges, the patient generally becomes withdrawn and uncommunicative. Intravenous therapy and other procedures may not be resisted or interfered with, but if complications such as phlebitis develop, they may go unreported.

As the patient enters the final stage of acceptance or resignation, the therapy is usually more readily accepted. However, a dying patient who is resigned to the inevitable outcome of the illness may react with various behavioral changes including the refusal of intravenous therapy and other treatments prescribed, because of a desire to die in peace (5).

FACTORS INFLUENCING PATIENT ANXIETY

The degree of anxiety experienced by a patient receiving intravenous drug therapy is influenced by several factors (4):

Nature of the underlying illness

The severity of the illness, as well as the abruptness of onset, duration, and degree of physical incapacity will affect the patient's overall response and thus his reaction to intravenous drug therapy. While any serious illness represents a threat to an individual's well-being, life-threatening conditions such as advanced cancer or extensive burns strain the individual's capacity to adapt and therefore are a source of severe stress because of the uncertain outcome as well as the often painful diagnostic tests and treatments (2). Severe trauma, burns and disfiguring surgical procedures necessitate a change in one's self-image, a long-term process which may continue far beyond the patient's discharge from the hospital.

Significance of the drug therapy itself and its relationship to the illness

When the intravenous therapy is considered routine, such as a keep-vein-open (KVO) infusion to insure a patent intravenous line in the event that medications are needed, or fluids and electrolytes given in the immediate pre- and postoperative periods, it is generally less frightening to the patient. However, when intravenous drugs represent an essential component of the treatment, such as an antineoplastic agent given to a cancer patient, or antibiotics used to treat a life-threatening infection, the drug therapy takes on increased significance in the eyes of the patient.

Patient's personal psychosocial resources

1. *Age.* An individual's age and developmental level affect his ability to understand and cope with

stressful situations. Infants and children who are unable to understand the nature of their illness and treatment can experience a greater fear of intravenous drug therapy. The special psychological needs of the pediatric age group are discussed in Chapter 6.

Patients whose mental and emotional ages are comparable to those of children, such as those with significant mental retardation and occasionally elderly persons with marked organic brain disease, react in a manner similar to that of children.

2. *Individual's Premorbid Personality.* How well a person was able to cope with stress prior to becoming ill can be an indication of how he will cope with both the current illness and the therapy.

3. *Family Relationships.* The nature of a person's relationships with his family will affect both the degree of anxiety he experiences during an illness and the amount of support the family can and will provide during this time.

4. *Presence of Other Concerns.* A hospitalized patient who is faced with unemployment, dependent children at home, marital or other problems will experience added anxiety during an illness. Stress from such concerns may be reflected in negative behavior such as lack of cooperation with the treatment.

5. *Previous Experience with Illness and Pain.* How well an individual is able to cope with the current illness is determined in part by how well previous life crises have been dealt with. In the absence of previous experience with serious illness, the presence of an unfamiliar environment with strange equipment can induce real and imagined fears. The amount of pain and discomfort anticipated from a test or procedure often exceeds that actually experienced.

Persons who have had past experience with illness and hospitalization, particularly long-term illness, have generally developed coping mechanisms enabling them to deal with stress. On the other hand, when several illnesses have occurred in rapid succession, the patient's adaptive capacity may be strained, causing him to overreact to even minor threats to his well-being.

If the patient has experienced prior illness which was associated with a significant amount of pain, how did he react to the pain? Whether the individual has a high or low pain threshold will influence his response to venipunctures.

How much does the person know about his illness and about his need for intravenous drug therapy? One of the greatest fears that an individual has is fear of the unknown (2). Most patients experience less anxiety and are thus better able to cooperate with their treatment when they are informed about their health problem and about any therapy they require.

6. *Patient's Relationship with the Members of the Health-Care Team.* The patient who has a positive view of members of the health team, trusts them, and is willing to communicate his concerns and feelings to them, will be able to cope with anxiety more effectively.

EFFECTS OF STRESS ON THE PATIENT

Individuals who are under considerable stress can experience exaggerated anxiety when faced with a painful or an otherwise threatening situation, such as the insertion of an intravenous cannula. This anxiety can provoke a vasovagal reaction of the autonomic nervous system, characterized by marked vasodilatation and a precipitous fall in arterial blood pressure, resulting in syncope or transient loss of consciousness. However, consciousness rapidly returns when the patient is placed in a recumbent position with legs elevated and the source of anxiety is relieved (11). Such a reaction, though generally of minor significance, may be avoided if early signs of fear and anxiety can be identified and measures taken to alleviate them.

Exaggerated anxiety can produce pulmonary edema in patients with advanced cardiac disease who are prone to develop congestive heart failure. Severe stress produces increased stimulation of the adrenal glands. The adrenal medulla secretes substances (catecholamines) which raise arterial blood pressure and increase heart rate and workload; the adrenal cortex increases secretion of its hormones (corticosteroids) and through several mechanisms (retention of sodium and chloride, decrease in intracellular potassium and increased production of antidiuretic hormone by the pituitary gland), marked fluid retention and vascular overload result. A patient with borderline cardiac compensation may not be able to tolerate an added fluid load, and pulmonary edema may develop as a result. Such cases have been documented in the literature (8).

Anxiety in the hospitalized patient may also be manifested as dependent, regressive behavior or as aggressive behavior. With the former the individual is often withdrawn and preoccupied with bodily functions (2). Anorexia, insomnia, and tremors are among the symptoms which may be seen. When aggressive behavior predominates, it may be expressed as a lack of cooperation with therapy or verbal expressions of dissatisfaction with the care. The patient receiving intravenous therapy might alter the flow rate, pull out the cannula or otherwise disrupt the system.

Helping the patient cope with stress

Since anxiety will be present to some extent in nearly every hospitalized patient, what measures can be instituted by the nurse to help him cope with the stress of the illness and hospitalization, as well as the intravenous therapy?

I. Establish and maintain a good interpersonal relationship with the patient. Such a relationship is fostered in institutions which provide primary patient care, where one nurse fulfills almost all the patient's nursing needs. However, even when nurse-patient contact is of short duration, such as with an intravenous therapy team, the nurse can lay the foundation for a trusting relationship, even in one visit. One means of accomplishing this is by acknowledging the patient by name upon entering his room and by introducing oneself to him. This enables the patient to view himself as a person rather than an object in the health-care system.

II. Eliminate fear of the unknown by providing information about the general aspects of the intravenous therapy, the drugs themselves and their relationship to his illness. The amount and depth of information given will of course be determined by the patient's physical, mental, and emotional state, as well as by his previous experience with intravenous therapy. In cases of acute illness, information too detailed can either be of little value or can actually increase the patient's anxiety.

A. When his condition allows, prepare him for what he is to expect and when. He should be made aware if the therapy is likely to be prolonged and to require periodic replacement of the cannula.

B. Be honest about the discomfort that will be experienced, acknowledging, but not emphasizing, that the venipuncture is not without some pain. While an occasional patient may be considered "suggestible," experiencing whatever symptoms have been mentioned to him, the majority of patients respond favorably and will place greater trust in the nurse when instructed about subsequent tests and procedures.

C. If time permits, it may be helpful to show certain equipment to the patient, particularly specialized equipment such as an infusion pump, which can be especially frightening. Understanding its purpose and benefits can reduce anxiety considerably.

D. Reinforce the instructions with written information when possible. Some hospitals provide their patients with a handbook on intravenous therapy (6). In addition to the general information about the venipuncture, the patient is advised what to do to keep the intravenous line patent and what things to avoid.

The concept of such a booklet is an excellent one, since it provides written reinforcement of the verbal instructions, which, in the midst of anxiety, can be misunderstood or forgotten. An institution can prepare its own booklet specific to the intravenous therapy procedures utilized. The value of such a booklet is enhanced by considering the educational and cultural background of the patient population served by the institution. There is a tendency to develop educational materials which exceed the reading and comprehension levels of some patients. The information is therefore lost to the patients who need it most. When a hospital serves patients with a broad range of educational backgrounds, it may be necessary to develop two booklets—one very basic and the other at a higher level. Or, if only one booklet is used, it should provide the most basic information in clear, simple terms without being condescending.

E. In addition to being instructed about the

general aspects of intravenous therapy, the patient should be given some information about the drugs he is receiving. While the specific information provided is once again determined by the person's condition and ability to understand, the following should be included when appropriate:

1. What does the patient already know or believe about intravenous drugs in general and the specific drug in particular? Making this determination can help to identify and alleviate fantasies he might have (13).

2. What is the drug actually being used for? What is the desired therapeutic response? Reinforcing a positive attitude about the expected effects of the drug can improve its effectiveness.

3. For approximately what length of time will the drug have to be given? For example, lidocaine, given to control arrhythmias in a patient with an acute myocardial infarction, may be needed for only a few days. Intravenous antibiotics administered for a systemic infection such as endocarditis may be required for up to six weeks.

4. What side effects might occur? While the patient should be prepared for adverse reactions that are likely, such as those associated with antineoplastic agents, he should also be given reassurance that measures will be used to alleviate such symptoms.

III. Be skillful in the care related to the intravenous therapy.

A. Performance of the venipuncture

1. Have all the equipment prepared in advance and on hand at the patient's bedside. Leaving the room during the procedure to get additional equipment may lead the patient to question the nurse's competence and promote anxiety as a result.

2. Provide privacy. Although performance of a venipuncture does not normally interfere with a patient's pattern of modesty unless a central vein is used, screening from neighboring patients and visitors can be helpful for highly anxious patients.

3. Keep the environment as comfortable as possible by eliminating distracting noises and maintaining a moderate temperature. A sufficiently warm room not only provides a feeling of comfort to the patient but by promoting dilatation and filling of the veins will facilitate selection and entry of the vein. Providing good lighting will likewise promote patient relaxation and comfort by increasing ease of cannula insertion.

4. When possible consider patient preference in selecting the insertion site (3). Most people wish to avoid use of their dominant arm in order to prevent restricted movement.

5. Approach the patient in a manner that will help to gain his confidence. An efficient, yet unhurried approach will reinforce a nurse's competence. A nurse who feels unsure of her abilities to skillfully perform a venipuncture will transmit that feeling to the patient. Only the most highly skilled individuals should insert an intravenous cannula in a child or an excessively apprehensive patient.

6. Minimize discomfort during the venipuncture by an adherence to details:

a) Select the best available vein and be sure it is maximally distended (see Chapters 3 and 4).

b) Avoid multiple punctures. Except in an emergency situation or in a comatose patient, no more than three successive attempts should be made to insert a cannula. If more sticks are necessary, the patient should be given a rest, or another person should be requested to try. If this also fails, the physician should be notified.

c) If alcohol is used as part of the skin disinfection procedure, wait until it dries before inserting the needle. This will reduce the stinging sensation felt as the needle enters the skin.

d) Insert the needle rapidly and at the correct angle (approximately 45 degrees when puncturing the skin) to further diminish the pain.

7. Follow a standardized technique for the

venipuncture and subsequent care of the insertion site. This insures consistency, particularly when numerous persons are responsible for performing these procedures, and diminishes the patient's anxiety by enabling him to know what to expect.

8. In securing the cannula and tubing, use tape that will prevent movement and dislodgement, yet will be easy to remove, such as silk or paper tape. When a considerable amount of hair is present, tape removal will be made more comfortable by shaving or using a depilatory on the area where tape will be in contact with the skin.

9. When an armboard is required:
   a) Pad it with a towel or use a contoured styrofoam-type board.
   b) Maintain the hand in a functional position, with fingers flexed over the end of the board and the wrist slightly extended. Contoured armboards promote this position.
   c) When securing it with tape, use two strips of tape with the sticky sides together on areas that are in contact with the skin.

B. Daily care and maintenance of the cannula
   1. Inform the patient of the amount of movement allowed on the side of the infusion and encourage movement within those limits. Some patients are unnecessarily fearful of moving even a small degree.
   2. Keep the call bell and other necessary items (water pitcher, tissues, etc.) on the side opposite the limb with the intravenous line (3). When a disability such as amputation, trauma, or CVA requires that the cannula be inserted in the patient's only usable arm, try to allow sufficient movement at least to enable access to the call bell when necessary.
   3. Encourage as much ambulation or wheelchair mobility as the patient's condition allows. Both comfort and mobility are promoted by the use of a heparin lock when only intermittent intravenous drugs are required. For patients who have a keep-open intravenous line with

fluid and tubing, provide a portable IV pole to enable ambulation.

THE PATIENT WITH SEVERE ANXIETY

While these measures are generally effective for most patients, some may continue to exhibit signs and symptoms of undue apprehension which will make the intravenous drug therapy more painful and perhaps even reduce its effectiveness. In this situation, it is helpful to try to determine the true source of the anxiety. If it is intravenous therapy itself, explore the patient's feelings with him, encouraging him to verbalize specific concerns such as fear of pain or complications. Acknowledgment of his concerns can often help to dissipate the anxiety.

If the apprehension is something other than the intravenous therapy (the illness, personal problems, etc.) as is often the case, likewise encourage him to ventilate his concerns. However, when this problem is one which is beyond the scope of the nurse's function and expertise, it should be brought to the attention of the physician, and, when indicated, a psychiatrist, social worker or other appropriate person should be consulted.

In a few instances, a patient may require tranquilizers during the initial portion or even throughout the duration of the therapy.

THE UNCOOPERATIVE PATIENT

The effectiveness of intravenous drug therapy is also dependent upon the cooperation of the patient. If he removes the cannula, alters the flow rate, or otherwise disrupts the delivery of the drug, the desired therapeutic response obviously will not be achieved. Why does a patient fail to cooperate with this or other aspects of his care? Lack of cooperation may be a result of a manifestation of the patient's reaction to stress or may be secondary to temporary or permanent alterations in mental status.

Patient's reaction to the stress of the illness and hospitalization

As discussed above, patients experiencing severe stress or crisis utilize a variety of defense mechanisms to cope with each stage of the crisis situation. Lack of cooperation may be seen while the patient is in the stages of denial and anger. Rather than focusing on the behavior itself, the nurse should try to recognize it as a symptom of stress and assist the patient in coping by actively listening and sharing the patient's concerns.

Alterations in mental status

Permanent mental impairment prevents a patient from understanding the illness and therapy required in spite of attempts to instruct him. Such impairments are present in mentally handicapped persons who, in spite of their chronological age, must be related to at their mental and emotional age, which is often that of a child. Mental impairments can also be associated with atherosclerotic cerebrovascular disease or chronic brain syndrome secondary to other organic causes and likewise affect the person's ability to cooperate. It is not uncommon for a confused geriatric patient to try to remove an invasive device, whether a urinary catheter, nasogastric tube or intravenous cannula. Efforts to prevent interference with the intravenous line or other device should initially be devoted to explaining its necessity and presenting basic information slowly, in a simple and direct manner (12). Such attempts may nonetheless prove unsuccessful in the severely confused patient. Occasionally, providing diversional activities such as television or magazines, along with more structured activities provided by the occupational or recreational therapist, may be helpful. Checking on the patient at regular, frequent intervals can sometimes provide sufficient reassurance to prevent the patient's obsession with removal of the intravenous device. Along with such measures, the intravenous line should be placed in a location that is less likely to interfere with movement (such as the forearm rather than the wrist or elbow) and should be well secured to make removal more difficult for the patient.

If all else fails and the elderly, confused patient continues to interfere with the intravenous therapy, a careful assessment of whether the medication(s) *must* be given by the intravenous route should be made. If the patient is able and willing to swallow, will the oral form of the drug be as effective? If not, can it be given intramuscularly if it is needed on a short-term basis only? If for pharmacologic or therapeutic reasons the medication must be administered to this patient intravenously, the nursing and medical staff are left with only three choices to assure security of the intravenous line:

1. Maintain constant attendance on the patient. Realistically, in the absence of critical care needs, very few health-care settings can provide continuous nursing supervision.
2. Sedate the patient. Mild sedation may be effective if intravenous drug therapy is needed for only a short duration, but may not be advisable on a long-term basis or in more acutely ill patients. Some of the potentially harmful effects which the physician must weigh against the benefits to be gained include respiratory depression, masking of signs and symptoms, and adverse behavioral changes.
3. Physically restrain the patient. Restraints should be reserved as a final measure (1). They are not advised as a general rule, not only because of the hazards associated with improper use, but also since they can increase agitation in some instances. However, since restraints may be required in some confused patients to insure their safety as well as the administration of needed intravenous medication, their use is justified if the proper safeguards are taken. A written order from the physician is essential and the following guidelines should be observed:
   a) Select the type of restraining device most suited to the individual patient. If the confused patient is primarily interested in getting out of bed, a jacket or waist restraint will be effective. Limiting the patient's movement will usually prevent accidental dislodgement of the intravenous cannula. For the patient who attempts to remove the intravenous device, but who is not combative, a mitt restraint on the opposite hand, or if needed, on both hands, can deter him. However, even mitt restraints may prove unsuccessful in more agitated patients. Soft limb restraints applied to both arms are appropriate, and, when used correctly, effective for such individuals. Restraints are not needed on a paralyzed limb, and in fact should be avoided, since they can impair circulation.
   b) Acknowledge the patient's concern about the use of restraints but explain that they are necessary for his safety (12).

c) Apply the restraining device properly as intended by the manufacturer. Restraints must be snug enough to prevent the patient from slipping out of them, yet loose enough to allow unrestricted circulation to the extremity. A wrist restraint that is loose when applied may tighten up due to patient resistance unless the correct type of knot is used. The device should not be applied either directly over or above the intravenous insertion site as it can create a tourniquet effect and obstruct flow of the intravenous fluid by causing blood to back-up into the cannula and clot (8). The restraint should be applied below the intravenous site, or an armboard should be used and the restraint fastened to the armboard.

d) Whenever restraints are in use, check the patient frequently to detect situations which signal impending injury. Limb restraints must be checked to insure that circulation has not been restricted and that the intravenous line remains patent. Jacket or waist restraints require monitoring to be certain that respiratory function is not compromised. Periodically, ideally at 1- to 2-hour intervals, the restraints should be removed to allow full circulation and range of motion to the extremity. The nurse is legally required to closely monitor any patient who is restrained. Failure to do so with resultant injury to the patient is regarded as negligence (9).

e) Thoroughly document the use of restraints in the patient's record. Written documentation should include justification for their use, type of device, sites and times applied and removed. When restraints are required for an extended length of time, a flow sheet might provide an efficient means of recording such data.

f) Avoid using the restraints for any longer than is absolutely necessary. They do not provide a substitute for good nursing care.

Temporary mental impairments which affect the patient's ability to cooperate with therapy can result from head trauma, neurosurgery, high fevers, altered metabolic states, alcohol or drug intoxication or withdrawal, or psychiatric disturbances. Such patients are often likely to be not only uncooperative but agitated and combative as well. Measures are usually required both to protect the patient and others from injury and to insure the administration of the intravenous medication. Depending on the cause of the mental changes, sedation may be ordered. In some patients this may be inadequate to control the agitation and for these and for patients in whom sedation is contraindicated, restraints are generally required, including those made of leather. When used, the same guidelines must be followed as those regarding soft restraints. Some additional precautions are also required.

1. Fasten the restraints securely enough to prevent the patient from freeing himself, yet allowing the staff to remove them rapidly if required. Restraints that lock with a key are generally not recommended unless the person responsible for the key is in constant attendance.

2. Ideally, an agitated patient in full restraints should receive constant nursing care (1). Even if sedation has been given, during the time required for it to take effect, the patient's resistance to the restraints may provoke injury. The nurse can reinforce the need for the restraints and can provide reassurance that they will be removed once he regains control of his behavior.

3. If a patient has eaten and then has been sedated, being restrained flat on his back can promote regurgitation and aspiration. Elevating the head of the bed often prevents this problem, but the nurse's presence is essential in case regurgitation does occur, to prevent aspiration.

4. When it is impossible for the nurse to remain in constant attendance, the patient must be checked at least every 15 minutes to insure that problems have not arisen. As soon as the patient's behavior is under control and his cooperation gained, the restraints should be removed.

OUTPATIENT CONSIDERATIONS

The psychological considerations discussed thus far have been in relation to patients receiving intravenous drug therapy on an inpatient basis. Since intravenous drugs are being given increasingly to outpatients, both in the clinic setting and at home, their special needs must be considered.

The intravenous drugs most commonly administered on an outpatient basis are the antineoplastic agents used in the treatment of cancer. Patients receiving a course of cancer chemotherapy may not require hospitalization, so they return daily to the clinic or physician's office to receive their medication until the course of therapy is completed. Being able to remain at home in one's own surroundings is beneficial to many patients, and by eliminating the stress associated with hospitalization, the patient is better able to cope with the illness itself.

Returning daily to the clinic to receive the medication, however, can produce additional strain on the patient and family, both psychologically and socially due to the time and expense involved in transporting the patient back and forth between the home and clinic. One solution is the administration of intravenous chemotherapy at home. This approach, though not suitable for all patients, has been made possible in part by the development of miniature infusion pumps. These allow small doses of drugs to be infused at very slow rates over a period of up to several days. Such devices are discussed in greater detail in Chapter 5. By being able to remain at home, the patient with a terminal illness is able to maintain a greater degree of independence for a longer period of time and is often able to resume some (and occasionally all) of his former activities.

The same benefits are derived by other patients who are able to receive various types of intravenous drugs at home. One such group that is now emerging involves patients requiring long-term intravenous antibiotics for major infections such as endocarditis or osteomyelitis (10). These may be required intermittently from four to six times per day, but other than the need for the drugs there is often no other reason for the patient to remain hospitalized. Other types of intravenous drugs, such as diuretics, which are often required on a regular basis (ranging from one or more times a week to daily), can also be administered in the home. With home intravenous therapy many patients are able to resume normal activities; some are even able to return to work or school during the course of the therapy (10).

Regardless of the type of drug being given, home intravenous therapy requires both instruction and psychological preparation for the patient and family and ongoing support and supervision by the community health nurse (7). The nurse is essential not only to perform the technical aspects of the therapy (such as cannula insertion and drug administration) but to assist the patient and family in coping with the condition and in maintaining a more normal life style, even when life expectancy is short.

Such support is now being provided to many terminally ill cancer patients through cancer home-care programs. Utilizing a multidisciplinary team approach, such programs provide direct care such as administering intravenous drug therapy, but place their major emphasis on giving psychological support to help the patient and family work through the grieving process and reach the final stage of acceptance.

REFERENCES

1. Anders, Robert L.: When a Patient Becomes Violent. *American Journal of Nursing,* 77(7): 1144–1148, July 1977.
2. Beland, Irene L., and Passos, Joyce Y.: *Clinical Nursing—Pathophysiological and Psychosocial Approaches* (3rd ed.), New York: Macmillan Publishing Company, Inc., 1975.
3. Butherus, Constance: Safety and Comfort Tips, *in* Bodnar, Andrew, and D'Agostino, Joanne: IV Therapy, Part II. *The Journal of Practical Nursing,* 27:24–27, September 1977.
4. Kaplan, Stanley M.: Psychological Aspects of Cardiac Disease. *Psychosomatic Medicine,* 118–233, May/June 1956.
5. Kübler-Ross, Elisabeth: *On Death and Dying.* New York: Macmillan Publishing Company, Inc., 1969.
6. Lee, Gladys, and Walker, Ted R.: A Handbook for I.V. Therapy Patients. *American Journal of I.V. Therapy,* 4:17–18, February/March 1977.
7. Michael, Sharon L.: Home I.V. Therapy. *American Journal of Nursing,* 78(7):1223–1226, July 1978.
8. Plumer, Ada Lawrence: *Principles and Practice of Intravenous Therapy* (2nd ed.), Boston: Little, Brown and Company, 1975.
9. Regan, William Andrew (editor): Restraints and Surveillance: Nurse's Legal Duty. *Regan Report on Nursing Law,* 17:2, July 1976.
10. Stiver, H. Grant, Telford, Gordon O., Mossey, Jana M., Cote, Dennis D., Van Middlesworth, Elizabeth J., Trosky, Sharon K., McKay, Norma L., and Mossey, Wilfred L.: Intravenous Antibiotic Therapy

at Home. *Annals of Internal Medicine,* 89(5):690–693, November 1978.

11. Thorn, George W., Adams, Raymond D., Braunwald, Eugene, Isselbacher, Kurt J., and Petersdorf, Robert G. (editors): *Harrison's Principles of Internal Medicine* (8th ed.), New York: McGraw-Hill Book Company, 1977.

12. Trockman, Gordon: Caring for the Confused or Delirious Patient. *American Journal of Nursing,* 78(9):1495–1499, September 1978.

13. Turco, Salvatore and King, Robert E.: *Sterile Dosage Forms—Their Preparation and Clinical Application,* Philadelphia: Lea and Febiger, 1974.

3 Preparation for the Establishment of the Intravenous Line

Except for drugs which are administered as a single dose via direct injection with a syringe and needle (a procedure generally performed by the physician), the administration of intravenous medications requires the establishment and maintenance of a patent intravenous line. As discussed in Chapter 1, the responsibility for venipuncture is increasingly being delegated to the nurse. Whether a member of an intravenous therapy team or a staff member providing primary patient care, the nurse must be highly skilled to insure both the psychological and physical well-being of the patient during the procedure.

For the insertion and maintenance of an intravenous line, the use of a systematic approach and adherence to established procedures is essential. While the nurse must follow the specific policies and procedures of the institution or nursing service, the following general guidelines can be utilized and adapted as indicated.

The steps required for the insertion of the intravenous line include:

I. Preparation
   A. Psychological preparation of the patient
   B. Physical preparation
      1. Setting up the fluid system
      2. Selecting the type of cannula
      3. Selecting the venipuncture site
II. Insertion
   A. Preparing the skin and performing the venipuncture
   B. Securing the cannula and dressing the site
   C. Establishing the correct flow rate

PSYCHOLOGICAL PREPARATION OF THE PATIENT

The explanations and reassurance given to the patient will foster his cooperation and promote success of the therapy. Patients who are very apprehensive or who are unable to understand the reason for the therapy, including infants and young children, can be more effectively managed if their psychological needs are anticipated. The guidelines in the previous chapter should be followed for adult patients while psychological needs specific to children are included in the pediatric section (Chapter 6).

SETTING UP THE FLUID SYSTEM

Preparing the fluid system and other equipment should be done before entering the patient's room in a specially designated clean area such as the medication room. This not only allows for greater accuracy and safety but can reduce the patient's anxiety as well.

In instances in which intravenous medications are required on an intermittent basis without the need for continuous infusion of fluids, an intermittent device such as a heparin lock (a winged-needle unit fitted with a resealable injection port) may be utilized. With such a device, a fluid system is not utilized since patency is maintained with a heparinized-saline flush. The use of these devices for the administration of drugs is discussed in Chapter 8.

For some patients, however, a continuous infusion of fluids or medications is required, or the physician may prefer that the patency of the cannula be maintained with fluids (referred to as KVO or a keep-vein-open IV). In such cases, choice of the type of fluid used remains the prerogative of the physician. However, the nurse must consider the compatibility of the fluid prescribed with any intravenous medication that the patient is receiving and call any potential incompatibility to the attention of the physician before the medication is administered. Since the scope of this text does not include intravenous therapy as such, the various types of fluids available will not be discussed. The means of assessing compatibilities, however, is discussed in Chapter 8.

The three components of the intravenous line include the fluid container, the administration set (tubing and adjunctive devices), and the cannula.

Types of containers

Intravenous fluids are available in both glass bottles and flexible plastic bags, each of which offers certain advantages. Recently, a semirigid plastic container has been introduced which combines features of each of the other two types.

GLASS BOTTLES

Glass bottles are available in sizes ranging from 150 to 1000 milliliters and as partially filled bottles containing from 50 to 750 milliliters. All glass bottles currently used are vacuum bottles designed with a rubber-stopper closure, through which the piercing pin of the administration set is inserted. The screwcap closure used in the past is no longer manufactured since it has been recognized that contamination can occur when the cap is removed to add drugs or attach the administration set (3, 26). As a result of a nationwide occurrence of septicemia in 1970 and 1971 associated with screwcap bottles, that type of system has been replaced with bottles incorporating rubber stoppers (15).

However, even bottles with rubber stoppers do not always provide a completely closed system, since air-venting is necessary. Bottles must be vented in one of two ways. Some are vented directly by means of an air tube within the bottle which goes through the rubber stopper and opens into the air. (Fig. 3-1, left). Since the air entering is not filtered, contamination is possible though unlikely. The other type of bottle has no direct air vent but uses an air inlet on the administration set (Fig. 3-1, right). Located between the drip chamber and piercing pin, it is covered with a bacterial retentive filter to reduce the chance of contamination.

Desirable features of glass bottles include their rigid construction, which makes them easier to manipulate when adding medications and attaching administration tubing and which allows fluid levels to be measured with greater accuracy. Being biologically inert, they do not generate particulate matter, and they are compatible with virtually all fluids and medications. The main disadvantage of bottles include their breakability, heavy weight, and amount of storage space needed. Disposal of empty bottles can also require considerable space.

FLEXIBLE PLASTIC BAGS

Flexible plastic bags have come into widespread use since their introduction into the United States in 1971 (26). Currently marketed by two Ameri-

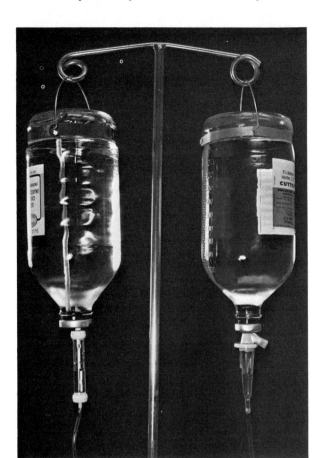

Fig. 3–1. (*Left*) Vented intravenous fluid bottle (McGaw Laboratories, Division of American Hospital Supply Corporation, Irvine, California 92714). (*Right*) Nonvented intravenous fliud bottle. Air enters the bottle via the inlet above the drip-chamber of the administration set. (Cutter Laboratories, Inc., Berkeley, California 94710)

can manufacturers, these containers, which are made of polyvinylchloride (PVC), offer such advantages as being lightweight, unbreakable, and easy to store and dispose of; also, because they collapse as the bag empties, no air venting is required (Fig. 3-2). Thus, they present a truly closed system, minimizing the risk of airborne contamination.

However, these containers are not without disadvantages. Their flexibility makes them a bit more cumbersome to manipulate and possibly more subject to touch contamination unless aseptic practices are rigidly followed (12, 21). Since they are not impervious to moisture, an outer wrap of polyethylene is required to prevent the

gradual loss of fluid while the container is being stored (13, 18). These plastic containers are not completely inert, and thus some components called plasticizers can be drawn or leached from the bag into the solution; and likewise, certain substances from the solution can be adsorbed onto the interior surface of the container (18). This has been associated particularly with insulin, though such adsorption has also been found to occur with glass bottles. While this phenomenon does not usually present a significant clinical problem, some investigators have recommended adding human serum albumin or plasma protein fraction to the container with the insulin to reduce the amount of adsorption (19).

Though it is known that particulate matter is present in fluids supplied in both glass bottles and plastic bags, studies differ as to which type of container has higher levels. Turco and Davis found many fewer particles in plastic containers they studied (25). In contrast, Needham and Luzzi obtained opposite findings (17). However, the high levels they noted in the plastic containers were generated after vigorous shaking of the containers and were found to be tiny balls of liquid plasticizer rather than true particles (7). Thus, it might be speculated that with ordinary use, the amount of particles or other substances may be quite low.

As with glass bottles, plastic containers are available in a full range of sizes including partially filled bags containing 50 to 100 milliliters. Since some drugs may not be compatible, data available from the manufacturer of the container should be consulted before a drug is added. Such information, when available, is also included in the drug information section of this book. Manufacturers information warn against the use of these bags in series connections; that is, connecting one bag directly to another. This is because residual air from the container that empties first can be drawn into the intravenous line and result in an air embolus.

Finally, since these containers have no vacuum, additive devices such as double needles cannot be used to add medications to the bag without the use of a special vacuum unit (26). The use of such units is discussed in Chapter 8.

SEMIRIGID PLASTIC CONTAINERS

Recently, a third type of intravenous fluid container has emerged, a semirigid plastic container which incorporates features of the two other types (Fig. 3-3). Constructed of a plastic material called polyolefin, the container when full is nearly as firm as a glass bottle, yet lightweight and unbreakable like other plastic containers. Unlike the material used in flexible bags, the plastic in this typ e of containe inert, virtually eliminating leaching of substances into the solution. Impermeable to moisture, it does not require an outer wrapper. As with other plastic containers, no air venting is required, so a closed system is maintained. As the container empties, the walls collapse symmetrically enabling a more accurate reading of fluid levels (Fig. 3-4). As with the other type of plastic container, these must not be used in series connections.

At present, the types of solutions and sizes available are somewhat limited, but will no doubt be expanded as usage increases.

All types of fluid systems currently available have both desirable and undesirable features. Thus, each institution must carefully weigh each factor and select a system which best suits its needs.

Inspection of the container for defects

Whether a glass or plastic container is used, it should be inspected before use to insure safety.

1. Verify the type and volume of solution. For safety, a 250-milliliter container is the largest one recommended for use with infants and young children.
2. Check the expiration date. Discard the solution if the expiration date has passed, even if there is no visible sign of contamination or deterioration.
3. With glass bottles, check all surfaces for chips or cracks. Hold the bottle up to a light and observe for sudden flashes of light which can indicate a microscopic crack. True defects must be distinguished from seams on the side or bottom of the bottle.
4. With flexible plastic containers, gently squeeze the bag to detect any leaks (Fig. 3-5).
5. Observe for clarity of the solution. Should any discoloration, cloudiness, or particulate matter be noted, discard the solution and report it to the pharmacy or responsible department so that other containers in the same lot can be checked.

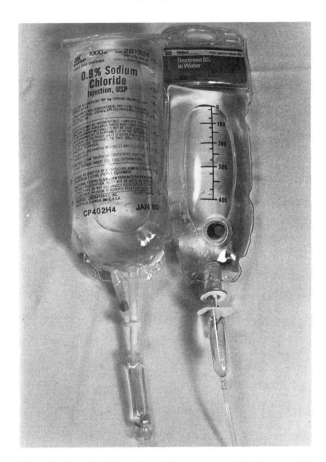

Fig. 3-2. Flexible plastic intravenous fluid containers. (*Left*) Viaflex, Travenol Laboratories, Inc., Deerfield, Illinois 60015. (*Right*) Life Care, Abbott Laboratories, North Chicago, Illinois 60064)

Preparation of the solution

Should any additive be required, prepare the admixture immediately before it is to be used, following the guidelines in Chapter 8. Whenever possible, avoid adding medications once the solution has begun infusing since incomplete mixing can result in the infusion of a concentrated amount or "bolus" of the drug. Once the solution has been prepared or if additives are not required, the administration set is attached to the container.

Attachment of the administration set

Most basic administration sets are similar except for variations necessitated by the type of fluid system used. Nonvented glass bottles require

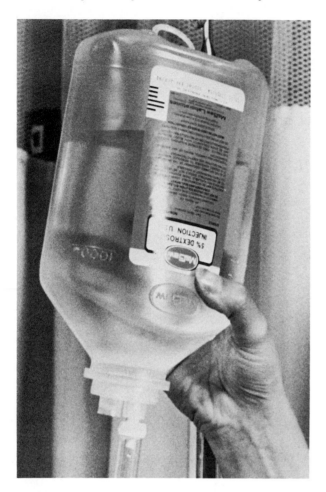

Fig. 3-3. Accumed semirigid plastic intravenous container combines features of both the glass container and the flexible plastic container. (Courtesy of McGaw Laboratories, Division of American Hospital Supply Corporation, Irvine, California 92714)

The drip chamber of each set is calibrated to deliver a specific number of drops per milliliter. Most standard sets provide 10, 15, or 20 drops per milliliter, depending on the manufacturer. It is essential to know the calibration of the system being used so that the flow rate can be accurately calculated and monitored. Microdrop sets are also available, which deliver 50 to 60 drops per milliliter. Such sets are used in the pediatric setting as well as for adults in whom fluid volumes and medication dosages must be precisely regulated. Standard sets can be modified to microdrop size by means of a special adaptor (20).

The flow control clamp may be of the roller or screw type. Both types provide a reasonably accurate rate of flow except when specific factors (discussed in Chapter 5) come into play. When set loosely to provide high flow rates, they are prone to slipping; so some individuals recommend use of a second clamp as an added safety measure (20). Some administration sets also include a metal or plastic slide clamp which is used to shut off the flow temporarily while changing the infusion container without altering the established flow rate. Because slide clamps do not allow precise rate adjustments, they should not be used to regulate the flow rate.

Injection sites, which enable the direct injection of a medication or the "piggybacking" of a secondary infusion, are available on most sets. They may consist of a latex rubber sleeve located near the distal end of the tubing or, more commonly, be the Y-type with a resealable rubber cap. Some sets incorporate two Y-sites, one near the lower (distal) end, the other near the upper end. A back-check valve may also be present to prevent backflow of fluid into the primary container while a medication or secondary infusion is being administered.

Additional features which are integrated into some sets include micropore filters and volume-control sets. The use of these and other devices is discussed in Chapter 8.

Attachment of the administration set to the container demands both adherence to aseptic technique and attention to specific details. The setting up of the intravenous fluid system should be done in a clean area away from heavy traffic. Hands must always be washed first. While specific techniques vary slightly according to the type of system used, the general procedure is as follows:

an air inlet while other types do not. Some sets can be used with all bottles of the same type (e.g., nonvented bottles) regardless of brand. Universal sets are available which can be adapted to several different types of systems. Since they contain an air vent, they can be used with all nonvented bottles; however, they can also be used with vented bottles as long as the latex diaphragm is left in place. They can be used with some plastic containers and drug additive containers as well (1).

Components of the basic administration set include the piercing pin, drip chamber, tubing, flow control clamp, injection site, and male needle adaptor.

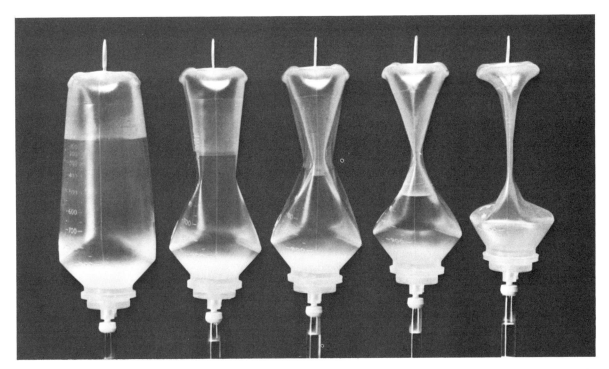

Fig. 3–4. Progressive symmetrical collapsing of Accumed container as it empties. (Courtesy of McGaw Laboratories, Division of American Hospital Supply Corporation, Irvine, California 92714)

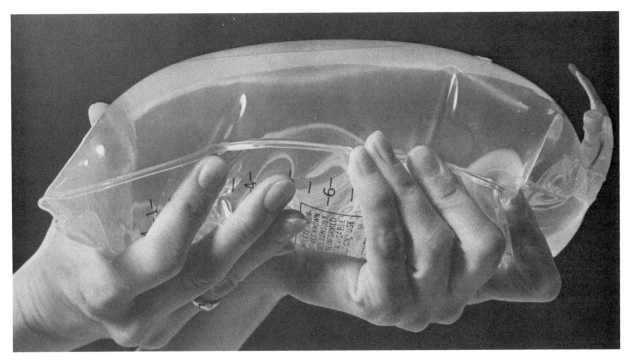

Fig. 3–5. Squeezing a flexible plastic container to check for leaks. (Travenol Laboratories, Inc., Deerfield, Illinois 60015)

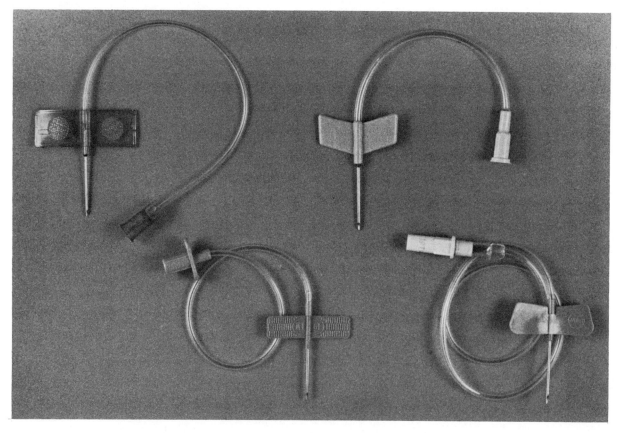

Fig. 3–6. Several types of winged-needle units. The side arms or wings facilitate both insertion and securing with tape. (*Clockwise from upper left*: Bard Hospital Division, C. R. Bard, Inc., Murray Hill, New Jersey 07974; The Deseret Company, Sandy, Utah 84070; McGaw Laboratories, Division of American Hospital Supply Corporation, Irvine, California 92714; Travenol Laboratories, Inc., Deerfield, Illinois 60015)

FOR GLASS BOTTLES

1. Remove the metal overseal cap and inner metal disc if present. If medications have been previously added by the pharmacy, remove the protective additive cap. Take care not to touch the rubber stopper (or latex diaphragm for vented bottles).
2. Close the clamp on the administration set to prevent nonfiltered air from being drawn into the bottle.
3. *Nonvented Bottles:* Firmly thrust the piercing spike straight through the center of the rubber stopper, taking care to avoid twisting or angling (1). As the spike is inserted, check for a hissing sound to verify that the vacuum was intact. If medications have been added, the vacuum will no longer be present.

    Vented Bottles: Remove the latex overseal with-out touching the rubber disc. The presence of the vacuum is confirmed by a hissing sound as the overseal is removed. Insert the piercing spike into the administration set site adjacent to the air-tube opening.
4. Invert the container and suspend onto a pole. The rising of air bubbles further documents that a vacuum was present.
5. Attach any adjunctive devices such as micropore filter to the distal end of the tubing. (See Chapter 8 for the specific use of filters.) If no filter is used, loosen the adaptor cover on the distal end of the tubing.
6. Squeeze the drip chamber until it is about one-half full.
7. Open the flow-control clamp to clear the air from the tubing. If any Y-injection sites or an in-line filter is present, invert each site as the fluid passes through and tap, if necessary,

to expel all air. Incomplete priming can allow air to enter the patient when the infusion is begun.

8. Close the flow-control clamp, and tighten the adaptor cap.

9. Label the container with the patient's name and room number; additives, including strength and amount; preparation date and time; bottle number; flow rate in milliliters per hour and drops per minute; the time the container is to start infusing and the time it should be completed; and the name of the person preparing and hanging the container.

FOR PLASTIC CONTAINERS

1. *Flexible Containers:* Remove the outer wrap, then remove the plastic protector or tear-tab from the administration port.

    Semirigid Containers: Tighten the blue screw top by turning it counterclockwise, and pull off with a sharp snapping motion. This also removes the clear plastic inner seal. Peel off the foil covering from the administration set site.

2. Close the clamp on the administration set and insert connector or piercing pin into administration port, taking care to avoid touch contamination of all exposed surfaces.

3. Invert the container and suspend onto a pole. Since there is no vacuum present, no air bubbles will be seen entering the container.

4. Follow remainder of steps (5 through 9) as described above.

SELECTING THE TYPE OF CANNULA TO BE USED

Once the fluid system is set up, the type of needle or cannula most suitable for the patient must be selected. Too often selection of the intravenous cannula is done by chance, the type being determined by whatever is handy at the time or the type most familiar to the person performing the venipuncture. However, since the safety and comfort of the patient must always take precedence over convenience, each individual involved in the insertion of intravenous lines must be thoroughly familiar with the basic types of cannulae as well as with their limitations and potential hazards. While the type selected is necessarily limited to one of those available in the institution, most hospitals stock each of the basic types.

Nurses responsible for performing venipunctures, particularly if on an intravenous therapy team, should be involved in decisions regarding the types of cannulae and other intravenous equipment selected for use within the institution.

The two basic types of intravenous cannulae are needles and plastic catheters. They can be further subdivided as follows:

I. Needles
   A. Straight needles
   B. Winged-needle units
   C. Intermittent winged-needle units (heparin lock)
II. Plastic Catheters
   A. Over-the-needle cannulae
   B. Through-the-needle catheters
   C. In-lying or cutdown catheters

The decision as to which kind of cannula is best suited to a given patient should be based on the type and expected duration of therapy as well as the patient's age and ability to cooperate. Ease of insertion and patient comfort are unquestionably desirable, yet the type of cannula meeting these needs may represent a poor choice from the standpoint of safety with a given patient, and, thus, to use it would compromise the overall well-being of the patient.

Needles

STRAIGHT NEEDLES

Straight needles, which are generally made of stainless steel or aluminum, represent the first type of infusion device available. When plastic cannulae were introduced and became popular, the use of needles diminished markedly. Recent studies, however, suggest a lower rate of infective complications with needles than with plastic cannulae (6, 24). Consequently, many institutions are resuming the use of needles for appropriate patients requiring short-term intravenous therapy via a peripheral vein.

Needles used for intravenous therapy range in size from approximately 14 gauge down to 25 gauge and vary in length from ¾ inch to about 2 inches. Current manufacturing methods provide a thin-wall construction in many needles, allowing an increased lumen and, therefore, a greater flow with the same outer diameter (20). This feature, along with a siliconized coating and a highly

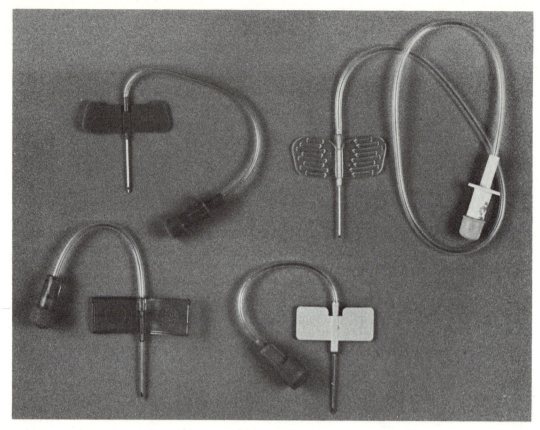

Fig. 3–7. Intermittent winged-needle units or heparin locks allow the maintenance of a patent intravenous line while eliminating the need for fluid containers and administration sets. (*Clockwise from upper left*: Abbott Laboratories, North Chicago, Illinois 60064; Cutter Laboratories Inc., Berkeley, California 94710; Jelco Laboratories, Raritan, New Jersey 08869; Bard Hospital Division, C. R. Bard, Inc., Murray Hill, New Jersey 07974)

sharpened, beveled tip, makes insertion less painful. The siliconized coating present on some needles is further believed to reduce its thrombogenic (clot-forming) potential, an essential consideration for all cannulae.

The rigidity of needles, however, limits the patient's mobility and causes more discomfort than other types of cannulae if used on a long-term basis. Because of the sharp, beveled tip, the risk of the needle moving and puncturing the vein with subsequent infiltration is high, particularly if it is inserted near an area of active movement such as at the antecubital fossa. Thus, straight needles are not suitable for highly agitated patients, patients with uncontrolled muscle movements (spasms, seizures, etc.), or infants and young children. Even with cooperative adults, straight needles may require rather frequent replacement, limiting their

value to short-term use. In fact, the short duration of use may be the factor responsible for the reduced complication rates.

WINGED-NEEDLE UNITS

An adaptation of the straight needle which makes it useful for a broader range of patients is the winged-needle unit or scalp-vein needle. This type of needle utilizes a short, usually small gauge needle with one or two plastic side arms or wings (Fig. 3-6). The wings both facilitate insertion by providing a firm handle to grip and allow the needle to be securely taped in place, thus helping to prevent movement and subsequent infiltration. These features make them ideal for infants and small children in whom scalp veins and small peripheral veins must be used. For neonates, a 25 to 27 gauge needle is used. A 21 to 25 gauge needle is suitable for older children, depending on their age and size and the type of fluids and drugs being administered. They are also well suited for elderly patients whose veins tend to be fragile or difficult to stabilize during venipuncture.

The winged needle is connected to vinyl tubing ranging in length from 3½ to 12 inches. When in use, the end of the tubing is connected to the adaptor end of the administration set. Units containing long tubing, up to 30 inches in length, are available for operating room or emergency use.

While winged needles are also somewhat prone to infiltration, their special features make them considerably more secure than straight needles. Since they are associated with a lower incidence of complications, many hospitals have made them the cannula of choice for short-term and even moderate-length therapy.

INTERMITTENT WINGED-NEEDLE UNITS

For patients not requiring continuous fluids, winged-needle units are also available with a resealable rubber injection port at the end of the tubing (Fig. 3-7). Also referred to as a "heparin lock," this type of unit is ideal for patients who require intermittent medications without a need for fluids. Eliminating the fluid container and tubing increases patient mobility and comfort and reduces expense (10, 23). Hanson found no greater incidence in complications in patients with heparin locks than those with keep-open intravenous lines; and, in fact, the rate of complications per patient day was actually lower with the heparin lock (10).

The patency of these units is maintained with a weak heparinized saline solution, instilled after each dose of medication or at regular intervals if no medication is being given. The use of the heparin lock for the intermittent administration of drugs is discussed in detail in Chapter 8.

Although studies suggest a lower rate of phlebitis with straight needles and winged-infusion units, phlebitis can still occur; and the frequency increases proportionately with the length of time the needle is left in place. Since the risk of such complications is diminished when the needle is replaced every 48 to 72 hours, this should be a routine procedure for all types of intravenous cannulae (8). Venous irritation can be further diminished by selecting a needle which is smaller

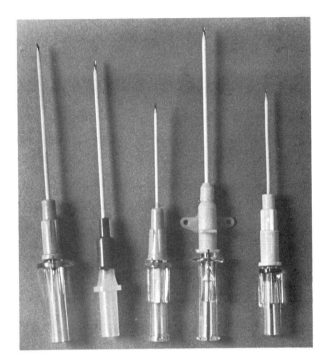

Fig. 3–8. Over-the-needle cannulae. (*From left*: Angiocath, The Deseret Company, Sandy, Utah 84070; radiopaque Teflon catheter, Jelco Laboratories, Raritan, New Jersey 08869; A-Cath, Bard Hospital Division, C. R. Bard, Inc., Murray Hill, New Jersey 07974; Vicra Quik-Cath, Travenol Laboratories, Inc., Deerfield, Illinois 60015; Abbocath-T, Abbott Laboratories, North Chicago, Illinois 60064)

in diameter than the lumen of the veins to insure good flow around it and the dilution of any fluid or drugs given.

Plastic catheters

OVER-THE-NEEDLE CANNULAE

The second major category of cannulae includes several different types of plastic catheters. One frequently used type is the over-the-needle cannula, which consists of a 1- to 3-inch catheter fused to a rigid hub. Like needles, it is available in a full range of sizes (Fig. 3-8). These cannulae are currently made of a variety of substances including polytetrafluoroethylene (Teflon), polyvinylchloride (PVC), or polyethylene.

The needle within the cannula is used for the venipuncture, and is then withdrawn once the catheter has been advanced over the needle into the vein. Current material and designs make severing of the catheter highly unlikely if proper insertion techniques are followed. However, should severing occur, most catheters are radiopaque to enable x-ray detection and subsequent removal.

Because the diameter of the catheter is slightly larger than the needle which entered the vein, leakage from the vein is minimized. Furthermore, the catheter is pliable, making it more comfortable for many patients; and since the blunt tip reduces the likelihood of puncturing the vein, the frequency of infiltration is much lower than with needles. Thus, it is appropriate for patients who are restless or agitated and in situations in which a secure intravenous line is required, such as for the uninterrupted administration of essential drugs that must be given via peripheral veins.

The over-the-needle cannula is also adaptable for patients requiring intermittent medications or a ready access to a vein without the need for continuous fluids. A sterile adaptor plug containing a resealable injection cap can be used to convert the cannula to a heparin lock (see Chapter 8, Fig. 8-22).

In special instances, an obturator with stylet can be inserted into the cannula to temporarily occlude the lumen and maintain its patency (Fig. 3-9). However, this device may allow some blood to collect between the inner surface of the cannula and the stylet if used for an extended period of time, and the fibrinous material that has accumulated can be pushed into the vein when the medication is administered (2). Thus, these devices should be used only in patients who are heparinized or for short-term use to keep the vein open when the administration tubing is disconnected (such as during an x-ray or other procedure or while transporting a patient).

THROUGH-THE-NEEDLE CATHETERS

Another type of plastic cannulae is the long, plastic catheter which is introduced into the vein through the needle. The first reported use in 1945 involved the insertion of an isolated segment of tubing through a separate needle (16). Such catheters are now fused to hubs for attachment to administration tubing. They are available in lengths ranging from 9 to 36 inches and in a variety of diameters (Fig. 3-10). Their major value is for the administration of drugs and fluid into a central vein. They may be used in pediatric pa-

tients when peripheral veins cannot be used, such as to administer irritating drugs and fluids, and in states of dehydration or shock. In the pediatric setting the 22 gauge size is most commonly used.

Through-the-needle catheters can be divided into two categories, depending on whether the needle remains within the system or is removed after insertion.

With the first type, after the catheter has been fully introduced into the vein, the needle is withdrawn from the vein and skin but remains over a segment of the catheter. A needle guard properly placed over the tip of the needle prevents the catheter from being punctured or severed by the needle once it is in place (Fig. 4-5I, p. 53). When insertion of such a catheter is performed by a highly skilled person using the correct technique, as discussed in the next chapter, the risk of shearing is low. However, severing of the catheter can occur during insertion if the catheter is pulled back through the needle; or it can occur after insertion if the needle guard is improperly placed.

Since the correct performance of this procedure by a highly skilled person cannot always be assured, a second type of catheter which eliminates this potential hazard was developed. Several such catheters are currently available which allow complete removal of the needle from the system once the catheter has been inserted (Fig. 3-11). Some of these catheters involve the initial insertion of a short introducer cannula, similar to a standard over-the-needle cannula. Once inserted, the needle is withdrawn, and the catheter is threaded through the introducer. This prevents shearing during insertion. Another model incorporates a split needle which is held together by a plastic sleeve. After the catheter has been inserted in the routine manner, the needle is withdrawn, the sleeve is peeled back, and the needle splits and is removed from the system. While some of these units are more cumbersome to insert, particularly during emergencies, such as resuscitative efforts, this inconvenience must be balanced against the hazard they seek to eliminate.

Since the through-the-needle catheter is smaller in diameter than the puncture wound from the needle, fluid can seep around it and create a potential portal of entry for organisms (20). Thus, proper dressing and subsequent maintenance of the insertion site is essential.

IN-LYING OR CUTDOWN CATHETERS

At times, when a patient's veins are inaccessible, percutaneous placement of a catheter is unsuccessful. In such instances a catheter can be inserted directly into a vein by means of a surgical incision known as a cutdown. Catheters used for this purpose are plain segments of tubing attached to a hub, as with other catheters, but come without any needle or introducer. They are always inserted by a physician.

Complications

As mentioned above, data from several studies suggest that complications, such as venous irritation and phlebitis, are frequently associated with plastic catheters (14) and seem to be higher than with needles even when changed every 48 hours (6, 24). However, the incidence of complications increases the longer the catheter remains in place.

Another factor believed associated with complications is the type of catheter material, although opinions differ as to the preferred ones. One study found that catheters constructed of a substance called fluoroethylenepropylene-Teflon (FEP-Teflon) resulted in a much lower incidence of venous irritation than those made of polyvinylchloride (PVC) or tetrafluorethylene-Teflon (TFE-Teflon) (24). Other investigators have recommended silicone rubber catheters because of a decreased likelihood of inducing clot formation (4). While the coating of catheters with silicone to prevent clotting has been advocated since 1955 (22), later studies by Hoshal and colleagues found that fibrin sleeves can form around siliconized rubber catheters as well as on those made of Teflon and polyethylene (11). This group noted significantly less fibrin sleeve formation around polyethylene catheters bonded with a substance called GBH (graphite-benzalkonium chloride-heparin sodium). Such conflicting findings indicate a need for more controlled clinical studies, not only on various types of catheter materials but on other factors suspected or known to be associated with infections in plastic catheters. Until more definitive conclusions can be drawn, some investigators recommend the use of needles, particularly scalp-vein needles, whenever feasible and confining the use of plastic cannulae to situations in which they are absolutely necessary (5, 9).

Situations necessitating the use of long, through-the-needle catheters include:

1. Monitoring of the central venous pressure
2. Infusion of hypertonic fluids requiring maximal dilution, such as hyperalimentation solutions
3. Administration of life-sustaining medications in emergency situations
4. Administration of medications which must be given via a central vein to prevent peripheral venous irritation

A comparison of the features of each type of cannula is found in Table 3-1. Regardless of the type of cannula selected, the risk of subsequent infection can be reduced by following the correct procedures during insertion. Adherence to proper aseptic technique can be fostered by the use of intravenous insertion kits (Fig. 3-12). Such kits contain the essential material for the insertion of the intravenous line. Some contain just the basic items including skin disinfectant, tourniquet, antiseptic ointment, gauze, or plastic bandages and tape. Other kits also include the cannula, either a winged-needle unit or short, over-the-needle cannula. A few through-the-needle catheters are also available in kit form. Such kits are not only useful for routine insertion and maintenance of the intravenous cannula but are of particular value in emergency situations.

SELECTING THE VENIPUNCTURE SITE

As with selecting the most suitable type of cannula, choosing the most appropriate site for the administration of intravenous drugs is essential to help achieve the desired therapeutic response and minimize complications.

General considerations

In theory, medications can be administered into any peripheral or central vein; but for reasons of accessibility and safety, those most commonly used are the superficial veins of the upper extremities (Fig. 3-13). Veins in the hand or forearm should be given first consideration unless the medication or fluid being given requires delivery into a central vein. Using a vein which can be readily visualized and palpated will foster easy in-

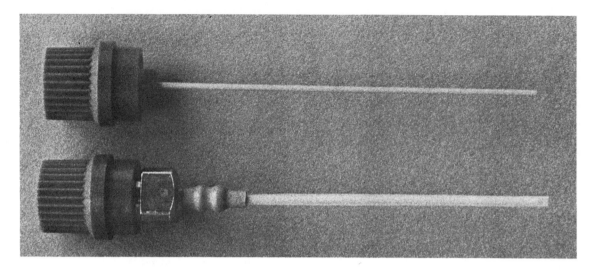

Fig. 3–9. An obturator with stylet will maintain the patency of a catheter on a short-term basis while the administration tubing is discontinued. (Jelco Laboratories, Raritan, New Jersey 08869)

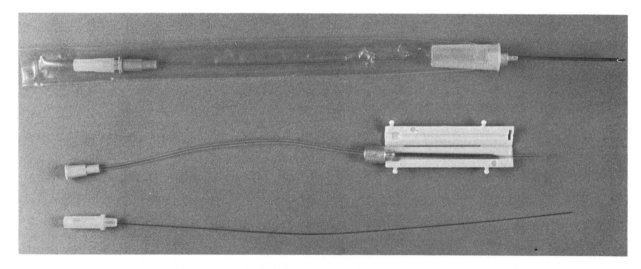

Fig. 3–10. Through-the-needle catheter. Since the needle will remain on the system after insertion, the tip must be covered with a rigid needle guard. (The Deseret Company, Sandy, Utah 84070)

sertion and promote the comfort of the patient. Avoiding areas of movement, such as the areas near the wrist and elbow joints, diminishes the chances of infiltration and often eliminates the need to use an armboard.

For infants and young children, the most commonly used sites are the scalp veins. When the cannula is properly secured, the likelihood of dislodgement is reduced. In older children, the sites used are the same as for adults. (See Chapter 6

for discussion of sites specific for infants and children.)

Except for situations in which all other sites have been exhausted, the use of veins in the lower extremities is not recommended. Diminished flow, particularly in shock states, inhibits effective delivery of the medications and creates the potential for phlebitis and thromboemboli. When upper extremity veins are not available, as in amputations or burns, some clinicians prefer to use a central

Table 3–1. COMPARISON OF DIFFERENT TYPES OF INTRAVENOUS CANNULAE

TYPE OF CANNULA	INDICATIONS FOR USE	ADVANTAGES	DISADVANTAGES
A. NEEDLES			
1. *Straight needles*	Cooperative, adult patients who require very short-term (1–3 days) therapy	Ease of insertion. Less likely to cause phlebitis	Rigid, difficult to secure so more prone to infiltration especially in active or agitated patients Less comfortable
2. *Winged-needle unit* (scalp-vein needle)	Short-term therapy for any patient, especially for infants and children; geriatric and other patients with fragile or rolling veins	Wings enable easy insertion and securing to prevent movement and dislodgement Less likely to cause phlebitis	Needle rigid and short so may infiltrate if patient very active or if needle not securely taped
3. *Intermittent winged needle unit* (heparin-lock)	Intermittent administration of drugs such as heparin, antibiotics; frequent blood sampling; or to keep vein open when no fluids are needed	Allows prompt access to the vein without giving fluids Economical; greater comfort and mobility for the patient	Will clot if not flushed with heparinized saline; part of clot can be injected into the patient when the next dose of drug is given
B. PLASTIC CATHETERS			
1. *Over-the-needle catheter*	Active or moderately agitated patients who require a secure venous line for uninterrupted delivery of drugs and/or fluids	Easy to insert More comfortable for the patient Less prone to infiltration than needles	More likely to cause phlebitis, particularly if not changed every 48–72 hours Can kink if inserted near an area of flexion (such as elbow)
2. *Over-the-needle catheter with resealable cap*	Patients on intermittent drugs without need for fluids, yet who require a secure device	Combines advantages of over-the-needle catheter with those of intermittent winged-needle unit (heparin lock)	Same as those of other over-the-needle catheters Will clot unless flushed with heparinized saline periodically
3. *Through-the-needle catheter*	Administration of hypertonic fluids or irritating drugs which must be given via a central vein to insure adequate dilution; for monitoring of CVP; emergencies in which life-sustaining drugs and fluids must be given rapidly and accurately	Very secure Available in many sizes and lengths so it can be inserted directly into a central vein or via a peripheral vein	Greater risk of infection and other complications especially when inserted into central vein Insertion requires a high degree of skill; incorrect insertion or guarding of needle can cause severing and embolization of catheter fragment
4. *In-lying* (cutdown) catheter	Patients in whom percutaneous access to veins is unsuccessful such as those in shock or cardiac arrest; those with sclerosed veins due to IV drug abuse; markedly obese patients	Provides access to superficial or deep veins May be the only means of establishing an intravenous line during emergencies Once inserted is very secure	Must be inserted by a physician Creates a surgical wound so the risk of infection is greater

vein. However, the hazards associated with central venous cannulation must be weighed against the potential risk of using the lower extremities. When the leg veins are used, the veins most commonly used are the dorsal venous network or the great saphenous vein (Fig. 3-14).

Although the peripheral veins, particularly those in the upper extremities, are the recommended sites for intravenous cannula insertion, it is sometimes necessary to insert a line into a cen-

tral vein. This is most often done when there is a need for central venous pressure monitoring, long-term drug therapy is required, or highly concentrated drugs and solutions are administered. Access to the central vein, the superior vena cava, is generally gained by threading a through-the-needle catheter from either the subclavian, internal jugular, or external jugular vein (Fig. 3-15). Because of the serious hazards associated with this procedure, including pneumothorax, arterial

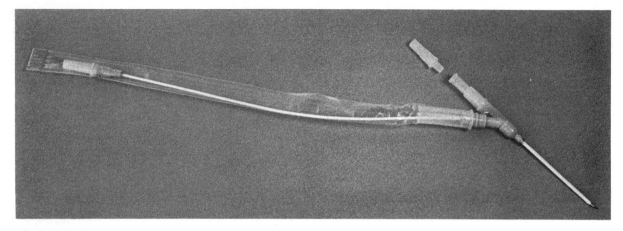

Fig. 3–11. Bard Advanset is one type of catheter which allows complete removal of the needle from the system, thereby reducing the risk of catheter severance and embolization. (Bard Hospital Division, C. R. Bard, Inc., Murray Hill, New Jersey 07974)

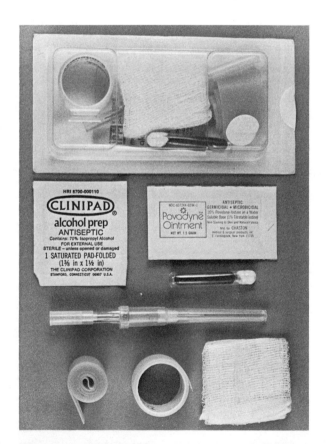

Fig. 3–12. IV Start Pak contains all the items needed for insertion of an intravenous cannula. (The Deseret Company, Sandy, Utah 84070)

puncture with resultant hemothorax, and brachial plexus palsy, this procedure is performed only by a physician. Occasionally, a central vein is reached by inserting a long catheter through a large peripheral vein, such as the cephalic or basilic. While less hazardous than the direct approach, this method is not without risk, and thus should be done only by a very skilled individual.

Specific factors in selecting the site

To select the most appropriate site, it is necessary to consider several other factors, some of which have also been examined in choosing the cannula. These factors are: the type of medication to be given, projected duration of therapy, accessibility of veins in the individual, and ability of the patient to cooperate with the therapy.

TYPE OF MEDICATION TO BE GIVEN

The majority of intravenous medications can be safely infused into the peripheral veins. If the needle or catheter is smaller than the lumen of the vein, there will be sufficient flow around it to insure adequate dilution as the fluid or medication is infusing.

Medications which are hypertonic or highly irritating require high-volume dilution to avoid systemic reactions as well as local venous irritation. Sometimes it is sufficient to dilute them before

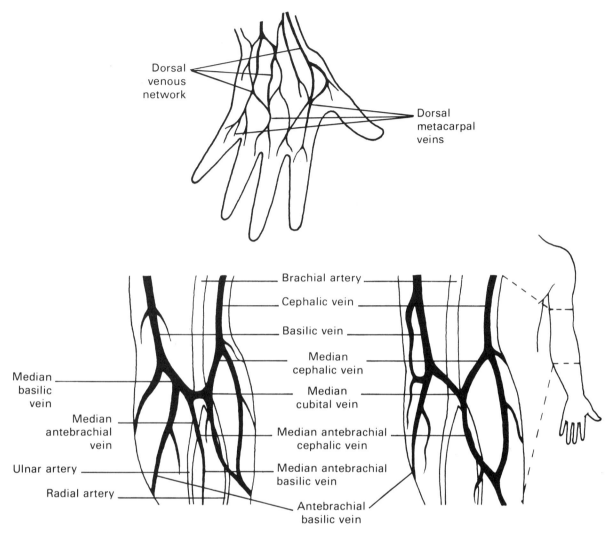

Fig. 3–13. (*Top*) The dorsal venous system of the hand. (*Bottom*) Two common configurations of the superficial veins of the inner aspect of the forearm.

administration and give them through a large peripheral vein. However, solutions such as protein hydrolysate and hypertonic sodium chloride should be administered only into a central vein. During states of shock or cardiac arrest, when peripheral blood flow is diminished, some drugs, including calcium chloride and epinephrine, are given centrally to achieve a more rapid response.

Some drugs with a potential for irritation or necrosis of surrounding tissue can be given peripherally provided that the presence of the needle or catheter within the vein has been properly established. Antineoplastic agents are an example.

Since the risk of infiltration is high, a winged-needle unit should be used only for single doses of such drugs and if the patient is cooperative. When repeated doses are required, a plastic catheter is preferable; and before each dose, the location of the catheter should be confirmed by aspirating with a syringe and needle.

If an existing intravenous line is unsuitable for the type of medication which has been ordered, another line must be inserted. When two or more intravenous medications are being administered, their compatibility must be considered. Using the appropriate diluent for each one, adequately spac-

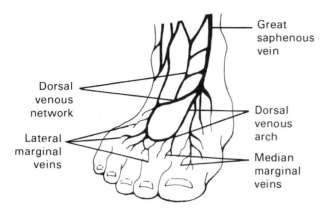

Fig. 3–14. Superficial veins of the foot and leg.

ing the doses, and flushing the line between doses may be sufficient. If the drugs must be given concurrently, however, a second intravenous line may have to be established to avoid incompatibilities.

PROJECTED DURATION OF THERAPY

For medications which are to be given as a single dose or for a few doses only and which do not require a central vein, any acceptable peripheral vein may be selected. When a medication is to be given over an extended period, as in long-term antibiotic therapy for generalized infections, many veins will probably be used since the site should ideally be changed every two to three days. Thus, care must be taken to preserve the veins by starting with the most distal sites and moving to more proximal veins as needed. Such situations demand greater attention to maintaining patency of the cannula by: (a) securing it well at the insertion site; (b) using an armboard, if needed, to prevent dislodgement through movement of the extremity; and (c) making sure that the infusion bottle is not allowed to run dry. While these all represent commonsense measures that each nurse is well aware of, they can sometimes be overlooked in the midst of a busy schedule.

AVAILABILITY OF VEINS IN THE INDIVIDUAL

While the anatomical distribution of veins is fairly consistent among most individuals, certain situations affect the accessibility of the veins most frequently used. Marked obesity may make access to peripheral veins extremely difficult if not impossible. The same is true for individuals who

have been habitual intravenous drug abusers and for patients with extensive burns or skin lesions. In these instances, it is usually necessary to either resort to a central vein or gain access to a peripheral vein through a cutdown.

Circulation to an extremity may be impaired as a result of amputation of part of that limb, immobility secondary to a CVA or other neurological disorder, an injury, or surgery such as a mastectomy. In such cases, use of the affected limb as an intravenous site should be avoided if possible. Intravenous drug therapy can present a dilemma in these patients. The affected side should not be used for physiological reasons; yet using the unaffected side can be detrimental psychologically if it restricts movement of the person's only usable arm. If the "good" arm must be used, every effort must be made to avoid selecting a vein in the hand or in the antecubital fossa which would restrict movement to the point of preventing the performance of essential daily activities, particularly eating.

When it becomes necessary to use the patient's affected side, special precautions are required. Check the infusion bottle to be sure that it is running and the site for evidence of swelling or irritation at least every two hours. If sensation is not impaired in that limb, instruct the patient to report any pain or swelling if he is able to do so. Further measures to promote good circulation include avoiding dependent positions for the extremity and encouraging exercise, active if possible.

When veins are equally accessible in both upper limbs in an individual, select a site on the nondominant side to avoid interference with daily activities.

ABILITY OF THE PATIENT TO COOPERATE
WITH THE THERAPY

Regardless of the appropriateness of the site chosen, successful intravenous drug therapy cannot be carried out if the patient is unwilling or unable to cooperate. Every nurse has cared for patients who have pulled out their intravenous cannula or who have in some way tampered with the needle or flow clamp so as to disrupt the infusion of the medication. Reasons for lack of cooperation and measures to counteract them have been discussed in some detail in the section on psychological factors (Chapter 2), but several points bear re-emphasis.

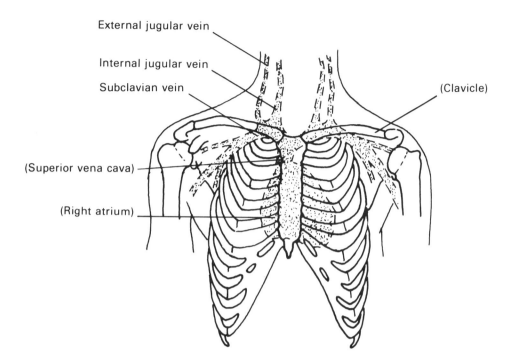

External jugular vein

Internal jugular vein

Subclavian vein

(Clavicle)

(Superior vena cava)

(Right atrium)

Fig. 3–15. Gross anatomy of the central venous system, showing large veins available for percutaneous introduction of intravenous cannulae. Related structures are in parentheses.

Patients who cannot understand the reason for the therapy include young children and people with altered mental status secondary to psychological or organic brain disease. They are often unable to cooperate despite all measures previously discussed. When intravenous drugs are required in these individuals, efforts must be directed toward preventing removal of the intravenous line. With very young children, use of a scalp vein reduces the likelihood of their tampering with it. With confused geriatric patients or other disoriented individuals, the mid-forearm is often the best peripheral site. By providing unrestricted use of that hand and arm, the intravenous line may prove less upsetting, and cooperation may be more readily gained. In such patients a central line may also be a good site since confused patients are often less aware of its presence.

Though restraints are generally used only as a last resort, they may be essential in this instance to insure administration of the medication. The most suitable type of restraining device should be selected. For patients who are confused but not combative, such as the elderly, a mitt restraint on the opposite arm will allow movement of the extremity without disruption of the infusion. Unfor-

tunately, even this may not be sufficient to deter the individual who is actively attempting to remove the intravenous cannula. Soft restraints applied to both arms would be appropriate for this individual, with care being taken that they are not applied directly over the cannula site, in which case they might create the situation they are attempting to prevent.

After assessment of these factors, the potential sites will have been narrowed down. In some patients only one location, and perhaps only one vein, will be acceptable; and thus, it must be used. With other patients who have many well-defined veins, all equally suitable, the final choice should be based on patient preference and comfort, allowing maximum mobility of the extremity.

A summary of the factors influencing the use of peripheral and central sites is found in Table 3-2. In spite of the importance of considering each of the criteria before establishing the intravenous infusion, the clinical situation at times makes such a thorough assessment impractical or impossible. In emergencies, such as during cardiopulmonary resuscitation, an intravenous line must be inserted as rapidly as possible; and thus, the most accessible location generally takes precedence. Following

Table 3–2. FACTORS IN THE SELECTION OF PERIPHERAL OR CENTRAL SITES FOR INTRAVENOUS INSERTION

FACTOR	PERIPHERAL VEINS		CENTRAL VEINS	
	Suitable	Unsuitable	Suitable	Unsuitable
Type of drug or solution	Most drugs Isotonic fluids	Irritating drugs or hypertonic fluids which require maximal dilution	Irritating drugs or hypertonic fluids	Drugs which if injected centrally could cause arrhythmias, shock or other complications
Duration of therapy	Short-term or intermittent therapy; is less hazardous	Long-term therapy, in which all available veins would be used up	Moderate to long-term continuous therapy	Short-term therapy; the patient is subjected greater risks
Accessibility of veins	Patients with adequate peripheral veins	Very obese patients; I.V. drug abusers; conditions which impair peripheral circulation	When peripheral veins inaccessible, especially if intravenous line is needed in an emergency	At times not accessible after repeated use (e.g. pacemaker). May be accessible, but increased risks due to location near lungs
Cooperation of patient	Extremity can usually be restrained sufficiently to allow insertion and maintenance of line	Disoriented or agitated adult or child may be more likely to attempt removal of intravenous line located in upper extremity	Central lines, especially subclavian, are less likely to be disrupted, once inserted	Patient must lie absolutely still during the insertion to prevet pneumothorax and other complications

successful resuscitation, the intravenous site can be relocated if necessary.

REFERENCES

1. Abbott Laboratories: How to Use a Universal I.V. Administration Set. *I.V. Tips,* North Chicago, Illinois: October 1975.
2. Abbott Laboratories: Intermittent I.V. Procedures. *I.V. Tips,* North Chicago, Illinois: October 1975.
3. Arnold, Thomas R., and Hepler, Charles D.: Bacterial Contamination of Intravenous Fluids Opened in Unsterile Air. *American Journal of Hospital Pharmacy,* 28:614–619, August 1971.
4. Bolasny, B. L., Shepard, G. H., and Scott, H. W., Jr.: The Hazards of Intravenous Polyethylene Catheters in Surgical Patients. *Surgery, Gynecology and Obstetrics,* 130:342–346, 1970.
5. Collins, Richard N., Braun, Peter A., Zinner, Stephen H., and Kass, Edward H.: Risk of Local and Systemic Infection with Polyethylene Intravenous Catheters. *New England Journal of Medicine,* 279:340–343, 1968.
6. Crossley, K., and Matsen, J. M.: The Scalp-Vein Needle: A Prospective Study of Associated Complications. *Journal of the American Medical Association,* 220:985–987, 1972.
7. Darby, Thomas D., and Ausman, Robert K.: Particulate Matter in Polyvinyl Chloride Intravenous Bags. (Cont.) (Letter) *The New England Journal of Medicine,* 290:579, March 1974.
8. Ferguson, Robert L., Rosett, Walter, Hodges, Glenn R., and Barnes, William G.: Complications with Heparin-Lock Needles. *Annals of Internal Medicine,* 85:583–586, November 1976.
9. Goldmann, Donald A., Maki, Dennis G., Rhame, Frank S., Kaiser, Allen B., Tenney, James H., and Bennett, John V.: Guidelines for Infection Control in Intravenous Therapy. *Annals of Internal Medicine,* 79:848–850, 1973.
10. Hanson, Robert L.: Heparin-Lock or Keep-Open I.V.? *American Journal of Nursing,* 76(7):1102–1103, July 1976.
11. Hoshal, Verne L., Ause, Robert G., and Hoskins, Phillip A.: Fibrin Sleeve Formation on Indwelling Subclavian Central Venous Catheters, *Archives of Surgery,* 102:353–358, April 1971.
12. Letcher, Kenneth I., Thrupp, Laurie D., Shapiro, David J., and Boersma, Johanna E.: In-Use Contamination of Intravenous Solutions in Flexible Plastic Containers. *American Journal of Hospital Pharmacy,* 29:673-677, August 1973.
13. MacDonald, Alan: Permeation of Water Vapour Through Plastic Containers for Intravenous Infusion Fluids. *The Journal of Hospital Pharmacy,* 32:174–176, September 1974.
14. Maki, Dennis G.: Preventing Infection in Intravenous Therapy. *Hospital Practice,* 11:95–104, April 1976.
15. Maki, Dennis G., Rhame, Frank S., Mackel, Donald

C., and Bennett, John V.: Nationwide Epidemic of Septicemia Caused by Contaminated Intravenous Products. *The American Journal of Medicine,* 60:471–485, April 1976.

16. Meyers, Lawrence: Intravenous Catheterization. *American Journal of Nursing,* 45(11):930–931, November 1945.

17. Needham, T. E., Jr., and Luzzi, L. A.: Particulate Matter in Polyvinyl Chloride Intravenous Bags. (letter) *The New England Journal of Medicine,* 289:1256, December 6, 1973.

18. Petrick, Robert J., Loucas, Spiro P., Cohl, Jerome K., and Mehl, Bernard: Review of Current Knowledge of Plastic Intravenous Fluid Containers. *American Journal of Hospital Pharmacy,* 34:357–362, April 1977.

19. Petty, Clayton, and Cunningham, Nelson L.: Insulin Adsorption by Glass Infusion Bottles, Polyvinyl Chloride Infusion Containers, and Intravenous Tubing, *Anesthesiology,* 40:400–404, April 1974.

20. Plumer, Ada Lawrence: *Principles and Practice of Intravenous Therapy* (2nd ed.), Boston: Little, Brown and Company, 1975.

21. Poretz, Donald M., Guynn, James B., Jr., Duma, Richard J., and Dalton, Harry P.: Microbial Contamination of Glass Bottle (Open-Vented) and Plastic Bag (Closed-Nonvented) Intravenous Fluid Delivery Systems. *American Journal of Hospital Pharmacy,* 31:726–732, August 1974.

22. Rappaport, A. M., Graham, R. K., and Kendrick, W. W.: The Use of Siliconized Polyethylene Tubing in Prolonged Intravenous Infusions. *Canadian Medical Association Journal,* 72:698–700, May 1, 1955.

23. Stern, Robert C., Pittman, Susan, Doershuk, Carl F., and Matthews, LeRoy W.: Use of a "Heparin Lock" in the Intermittent Administration of Intravenous Drugs. *Clinical Pediatrics,* 11:521–523, September 1972.

24. Thomas, Edward T., Evers, William, and Racz, Gabor B.: Postinfusion Phlebitis. *Anesthesia and Analgesia,* 49:150–159, 1970.

25. Turco, Salvatore J., and Davis, Neil M.: Particulate Matter in Intravenous Infusion Fluids—Phase 3. *American Journal of Hospital Pharmacy,* 30:611–613, July 1973.

26. Turco, Salvatore and King, Robert E.: *Sterile Dosage Forms—Their Preparation and Clinical Application,* Philadelphia: Lea and Febiger, 1974.

4 Insertion of the Intravenous Line

Once the initial preparations have been completed, the fluid system, cannula, and other needed equipment are brought to the patient's bedside. The final steps involved in initiating an intravenous line include selecting the specific vein, disinfecting the skin, performing the venipuncture, and securing the cannula and dressing the site.

SELECTING THE VEIN

While the general site has been chosen based on the factors discussed in the previous chapter, the specific vein and the entry site are located only after a careful inspection and palpation of veins in the limb selected. This can be accomplished more readily after application of a tourniquet to distend the veins. The tourniquet can consist of either rubber tubing, a flat rubber strip (sometimes available with self-adhering ends), or a blood pressure cuff. Tourniquets are often disregarded as a potential source of infection; but when used repeatedly on many patients, cross-contamination can occur.

Apply the tourniquet several inches above the venipuncture site, making sure that it is not obstructing arterial flow. Rubber tourniquets which must be tied should be secured with a loop rather than a knot so that they can be rapidly removed by pulling one end (Fig. 4-1). In individuals with veins which are sclerosed, care must be taken that the tourniquet is not left on too long lest the pressure increase, making them hard and difficult to enter (18). Thus, in some cases it might be best to avoid using a tourniquet.

Additional measures may be used to achieve maximal distention of the vein:

1. Keep the limb in a dependent position prior to application of the tourniquet.
2. If the environment is cool, apply a warm towel to the area for 10 to 20 minutes.
3. Lightly tap the limb over the vein.
4. Ask the patient to alternately tightly close and open his fist several times.

In most instances these measures produce sufficient venous engorgement to enable successful venipuncture.

SKIN PREPARATION

Both the extent and the type of skin preparation required remains somewhat controversial, but the need for removal of potentially harmful organisms cannot be denied. It is generally agreed that a quick wipe with an alcohol pad is ineffective in eliminating pathogenic organisms from the insertion site.

Resident bacteria, which comprise the permanent inhabitants of an individual's skin, are relatively difficult to remove; yet fortunately, few are generally pathogenic. Transient bacteria, those that are constantly being acquired through contact with the environment, are abundant on the hands and other exposed skin surfaces. While they are less resistant to removal, pathogenic varieties are common; and thus, they represent a potentially greater threat whenever the skin is punctured. In a hospital environment where numerous pathogens abound, prolonged exposure may result in colonization of many of these normally transient organisms in personnel and patients alike (22). Thus, meticulous skin disinfection should be carried out prior to any procedure in which the integrity of the skin is disrupted.

While this discussion is concerned primarily with disinfection of the skin of the patient, the individual performing the venipuncture, who represents a potential transmitter of pathogenic organisms, must not be neglected. Handwashing is a procedure that is so routine to health-care personnel, particularly nurses, that it would seem almost unnecessary to mention it. Yet, inasmuch as habitual practices can become haphazard when not given attention, the need for thorough handwashing using a standard technique must be re-emphasized. Developing a conscious awareness of this will help to insure that adequate handwashing is carried out both before approaching the patient and after performing the procedure.

Basic skin disinfection is essential even for venipunctures performed solely for the collection of venous blood samples. The more detailed procedure described below is essential for insertion of intravenous cannulae, since such devices represent a prime source of entry for any organisms inhabiting the skin around the insertion site.

Skin disinfection has been directed toward three areas:

1. Removal of hair

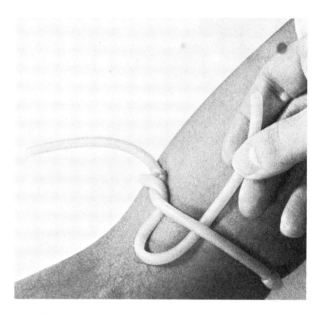

Fig. 4–1. When correctly applied, a tourniquet can be removed rapidly by pulling one end.

2. Defatting of the skin
3. Antisepsis of the skin

Removal of hair

The removal of hair, generally by shaving, has traditionally been considered essential to insure the removal of all organisms. However, current evidence suggests that hair does not harbor different or more organisms than skin, and methods which effectively disinfect the skin likewise disinfect the hair (16). Furthermore, the use of a razor creates microabrasions and occasionally nicks which can provide access for bacterial entrance (22). Thus, hair need not and perhaps should not be routinely removed. When abundant hair makes cannula insertion difficult, consideration should be given to the use of chemical depilatories or trimming with scissors rather than shaving (19). When prevention of the discomfort due to later removal of the tape is the primary reason for shaving the hair, it might suffice to remove only the hair around the site where the tape will be placed and to avoid the site where the cannula will be inserted.

Defatting of the skin

In the past it has been thought that the resistance of resident bacteria to removal from the skin was due to skin oils or secretions from sebaceous glands (9). Consequently, agents such as ether and acetone, which have a fat-solvent action, were widely recommended in the hope of aiding bacterial removal. More recent studies, however, suggest that grease, oil, and sebum do not provide a source of attachment for bacteria (22). Therefore, the use of those agents seems unnecessary and, in view of their inflammability, probably unwise.

Antisepsis of the skin

The perfect agent for disinfecting the skin has not yet been found. Such an antiseptic should be bactericidal, fungicidal, and sporicidal, and yet pose a minimal risk of irritation, burning, or allergic reactions. Agents containing hexachlorophene (pHisoHex, Septisol) which require several days of repeated use to achieve antisepsis, would be unsuitable for one-time procedures such as venipuncture. Compounds such as benzalkonuim chloride (Zephiran), which were once in widespread use, are now known to be able to support the growth of organisms such as *Pseudomonas* and thus are not recommended (16). A newer agent, chlorhexidine (Hibiclens) can also become contaminated with *Pseudomonas* and *Proteus* and is thus not the agent of choice (22).

Of agents currently available, the most effective are the iodine preparations, which include tincture of iodine and the iodophors. Since they are more likely to produce skin reactions, inquiry should be made before they are used regarding any history of allergy to iodine. Although a patient may not realize that he is allergic to iodine, he may be aware of an allergy to certain types of seafood including shellfish.

Tincture of iodine (2 percent iodine in 70 percent alcohol) is probably more effective than the iodophors but presents a greater likelihood of skin reactions (11, 22). When it is utilized, the skin should be scrubbed with moderate friction, using a circular motion starting at the insertion site and moving outward (21) (Fig. 4-2). After allowing the skin to dry for 30 to 60 seconds, rinse with 70 percent alcohol to prevent skin irritation.

The iodophors such as povidone iodine (Betadine) are a combination of iodine and an organic compound. They are applied in a similar manner but should *not* be rinsed off with alcohol since that would inhibit their effectiveness. They should be allowed to dry for two to four minutes. It is believed that their action persists as long as their yellow color is visible (22). For ease of administration, iodophors are available in the form of prep pads, applicator sticks, and crushable capsules, all of which are not only less messy but eliminate the bulky, large volume containers which are prone to contamination.

For individuals who are sensitive to any iodine-containing preparation, 70 percent alcohol is an effective agent if applied with sufficient friction for at least one minute.

Once the skin has been disinfected, it is essential that the site not be touched. While such a recommendation represents common sense, in actual practice it is not uncommon to observe an individual cleanse the skin and then palpate the prepared site to locate the vein. The importance of avoiding such a practice cannot be overemphasized.

PERFORMING THE VENIPUNCTURE

Procedures vary, depending on the type of cannula used; but all represent a variation of the basic technique for inserting a needle.

Straight needle

1. Connect the hub of the needle to the administration tubing using aseptic technique and flush with solution to expel all air. If blood samples are required, a syringe is attached to the needle; and once the needle is in place, the blood is withdrawn. After the needle is securely in the vein, the administration tubing is then attached. Some individuals prefer to use this technique even when a blood sample is not needed since the larger, firmer "handle" allows easier manipulation of the needle. As a general rule, however, this method is rarely used.
2. Anesthetizing the site is usually unnecessary unless the needle is 16 gauge or larger. In fact, the stinging associated with infiltration of the anesthetic can be more painful than the needle prick itself.
3. Firmly hold the patient's arm or hand to prevent sudden movement when the skin is punctured. With the thumb below the insertion point, exert slight pressure to pull the skin taut and to stablize the vein.

4. Holding the needle bevel side up and with the needle shaft at a 45-degree angle to the skin, quickly and firmly enter the skin and underlying tissue at a point about one-half inch below that where the needle will enter the vein.

5. Lower the needle shaft until it is almost parallel with the skin and pierce the vein. The resistance encountered as the vein is entered is sometimes felt as a snapping sensation (3). A flashback of blood into the tubing or syringe further documents the needle's presence within the vein.

6. Lifting the needle slightly, advance it with caution until it is securely within the vein. This lifting movement decreases the likelihood of puncturing the posterior wall of the vein (2).

7. Release the tourniquet and open the clamp on the administration tubing to initiate the flow of solution. Check for a free flow while observing for any signs of infiltration. Some individuals prefer to open the flow clamp slightly *before* beginning the venipuncture, bending the tubing between two fingers to stop the flow. After the venipuncture has been accomplished, the tubing is released to reestablish the flow (18).

If the syringe method is used, once the presence of the needle in the vein is verified, the blood sample is withdrawn as required. Then, while the needle hub is held securely to prevent dislodgement, the syringe is removed and the administration set is quickly attached.

SECURING THE CANNULA AND DRESSING THE SITE

1. Anchor the needle securely by placing a piece of tape over the needle hub and shaft but not over the insertion point. Such taping is essential to reduce the chance of infiltration, irritation, and phlebitis due to any to-and-fro movement of the needle. For additional security, place a narrow piece of tape with the adhesive side up beneath the needle hub. Bring each end up, crisscrossing them in chevron fashion over the needle.

2. Loop the tubing back and tape it separately. Use of a single strip of tape over both the cannula and tubing is not recommended, as dislodgement can occur when the tubing is changed.

3. Apply an antiseptic iodophor ointment to the

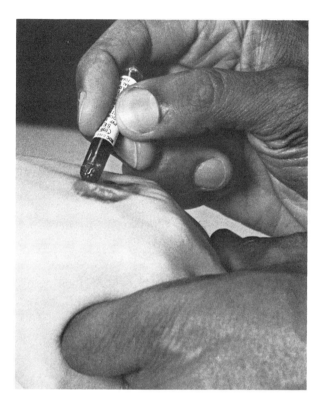

Fig. 4–2. Disinfection of the skin. Using a circular motion, begin at the insertion site and move outward.

insertion site and cover with either a 2-by 2-inch gauze pad or a plastic adhesive bandage. The latter allows the site to be easily inspected, cleansed, and redressed without removal of all the tape and thus promotes daily cannula care and reduces the likelihood of complications (5).

4. Record on the tape the date and time of insertion as well as the name of the person inserting the intravenous line.

5. When the cannula is inserted near an area of active movement, such as a joint or the dorsal surface of the hand, or if the patient is unable to cooperate, the site should be immobilized with an armboard. (Special techniques for immobilizing limbs in infants and children are discussed in Chapter 6.) To prevent deformities, the limb should be placed in a functional position with the hand and fingers slightly flexed. Contour armboards are available which promote proper positioning. To secure it, apply wide strips of tape at both ends of the board, making certain that pressure is not applied on the cannula site. Patient comfort

and safety can further be promoted by:

    a. Limiting the length of the armboard to the involved joints. When the cannula is in the hand or wrist area, do not immobilize the elbow joint.

    b. Padding the armboard with a towel or other soft material.

    c. Using double tape (placing two strips of tape with the adhesive sides together) on the areas which will be in contact with the patient's skin. This both decreases the chance of skin irritation and prevents discomfort due to pulling of hair and skin when the tape is removed.

    d. Removing the armboard at least once daily to allow movement of the fingers and wrist while avoiding dislodgement of the needle.

6. Adjust the flow rate as described in the next chapter.

Winged-needle unit (Fig. 4-3)

To insert a winged-needle unit or scalp-vein needle, follow the same basic steps as with a straight needle with the following exceptions:

1. The procedure which is most often recommended involves connecting the administration set first and flushing it with fluid to clear the tubing and needle of air (1, 17, 18). With the other method, the winged-needle unit is inserted before being connected to the administration tubing, in which case the adaptor cover is kept in place (15).

2. Hold the needle by grasping the two wings together with thumb and forefinger and perform the venipuncture as described in Steps 3 through 7 above.

3. After the needle has been advanced well into the lumen of the vein and the flow of solution has been initiated, secure the needle by using either of two methods. One is the chevron method described above. In this instance, the tape is crisscrossed over the two wings. The needle tubing is then coiled on top of the wings and secured with another piece of tape (15). The other technique involves applying separate short pieces of tape over each wing and a third strip perpendicularly across the top. The tubing is coiled and taped in place. The site is dressed, using an antiseptic ointment and small bandage as with a straight needle.

Intermittent winged-needle unit

The procedure for insertion of an intermittent unit or heparin lock is similar except for a few points.

1. After cleansing the rubber injection site with alcohol, insert a needle and syringe filled with saline or sterile water and flush the unit to clear the air (14).

2. With the needle and syringe kept in place, insert the needle into the vein, as with a standard winged-needle unit, by grasping hold of the wings.

3. To verify the presence of the needle in the vein, pull back the plunger to aspirate blood.

4. Inject some of the solution remaining in the syringe. If a sudden swelling or pain at the site is noted, the needle has infiltrated and must be removed.

5. If it has not infiltrated, withdraw the needle and syringe; then flush the unit with heparinized saline. Less than one-half milliliter of solution is required to flush a standard unit. While many strengths of heparinized saline have been advocated, it is generally recommended that the weakest strength capable of maintaining patency without altering coagulation times be used (8). It has been demonstrated that a concentration of 10 units of heparin per milliliter of saline instilled after every dose of medication or at least every eight hours can meet these criteria (12).

When an intermittent winged-needle unit is not available, a standard winged-needle unit can be converted into a heparin lock through the use of a sterile adaptor plug designed for that purpose. The adaptor plug is connected to the end of the needle tubing. After the unit has been inserted into the vein in the standard manner, the unit is then flushed and maintained with heparinized saline as described above (4).

Over-the-needle cannulae

As discussed in the previous chapter, several investigators have noted an increased risk of infective complications associated with plastic catheters (16, 20). Thus, their insertion requires even more diligent adherence to aseptic techniques than does the insertion of needles. Disinfection of the skin should include all of the measures described

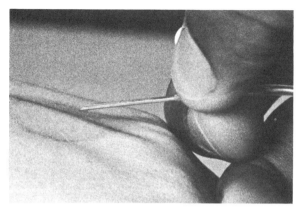

A. Hold the unit bevel up by grasping the wings together and insert into the skin at approximately a 45-degree angle.

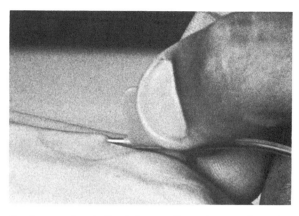

B. Lower the shaft of the needle and enter the vein, looking for a flashback of blood to verify successful venipuncture.

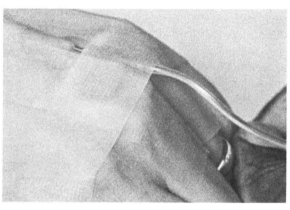

C. After advancing the needle fully within the vein, lower the wings and secure with tape over each wing (parallel to the tubing) and place a third strip perpendicularly across the top.

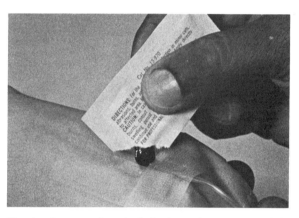

D. Apply an antiseptic iodophor ointment to minimize the likelihood of infection.

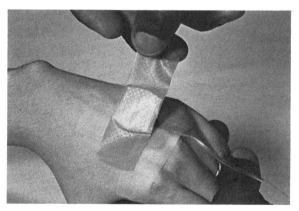

E. Cover the site with a sterile plastic bandage to simplify daily inspection and redressing of the insertion site.

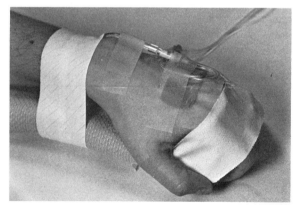

F. Coil the tubing and tape securely; apply an armboard to prevent excessive movement and dislodging of the needle.

Fig. 4–3. Insertion of a winged-needle unit (scalp-vein needle).

above. As an additional precaution, it has been recommended that sterile gloves be worn (11). While this is certainly advisable, the procedure can be safely carried out without them if aseptic practices are diligently followed.

A few over-the-needle units are packaged with a syringe attached, but most units are available instead with a sight chamber and a hub cover to enable rapid visualization of the blood flashback and to provide a firm handle, decreasing the chance of touch contamination of the cannula during insertion. To insert the cannula, the following steps are carried out (Fig. 4-4):

1. With the tourniquet in place to distend the vein, hold the flash chamber of the unit; and keeping the needle at a 45-degree angle to the skin, insert as with a straight needle.
2. After the needle has been placed at least one-half inch within the vein, stabilize the needle hub with one hand; and using the other hand, gradually advance the catheter over the needle until it is the desired distance within the vein. Once the catheter is in place within the vein, *never* readvance the needle, as it can puncture the catheter, introducing the risk of shearing.
3. After proper placement of the catheter, release the tourniquet, withdraw the needle while stabilizing the catheter hub, and attach the administration tubing. To prevent leakage of blood before the tubing is attached, a method which has been referred to as the "Dutch-Boy" technique can be employed (10). This involves applying slight pressure directly over the vein with one or two fingers to temporarily interrupt the backflow of blood until the tubing can be attached (18).
4. Open the flow-control clamp, observing for signs of infiltration, and adjust the flow rate as discussed in the next chapter.
5. Tape the catheter securely using the crossover or chevron method. One catheter unit model is designed with small wings attached to the hub, which allows an easy and secure means of taping.
6. Apply antiseptic ointment and a small gauze pad or plastic adhesive bandage to the insertion site. Secure with a strip of tape.
7. Loop the tubing and apply a separate piece of tape.
8. Record the date and time of insertion, size of

catheter, and name of person inserting the cannula on the tape.

If the catheter is to be used as an intermittent unit or heparin lock, insert in the same manner, but attach an intermittent adaptor plug instead of the administration tubing. Flush with heparinized saline immediately to prevent clotting.

Through-the-needle catheters

The insertion of long catheters which advance through the needle requires a more exacting procedure than with needles or short, plastic cannulae since their placement has been found to be associated with more local trauma and bacterial colonization than other types of cannulae (6, 18). Thus, their insertion should be limited to highly skilled individuals. In hospitals in which nurses or other nonphysicians are responsible for initiating intravenous lines, it is recommended that a specific order be obtained from the physician when this type of device is to be inserted.

Because of the increased likelihood of infection noted with long, plastic catheters, skin disinfection must be even more exacting than with insertion of other types of cannulae (6). Sterile gloves should always be worn, and the use of sterile drapes is desirable. Specific procedures for insertion will vary slightly depending on the type of device used. The manufacturer's guidelines included with each catheter should be known and followed. The general procedure for units in which the needle remains on the system after insertion is as follows:

1. Holding the needle at the hub, perform the venipuncture by carrying out the same steps as with a straight needle (Steps 1 to 6).
2. Once the needle is well within the vein, hold the hub securely and slowly advance the catheter into the vein. Some catheters are enclosed in a thin, plastic sleeve as a further precaution against contamination.
3. Continue to introduce the catheter until the desired length is within the vein. Once advancement has begun, NEVER PULL BACK THE CATHETER as the risk of its being sheared off by the needle is high. If attempts to advance the catheter are unsuccessful, the needle and catheter MUST BE WITHDRAWN SIMULTANEOUSLY and a new unit used for a subsequent attempt.
4. When the catheter has been successfully

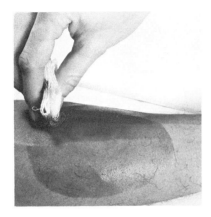

A. Disinfect the skin using an iodophor preparation.

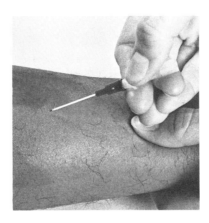

B. Holding the clear flash chamber, insert the needle at a 45-degree angle.

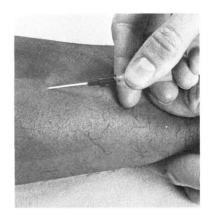

C. After entering the skin, lower the needle shaft until it is nearly parallel with the skin.

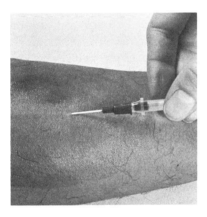

D. Enter the vein, watching for a flashback of blood in the site chamber.

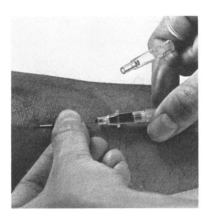

E. Gradually advance the catheter over the needle, until it is fully within the vein. NEVER readvance the needle once the catheter is in place.

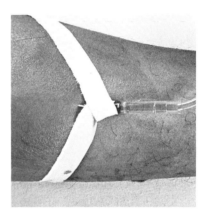

F. After removal of the needle, attach the administration tubing in and secure the cannula with tape; use the chevron method.

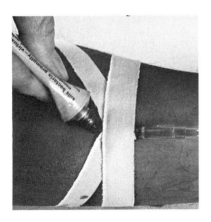

G. Apply an antiseptic iodophor ointment to the insertion site.

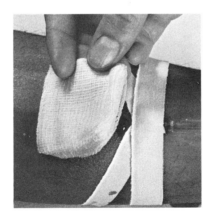

H. Cover with a sterile gauze pad.

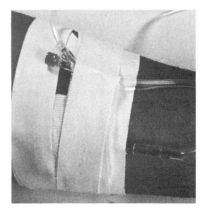

I. Tape securely; loop the tubing and tape.

Fig. 4–4. Insertion of an over-the-needle cannula.

49

placed, release the tourniquet. While holding the catheter hub securely, withdraw the needle until it is completely outside of the skin, leaving approximately ⅛ to ¼ inch of catheter exposed.

5. Using a sterile gauze pad, apply pressure over the site briefly to prevent bleeding (18).

6. Attach the rigid guard over the needle tip to prevent bending and severing of the catheter. Units in which the plastic guard is long enough to cover the entire needle from the hub to beyond the tip provide the greatest margin of safety. Those designed with smaller guards require special care to insure that the needle tip is completely covered. Taping a wooden tongue depressor to the needle and exposed portion of the catheter is recommended by some individuals as an added precaution (18). Incorrect shielding can result in severing of the catheter near the insertion site and possible subsequent embolization of the fragment. Although their radiopacity generally enables x-ray detection of the embolized catheter, removal is sometimes unsuccessful. More detailed information about the occurrence and treatment of this complication is given in Chapter 7.

While the incidence of catheter embolization is fortunately quite low, the occurrence might be reduced further by the use of through-the-needle units in which the needle is completely removed from the system. Insertion techniques vary according to the design of the unit. As mentioned in Chapter 3, this type usually incorporates a separate placement cannula. The over-the-needle cannula is inserted first in the standard manner. After withdrawal of the needle, the catheter is inserted through the introducer cannula, either via a Y-type connection or by means of a separate unit that locks into place. Because no needle is present either during insertion of the catheter or afterward, the shearing hazard is virtually eliminated. However, since two foreign bodies, both the inner and outer catheters, remain within the vein, there may be an added risk of infection.

Another type of unit utilizes a split needle. The needle and intracatheter are introduced using the same technique as for standard through-the-needle catheters. Thus, severing can still occur during insertion unless care is taken to avoid pulling back the catheter. After the needle is withdrawn from the vein, the plastic sheath covering the needle is removed, and the needle is split in half and removed from the system.

A drawback of many of the units which enable complete removal of the needle from the system is that their insertion technique is somewhat more complex, which can be a disadvantage in emergency situations. However, it would seem that the hazard they seek to eliminate would justify continued research into the perfection and simplification of their design.

Central venous catheterization

The insertion of a catheter into a central vein is always performed by a physician, but the nurse frequently assists with the procedure and is responsible for maintaining the patency of the cannula and the follow-up care of the insertion site. Therefore, a discussion of this procedure is included here.

When placement of a catheter into a central vein is required for the administration of medications or fluids, it can be done in adults by passing a long, through-the-needle catheter by means of a peripheral vein until the tip is within a central vein. Because of the great length of the catheter required, this method can present an increased risk of vein irritation and infection. Insertion can also be hindered by kinking of the catheter, causing it to double back onto itself or be misdirected into another vein.

Therefore, in most instances, central venous catheterization is accomplished directly into a central vein such as the subclavian or internal or external jugular. Since the procedure is lengthier and involves more discomfort than with a peripheral venipuncture, greater attention must be given to psychological preparation of the patient whenever possible. Such a preparation should include information about what the procedure involves, positioning, skin prep, wearing of sterile attire, including gown, mask, and gloves, by the physician, and discomfort associated with the administration of the anesthetic and the actual needle insertion (18). The presence of the nurse throughout the procedure can allay some of the patient's apprehension and help to elicit his cooperation. Additional nursing responsibilities include monitoring vital signs on critically ill patients and observing for respiratory distress, vagal reactions, and other complications.

The *subclavian vein* can be entered from either below or above the clavicle. Clinicians disagree as to which approach minimizes both risk of complications and patient discomfort (7, 13). Since the infraclavicular approach remains the more widely used of the two in many institutions, this is the one that will be described (Fig. 4-5).

1. To promote maximal filling of the vein, the patient is placed in a Trendelenburg position with a rolled towel placed along the axis of the spine. The head is turned away from the side being used.

2. Strict aseptic technique must be followed throughout, including the wearing of sterile gloves, gown, and a mask by the person inserting the catheter. It is advisable that other individuals standing nearby also wear masks. Shaving of the skin and use of a defatting agent are recommended by some clinicians but remain controversial (7). However, the need for disinfection of the skin with an agent such as tincture of iodine or an iodophor cannot be disputed. After the skin has been disinfected, a wide area around the insertion site is covered with sterile drapes.

3. Unless the patient is comatose and unresponsive to pain, the insertion site and underlying tissues are infiltrated with a local anesthetic. Lidocaine (1 to 2 percent) is the agent most often used.

4. Using a large, usually 14 gauge, needle with a 2- to 5-milliliter syringe attached, the physician inserts the needle under the midclavicle directing the needle horizontally toward the supraclavicular notch.

5. As the needle is advanced, slight negative pressure is applied to the syringe until a flashback of blood is obtained signaling puncture of the vein. The needle is then advanced an additional few millimeters to make certain that the bevelled tip is well within the vein. Should bright, red blood enter the syringe without application of negative pressure, the chance of puncture of the subclavian artery is likely, requiring withdrawal of the needle and application of firm pressure over the puncture site well under the clavicle for at least five minutes.

6. Once the presence of the needle within the subclavian vein is ascertained, the syringe is detached while the patient is asked to perform a Valsalva maneuver (exhaling against a closed glottis). If the patient's condition prevents him from doing this, the same effect is achieved by compressing his abdomen (13). This measure along with temporarily covering the opening of the needle with a gloved finger helps to decrease the chance of air embolism (2).

7. Holding the needle securely, the catheter (generally 16 gauge and 8 to 12 inches long) is threaded through the needle. With the bevel of the needle in a downward position to facilitate the catheter's movement inferiorly into the vena cava, the catheter is gradually advanced its full length. If advancement is unsuccessful, the needle and catheter MUST BE WITHDRAWN SIMULTANEOUSLY. THE CATHETER MUST NEVER BE PULLED BACK THROUGH THE NEEDLE due to the risk of severing as described above. As an additional precaution in the event of severing and embolization, all catheters inserted into a central vein must be radiopaque.

8. The administration tubing is immediately connected to the catheter hub and the flow established to maintain catheter patency. To further document free flow in both directions, the fluid bottle is temporarily lowered to obtain a sudden flashback of blood (7). The solution should again flow freely as soon as the bottle is raised.

9. The needle is then withdrawn allowing about 1 centimeter of catheter between the needle tip and the skin. A rigid needle guard must be properly applied over the needle tip to prevent severing of the catheter.

10. To prevent dislodgement or kinking, the catheter is generally sutured in place with 3-0 silk.

11. Antiseptic ointment such as an iodophor is applied to the insertion site, and a dressing is applied. A sterile 2- by 2-inch or 4- by 4-inch gauze pad both is placed below and on top of the catheter at the insertion site. The use of preslit dressings which can encircle the catheter are helpful with a standard guaze pad on

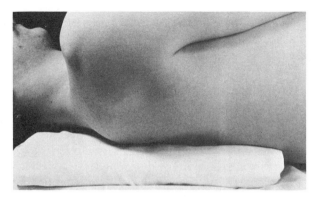

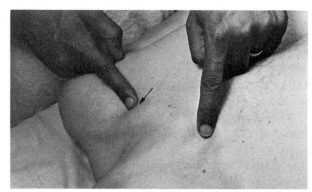

A. The patient is placed in a Trendelenberg position with a rolled towel along the axis of the spine.

B. Measuring from the sternal notch, the insertion point is located, one-half to two thirds the distance along the clavicle.

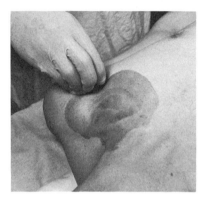

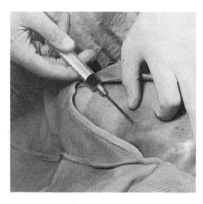

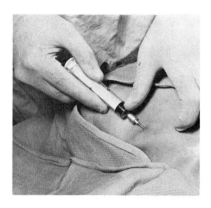

C. Wearing sterile attire, the physician disinfects the patient's skin with an iodophor preparation.

D. After the area is anesthetized, a 14 gauge needle is inserted under the midclavicle and directed horizontally toward the sternal notch.

E. While slight negative pressure is applied on the syringe, the needle is advanced further at the same angle.

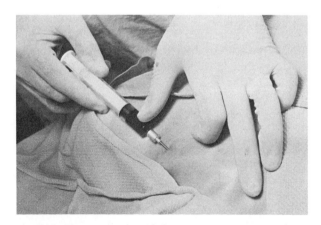

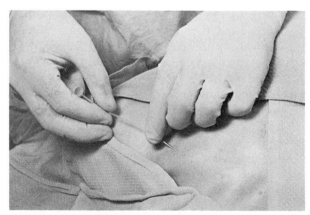

F. Entry into the vein is signaled by blood entering the syringe.

G. The syringe is detached and the catheter is quickly threaded through the needle. Once advancement of the catheter has begun, it must NEVER be pulled back through the needle, since severing can occur.

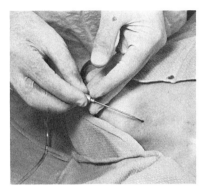

H. The administration tubing is quickly attached, the flow of fluid is established, and the needle is withdrawn from the skin.

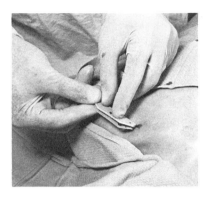

I. A rigid needle guard is applied over the entire needle to prevent shearing of the catheter.

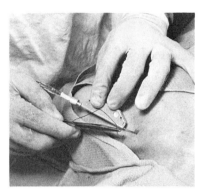

J. Suturing of the catheter to the skin is a further means of preventing dislodgement.

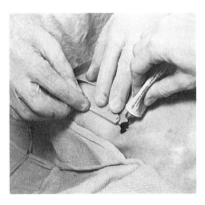

K. An antiseptic iodophor ointment is applied to the injection site.

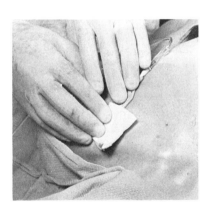

L. Sterile gauze pads are placed over the site.

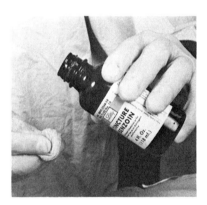

M. Application of tincture of benzoin to the surrounding skin helps to minimize skin irritation and to promote adherence of the tape.

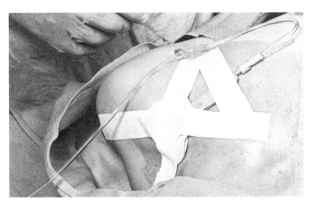

N. Adhesive tape is placed over the dressing and needle guard.

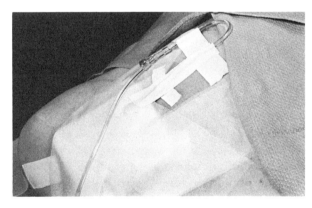

O. Wide strips of tape are applied to the entire area, with separate pieces placed over the junction of the catheter hub and tubing to prevent separation.

Fig. 4–5. Subclavian vein catheterization.

top. Tincture of benzoin is applied around the edges to minimize skin irritation and promote adherence of the adhesive tape. After the benzoin has become slightly tacky, several strips of adhesive tape are applied. Whether or not the dressing should be totally occlusive remains the subject of controversy. Some individuals advocate occlusive dressings (7, 18), while others suggest that such dressings may actually create a favorable climate for germ growth since they produce a moist, airless environment (16).

12. As with other intravenous catheters, the insertion date, time, and catheter size should be marked on the tape.

Of the hazards associated with subclavian catheter insertion, pneumothorax is the most common. Hydrothorax, due to infiltration of the intravenous fluid into the chest cavity, and hemothorax, due to laceration of the vein or arterial puncture, can also occur (2). Thus, a chest x-ray should always be done following insertion or even when an insertion attempt is unsuccessful.

The technique for subclavian catheterization using the supraclavicular approach is essentially the same except that no pillow or towel is used behind the back, and the needle is inserted above and behind the clavicle.

Because of the serious complications associated with catheter insertion into the subclavian vein, the *jugular veins* are preferred by some clinicians for central venous lines. They also represent a common site in infants and young children. While the occurrence of pneumothorax is avoided with this site, other complications, though rare, can occur. The major one is misdirection of the catheter superiorly. Any air entering could rapidly embolize to the brain. For this reason, the head should always be tilted downward 20 to 30 degrees during the insertion (2). Coiling the catheter upward can also result in complications such as thrombophlebitis if a hypertonic or irritating solution were administered, due to inadequate dilution. To prevent such a problem, an x-ray should be done following insertion to document correct placement of the catheter.

While less risky than use of the subclavian vein, jugular placement has the disadvantage of making dressing application difficult. If measures such as a tongue depressor are used to prevent kinking or

dislodgement of the catheter, movement of the patient's head will be restricted. This should be taken into consideration if long-term intravenous therapy is required for an alert and active patient.

Surgical cutdown

Access to a vein may be gained surgically if the percutaneous approach has been unsuccessful. This procedure can be used to place a catheter in either a central vein or a superficial or deep vein in an extremity (2). The same degree of asepsis must be followed as with any bedside surgical procedure. Following insertion of the catheter, which is sutured in place, an antibiotic ointment containing bacitracin, neomycin, and polymyxin should be applied to the site, followed by a sterile dressing (16).

The nurse's role in this procedure includes preparing the patient and remaining with him while it is being performed, assisting the physician, and follow-up care of the cutdown site to prevent infection.

REFERENCES

1. Abbott Laboratories: How to Make the Venipuncture. *I.V. Tips*, North Chicago, Illinois, November 1977.

2. Abbott Laboratories: *Needle and Cannula Techniques*, North Chicago, Illinois; 1971.

3. Adriani, John: Venipuncture. *American Journal of Nursing*, 62:66-70, March 1962.

4. Augspurger, E. F., and Davis, Leon F.: Heparin Lock Intravenous Technique. *Journal of Oral Surgery*, 32:786, October 1974.

5. Cantrell, Mary, Shoup, Larry K., Cole, Lois, and Kamm, Judy: Improved Techniques in I.V. Therapy Reduce Contamination Hazards. *American Journal of I.V. Therapy*, 2:46–50, August/September 1975.

6. Collin, Jack, Collin, Christine, Constable, F. L., and Johnston, I. D. A.: Infusion Thrombophlebitis and Infection with Various Cannulas. *The Lancet*, 2:150-152, July 26, 1975.

7. Daly, John, Ziegler, Barbara, and Dudrick, Stanley: Central Venous Catheterization. *American Journal of Nursing*, 75(5):820–824, May 1975.

8. Deeb, Edmund N., and DiMattia, Philip E.: How Much Heparin in the Lock? *American Journal of I.V. Therapy*, 3:22–26, December/January 1976.

9. Evans, C. A., Smith, W. M., Johnston, E. A., and Gilbett, E. R.: Bacterial Flora of the Human Skin. *Journal of Investigative Dermatology*, 15:305, 1950.

10. Freshwater, M. Felix: "Dutch Boy" Technique Helps During I.V. Insertion. *RN*, 39:ICU/CCU 8, January 1976.

11. Goldmann, Donald A., Maki, Dennis G., Rhame, Frank S., Kaiser, Allen B., Tenney, James H., and Bennett, John V.: Guidelines for Infection Control in Intravenous Therapy. *Annals of Internal Medicine,* 79:848–850, 1973.

12. Hanson, Robert L., Grant, Alan M., and Majors, Kenneth R.: Heparin-Lock Maintenance with Ten Units of Sodium Heparin in One Milliliter of Normal Saline Solution. *Surgery, Gynecology and Obstetrics,* 142:373–376, March 1976.

13. James, Paul M.: Central Venous Cannulation. *Hospital Medicine,* 13:106–120, May 1977.

14. Kimmell, Rosemary: Keys to Using the Heparin Lock. *Nursing '74,* 4:52–53, November 1974.

15. Kurdi, William J.: Refining your I.V. Therapy Techniques. *Nursing '75,* 5:41–47, November 1975.

16. Maki, Dennis G., Goldmann, Donald A., and Rhame, Frank S.: Infection Control in Intravenous Therapy. *Annals of Internal Medicine,* 79:867–887, 1973.

17. Milgram, Elias: Starting an I.V. in Small Veins. *Hospital Physician,* 40–41, February 1974.

18. Plumer, Ada Lawrence: *Principles and Practice of Intravenous Therapy* (2nd ed.), Boston: Little, Brown and Company, 1975.

19. Seropian, Richard, and Reynolds, Benedict, M.: Wound Infection after Preoperative Depilatory Versus Razor Preparation. *American Journal of Surgery,* 121:251–254, March 1971.

20. Thomas, Edward T., Evers, William, and Racz, Gabor B.: Postinfusion Phlebitis. *Anesthesia and Analgesia,* 49:150–159, 1970.

21. Ungvarski, Peter: Parenteral Therapy. *American Journal of Nursing,* 74:1974–1977, December 1976.

22. White, John J., Wallace, Craig K., and Burnett, Lonnie S.: Skin Disinfection. *Hopkins Medical Journal,* 126:169–176, 1970.

5 Establishment and Maintenance of Flow Rate

Maintenance of the correct flow rate represents one of the major nursing responsibilities in intravenous therapy. Both intravenous fluids and medications must be infused at an appropriate rate and in a constant and accurate manner to achieve the desired therapeutic response and to prevent complications. Turco reminds us that "inaccurate infusion rates are incompatible with rational drug therapy" and can result in serious hazards to patients (19, p16). These hazards include drug toxicity, delayed response to the drug, pulmonary edema, metabolic disturbances, and heightened potential for venous irritation and phlebitis (19). Other complications that can occur when the flow rate deviates markedly from the desired rate are air embolism from a container which has unexpectedly run dry, and a clotted cannula due to cessation of fluid flow. Thus, the nurse must first be aware of the correct infusion rate for each drug and fluid given to a particular patient and, secondly, must insure that the appropriate rate is maintained.

For fluid and electrolyte replacement, the physician will generally specify the length of time in which a certain volume is to be administered. In such instances it is essential not only to insure that the fluids are infused within the specified time period, but to keep the flow rate constant throughout that time period. Attempts should not be made to "catch up" when fluids get significantly behind schedule, since rapid infusion rates can result in fluid overload and pulmonary edema, particularly in patients with compromised cardiovascular states or renal impairment. Even when the prescribed rate is being maintained, all patients should be monitored for signs of fluid overload. These complications are discussed in greater detail in the next chapter.

The rate of administration of intravenous medications is governed by the pharmacologic properties of the medication, the specific mode of administration (continuous infusion, intermittent infusion, or injection), and the patient's condition and response. Significant deviations in the flow rate can result in the complications mentioned above. Specific guidelines for the rate of administration of each medication are provided in the drug information section in the back of this book.

Fluids administered solely to maintain the patency of the intravenous line (to keep the vein open or KVO) should be given as slowly as possible while avoiding clotting of the cannula. Rates of approximately 10 milliliters per hour will generally suffice for fluids infused by gravity. With lower rates venous pressure will cause blood to back up into the cannula and clot (20). However, rates of 1 milliliter per hour or less can be used with infusion pumps, depending on the amount of pressure generated.

FACTORS AFFECTING FLOW RATES

Flow rates are affected by a number of factors which should be given consideration, especially with fluids infused by gravity.

Factors related to the fluid and container

1. Characteristics of the fluid given, including viscosity and temperature, will affect the flow rate. When another solution or drug is added, the rate should be readjusted. Refrigerated solutions should be brought to room temperature if possible before infusing to avoid diminished flow and patient discomfort due to venous spasm (15, 18).
2. Due to a greater head pressure (the pressure exerted by the fluid within the container), a full container will flow faster than one which has partially emptied. Thus, to maintain a constant, accurate rate, periodic readjustments are necessary as the container empties.
3. The height of the fluid container in relation to the patient affects the flow rate. The fluid container is usually placed about 30 to 36 inches above the patient. Raising the container increases the flow rate. The rate may also vary according to the position of the patient. For example, it is generally faster when the patient is recumbent than when sitting.

Factors related to the flow control clamp

1. Depending on its design, the clamp may slip and loosen, resulting in a very rapid or runaway infusion. The rate may also vary as a result of distortion of the plastic tubing due to

pressure of the clamp against the tubing, a phenomenon known as cold flow (18).
2. Any marked tension or stretching of the tubing can render the clamp ineffective (1). This can occur if the patient turns in bed, particularly if the tubing is too short.

Factors related to the cannula and intravenous line

1. The size of the cannula limits the maximum attainable flow rate. When the flow is to be rapid, a large gauge needle or catheter should be selected.
2. The flow can be markedly altered by the position of the cannula within the vein. If the bevel of the needle is pushed against the wall of the vein, the flow will diminish or stop (15). Likewise, reduction or cessation of flow can occur if a plastic catheter bends or kinks due to patient movement. If the flow rate is adjusted while the catheter is in the bent position, the rate will suddenly increase when the position changes and the obstruction is relieved. Thus, closer monitoring is indicated when the cannula is located near an area of active movement such as a joint. If movement of a joint or limb results in marked changes in flow rate, the site should be immobilized with an armboard.
3. Clotting of the cannula interrupts the flow. As discussed in the next chapter, a clotted cannula should never be forcefully flushed but rather should be replaced with a new one, because of the danger of causing an embolus.
4. The drop calibration of the administration set being used will limit the maximum attainable flow rate. Standard sets which deliver 10, 15, or 20 drops per milliliter will allow high flow rates. Sets delivering microdrops will provide 50 or 60 drops per milliliter. Because of the small size of drops produced, the sets cannot deliver a total flow rate equal to that of a standard set. With flows above 100 milliliters per hour (100 drops per minute), the drops become difficult to count and accuracy is lost. Thus, microdrop-type administration sets should generally be reserved for drugs and fluids that are to infuse at rates below these.
5. Pinched or bent tubing or an obstructed air inlet or vent will cause flow to decrease or stop.
6. Devices such as micropore filters, particularly

0.5 micron in size or smaller, diminish the flow rate (18).

Other factors

Patients, for a variety of reasons, may occasionally manipulate the flow control clamp or otherwise tamper with the intravenous line, thus altering the established flow rate.

CALCULATION OF FLOW RATES

Since intravenous medications and fluids must be administered with precision, the desired flow rate should be calculated and recorded each time a new container of fluid or dose of medication is administered. Recording the rate on each container promotes accuracy and saves considerable time should subsequent readjustments be necessary.

Flow rates are expressed as volumes of fluid delivered per unit of time, usually as milliliters per hour or drops per minute. The flow rate expressed in milliliters per hour represents a more accurate means of monitoring the volume delivered over a period of time. This rate is calculated by dividing the volume of fluid to be infused (in milliliters) by the infusion time (in hours).

However, to monitor the flow at frequent intervals and make periodic adjustments as needed, it is desirable to also express the flow rate in drops per minute. To calculate the rate in drops per minute, it is necessary to know:

1. The volume of fluid to be infused
2. The total infusion time
3. The calibration of the administration set utilized; that is, the number of drops per milliliter it delivers (this information is found on the administration set package)

A rapid means of determining flow rate is by using an IV calculator or a conversion table. These are available from the manufacturers of intravenous fluids. Using either a circular or linear design, the three variables are located on the dial or rule and the answer is quickly obtained.

In the absence of such handy devices, the flow rate can also be determined with ease by using the following formula: Divide the volume of fluid ordered (in milliliters) by the length of time it is to infuse (in minutes) and multiply by the calibration of the administration set used (number of drops per milliliter) (1). As mentioned above,

most standard administration sets provide 10, 15, or 20 drops per milliliter, while those calibrated in microdrops deliver 50 or 60 drops per milliliter. Expressed as an equation, the above formula would be:

Flow rate (in drops/min.) =

$$\frac{\text{volume of fluid (in ml.)}}{\text{time it is to infuse (in min.)}} \times \frac{\text{calibration}}{\text{(drops/ml.)}}$$

For example, if 1000 milliliters of fluid is to be infused in eight hours, using an administration set which delivers 15 drops per milliliter, then:

$$\text{Flow rate} = \frac{1000 \text{ ml.}}{480 \text{ min.}} \times 15 \text{ drops/ml.}$$

Flow rate = 31 drops/minute

If a medication which is dissolved in 120 milliliters of fluid is to be administered over a two-hour period, but with a microdrop administration set which delivers 60 drops per milliliter, then:

$$\text{Flow rate} = \frac{120 \text{ ml.}}{120 \text{ min.}} \times 60 \text{ drops/ml.}$$

Flow rate = 60 drops/minute

Another rapid method of calculating the flow rate starts with the volume of fluid to be administered over an hour (15). With administration sets that deliver 10 drops per milliliter, divide the hourly volume by 6. With administration sets that provide 15 drops per milliliter, divide the hourly volume by 4. With sets that deliver 60 drops per milliliter, the hourly volume or number of milliliters per hour equals the number of drops per minute.

Once the flow rate has been calculated, the rate in gravity infusion systems is set by adjusting the flow control clamp. To verify its constancy, it should be rechecked in 10 to 15 minutes; thereafter, it should be checked hourly.

The ability to regulate the rate is affected by not only the factors discussed earlier, but by the type of flow control clamp as well. Slide clamps which are found on some administration sets are intended to be used to stop the flow temporarily while the container is changed without interference with the established rate setting. Thus, they should *not* be used to regulate the flow rate. To set and maintain specific flow rates, administration sets contain either a screw clamp or a roller clamp. Both types permit a range of rate adjustment with a reasonable degree of accuracy, but the roller design is somewhat easier to manipulate with one hand. A relatively new roller design, in which the tubing fits into a groove, compresses the tubing along the lateral edges instead of at the center. This has been shown to provide a more constant flow with less frequent need for readjustment than standard roller clamps or screw clamps (8).

Nonetheless, even the newer manual flow clamps cannot insure a complete degree of accuracy because of the many factors affecting flow rate in a gravity-feed situation. One group of investigators found considerable rate deviations among administrations sets (4). Even when the drop *rate* is maintained with some consistency, the total volume infused may be inaccurate due to variations in drop, *size.* There may be minor differences in the calibration of drop size from one set to another of the same manufacturer. Other factors responsible for alterations in drop size are type of solution and infusion rate (7). Smaller drops are formed by solutions such as total parenteral nutrition (TPN) solutions which have a higher specific gravity. It has been shown that the faster the rate, the larger the volume of drops formed with the same set. Thus, if rapid rates are maintained for a long period, the total volume infused should be checked at frequent intervals and the rate readjusted as needed.

A simple device is currently available which enables more accurate regulation of the flow rate with gravity-fed infusions. Known as the Dial-a-Flo, it can regulate flow between 5 and 250 milliliters per hour and is more consistent and dependable than a standard flow clamp (Fig. 5-1). It consists of a disc with a rotating calibrated dial between two short segments of tubing. One end attaches to any standard administration set; the other end is then connected to the hub of the intravenous cannula. To use it, the device must first be calibrated to the specific administration set being used. To calibrate:

1. Set the dial at 60 milliliters per hour, which equals 1 milliliter per minute.
2. Open the flow control clamp on the administration tubing to its maximum position.
3. Adjust the height of the container to approximately 3 inches above the patient's mid-axillary line.
4. Count the drop rate (number of drops per

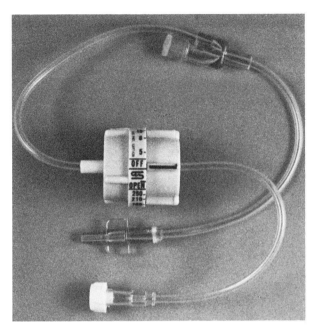

Fig. 5-1. Dial-a-Flo. This simple device allows greater accuracy in flow rate regulation with gravity-fed infusions. (Sorenson Research Company, Salt Lake City, Utah 84115)

minute) via the drip chamber. Raise or lower the fluid container as needed until the rate equals the number of drops that the set normally delivers (e.g., 15 drops per minute for sets delivering 15 drops per milliliter).
5. After calibrating, rotate the dial to set the desired infusion rate in milliliters per hour.

While offering a simple, economical means of regulating flow, this device is limited to standard solutions and cannot be used with very viscous fluids such as certain TPN solutions and blood.

Another device designed to achieve the same function has been described by a group of investigators from Israel (11). Referred to as an infusion flow stabilizer (IFS), it is a small disposable plastic cylinder which is added to a standard intravenous line. Unlike the Dial-a-Flo, it is connected directly to the fluid container, and the administration set plugs into its lower end. The desired flow rate is set by adjusting a screw, and the rate is maintained by means of a float valve within the chamber which regulates the amount of fluid passing. Air passage is prevented by an automatic shutoff below the float valve.

Although such devices can reduce most of the flow rate deviations found to be associated with gravity infusion, there remain many instances in which absolute accuracy must be insured in the administration of drugs and fluids. In addition to the potentially serious problems that can result from infusion of drugs and fluids at an inaccurate rate, manually controlled flow presents other disadvantages. Greater expense can be incurred in the long run due to added volumes of fluid required either as a vehicle for the medications or to maintain patency of the vein. Clotted cannulae due either to a flow that has stopped or a container that has run dry can result in the need for frequent restarting of the infusion and added discomfort to the patient. Many or all of these problems can be eliminated through the use of infusion controllers and pumps.

CONTROLLERS

The controller is an electronic device used to regulate intravenous flow rates. It physically resembles pumps yet operates by a completely different mechanism. Controllers or infusion-rate regulators rely on gravity rather than exert any pressure (19). The rate is regulated either by electronically monitoring the drop rate, as in the IVAC 230* or by regulating the passage of fluid through the tubing by means of a magnetically activated metal ball valve which synchronizes with a drop detector (10), as in the Epic 100.† Controllers are limited by the fact that drop rate is not a completely accurate reflection of volume infused due to variations in drop size as discussed above. In spite of such variations, controllers can be of value with a wide range of fluids and medications.

Since the design of controllers is mechanically simpler than that of pumps, they can be assembled easily and rapidly and should require less frequent maintenance. They are also more economical to operate and thus are appropriate for a large percentage of infusions which do not require the accuracy of pumps. The Epic 100 costs considerably less than pumps, though a special administration set is required. The IVAC 230 is somewhat higher in price but can be used with any standard administration set, which may offset the extra cost in the long run.

*IVAC Corporation, LaJolla, California 92038
† Burron Medical Products, Inc., Bethlehem, Pennsylvania 18018

INFUSION PUMPS

In contrast to controllers, pumps operate by exerting pressure either on the intravenous tubing or on the fluid itself (2). Since they pump against pressure gradients, a constant infusion rate and volume can be maintained even with fluctuations in the patient's venous pressure. In addition, pumps can infuse large volumes of fluid through a micropore filter (10).

To produce the pumping action, one of two basic mechanisms is utilized: either a peristaltic action or a piston-cylinder action.

Peristaltic action

Peristaltic pumps move the fluid by exerting an externally applied force on the administration tubing. The fluid delivery rate is generally expressed in drops per minute. To compress the tubing, peristaltic pumps can employ either a linear or a rotary device.

LINEAR DEVICES

The linear type consists of a tubular pumping chamber incorporating fingerlike projections which alternately advance and retract, pressing the tubing against a stationary surface. Thus, the fluid is propelled forward in wavelike motions (19). The LaBarge 2051 (Fig. 5-2) and the IVAC 530 (Fig. 5-3), which have a linear mechanism, can be used with standard administration sets. The Sigmamotor Sigma 5000 (Fig. 5-4), utilizes a special calibrated tubing which has a silastic pumping chamber designed with a spring-operated "flood stop" which occludes the tubing whenever the pump door is open. This prevents the fluid from accidentally infusing at full speed in case the tubing should become disengaged. However, if it is taken out of the pump, the tubing will allow gravity flow.

ROTARY DEVICES

Rotary pumps consist of roller fingers mounted onto a rotating disc. Administration tubing which is specific for each model contains an integrated pumping chamber, usually made of silicone rubber. As the disc rotates, the rollers alternately press and release the pumping chamber, moving the fluid forward (Fig. 5-5) (2, 12). The flow rate, which is expressed in milliliters per hour, is determined by the caliber of the pumping chamber

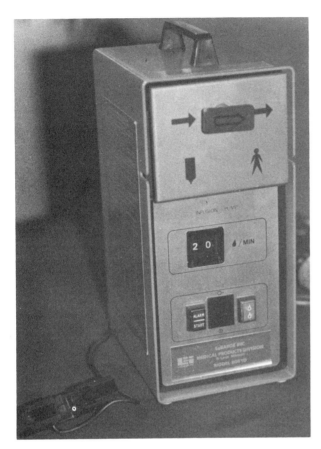

Fig. 5-2. LaBarge 2051 peristaltic infusion pump uses a linear mechanism. (Courtesy of LaBarge, Inc., Medical Products Division, St. Louis, Missouri 63102)

Piston-cylinder action

With piston-cylinder pumps, the pumping mechanism is provided by a piston or moving diaphragm which exerts pressure on the fluid within a cylinder (19). A given amount of fluid is expelled from the cylinder with each cycle and, thus, the mechanism is often referred to as volumetric. (The Sigmamotor Sigma 5000 and the Extracorporeal 2100, although peristaltic models, are also calibrated in milliliters per hour and can be referred to as volumetric too. However, in most in-

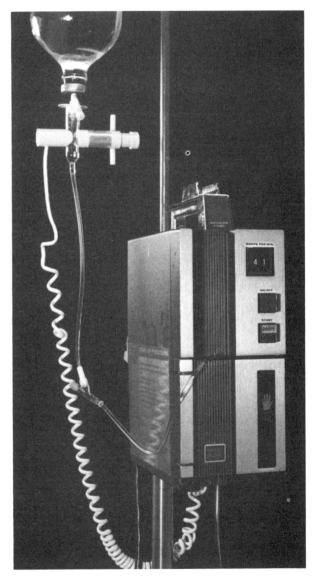

Fig. 5-3. IVAC 530 peristaltic infusion pump set up with standard administration tubing and drop sensor in place (IVAC Corporation, LaJolla, California 92038)

tubing used and the speed of the rotor (2). With some models, several different sizes of tubing are required to achieve a complete range of flow rates. Thus, each time significant changes in rate are required that cannot be accommodated by the tubing being used, it is necessary to replace it with the size that will deliver the desired flow rate. However, one model, the Extracorporeal 2100 (Fig. 5-6) can deliver a full range of flow rates from 0 to 999 milliliters per hour with one size tubing. This feature, plus a totally closed system with the pumping chamber integrated into the administration set, represents a significant improvement over earlier rotary pump designs. By eliminating unnecessary connections and decreasing the number of manipulations required, the chance of touch contamination is reduced. With most rotary models, if the pump has to be temporarily disconnected, the administration tubing will allow gravity flow.

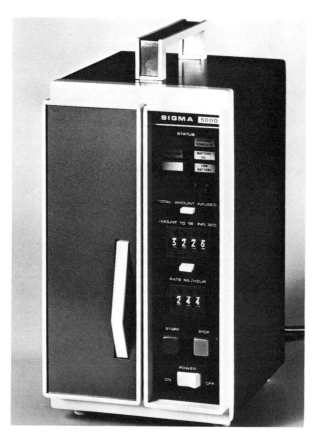

Fig. 5–4. Sigma 5000, although using a peristaltic mechanism, is considered volumetric in that fluid delivery is calibrated in milliliters per hour. (Courtesy of Sigmamotor, Inc., Middleport, New York 14105)

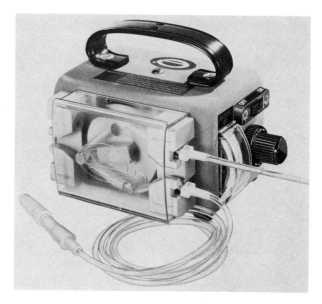

Fig. 5–5. Holter 911. Rotary pumps utilize rollers mounted on a disc. Fluid is propelled by the compression and release of the tubing as the disc rotates. (Courtesy of Extracorporeal Medical Specialties, Inc., King of Prussia, Pennsylvania 19406)

stances the term "volumetric" is used to refer to pumps which employ a piston-cylinder mechanism). With this type of pump, the flow rate is determined primarily by the frequency of movement by the piston or diaphragm as well as by the size of the cylinder (2). Two types of pumps employ a piston-cylinder action: syringe pumps and volumetric pumps.

SYRINGE PUMPS

The syringe pump represents one of the earliest types of pumps in clinical use (10). It consists primarily of a motor-driven syringe, the plunger of which is depressed at a constant preset rate to eject the drug (Fig. 5-7). The rate at which the plunger is advanced and the size of the syringe determine the flow rate and total volume that can be infused. Once the syringe has emptied, most

require manual refilling or replacement. A few models can accommodate two syringes so that after one has emptied, it can be refilled either manually or automatically from a fluid reservoir, while the second one is pumping. This enables maintenance of continuous flow.

Due to the relatively small volume that can be accommodated (usually a maximum of 50 milliliters) and the extremely slow yet constant flow rates (can be as low as 0.1 milliliter per hour for clinical use), syringe pumps are particularly suited for pediatric use as well as for critical care settings in which small volumes of concentrated drugs must be administered slowly over an extended period of time. Two models which are appropriate for these and other general clinical applications are the Sage 242* and the Harvard 2620 (Fig. 5-8).

In contrast, some syringe pumps have been designed for a specific drug or laboratory function. For example, there are pumps designed for administration of oxytocin, which must be given with great precision for the induction of labor.

*Sage Instruments, Division, Orion Research Inc., Cambridge, Massachusetts 02139

Currently available models include the 700 Obstetrical Infusion Pump[†] and the Oxytocin Infusion Pump Model 909.[‡] While their operation is similar to that of other syringe pumps, they can easily be set to deliver the desired dosage rate of oxytocin. Specific considerations for the administration of oxytocin are included in the drug information section in the back of this text.

Specially designed pumps are available for the administration of heparin during hemodialysis (Sage Model 240) and for diagnostic studies such as dye dilution for the determination of cardiac output during cardiac catheterization (Sage Model 367 and Harvard Models 2603 and 2604).

Many syringe pumps are designed to be placed on top of a table or stand, which limits their portability. However, some newer clinical models can also be attached to an IV pole, a feature which increases their versatility.

VOLUMETRIC PUMPS

Also utilizing a piston-cylinder action are volumetric pumps, in which a specialized pumping chamber is incorporated into the administration tubing. The pumping chamber consists of a metered chamber or cassette with a diaphragm, valve, or plunger. Flow is controlled by the pistonlike movement of the plunger, which in one phase of the cycle draws a measured volume of fluid into the cassette chamber (filling phase) and then ejects or delivers the fluid into the distal tubing (delivery or infusion phase). Currently available volumetric pumps include the IVAC 600,[*] the Abbott/Shaw LifeCare pump (Fig. 5-9), the Valleylab 5000,[†] and the IMED 922 (Fig. 5-10), which is virtually the same as the McGaw VIP.[‡]

Setting up and changing the tubing on a volumetric pump generally requires more time than with other types. When priming the administration set, special care must be taken to insure removal of all air bubbles from the pumping chamber since most models will not pump air. This feature, along with an empty container detector, provides a safeguard against air emboli. If any air

[†] Corometrics Medical Systems, Inc., Wallingford, Connecticut 06492
[‡] Berkeley Bio-Engineering, Inc., San Leandro, California 94577
[*] IVAC Corporation, LaJolla, California 92038
[†] Valleylab, Boulder, Colorado 80301
[‡] McGaw Laboratories, Irvine, California 92714

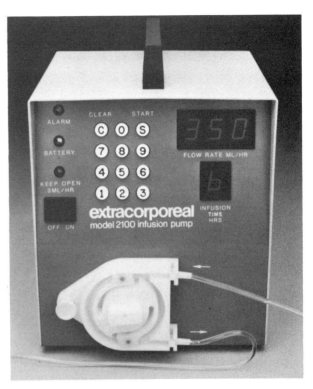

Fig. 5-6. Extracorporeal 2100. Unlike some rotary pumps, this model can deliver a wide range of flow rates with one size tubing. (Courtesy of Extracorporeal Medical Specialties, Inc., King of Prussia, Pennsylvania 19406)

enters the pump chamber during operation, some models will immediately stop fluid delivery and activate an alarm. Others continue pumping, but the air remains trapped within the pumping chamber, altering the volume of fluid delivered with each stroke and thus resulting in an inaccurate flow rate.

On the average, volumetric pumps tend to cost slightly more than peristaltic models, and the special administration sets required are somewhat higher priced, making them more expensive to operate. However, their greater accuracy and inability to pump air can justify the added expense in many clinical situations.

Specialized pumps and infusers

The standard infusion pumps described above are well suited for the delivery of most drugs but particularly for those given on a short-term basis. However, when drugs must be administered con-

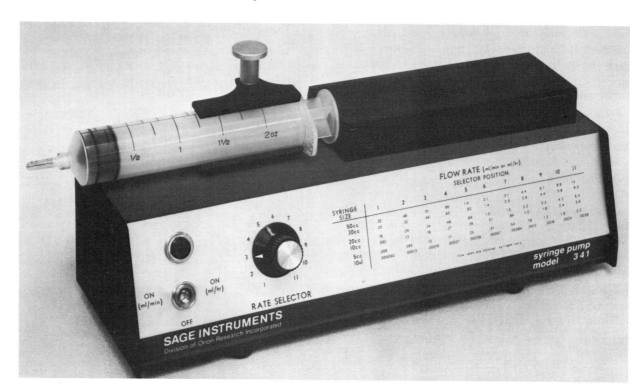

Fig. 5–7. Sage 341. Syringe pumps enable a broad range of flow rates by using various size syringes. (Courtesy of Sage Instruments. Division, Orion Research, Inc., Cambridge, Massachusetts 02139)

tinuously at a very slow rate and over an extended period of time, standard pumps present drawbacks. Most pumps require that the drug be diluted in a rather large volume of fluid; and except for serving as a vehicle for the drug, the fluid is often not needed; and in some cases, it is undesirable or contraindicated. Furthermore, some drugs, particularly certain cancer chemotherapeutic agents, are most effective when given very slowly over a period of several days. Most types of pumps cannot deliver the extremely slow rates required. While some syringe pumps can achieve such rates and also allow minimal dilution of the drug, their size and weight generally make them impractical for use outside the hospital. Thus, it is usually necessary for patients to be readmitted to the hospital for several days whenever a course of chemotherapy is given, usually at three- to four-week intervals.

The need for such inconvenience and expense is being reduced by the development of unique infusion devices, a few of which are now available for patient use. Such devices can enable patients to receive intermittent chemotherapy and long-

term therapy with certain other drugs such as heparin and antibiotics safely at home. This is not only highly desirable psychologically but can save the patient time and expense by eliminating the need for repeated or prolonged hospitalization.

MINIATURE INFUSION DEVICES

The *AR/Med®* *infusor* is a small, 6.2 cm. by 13.3 cm. by 2.5 cm. (2½ in. by 5 in. by 1 in.) disposable unit which weighs only 100 grams (3½ ounces) when full and is designed for the continuous intravenous administration of drugs over several days (Fig. 5-11). It is unique in that it uses the elastomeric energy of the drug-containing reservoir as its energy source rather than any external driving force, such as gravity or electricity (9). The drug cartridge which locks into the control unit to activate fluid flow contains an inflatable reservoir which has a capacity of 25 milliliters of solution. Other components of the system include a precalibrated valve, a 0.2-micron bacterial filter, and noncollapsible tubing. Capable of delivering very low flow rates, ranging from 0.4 to 2.0 milliliters per hour, this infusor enables the use of a very small gauge cannula, an important consideration in both patient comfort and reduction of venous irritation.

Since filling of the cartridge requires strict aseptic technique, it should be done under a laminar flow hood, ideally by a pharmacist. Once the infusor has been set up and attached to the patient (usually on the upper arm), it is connected to the hub of the intravenous cannula. If a loading dose is required, a loading valve is activated, permitting infusion of the desired volume at a rate of 3 milliliters per *minute.* The maintenance flow rate is then set; and since the rate varies only minimally once set, the risk of rapid infusion is virtually eliminated. The design also minimizes the likelihood of air embolism, even if the cartridge empties completely (9).

When chemotherapy is to be carried out on an outpatient basis, the unit is initially set up and the flow rate adjusted, if necessary, in the hospital or clinic. The patient is given additional prefilled

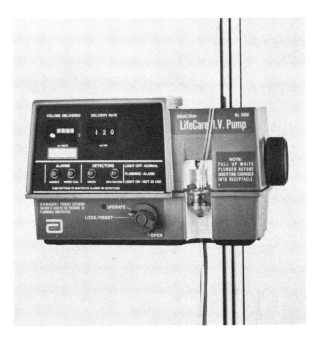

Fig. 5–9.   Abbott/Shaw LifeCare Pump. Volumetric pumps incorporate a cassette-type pumping chamber which utilizes a pistonlike movement to advance the fluid. (Abbott Laboratories, North Chicago, Illinois 60064)

cartridges to enable several days of uninterrupted therapy. The nurse can play a significant role in preparing the patient for home therapy. It is essential that the patient be thoroughly instructed in how to change the cartridge using sterile technique, how to observe for signs of infiltration and infection, and how to report these and other problems to the appropriate individual, as well as specific information and precautions about the drug being administered. As an added safeguard, such patients would benefit from support and supervision at home by a community health nurse.

This infusor has been approved for commercial use but is manufactured and distributed only in limited quantities. Therefore, any inquiries regarding availability and indications for use should be made directly to the manufacturer.

The *Watkins USCI CHRONOFUSOR* * is another type of miniature, self-contained infusion pump. Weighing less than 1 pound (426 grams), it can easily be worn using a harness by ambulatory patients. It is designed for continuous intravenous or intra-arterial infusions of cancer chemothera-

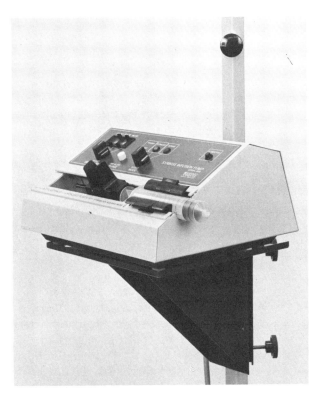

Fig. 5–8.   Harvard 2620. Syringe pumps allow the infusion of small volumes of concentrated drugs over an extended period of time. (Courtesy of Harvard Apparatus Company, Inc., Millis, Massachusetts 02054)

*United States Catheter and Instrument Corporation, a division of C. R. Bard, Inc., Billerica, Massachusetts 01821

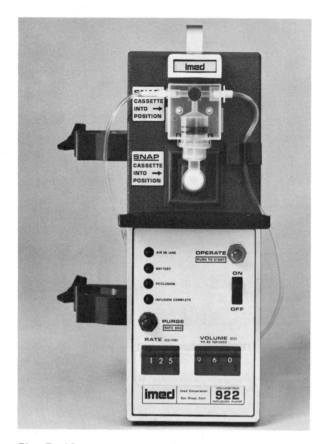

Fig. 5-10. IMED 922 volumetric pump uses a syringe chamber cassette. The battery can operate for up to 100 hours without recharging, thus increasing portability. (Courtesy of IMED Corporation, San Diego, California 92131)

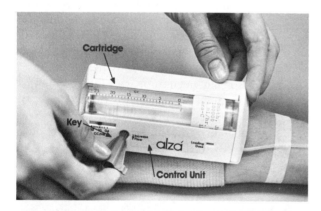

Fig. 5-11. AR/MED infusor. The compact design and very low flow rates enable continuous administration of drugs over several days at home. (Courtesy of ALZA Corporation, Palo Alto, California 94304)

peutic agents, heparin, or antibiotic solutions. A miniature roller pump with a spring mechanism is driven by a hand-wound chronometric motor. The unit also contains a disposable reservoir bag which has a capacity of 25 to 40 milliliters. Infusing at the rate of 0.2 milliliters per hour (or 5 milliliters per day), it can hold a four- to seven-day supply, enabling outpatients to receive therapy at home and return once or twice a week to receive a new supply of the drug.

Several other types of miniature, self-contained pumps and infusors are also available. Among these are Sage Instruments Model 216, a battery-operated pump with a 10-milliliter capacity (Fig. 5-12). The minimum flow rate is 1 milliliter per *day;* the maximum is 4 milliliters per *hour* for drugs which must be administered over a shorter period of time.

Another battery-operated model is the ML6-4 Ambulatory Infusion Pump,* which utilizes a disposable 50-milliliter infusate bag and tubing set. The flow rate can be adjusted via a separate meter to deliver from 4 to 20 milliliters per 24 hours. The battery will operate the pump for up to seven days without recharging. A similar model, the ML6-8, is designed for total parenteral nutrition (TPN). Allowing flow rates of 600 to 3000 milliliters per 24 hours, it permits connection to standard plastic fluid containers. A vest-type harness allows both the pump and fluid bags to be worn on the body, thus enabling unrestricted ambulation.

Still another type has a quartz crystal control. It has a 2-milliliter capacity, which can be administered at either of two flow rates; 2 milliliters in 8 hours or 2 milliliters in 24 hours. While less versatile in terms of volume capacity and range of flow rates, it has the advantage of being unaffected by small gauge cannulae or by back pressures (14).

The miniature infusion systems discussed above as well as others currently being developed represent a new dimension in the treatment of patients requiring long-term intravenous drug therapy. As their design becomes refined, their applications will become broader; and an increasing number of patients may be able to receive intravenous therapy in the home setting.

*CORMED, Inc., Middleport, New York 14105

IMPLANTABLE INFUSION PUMPS

At times it is desirable to give continuous intravenous medications for as long as months at a time. An example is the need for chronic anticoagulation by patients with recurrent thromboemboli and those at high risk following prosthetic heart valve implantation or heart transplantation. Heparin is believed by many investigators to be more effective and, in some respects, safer than oral anticoagulants. Because of problems associated with standard intravenous administration, e.g., infection and bleeding due to excessive dosages, a totally implantable pump has been developed, known as the Infusaid.* It resembles a cardiac pacemaker in size, shape, and location of implantation. The device is a two-chambered bellows apparatus—the inner chamber contains the solution to be infused; the outer holds a volatile liquid, which, upon expansion in its outer chamber, provides the driving force of the unit, expelling the solution into the administration catheter (17).

When the supply is depleted (one to three months), the inner chamber is refilled via a percu-

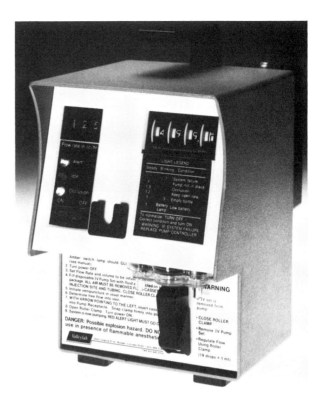

Fig. 5–13. Valleylab 5000. When an alarm is activated, the light legend on the front enables rapid determination of the problem. (Courtesy of Valleylab, Boulder, Colorado 80301)

taneous needle. The pump and catheter are surgically removed when therapy is complete. This pump has been used successfully in a patient for one year, and clinical investigations are continuing. For further information about this promising development, the manufacturer should be consulted.

CRITERIA FOR PUMP SELECTION

The responsibility for pump selection and operation may be delegated to one or more hospital departments, depending on the institution's needs and preferences. In some instances, it is the nursing service; in others, it is the pharmacy department or medical service. Regardless of which department assumes primary responsibility, the nursing service, because of its intimate involvement in pump usage, must also be actively involved in their selection. With several different pump mechanisms and so many models of each available, selecting the most appropriate pump for

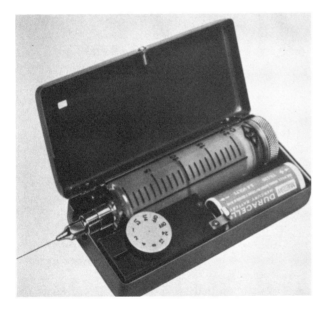

Fig. 5–12. Sage 216. Portable battery-operated pumps allow intravenous drug administration for ambulatory patients. (Courtesy of Sage Instruments, Division, Orion Research, Inc., Cambridge, Massachusetts 02139)

*Metal Bellows Corporation, Sharon, Massachusetts 02067

a given clinical situation can be difficult. To insure a wise choice, several criteria for selection should be followed:

1. Consider the needs of the hospital or institution. What is the usage rate of drugs which should be given by infusion pump or controller? Categories of drugs for which pumps are generally recommended include anticoagulants, potent antihypertensives, cancer chemotherapy agents, cardiovascular drugs including antiarrhythmics, vasopressors and others used in shock states, cortiocosteroids, TPN solutions, immunosuppressives, muscle relaxants, and oxytocics. Some individuals also recommend that pumps be used to administer intravenous anesthetics, alkalizers such as tromethamine (THAM), or sodium bicarbonate, antibiotics, electrolytes, osmotic diuretics, and plasma expanders (19).

   On what clinical services or speciality units are the above drugs most frequently used? In most hospitals these units include critical care units, medicine, surgery, pediatrics, obstetrics, oncology, hemodialysis, and anesthesia. Usage may be higher in pediatrics when accuracy in delivering concentrated drugs and fluids is even more critical. Data regarding drug usage within an institution should be available from the pharmacy department.

2. Investigate the characteristics of various brands of pumps and compare with a checklist of essential and desirable features. It is generally agreed that despite the type of mechanism employed, all standard pumps should provide the following features. Most criteria, with a few exceptions, also apply to specialty pumps.

   a. Wide range of flow rates, ideally from one to several hundred milliliters per hour. With syringe pumps the flow rate is quite variable. Some are capable of delivering rates as low as 0.1 milliliter per hour or as high as several hundred milliliters per hour.

   b. Maintenance of a constant and accurate flow. There should be no more than a ±2 to 4 percent variation from the set rate.

   c. Both audible and visible alarms that are triggered by an empty bottle (or syringe) and by occlusion of the tubing. When an alarm sounds, the flow should temporarily stop until the problem is corrected. In several volumetric models, the pump will revert to a keep-open rate of 1 to 4 milliliters per hour if the bottle empties. The pump eventually turns off when air reaches the pump chamber. Such alarms are essential to reduce the risk of air embolism, a problem which can be much more hazardous with pumps than with gravity flow due to the pressure they exert.

   Several types of alarms can be utilized. Some consist of a photoelectric sensor to monitor the drops as they fall within the drip chamber. Others monitor the fluid level in the container or syringe, while still others rely on the weight of the container to determine when the container is empty. Occlusion may be signaled by absence of any drops in the drip chamber or by pump pressure exceeding a maximum limit. One model (Abbott/Shaw LifeCare; see Fig. 5-9) has an infiltration detector which activates an alarm should a sudden change in skin temperature occur due to extravasation of cool fluid into the tissue.

   Some models have only one alarm light which is activated for any type of malfunction. This requires the nurse to "troubleshoot" to determine the cause of the problem. Other pumps have several lights, each indicating a different problem. One model (Valleylab 5000; Fig. 5-13) also has a written legend on the front of the pump to enable rapid determination of the problem.

   d. Simplicity of operation including ease of priming and setting the flow rate. Pumps requiring fewer steps and less time to set up reduce the likelihood of operator error.

   e. Line-powered at voltages of 95 to 135 volts (19).

   f. Electrical safety insured. Many patients for whom infusion pumps are used also require the use of other electrically powered equipment, such as cardiac monitors, respirators, and hemodialysis machines. The greater the number of line-powered devices connected to a patient, the greater the potential for electric shock should any stray leakage current be present. Thus, to minimize any electrical hazard to the patient and personnel alike, all infusion pumps and controllers must meet basic standards of electrical safety. The pump should be designed to meet Underwriter's Laboratories (UL) standards insofar as ground leakage is concerned. (The level should not exceed 10–25 microamperes.) Exposed surfaces should be constructed of non-conductive material such as plastic or, if metal, coated with several layers of baked-on enamel.

g. Reliable performance with minimal need for repairs. The more time taken up for maintenance, the less time that will be available for performing its function.

3. In addition to the above criteria for pump performance, there are several other features that, while not strictly required, are highly desirable and should be given consideration in the selection of a pump. Such features include:

a. A one-piece, closed administration set (10). Those that require attachment of a separate pumping chamber or a standard administration set increase the risk of touch contamination and infection. Sets which are available with integrated micropore filters are desirable for the same reason.

b. An administration set which allows conversion to gravity flow. If the pump is no longer required or if it must be temporarily disconnected, such as to move a patient, gravity flow will maintain patency of the line. Otherwise, the administration set would have to be changed, requiring added time and expense. Syringe pumps should enable manual injection of the drug if required.

c. Automatic conversion to a keep-open rate when the container empties. This allows the nurse sufficient time to return to change the container before the cannula clots.

d. Optional battery power with an automatic switchover from line to battery operation in the event of a power failure. It is also desirable to have a low battery alarm which activates when the battery needs charging.

e. A relatively lightweight and compact design. It should also have a clamp for attachment to an IV pole. These features, along with battery power, enable portability.

f. Low noise and vibration level (10). This is particularly important in a critical care unit since multiple pieces of electronic equipment, each generating monotonous sounds,

can be a source of stress and, in some instances, can be a significant factor in evoking transient psychotic reactions (13).

4. After the general features of many pumps have been investigated and compared using the above criteria, a clinical evaluation should be conducted of models which best fit the needs of the institution. Ideally, the trials should include side-by-side comparative evaluations by individuals who will be using the pumps. A written evaluation guide or questionnaire is helpful in eliciting the kind of information required and in providing written documentation of test results (16).

5. Because the purchase of infusion pumps represents a major expenditure for an institution, the purchase price and operating costs must be given consideration. Many pump models can be leased rather than purchased; some have a lease-purchase option, while others offer a supply-usage plan in which the pumps are provided free if a minimum number of pump administration sets are purchased monthly (16). Hospital officials who are responsible for procurement of equipment should investigate the various purchase and lease plans as well as provisions for preventive maintenance and service before deciding on a particular pump.

INFUSION PUMP PROGRAMS

Opinions differ as to which hospital department should assume responsibility for procuring, dispensing, and monitoring the use of infusion pumps. The nursing service represents the major department which must be intimately involved in any infusion pump program since it is the nurse who is responsible for the accurate administration of the drug or fluid (even if the drug or fluid is prepared by the pharmacy) and for monitoring the use of any adjunctive equipment. Even when the equipment has been set up by another department, it is the staff nurse who must insure its correct function throughout the duration of the infusion and safeguard the patient against any complications.

Many individuals believe that a pump program should also include the active involvement of pharmacists by virtue of their greater knowledge of drugs, dosage, and compatibilities and their role as resource persons for physicians and nurses (19). This is a valid and reasonable expectation. Others, however, suggest that the involvement of pharmacists should be limited to an advisory role rather than include direct responsibility for purchase, distribution throughout the hospital, or maintenance (3).

Pump usage will also involve the medical service, either directly or indirectly, since the physician has the overall responsibility for each aspect of the patient's treatment. Some institutions require a written order by the physician both to initiate and discontinue an infusion pump (16). However, with appropriate policies and guidelines specifying situations in which an infusion pump is required or recommended, it would seem appropriate that in most instances this decision be a matter of nursing judgment.

Other departments which may be included in a pump program are the central supply department, which may be utilized for storage, dispensing, and routine cleaning, and the hospital's bioengineering or maintenance department, which is responsible for preventive maintenance and repair of pumps unless these services are provided by the manufacturer.

An alternative to delegating the responsibility for use of infusion pumps among several departments, which can result in duplication or omission of services, is to have pumps controlled by the intravenous therapy team or by a separate infusion pump team (16). The latter method might be preferable in large hospitals in which pump usage rates are very high. However, in general, combining all infusion-related services, including starting infusions, changing dressings and administration sets, and setting up and monitoring the use of infusion pumps, under one team is a means of centralizing all aspects of intravenous therapy and might represent a more efficient use of personnel and equipment. Members of such a team should include nurses, a pharmacist or pharmacy technician, and a biomedical engineer or electronics technician.

In spite of increasingly sophisticated designs, infusion pumps, like any electronic equipment, can be subject to operational problems. In many cases, such problems arise from operator error, due either to carelessness or to ignorance of pump operation (5). To minimize their occurrence, the need to familiarize all personnel with the correct use of pumps cannot be overemphasized. Thus, regardless of whether an institution utilizes a team approach for management of infusion pumps or whether all nurses are responsible for setting up and monitoring pumps when required for their patients, each nurse should be thoroughly familiar with all aspects of pump operation. An initial inservice training program is essential for all staff members who are responsible for pump operation. Provision must also be made for periodic refresher programs, particularly for areas in which the rate of pump usage is low. Pump operation manuals containing the manufacturer's guidelines should be accessible to all personnel (2).

Maintaining the nursing staff's familiarity with all facets of pump usage is more realistically accomplished if the fewest types of pumps are used. The purchase of several different brands of pumps can result in considerable confusion for the staff, prevent a good working knowledge of the special features of each model, and increase the likelihood of operator error (5). If a hospital has need for more than one type of pump mechanism, such as controllers, syringe pumps and either peristaltic or volumetric pumps, then ideally no more than one brand of each basic type should be purchased unless a special purpose pump will be confined to one particular hospital location (such as labor and delivery or a hemodialysis unit).

NURSING IMPLICATIONS

In spite of proper training of personnel, a variety of problems can be encountered in using pumps, and the nurse should be acquainted with preventive as well as corrective measures.

Occasional malfunctions including false alarms

Though infusion pumps are a valuable adjunct to patient care, they do not replace the need for good nursing assessment and intervention. Patients requiring therapy via infusion pumps must be checked frequently (and perhaps as often as patients receiving gravity-fed infusions) to insure that the pump is functioning correctly, that the proper flow rate is being maintained, and that infiltration has not occurred.

Infection

Infection remains one of the most likely complications. Strict aseptic technique must be maintained when setting up or changing the pump administration set. If the pump administration set requires the use of a standard set or if an adjunctive device such as a filter is used, connections must be tight. Pump administration sets and other disposable components should be changed every 24 hours and labeled with the date and time of change. The infusion site should be inspected daily for evidence of infection as discussed in Chapter 7.

Air embolism

Air embolism is another potential hazard. Administration sets must be carefully primed to remove all air. Pumps utilizing a peristaltic mechanism can conceivably pump air if it enters the tubing below the drip chamber, such as via a puncture of the pump chamber tubing. To eliminate the possibility of such an occurrence, some manufacturers recommend the use of a micropore filter to trap or vent any air present in the line. Check each manufacturer's guidelines as to whether a filter is suggested and, if so, what micropore size is required.

Flow rate inaccuracies

Flow rate inaccuracies may be due to several mechanisms.

1. With peristaltic pumps which count drop rate, inaccuracies can occur as a result of the varying size of drops formed which, as mentioned above, can cause marked differences in volume delivered. To prevent, check the volume delivered after the first half hour and hourly thereafter, making adjustments as needed.
2. With volumetric models, air trapped in the cassette chamber results in the delivery of an inaccurate volume of fluid. This can be avoided by careful priming of the administration set and removal of any air bubbles entering afterward, such as those produced by release of a gas from the fluid (5).
3. A malpositioned drop sensor can also result in rate errors. If placed too high or if the chamber is overfilled, drops will be missed; if positioned too low, splashes can be counted as

drops. Place the sensor in the correct position as recommended by the manufacturer. Prevent any tilting of the drip chamber, a problem which is more likely with plastic containers. Keep the drip chamber clean to prevent the formation of fluid residues which could affect the photoelectric sensors.

Occlusion

Occlusion of the tubing, clogged filters, or infiltration can cause the pump pressure to reach the maximum level. This can rupture connections or the filter. If the cannula has infiltrated, the infiltration will be rapid and extensive due to the high pressure. To prevent such problems, avoid pinching the tubing in the bedrails or other pieces of equipment. Coil and tape the distal segment of tubing correctly to avoid kinking (see Chapter 4). Change the micropore filter at least every 24 hours or more often if recommended by the manufacturer. Check the cannula site frequently for signs of infiltration. The occlusion alarm may not always be reliable if the alarm pressure setting is too high (5).

Crushing of the tubing

Crushing of the tubing can occur with models that use a standard administration set. To avoid, reposition the tubing approximately 2 to 3 inches either forward or backward every few hours so that the same segment will not always be in contact with the pump mechanism (2).

Opaque fluids

Opaque fluids, including blood and fat emulsions, cannot be administered with some pumps since they cannot be detected by the drop detector. Be aware of the manufacturer's specifications about this. Other models cannot be used to pump blood because they can cause hemolysis (2).

Artifacts in electrocardiographic (ECG) recordings

Artifacts in electrocardiographic (ECG) recordings can be produced by some controllers (IVAC 200 and 230). When a patient in whom a controller is being used requires periodic ECG tracings, the staff must be trained to distinguish artifacts from arrhythmias in order to prevent incorrect diagnosis and treatment. The problem can often be avoided by maintaining good electrode contact (5).

The alarm

The alarm can be disabled by silencing the audible component. This can cause problems or malfunctions to go undetected. To be of value, the alarms should always be turned on. If an alarm is activated, it can be *temporarily* silenced while the cause of the problem is being assessed. Once the problem is corrected, reset the pump mechanism and alarm. Failure to do so may keep the pump turned off or running at a keep-open rate.

Dislodgement of tubing or cassette

The patient may either accidentally or deliberately dislodge the tubing or cassette from its correct position or manipulate the flow-rate settings. For patients who are alert and cooperative, a careful explanation of the purpose of the pump will generally prevent any interference with it. Confused and combative patients may require sedation or restraints (see Chapter 2).

Electrical or mechanical malfunction

Electrical or mechanical malfunction may occur due to inadequate cleaning or faulty handling. Be aware that like any piece of electronic equipment, infusion pumps must be treated with great care. Each pump should be inspected by the hospital's bioengineering department prior to use. All pumps also require periodic preventive maintenance (6). Should any electrical or mechanical problem be suspected, remove the pump from the patient area and follow the hospital's procedure for having it inspected and serviced.

As pump technology becomes more sophisticated, its applications will become broader. Future pumps may have the capability of automatically infusing set doses of medications intermittently at scheduled intervals or according to change in certain physiological parameters (blood pressure, blood chemistries, etc.) (12). For the present, however, the nurse is responsible for administering each dose of medication in the correct manner and at an appropriate rate. Whether a drug is infused via pump or by gravity, the maintenance of the proper flow rate remains one of the major nursing responsibilities in regard to intravenous drug therapy. Other responsibilities, which are directed toward prevention of complications, are discussed in Chapter 7.

REFERENCES

1. Abbott Laboratories: Factors Affecting I.V. Flow Rates. *I.V. Tips,* North Chicago, Illinois, August 1976.
2. Beaumont, Estelle: The New I.V. Infusion Pumps, *Nursing '77,* 7:31-35 July 1977.
3. Cohen, M. R.: Intravenous Infusion Pumps: The Pharmacist's Role. *Hospital Pharmacy,* 11:456, 479, November 1976.
4. Demoruelle, J. L., Flow Rate Maintenance and Output of Intravenous Fluid Administration Sets. *American Journal of Hospital Pharmacy,* 32:177, 1975.
5. Emergency Care Research Institute (ECRI): Infusion Pumps. *Health Devices,* 9:111-115, February 1978.
6. Emergency Care Research Institute (ECRI): Maintenance of Infusion Pumps. *Health Devices,* 4:217-221, July 1975.
7. Ferenchak, Paul, Collins, John, and Morgan, Alfred: Drop Size and Rate in Parenteral Infusion. *Surgery,* 70(5):674-677, November 1971.
8. Fonkalsrud, Eric W., Carpenter, Karon, and Adelberg, Marvin: A New Even-Flow Intravenous Infusion Clamp. *Archives of Surgery,* 102:530-531, 1971.
9. Herbst, Suzanne F.: A New Approach to Parenteral Drug Administration. *American Journal of Nursing,* 75:1345, August 1975.
10. Kitrenos, Jack G., Jones, Maurice, and McLeod, Don C.: Comparison of Selected Intravenous Infusion Pumps and Rate Regulators. *American Journal of Hospital Pharmacy,* 35:304-310, March 1978.
11. Laufer, Neri, Brun, Dan, Perel, Azriel, and Freund, Herbert: A New Infusion Flow Stabilizer. *Archives of Surgery,* 112:53-54, January 1977.
12. Monahan, John J., and Webb, John W.: Intravenous Infusion Pumps—An Added Dimension to Parenteral Therapy. *American Journal of Hospital Pharmacy,* 29:54-59, January 1972.
13. Parker, Donald, and Hodge, James: Delirium in a Coronary Care Unit. *Journal of the American Medical Association,* 201:132-133, August 28, 1967.
14. Parsons, J. A., Rothwell, D., and Sharpe, J. E.: A Minature Syringe Pump for Continuous Administration of Drugs and Hormones: The Mill Hill Infuser. *Lancet,* 1(8002):77-78, January 8, 1977.
15. Plumer, Ada Lawrence: *Principles and Practice of Intravenous Therapy* (2nd ed.), Boston: Little, Brown and Company, 1975.
16. Robinson, Lawrence A., and Vanderveen, Timothy

W.: Pharmacy-Based Infusion Pump Program. *American Journal of Hospital Pharmacy,* 34:697-705, July 1977.

17. Rohde, Thomas D., Blackshear, Perry J., Varco, Richard L., and Buchwald, Henry: One Year of Heparin Anticoagulation: An Ambulatory Subject Using a Totally Implantable Infusion Pump. *Minnesota Medicine,* 60:719-722, October 1977.

18. Turco, Salvatore J.: Inaccuracies in I.V. Flow Rates.

American Journal of I.V. Therapy, 3:28-30, June-July 1976.

19. Turco, Salvatore J.: Pressure for Precision, a Progress Report on I.V. Infusion Pumps. *The American Journal of I.V. Therapy,* 4:13ff., October–November 1977.

20. Turco, Salvatore, and King, Robert E.: *Sterile Dosage Forms—Their Preparation and Clinical Application,* Philadelphia: Lea and Febiger, 1974.

6 Special Considerations for Pediatric Patients

Donnajeanne Bigos Lavoie, RN, MSN

Assistant Professor, College of Nursing, Department of
Maternal and Child Health, Howard University,
Washington, D.C.; Neonatology Nurse Consultant;
formerly Neonatology Nurse Clinician, Children's
Hospital National Medical Center, Washington, D.C.

Although the basic principles regarding administration of intravenous drugs and the management of delivery apparatus are essentially the same for patients in all age groups, special psychological, anatomical and physiological considerations necessitate certain modifications in practices and techniques for the pediatric population.

The specific social and emotional needs of the child receiving intravenous drug therapy depend upon the stage of psychosocial development that the infant or child is in at the time. Anatomical differences, primarily those of size, affect the type of intravenous cannula and other equipment used and the selection of the venipuncture site as well as the range of drug dosage. The therapeutic dose range is also modified by physiological factors, particularly immaturity of certain organ-systems in the neonate and young child. The nurse who is responsible for any aspect of intravenous drug therapy in the pediatric patient must be keenly aware of such differences to insure that the drug therapy will be both safe and effective. Each of these aspects is dealt with in detail in this chapter.

PSYCHOLOGICAL CONSIDERATIONS OF INTRAVENOUS DRUG THERAPY IN PEDIATRIC PATIENTS: SOCIAL AND EMOTIONAL NEEDS

Illness and hospitalization create in children a series of real, imaginary or potential threats. The level of anxiety and fear experienced depends upon such factors as age and developmental level, previous experience with similar threats and/or fears, level of ego strength and cognitive functioning, amount and type of relevant information possessed, and amount and type of support received from others, especially trusted adults (i.e., parents). The nurse must obtain information relating to these factors in order to develop a meaningful relationship with the child and a working knowledge from which to form a baseline for a nursing care plan. A nursing history with data obtained from the parents, as well as direct observation and assessment of the child, are means of obtaining and organizing this information to allow efficient utilization in the planning and implementation of care.

The threats, fears and anxieties the child might have can be classified into five categories, each of which may be experienced to varying degrees, depending upon the above-mentioned factors. These fears include: (1) bodily injury in the form of discomfort, pain, mutilation or death; (2) separation from parents (trusted persons) as well as from a familiar environment, routines and peers; (3) the strange and unknown, with its possibility of surprise; (4) uncertainty about limits set or expected acceptable behavior; (5) relative loss of control, autonomy, independence, competence and self-confidence. Generally any procedure may generate increased fear in anticipation of pain. A procedure involving a needle increases this fear.

Nursing implications specific to intravenous therapy

To minimize stress, help the child to cope with fears, and promote cooperation, the nurse must provide emotional support, psychological preparation and explanations. Explain the purpose and nature of the procedure in terms the child will understand. The explanation should be based upon the child's age, developmental stage and level, and what he already knows or expects.

YOUNG INFANTS (1 TO 3 MONTHS)

Young infants possess a built-in stimulus barrier that causes reaction delays and possibly reduces sensitivity to painful stimuli. Their intellectual level and lack of experience tend to minimize fear and anxiety. However, restricted movement, prolonged discomfort and deep painful stimuli do cause distress. Gentle handling, stroking and a soothing voice can provide some comfort during and after the procedure.

OLDER INFANTS (UP TO 12 MONTHS)

Older infants generally anticipate pain and will cry, wiggle and struggle. Parents may be helpful in comforting children of this age, gently supporting them by stroking them and verbally reassuring them in a soothing voice.

TODDLERS (1 TO 3 YEARS) AND PRESCHOOL CHILDREN (3 TO 5 YEARS)

In children of these ages, the meaning of the procedure may be affected by previous experiences and fantasies, as well as by cognitive functioning. Language limitations may result in physi-

cal expressions of fear, such as crying, striking at the nurse or moving away. The child can be supplied with a syringe (without a needle), administration tubing, bandage, tourniquet, armboard, etc. to allow him to examine and use them on himself, a doll, puppet or the nurse. Tell the child there will be pain and when it will occur. Tell him that he may cry if he wants to during the procedure but that he must keep the extremity still, and that someone will be with him (parent or nurse) during the procedure.

SCHOOL-AGE CHILDREN (6 TO 12 YEARS)

At this age, the child has the intellectual capacity to understand the purpose of the procedure and the technique used. He will be able to cooperate when he knows what is expected of him. Tell him that his important task or "job" during the procedure is to remain still and to avoid moving the extremity being used. Allow him time to verbalize his fears and concerns. Equipment and dolls may also help the child to work out some of his fears. At this age, the child may prefer seeing simple anatomical pictures or drawings, or reading about the procedure.

During the preparation period, allow the child to play with, manipulate and examine the equipment that will be used. Provide appropriate explanations. Proper timing is an important factor. Do not tell the child so far in advance that he worries an unnecessarily long time, but allow him enough time to absorb what he is being told and to work through some of his feelings.

ADOLESCENTS (13 YEARS TO ADULT)

The information given to the adolescent is generally the same as that given to an adult. Consider that the adolescent may be concerned about body image and threatened by illness and helplessness. The explanation about the procedure should be as detailed as necessary.

Providing support

While explaining the procedure, the nurse must continue to provide support and reassurance and to encourage the child to express his version of what is going to occur. At this time, increase his sense of mastery by allowing him some choice whenever possible, such as determining what side to use or identifying how he wants to help. This is especially important when dealing with a child who may require repeated venipunctures. Listen to what he says—"This is the best place"—indeed, it may be. Acknowledge the child's fears. Accept his fears by letting him know it is all right to be afraid and to cry.

Provide the parents with support and encouragement by first determining what they already know about the procedure and what they have told the child; reinforce what they have been told and correct any misunderstandings they may have. Encourage parents to remain with the young child when the procedure is being explained to him and to act as a liaison between nurse and child when information is needed. Stress the importance of their role of comforting their child, physically and emotionally, both during and after the procedure. Rarely, a parent's presence may actually intensify a child's anxiety. A nursing assessment of parent-child interaction will help to determine whether the parent's participation will be helpful to the child. Be certain that the parents are prepared for the procedure and for their role if they are to be present.

Because it is often a traumatic procedure for the child, even when he is prepared, the insertion of an intravenous cannula should be done in the treatment room. Having uncomfortable procedures done in another area allows the child to associate his bed and room with some comfort and security. Additionally, other children who are unprepared are spared needless exposure to the procedure.

During insertion of the cannula, the nurse should continue to give the child support and to explain what is happening and how he is to behave. If a parent is present, she or he should not be expected nor allowed to do anything but comfort and support the child.

Following the procedure, the nurse can continue this support by praising his behavior as appropriate or by helping him to understand how he could have been of more help. The child should be provided with opportunities to talk about or "play out" any feelings he may have. Since the child may be restrained or positioned in bed, appropriate stimulation, activity and diversions should also be provided. Unless movement is otherwise contraindicated, however, the intravenous line itself should not restrict the child to bed. With adequate taping and support of the extremity (such as an armboard), the child should be allowed out of bed and encouraged to participate in play activities. The infant and young child may find great comfort in being held and cuddled following the procedure if this is not otherwise contraindicated.

Restraints or protection devices may be necessary when an infant or child is totally uncooperative and attempts to pull out the cannula (Fig. 6-1). However, with proper psychological and emotional support as well as an explanation of the reason for the intravenous line, the need for such restraints is generally minimized.

SELECTION OF THE CANNULA

In pediatrics, selecting the equipment to be used for intravenous infusion is basically the same as with adults, (see Chapter 3) with variations specific to the age and size of the child and to the infusion site. State laws and institutional policies determine whether a nurse can insert intravenous lines in peripheral sites in infants and children.

Winged-needle unit

The winged-needle unit is frequently used (see Fig. 3-6, p. 28). The neonate may need a 25–27 gauge needle, whereas the older child may accommodate a 23–25 gauge needle, depending upon age, size, and fluids to be administered. When the winged-needle is used, it is frequently easier to determine entry into the vein by attaching to the end of the tubing a 5 milliliter syringe containing 2.0 to 2.5 ml. normal saline, or an appropriate flush solution such as dextrose and 1/3 normal saline. (Flush the needle and catheter prior to entry into the vein.) This is beneficial because in the neonate and small child, venous pressure cannot be relied upon to cause sufficient backflow of blood through a small needle to confirm venous entry. As the needle is inserted, the syringe is gently aspirated. Blood return indicates entry into the vein. Once blood is obtained, gently inject 0.1 to 0.2 ml. saline into the vein to clear the tubing and needle. This pull-push maneuver is continued periodically during taping to assist in determining dislodgement of the needle or obstruction of flow because of taping. Tape and secure the needle as described in Chapter 4 or according to physician preference. Useful practices include: (1) placing a small pad under the device at the hub of the needle, between it and the skin to prevent the needle from being forced through the vein during taping, and (2) securing the tubing so as not to cause pressure on the skin. The Ranfac Preemie Needle,* a 27 gauge needle with a flat undersurface, is frequently used in premature infants and small neonates. When securing the needle after insertion, cut a hole in a square piece of tape and place this over and around the needle. A pair of surgical tweezers is useful in handling the needle during insertion.

In-lying (cutdown) catheter

A 22 gauge catheter is generally used for a cutdown in pediatrics. Other equipment is essentially the same as for adults. When umbilical vessels are the sites being considered, the vessel used, arterial or venous, determines the type of catheter. For an arterial catheterization, Argyle Umbilical Arterial Catheters† are available; however, a No. 3.5 French catheter for infants under 1500 grams or a No. 5 French catheter for infants over 1500 grams may be preferred. For a venous catheterization, a polyvinyl feeding tube with side holes is used.

A pediatric infusion set (volume-control set) should be used with all children under the age of 12 years. Such a set consists of a closed, volume-control or burette chamber which allows only 50 to 100 milliliters of fluid at a time to be accessible for infusion, and a mini- or microdropper, a device that reduces the drop size from the control chamber to 1/50 or 1/60 of a milliliter (normal drop size is 1/10 to 1/15 of a milliliter). A 250-milliliter container only should be used to fill the volume control chamber in *any* pediatric patient receiving less than 100 ml per hour.

Other equipment includes a soft, well-padded pediatric armboard or covered sandbag and gauze bandage to secure and restrain the extremity (Fig. 6-2), and a small tourniquet or rubber band. Three-way extension tubing, to be added to the original administration set should be available for convenience and minimal delay should it be needed unexpectedly. Additional restraining devices that may be needed include bath blanket, extremity restraints (Fig. 6-1), or a covered sandbag. The type used depends upon the age of the child, his

*Randall Saichney Corp., Avon Industrial Park, Avon, MA 02322
†Sherwood Medical, 1831 Olive Street, St. Louis, MO 63103

understanding and cooperation, and the site selected for infusion.

INFUSION SITES

Sites used for intravenous infusions in children include many of the same locations used in adults (see Chapter 3).

Extremities

Dorsal hand veins are often the preferred sites because their use allows the child to remain mobile. If possible, avoid using the dominant hand or the hand the child prefers for thumb-sucking. To visualize the dorsal hand veins more easily and to stabilize the vein during insertion, the operator grasps the child's hand by placing the index and middle finger of the corresponding side in the child's palm and the thumb over the proximal ends of the child's fingers (Fig. 6-3).

Dorsal foot veins and veins of the *flexor surfaces of the wrist* are the same as in the adult. In infants, the only tourniquet that may be necessary is the secure hand grasp of an assistant around the extremity of the child. Frequently, the tourniquet is one part of the procedure most objected to by the child. To decrease the discomfort of the tourniquet, soft clothing or a tissue is placed between the child's skin and the tourniquet. Before the venipuncture is attempted, the extremity must first be immobilized by taping it to a padded splint or covered sandbag (see Fig. 6-2).

Any extremity used should be secured in such a way as to prevent circulation compromise and to provide access to site of infusion.

The *antecubital fossa* is generally not very satisfactory for use in infants and small children because subcutaneous infiltration is common due to difficulty in immobilization of the needle and extremity. When the older child is able to cooperate, the technique is the same as in the adult. The arm must be immobilized with a padded armboard, splint or covered sandbag. If possible, allow the child to select the arm to be used. With adequate taping of the needle, the child should be free to move about and participate in other activities.

Peripheral vein cutdown is similar to the procedure in adults, i.e., usually a large leg vein is used. When the saphenous vein is used, the foot should be secured to a covered sandbag or padded splint prior to starting the sterile procedure (Fig. 6-4).

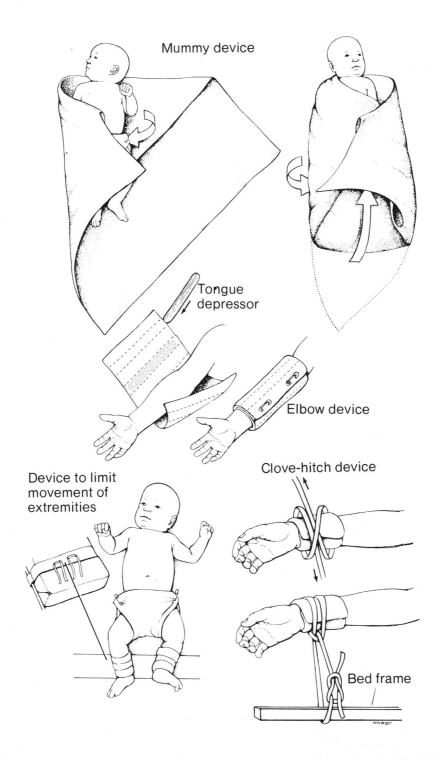

Fig. 6-1. Restraining techniques. (Brunner, L. S., and Suddarth, D. S., *The Lippincott Manual of Nursing Practice*, Philadelphia, J. B. Lippincott, 1978)

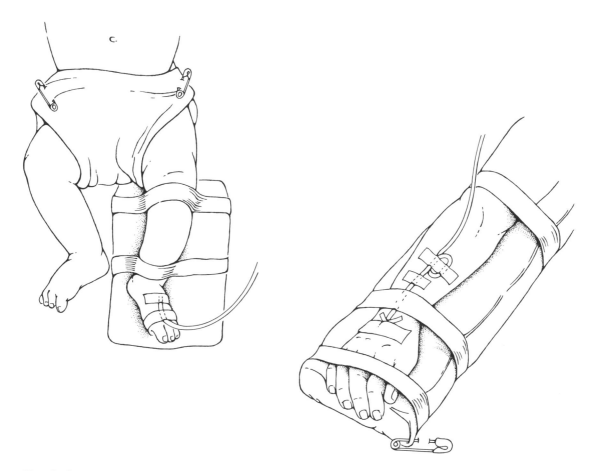

Fig. 6-2. Methods of restraining the arm and leg for intravenous infusions. *(Left)* Infant's leg taped to sandbag for immobilization. *(Right)* Restraint of arm when hand is site of infusion. (Redrawn from Brunner, L. S., and Suddarth, K. S., *The Lippincott Manual of Nursing Practice* [2nd ed.], Philadelphia, J. B. Lippincott, 1978)

This method should be used only in infants and young children who may require prolonged intravenous infusion and antibiotic therapy or when it is impossible to enter a vein with a needle.

The two intravenous infusion sites specific to infants are scalp veins and umbilical vessels in the sick newborn.

Scalp veins

The most commonly used scalp veins are the superficial temporal, supraorbital, posterior auricular and facial veins. Before the procedure is started, the infant is wrapped in a mummy restraint with his head held firmly against the table (with care being taken by the assistant not to obstruct the child's breathing with her hand). The scalp hair at the site is shaved, with a margin for

taping. A rubber band placed around the cranium can be used as a tourniquet. To allow for easier release of the tourniquet, a second rubber band is placed crosswise under the tourniquet. To release the tourniquet, grasp the unstretched rubber band, pull out and cut tourniquet (Fig. 6-5). Check periodically to see that the tourniquet has not slipped down to compress the infant's eyes. Once the infusion has been established, the needle is secured and the insertion site is covered with either small sterile gauze dressing or adhesive bandage. Avoid overtaping that will prevent early observation of infiltration. In addition to the hazards discussed in Chapter 7, infiltration can cause facial and head asymmetry, which is very disturbing, especially to the parents. Once the needle is secured, tape the administration tubing onto the head, being careful

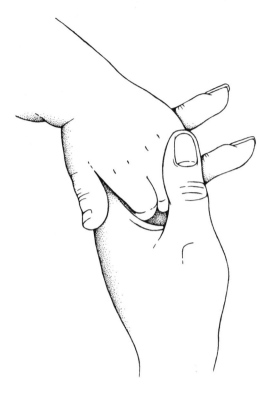

Fig. 6-3. The child's hand must be held securely during the insertion of an intravenous appliance. (Redrawn from Hanid, T. K.: Intravenous Injections and Infusions in Infants. *Pediatrics,* 56(6):1080, December 1975)

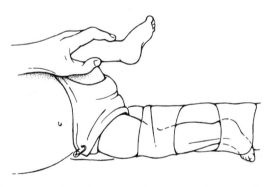

Fig. 6-4. Positioning and taping the leg for a cutdown incision. (By permission of Silver, H. K.: et al.: Handbook of Pediatrics, Los Altos, CA: Lange Medical Publications, 1977 [redrawn])

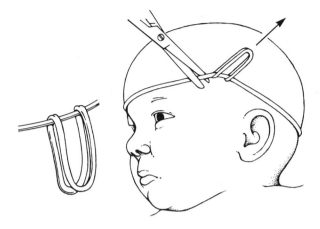

Fig. 6-5. Rubber band scalp tourniquet technique. (Redrawn from Brunner, L. S., and Suddarth, D. S., *The Lippincott Manual of Nursing Practice* [2nd ed.], Philadelphia, J. B. Lippincott, 1978)

to avoid pressure on the skin from the tubing. Cover the needle with a small plastic or paper medicine cup and tape in place to protect it from the infant's normal movements (Fig. 6-6). Avoid using infusions of hypertonic parenteral solutions such as 50 percent glucose, as infiltration may result in tissue sloughing and necrosis. Phlebitis frequently occurs after a few days when this infusion site is used.

Umbilical vessels

Indications for umbilical vessel catheterization include exchange transfusion, monitoring arterial blood pressure, administration of parenteral fluids and medications, blood withdrawal for biochemical analysis (umbilical artery is the most reliable unless the venous catheter tip is passed through a patent foramen ovale into the left atrium), and compromised pulmonary function. This route should not be used for the sole purpose of intravenous fluid administration. Generally, successful catheterization can be accomplished through the third day of life and the catheter can be left in place 3 to 7 days. The advantage of this procedure is that it can be used for emergency correction of acidosis, hypoglycemia and hypovolemia soon after birth when peripheral administration is not possible. Complications occurring with this route include infection, as umbilical cellulitis, sepsis or multiple abscesses (higher frequency with venous catheter); thrombosis, and vasospasm resulting in blanching or cyanosis of the lower extremities (with arterial catheter). (Evans and Glass, p. 5). Other complications are vascular perforation, emboli and hemorrhage. Complications occur about four times more frequently with venous than with arterial catheterization. The advantages must outweigh the risks when this route is considered. Arterial catheterization is preferred for di-

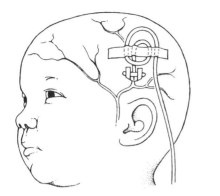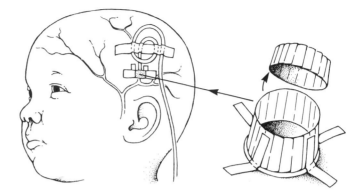

Fig. 6-6. Technique for dressing and securing a scalp-vein needle. *(Left)* Venipuncture of scalp vein. *(Center)* The needle is secured. *(Right)* Paper cup taped over venipuncture site for additional protection. (Redrawn from Brunner, L. S., and Suddarth, D. S., *The Lippincott Manual of Nursing Practice* [2nd ed.], Philadelphia, J. B. Lippincott, 1978)

luting potentially cardiotoxic and thrombophlebitic effects of drugs.

When an umbilical vessel catheterization is done, it should be carried out as a surgical procedure. The infant should be placed under a radiant heater for warmth. Resuscitative equipment should be available—oxygen, suction, breathing bag, laryngoscope and endotracheal tubes. Special catheter trays are available for this procedure. Monitoring of heart rate and respirations should be continual throughout the procedure. All four extremities must be gently and securely restrained. Since arteriospasm may occur during catheterization, observe for any blanching of the legs during the procedure. Be prepared to warm the legs if spasm continues; parenteral tolazoline (Priscoline) may be needed (see drug information section). If heparin is used during therapy to avoid thrombus formation, the catheter should not be removed for 6 hours following heparin in-

fusion to avoid hemorrhage. An x-ray should be taken following catheterization to determine catheter location. The catheter must never be flushed if blocked, as this may dislodge a thrombus that could enter the circulation.

Umbilical vein catheter. The tip of the catheter should be in the inferior vena cava through the ductus venosus.

Umbilical artery catheter. The most frequently used location of the catheter tip is just above the aortic bifurcation (Fig. 6-7) at L_4–L_5 in order to prevent compromised circulation to gastrointestinal tract and kidneys.

The reader is referred to the following for in-depth discussions of umbilical vessel catheters: (1) Evans, H. E., and Glass L.: *Perinatal Medicine.* New York: Harper and Row, 1976; and (2) Evans, M.: Adaption of the infant at birth and intervention techniques for distressed neonates. *Journal of Nurse Midwifery,* 20 (4):18–28, Winter 1975.

REMEMBER:

1. All infusion site taping should be done so as not to obscure the site or prevent observation for any infiltration or local reaction. (signs of infiltration as well as its prevention are discussed in Chapter 7).
2. All dressings should be completely changed at least every 24 hours if a catheter is used; all tubing and fluid containers should be changed every 24 hours. (Brunner and Suddarth, pp. 1413–1414).
3. The child's condition should be assessed continually during the procedure for any change or sign of distress.
4. Comfort and support measures should be maintained during the procedure.

MAINTENANCE OF FLOW RATE

During intravenous fluid therapy, one of the most important responsibilities of the nurse is to control the flow rate of the infusion. The flow

rate must be accurate and constant to insure maintenance of proper fluid balance and to prevent overhydration.

A very small amount of excess fluid can cause fluid and electrolyte imbalances in infants and young

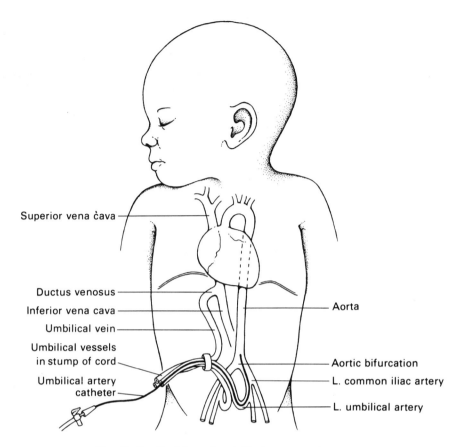

Superior vena cava

Ductus venosus

Inferior vena cava

Umbilical vein

Umbilical vessels
in stump of cord

Umbilical artery
catheter

Aorta

Aortic bifurcation

L. common iliac artery

L. umbilical artery

Fig. 6–7. Position of umbilical artery catheter.

children. Certain criteria are used to assess the status of hydration and to evaluate the results of parenteral fluid therapy. It is a nursing responsibility to accurately observe and record these criteria.

1. *Intake.* Keep an hourly record of the kind and amount of fluid the child has received, the amount of fluid absorbed in the last hour and a running total; rate of flow (count number of drops per minute); amount of fluid remaining in the bottle/chamber; and amount of fluid added to the chamber. The amount of fluid remaining in the bottle should be adequate for the amount needed in the chamber for the next hour.

The flow rate should be regulated when the infant is at rest. If he is crying the tension of his muscles will constrict the blood vessels causing changes in venous pressure, and the fluid will flow more slowly. When he quiets down, the flow rate will increase. A constant flow or infusion rate must be maintained, as a fluctuating rate may result in erratic blood glu-

cose values or overhydration which may lead to congestive heart failure and pulmonary edema in the sick neonate (Table 6-1). In addition to the drop control device on pediatric infusion sets such as the Soluset,* infusion pumps are useful to assist in controlling the flow rate. An infusion pump *must* be used with an umbilical arterial catheter to maintain an infusion pressure greater than aortic pressure. When an infusion pump is used with a small gauge needle in an infant or small child, carefully observe for early signs of infiltration, as the pumps may continue to infuse fluid at the preset rate. Report immediately to the physician any suspected infiltration or major changes in flow rate and hourly intake (changes of 50 percent of prescribed amount). (Detailed information regarding use of infusion pumps is given in Chapter 5.)

2. *Output.* Record urinary output either by catch-

* Abbott Laboratories, North Chicago, IL. 60064

ing urine in receptacle, weighing diapers (for accurate measurement), or identifying "wet diaper" (for less accurate measurement). (To weigh diapers: Weigh a dry diaper—preferably a plastic-backed disposable—and record prior to applying to infant. After infant has voided, weigh the diaper again. If the weight is measured in grams on a diabetic food scale, 1 gram will equal 1 ml. urine.) Urine specific gravity or osmolality is to be measured periodically (every 4 to 8 hours or as prescribed). Report any significant changes or repeated high or low values (see Appendix for normal urine output values). Record any drainage, stools, or vomiting, including amount and characteristics. Keep an accurate record of amount of blood withdrawn from the neonate (for lab studies, etc.), as replacement may be necessary.

3. *Accurate Weight.* An accurate record of weight is often essential for proper evaluation of the child's condition and/or response to therapy. When weighing an infant or child, note the time and any clothing. Use the same scale each time. Report any acute loss or gain (5 percent) to the physician immediately.

4. *Evaluate the general condition* of the infant or child. Note especially activity or behavior,

Table 6-1. SIGNS OF CONGESTIVE HEART FAILURE IN THE INFANT AND OLDER CHILD

INFANT	OLDER CHILD
Tachycardia	Fatigue
Feeding difficulties	Effort intolerance
Poor weight gain	Anorexia
Excessive perspiration	Abdominal pain
Irritability	Cough
Weak cry	Breathlessness at rest
Noisy, labored respirations with subcostal and costal retractions	Hepatomegaly
	Cardiomegaly
Flaring of nares and sternal retractions	Distended external jugular veins
Hepatomegaly	Edema—legs, face, etc.
Cardiomegaly	Orthopnea
Gallop rhythm	
Sudden increase in weight that decreases with diuretics	
Edema—generalized, involving eyelids, sacrum, legs, etc.	

From Vaughan, V. C., and McKay, R. J. (editors): *Nelson's Textbook of Pediatrics* (10th ed.). Philadelphia: W.B. Saunders, 1975, pp. 1088, 1089.

TABLE 6-2. SIGNS AND SYMPTOMS OF FLUID IMBALANCE IN INFANTS AND CHILDREN

DEHYDRATION	OVERHYDRATION
(LOSS OF BODY WATER RESULTING FROM NEGATIVE WATER BALANCE AND LOSS OF ELECTROLYTES)	(RESULTS FROM THE BODY'S RECEIVING MORE FLUID THAN IT CAN EXCRETE)
1. Decreased urine output	1. Headache
2. Increased urine concentration (specific gravity or osmolality)	2. Abdominal cramps
3. Dry mucous membranes	3. Lethargy
4. Dry skin, decreased skin turgor	4. Muscle twitching
5. Skin cold and clammy to touch (seen in hyponatremic dehydration)	5. Excessive weight gain
6. Lack of tear formation	6. Flushed skin
7. Increasing hematocrit	7. Increasing pulse rate
8. Thirst	8. Increased blood pressure
9. Fever	9. Increasing urine volume
10. Lethargy	10. Edema, beginning in the feet and progressing to the body (infants—periorbital, sacral, and occipital areas, then the feet and body)
11. Irritability (usually seen in hyponatremic dehydration)	11. Chest retractions
12. Hypotension	12. Rales
13. Increased pulse rate	13. Cough and shortness of breath
14. Increased urine sodium concentration	14. Increased respiratory rate
15. Increased BUN	15. Increased oxygen need
16. Sunken eyeballs	16. Syncope
17. Sunken anterior fontanelle (up to 18 months of age)	17. Increased arterial PCO_2
18. Decreased weight	
19. Acidosis	
20. Circulatory failure	

change in vital signs, elevated or subnormal temperature, decreased skin turgor, sunken or bulging fontanelles or diarrhea (see Table 6-2).

5. *Laboratory studies.* Insure that laboratory studies requested are being done. Be aware of their results in relation to normal and expected results for the child. Notify the physician as is appropriate.

GUIDELINES FOR PREVENTING FLUID OVERLOAD

Certain precautions must be taken to prevent fluid overload, because the child's heart and circulatory system are smaller than the adult's. Too much fluid would quickly overload the system and cause congestive heart failure and pulmonary edema.

1. Maintenance of a constant flow rate with an infusion pump. By this device, flow rate can accurately be adjusted to a few drops per minute while patency of the intravenous line is maintained.
2. Pediatric infusion set (volume-control set). This allows only 50 to 100 milliliters of fluid to be accessible in the chamber at a time. Be certain that the clamp between volume-control chamber and bottle is securely closed.
3. Mini- or microdropper reduces the size of the drop from the control chamber.
4. All parenteral fluids should be ordered in milliliters per hour, not only drops per minute.
5. Never place more than one-third the daily requirement in the chamber at any one time for infants and small children.
6. Only 250-milliliter reservoir containers should be used for infants and children.

During parenteral fluid therapy, insure that the child is comfortable. Frequently check restraints to see that they have not loosened or become too tight. Change the child's position periodically and give skin care; provide passive exercise, if appropriate. Frequently the child receiving parenteral therapy receives nothing by mouth, so oral hygiene is a comforting and essential measure. Continue to provide diversional activity as appropriate for the age and condition of the child.

The nurse should be aware that intravenous fluid and drug therapy in itself is a risk. The size of the veins of an infant or small child, the difficulty of adequate restraining, the already compromised patient, and the infusion fluid, all set up a situation that may result in infiltration or other complication that may be unavoidable even with superior nursing management and care.

FLUID AND ELECTROLYTE BALANCE IN CHILDREN

When intravenous medications are administered to an infant or child, fluid and electrolyte balance becomes an important consideration. The composition of the intravenous solution in which the drug will be delivered, the electrolyte composition of the drug, and the composition of the diluent used to prepare the drug from a powder must all be calculated into the child's fluid and electrolyte allotments each day to prevent fluid and electrolyte overload. It is a well known fact that such an overload can occur more quickly and have potentially greater consequences the smaller the patient. Children with renal or cardiac disease who have pre-existing problems in handling electrolytes and fluids are in an even more delicate balance. Frequently used drugs that contain considerable amounts of electrolytes are cephalothin sodium (Keflin), and sodium and potassium penicillin (consult the Drug Information section for the milliequivalents of sodium or potassium contained in each unit e.g., grams, milligrams, units, of drug). In addition, a drug requiring 1 milliliter or more of dilution prior to injection, that is given frequently, will add a significant amount of fluid to a child's intake over a 24-hour period. These issues make it necessary to include a thorough discussion of fluid and electrolyte balance.

Body composition of infants and young children, in terms of proportions of water and fat, differs from that of older children and adults. In addition, newborns lose from 3 to 10 percent of body weight in the form of water during the immediate postpartum period. (The normal newborn usually loses 3 to 5 percent while the premature infant may lose up to 10 percent.) Total body water and proportions of intracellular volume and extracellular volume decline during infancy. Adult values of body water proportions are reached after the first year of life. The proportion of extracellular fluid to intracellular water is greater in the infant than the older child and adult. Intracellular fluid in the infant is approximately 35 percent (30 to 40 percent) of body weight; at 1 year of age it is 40 to 45 percent of body weight, proportionately changing little with age. Extracellular fluid in the infant is approximately 45 percent of body weight; at 1 year of age, it is 25 to 28 percent of body weight; at two years of age, 20 to 25 percent (Winters, p.100).

In infants and young children, the water turnover rate per unit of body weight is three or more times greater than in the adult, due to several factors:

1. The young child has a larger surface area in relation to weight, which results in greater insensible losses of water than in the adult.
2. The metabolic rate in the child is higher than in the adult; thus more water is required to carry out metabolic activities.

3. Immature kidney function may impair the infant's ability to concentrate urine; thus greater volumes of water are excreted in the urine.

The rate of water turnover in infants and small children makes any dehydration mechanism more serious as related to renal transport and excretion of drugs. Maintaining normal fluid and electrolyte balance in infants and young children can influence the outcome of an underlying condition. Intravenous fluid therapy is essential with a serious illness which involves severe vomiting, diarrhea, dehydration, blood loss, or loss of consciousness, or when there is a need to provide high blood levels of a drug. The functioning and regulatory mechanisms of several body systems are critical in establishing and maintaining electrolyte balance. These systems include cardiovascular, renal, pulmonary, and endocrine (specifically adrenal, pituitary and parathyroid). Since electrolyte balance is also affected by intravenous fluid therapy, intravenous fluid infusion must be scheduled in specific blocks of time, such as 6, 12, or 24 hours. This allows for regular clinical and biochemical evaluation of the child and his response to therapy. The readjustment of fluid composition, additives and/or flow rate can then be accomplished as required.

To calculate maintenance fluid requirements, three alternatives are available using different body parameters and dosage criteria:

1. *Body weight and age* (Tables 6-3 and 6-4). ml./kg./24 hours—maintenance fluid
2. *Surface area*—determined from weight and length by using a nomogram. (See Appendix.) 1200–1500 ml./m²/24 hours—maintenance fluid
3. *Metabolic rate*—based upon metabolic rate and basal caloric expenditures in 24 hours (not as commonly used)

Maintenance electrolyte requirements

Parenteral fluids generally cannot provide the child with normal caloric requirements; thus 5 percent dextrose can be added to provide some calories and minimize breakdown of fat stores. Basal calories have to be supplied. Solutions of 10 percent glucose are frequently administered to partially meet this requirement. Solutions of dextrose greater than 5 percent, when administered at infusion rates sufficient to meet water requirements in infants, may result in loss of dextrose in urine. This in turn causes an osmotic diuretic effect that may increase water requirements.

Management goals for fluid and electrolyte therapy

In the fluid and electrolyte management of infants and young children receiving parenteral fluid therapy, three areas are to be considered (Vaughan and McKay, p. 250):

1. *Replacement of pre-existing deficits* which may occur from inadequate intake or excessive losses, as in diarrhea. The aim is to estimate and to correct these deficits as quickly and safely as possible and to return serum and extracellular fluid volume to normal to relieve or prevent shock and restore adequate renal function. Intracellular fluid volume is restored more slowly, 8 to 24 hours after the child's condition has improved. Losses are expressed in terms of body weight; that is, in ml. or mEq/kg. body weight.
2. *Provision of maintenance requirements,* to maintain the child in normal balance and prevent deficits. Normal requirements are a result of normal expenditures of water and electrolytes, through urine, sweat, feces and lungs, as a result of normal metabolism. There is a close relationship between maintenance requirements and metabolic rate; thus requirements are ideally calculated in terms of caloric expenditures.
3. *Correction of ongoing losses* which may occur during therapy, usually via the gastrointestinal tract as diarrhea, vomiting or the removal of secretions. Replacement should be similar in type and amount to what is being lost, and is calculated as milliliters of fluid or milliequivalents of electrolytes. Specific fluid and electrolyte therapies may be required for treatment of certain conditions, such as salicylate intoxication in which case alkalinization and induction of diuresis is used therapeutically to increase salicylate excretion in the urine.

Although the nurse is not responsible for prescribing intravenous fluids, a basic understanding of their composition and uses is essential to total nursing care and allows the nurse to make more accurate patient assessments (Table 6-5). Com-

TABLE 6-3. AVERAGE MAINTENANCE REQUIREMENTS FOR FLUID AND ELECTROLYTE THERAPY

	H$_2$O (ml/kg)	Na$^+$ (mEq/kg)	K$^+$ (mEq/kg)	Carbohydrate (g/kg)
Premature	50–70	1.5–2.0	1.5–2.0	2–3
Newborn	40–60	0.8–1.0	0.8–1.0	2–3
4–10 kg	120–100	2.5–2.0	2.5–2.0	5–6
10–20 kg	100–80	2.0–1.6	2.0–1.6	4–5
20–40 kg	80–60	1.6–1.2	1.6–1.2	3–4
Adult total	2500–3000	50	50	100–150

As formulated, the maintenance requirements do not include allowances for such complicating factors as fever, excessive sweating, excessive insensible loss through hyperventilation, or impaired renal function. Appropriate adjustments of water and electrolyte requirements should be made under any of these circumstances.
Reproduced with permission from Silver, H. K., et al.: *Handbook of Pediatrics* (12th ed.). Los Altos, CA: Lange Medical Publications, 1977, p. 60.

mon abnormalities of fluid and electrolyte metabolism are given in Table 6-6.

TOTAL PARENTERAL NUTRITION (TPN)

Total parenteral nutrition (TPN) is a method of providing complete nutrition by way of continuous intravenous infusion.

In many institutions caring for infants and children, total or peripheral parenteral nutrition has become commonplace. This has occurred because of documented success, improvements in nutritional fluids, and advances in equipment design. Indications for the use of TPN in pediatrics include gastrointestinal problems, e.g., chronic diarrhea, malabsorption syndrome, esophageal atresia or obstruction, and omphalocele; prematurity with very low birth weight; malnutrition or failure to thrive; and conditions that result in excessive nutritional needs, e.g., burns, neurosurgical procedures, large wound infections and cancer. The infusion consists of a hypertonic solution of glucose, a nitrogen source, water, minerals, electrolytes and vitamins to promote growth. The percentage of glucose is gradually increased to 20 percent based upon the child's tolerance. With the advent of Intralipid,* a high-calorie, low-osmotic, fat-containing solution, the hypertonic solution of glucose may be used less frequently (see Intralipid, page 324, Drug Information Section).

As with adults receiving TPN, a central vein is required to insure adequate dilution of the solution. In infants and small children, the catheter is usually inserted into the vena cava through the internal jugular or external jugular (most common) vein. The free end of the catheter is passed through a subcutaneous tunnel and secured in place at the parietal scalp (Fig. 6-8). This method prevents displacement of the catheter by the child's movements and contamination from nasal and oral secretions. The site is dressed as with the central venous catheter in adults. The dressing is labeled with the date the catheter was inserted and the type of catheter used.

To decrease the risk of air embolism as well as bacterial and particulate contamination, a micropore filter should be used with any TPN infusion. The use of an infusion pump is also essential to maintain a constant flow rate and prevent backflow of blood into the tubing where central venous pressure is increased from the infant's crying (Fig. 6-9). (See Chapter 5 for more information about maintenance of flow rate and the use of infusion pumps.)

The infusion rate *must* be kept constant. Check the infusion rate every one-half to one hour. Variations in flow rate should not exceed 10 percent of the ordered rate per hour. A sudden increase in infusion rate may cause pulmonary edema, hyperglycemia and osmotic diuresis. Hyperglycemia and resultant osmotic diuresis lead to dehydration because excretion of glucose requires an accompanying excretion of free water. A sudden decrease in infusion rate may lead to hypoglycemia. This occurs because the body's increased insulin secretion (a response to the increased glucose concentration resulting from the large quantities of glucose in the TPN solution) continues after the glucose concentration is decreased.

Other nursing measures that are critical in caring for the child receiving TPN include:

1. *Careful monitoring of total intake and output* including stools, emesis, and gastric drainage. Record any oral intake with a caloric count.
2. *Daily weights*—weigh the child at the same time each day; use the same scales and insure that the child is wearing the same amount of clothing. A steady weight gain is indicative of a positive response to therapy. Measure the infant's head circumference and length weekly as they also indicate growth.
3. *Monitoring for loss of glucose in urine and stool*—frequent Dextrostix (every voiding, every 4 hours, or daily), urine and stool Labstix, Clinitest on every stool.
4. *Checking of urine every voiding for a specific quantity of protein.*
5. *Monitoring temperature*—temperature changes may indicate infection.

Infection, occurring both at the catheter insertion site and as sepsis, remains one of the major complications. In an attempt to prevent contamination and reduce the possibility that infection will develop, specific precautions are necessary. Change the solution bottle, administration tubing and filter at least once a day, being careful not to contaminate any connections. Secure connections with adhesive tape to prevent accidental separation of tubing. Label with date and time tubing is changed. Culture the filter each time it is changed, to detect microbial contamination prior to the development of clinical signs. Change the dressing at the catheter insertion site at least three times a week using strict aseptic technique as described in cannula care for adults (see Chapter 7).

Constant and careful observations must be maintained for detection of other complications of therapy. Insure that the TPN line is not used for any other reason, including medications, to reduce the chance of both incompatabilities and infection. Most of the major complications result from the presence of the cannula (Brunner and Suddarth, p. 1419):

1. Thrombosis of blood vessels
2. Dislodging or plugging of the catheter
3. Local skin infection
4. Erosion of vessels

Table 6–4. AVERAGE MAINTENANCE FLUID REQUIREMENTS FOR INFANT BASED ON DAILY WEIGHT

	LOW BIRTH WT. (ml/kg/24 hr)	TERM (ml/kg/24 hr)
Day 1	60–100	
Day 2	100–120	50–80
Day 3	120–140	
>Day 3	150–180	120

Adapted from Schaffer, A. J., and Avery, M. E.: *Diseases of the Newborn* (4th ed.). Philadelphia: W. B. Saunders, 1977, p. 26.

5. Cardiac arrhythmia
6. Leaking from around the catheter or holes in catheter
7. Air embolus
8. Extravasation of fluid

Metabolic complications include:

1. Hyperglycemia—osmotic diuresis and dehydration
2. Hypoglycemia
3. Metabolic acidosis
4. Abnormal amino acids
5. Electrolyte imbalance
6. Persistant glycosuria
7. Postinfusion hypoglycemia

Meticulous physical care must be maintained in conjunction with TPN therapy to insure that the child will be as comfortable as possible. Provide good skin care, especially in the infant and whenever there is diarrhea. Oral hygiene will provide comfort when the child is not taking anything by mouth. Restraints should be checked frequently to insure that they have not become too tight and restricting, or too loose (thus enabling their removal), and that there is no irritation.

TPN therapy in itself may create undesirable psychological problems. Maternal separation can be minimized by encouraging the parents to visit the infant or child as often as possible and to become involved in his care to the fullest possible extent. Encourage them to hold, cuddle and comfort the child if there are no contraindications. Support the parents, allowing their participation to increase as their tolerance permits.

Lack of oral stimulation may result in lack of

TABLE 6–5. COMPOSITION AND USES OF FREQUENTLY USED PARENTERAL FLUIDS

FLUID	CALORIES PER LITER	ELECTROLYTES, mEq./liter			USE
		Na	K	Cl	
Water with 5% dextrose	170	0	0	0	1. Correction of water deficits in excess of salt, due to inadequate water intake and/or excessive water losses in urine or perspiration
Water with 10% dextrose	340	0	0	0	2. Promotion of sodium diuresis following the excessive use of electrolyte solutions
					3. Prophylaxis and treatment of ketosis in starvation, diarrhea, vomiting, or high fever
0.9% NaCl (normal saline)	0	154	0	154	Correction of dehydration
0.45% NaCl (½ normal saline)	0	77	0	77	
5% dextrose and 0.2% NaCl in water	170	34	0	34	Standard solution for initial therapy, e.g., after surgery or before lab results are available, etc.
Ringer's solution	0–340	147	4	155.5	1. Hypotonic dehydration (also contains Ca 4 mEq./L.) 2. Mild alkalosis 3. Hypochloremia
2.5% dextrose in 0.45% NaCl	85	77	0	77	Repair of dehydration while still providing calories and water
5% dextrose in 0.45% NaCl	170	77	0	77	
Ringer's lactate	0–340	130	4	109	1. Dehydration of any type 2. Restoration of normal fluid balance following distributional shifts of extracellular fluid due to burns, fractures, infection, etc. 3. Moderate metabolic acidosis as occurs with infant diarrhea, mild renal insufficiency.

mastery of the sucking-swallowing reflex as well as loss of the sucking reflex. Establish a schedule of allowing the infant to suck on a pacifier at intervals, associated if possible with being held and comforted. Lack of attention, stimulation, and body contact can easily be prevented by developing a nursing care plan that allows time for positive attention and stimulation during routine procedures, such as the bath, and at specific times during the day. Place colorful and attractive objects such as mobiles within sight and touch, and a music box within hearing (Fig. 6-9). Gently touch, stroke and hold the child. If his physical condition permits, moving the older child out of his room into other areas, out of bed if possible, will decrease mobility deprivation.

Peripheral hyperalimentation, which involves administration of a solution of 10 to 15 percent dextrose, proteins, electrolytes and vitamins via a peripheral vein, as an alternative form of total parenteral nutrition, used when a child needs to be maintained on intravenous infusions for a short time or where normal alimentation needs to be supplemented. The solution is calculated to include 60 to 130 calories per kilogram and 150 to 250 milliliters per kilogram. If possible, avoid using the flexor surfaces of the wrist and dorsum of the foot as cannula insertion sites. Check the skin at the infusion site frequently to note any early extravasation, which can cause cutaneous sloughing and damage to underlying tendons. Septic complications are rare, however, metabolic complications are the same as for total parenteral nu-

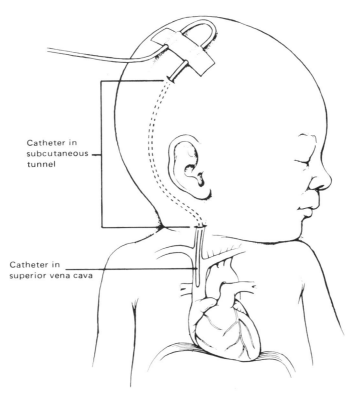

Fig. 6-8. Central venous catheterization using the subcutaneous tunnel. (From Brunner, L. S., and Suddarth, D. S., *The Lippincott Manual of Nursing Practice* [2nd ed.], Philadelphia, J. B. Lippincott, 1978)

trition. Phlebitis and local complications of extravasation are frequently seen.

INTRAVENOUS DRUG ADMINISTRATION IN PEDIATRICS

The basic principles that apply to intravenous drug administration for any patient are discussed in Chapter 8.

Many medications are not approved for pediatric use, especially for children under the age of 12 years. Because of lack of testing, their safety and efficacy in children has not been adequately established; thus dosages are not available. Children who are deprived of such drugs are considered *therapeutic orphans* (Shirkey, p. 62).

The therapeutic response in the pediatric patient, and therefore the dosage of drug prescribed, depend upon several factors. As with fluid and electrolyte therapy, body weight and surface area are the critical measurements in determining drug dosage. Dosages are usually based on kilograms of body weight and occasionally on square meters (M^2) of body surface area.

The age of the infant and young child is another important consideration. Drug dosage depends upon the course of the drug within the body, which involves route of administration, delivery, action at cell level, metabolism, and excretion; these functions are related to organ maturity and metabolic rate. Organ systems that must be considered in individualizing drug dosages are hepatic and biliary, central nervous system, renal, cardiovascular, pulmonary and gastrointestinal. Premature infants and neonates may require a reduced dosage because of deficient or absent detoxifying enzymes, decreased efficiency in renal function, and altered blood-brain barrier and protein-binding capacity. Also, since infancy is a period of rapid growth, all organs are maturing at different rates, so drug metabolism in infants is

TABLE 6-6. COMMON ABNORMALITIES OF FLUID AND ELECTROLYTE METABOLISM

SUBSTANCE	MAJOR FUNCTION	ABNORMALITY	CAUSE	CLINICAL MANIFESTATION	LAB DATA
Water	Medium of body fluids, chemical changes, body temperature, lubricant	Volume deficit	1. Primary—inadequate water intake 2. Secondary—loss following vomiting, diarrhea, excessive gastrointestinal obstruction, etc.	Oliguria, weight loss, signs of dehydration including: dry skin and mucous membranes, lassitude, sunken fontanels, lack of tear formation, increased pulse, decreased blood pressure	Concentrated urine azotemia, elevated hematocrit, hemaglobin and erythrocyte count
		Volume excess	1. Isotonic—due to clinical edematous states such as congestive heart failure; renal disease 2. Hypotonic—due to retention of water in excess sodium	Weight gain, peripheral edema, signs of pulmonary congestion	Oliguria, concentrated urine with reduced sodium chloride concentration
Potassium	Intracellular fluid balance, regular heart rhythm, muscle and nerve irritability	Potassium deficit	1. Excessive loss of potassium due to vomiting, diarrhea; prolonged cortisone, ACTH or diuretic therapy; diabetic acidosis 2. Shift of potassium into the cells such as occurs with the healing phase of burns, recovery from diabetic acidosis	Signs and symptoms variable, including weakness, lethargy, irritability, abdominal distention and eventually cardiac arrhythmias	Low plasma K+ level (may be normal in some situations) polyuria with very dilute urine, hypochloremic alkalosis
		Potassium excess	Excessive administration of potassium-containing solutions, excessive release of potassium due to burns, severe kidney disease, adrenal insufficiency	Variable, including: listlessness, confusion, heaviness of the legs, nausea, diarrhea, ECG changes, ultimately paralysis and cardiac arrest	Elevated potassium plasma level
Sodium	Osmotic pressure, muscle and nerve irritability	Sodium deficit	Water intake in excess of excretory capacity; replacement of fluid loss without sufficient sodium; adrenal insufficiency; malnutrition	Headache, nausea, abdominal cramps, confusion alternating with stupor, diarrhea, lacrimation, salivation, later hypotension; early polyuria, later oliguria	Low sodium plasma level oliguria with concentrated urine except in severe K+ depletion or simple overhydration
		Sodium excess	Inadequate water intake especially in the presence of fever or sweating; severe, watery diarrhea; hyperventilation in warm, dry air; diabetes insipidus	Thirst, oliguria, weakness, muscular pain, excitement, dry mucous membranes, hypotension, tachycardia, fever	Elevated Na+ plasma level, high sp.gr. of urine

(Continued)

TABLE 6–6. COMMON ABNORMALITIES OF FLUID AND ELECTROLYTE METABOLISM—Continued

SUBSTANCE	MAJOR FUNCTION	ABNORMALITY	CAUSE	CLINICAL MANIFESTATION	LAB DATA
Bicarbonate	Acid-base balance	Primary bicarbonate deficit	Diarrhea (especially in infants); diabetes mellitus; starvation; infectious disease; shock or congestive heart failure producing tissue anoxia	Progressively increasing rate and depth of respiration—ultimately becoming Kussmaul respiration, flushed, warm skin, weakness, disorientation progressing to coma	Urine pH usually less than 6 Plasma bicarbonate less than 20 mEq./L. Plasma pH less than 7.35
		Primary bicarbonate excess	Loss of chloride through vomiting, gastric suction, or the use of excessive diuretics; excessive ingestion of alkali	Depressed respiration, muscle hypertonicity, hyperactive reflexes, tetany and sometimes convulsions	Urine pH usually above 7.0, plasma bicarbonate above 25 mEq./L. (30 mEq./L. in adults) plasma pH above 7.45

From Brunner, L. S., and Suddarth, D. S.: *The Lippincott Manual of Nursing Practice*, (2nd ed.). Philadelphia: J. B. Lippincott, 1978, pp. 1405–1406.

different from that in older children and adults. For example (Waechter and Blake, pp. 115–16):

1. The quantity of oxidizing enzyme produced in the liver for metabolism is low in the newborn. Thus, a prolonged and elevated blood level of the drug may occur. This must be considered when using barbiturates.
2. By the third day of life, liver enzymes in the full-term baby are only about one-third as active as those of the adult. However, the biliary flow is low, thus resulting in prolonged effects of drugs excreted by the biliary tract, such as digitoxin and nafcillin.
3. Drugs that are mainly excreted by the kidney (e.g., kanamycin), must be given with special care with regard to dosage to infants under four weeks of age, because of decreased efficiency in renal function.
4. Drugs that affect bilirubin binding capacity with serum albumin, such as sulfonamides and novobiocin, increase the risk of kernicterus. Chloramphenicol is detoxified by the same mechanism as bilirubin; therefore, if the enzymes are not sufficient, the infant becomes toxic.
5. It should also be remembered that the neonate is more susceptible to respiratory depression due to anesthetics and has an increased sensitivity to such drugs as phenobarbital, morphine sulfate, and chlorpromazine, showing exaggerated responses to these drugs.

Body composition in relation to water and fat solubility ratios, membrane permeability, and protein-binding capacity determine drug concentration within the body (Waechter and Blake, p. 114). Solubility of the drug affects its distribution within the body, and distribution changes occur with increasing age because of the changing ratio of water and fat.

Although allergic reactions to drugs are less frequent in infants and young children than in adults, they do occur. The nurse must know the common signs and symptoms of drug reactions, such as skin rashes, temperature variations, unusual behavior and/or anaphylaxis. (see Chapter 8 for more details). Drugs may also cause changes in urine color and feces or interfere with lab tests. All symptoms must be promptly recorded and reported to the physician, and emergency equipment should be readily available. Remember that the child often cannot verbally communicate signs of distress that indicate overdosage or idiosyncrasy; he must rely upon the careful and accurate observations of the nurse.

The techniques of intravenous drug administration, including rate, modes, proper dilution and incompatibilities that can occur with other drugs, should be known. Untoward and toxic effects, precautions and contraindications should be part of the nurse's working knowledge. The reason a certain drug is being given and the response expected must be known. The nurse must be fa-

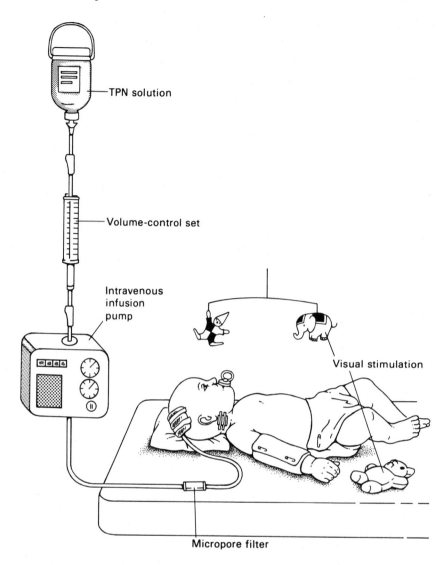

TPN solution

Volume-control set

Intravenous
infusion
pump

Visual stimulation

Micropore filter

Fig. 6-9. Delivery system used for total parenteral nutrition (TPN). (Adapted from Brunner, L. S., and Suddarth, D. S., *The Lippincott Manual of Nursing Practice* [2nd ed.], Philadelphia, J. B. Lippincott, 1978)

miliar with appropriate dosages of specific drugs and be alert to a drug prescription that would be inappropriate for a given child. Should an unusual or inappropriate dosage be noted, inquiry must be made. (For example, the *pediatric* dosage of digoxin should be 0.02 mg.; an order for 0.2 mg. must be questioned. See Chapter 1 for legal implications.) This is especially important when dealing with the pediatric patient, as drug dosages may not be standardized and must be regulated according to the size of the child.

The general principles regarding modes of in-travenous drug administration are the same as in adults (see Chapter 8). Heparin lock for children receiving intermittent intravenous medications is a standard winged-needle unit (scalp-vein needle attached to plastic tubing with a rubber injection site), maintained to assure patency and sterility. The piggyback technique is generally not recommended in infants and children because of the increased risk of uncontrolled fluid infusion. If it is used, meticulous care should be taken to prevent overhydration. This technique is more likely to result in contamination.

Drug dosage's can be calculated according to one of several formulas. Calculations based on weight and age and using adult dosages have limitations. Calculations using surface area are accepted, but may be confusing. Drug literature giving the recommended dose per kilogram (or pound) of body weight is the most accurate source of pediatric dosage information.

The following rules may be used as an *estimate* of the pediatric dosage based on adult dosage:

1. Clark's weight rule (for child of 2 years or more)

$$\frac{\text{weight in lbs}}{50} \times \text{adult dose}$$
$$= \text{approximate child dose}$$

2. Fried's rule (for infant under 1 year)

$$\frac{\text{age in months}}{150} \times \text{adult dose}$$
$$= \text{approximate infant dose}$$

3. Young's rule (for child of 2 years and older)

$$\frac{\text{age in years}}{\text{age in years} + 12} \times \text{adult dose}$$
$$= \text{approximate child dose}$$

4. Methods using surface area

$$\frac{\text{Surface area in square meters}}{1.75} \times \text{adult dose}$$
$$= \text{approximate child dose}$$

$$\frac{\text{Surface area of child}}{\text{Surface area of adult}} \times \text{adult dose}$$
$$= \text{approximate child dose}$$

Surface area in square meters × dose per
square meters = approximate child dose

Generally, intravenous drugs are given by infusion or injection (slow push) in pediatric patients. Details about how to administer each mode are included in Chapter 8. Nursing implications for specific drugs are found in the Drug Information section in the back of this book.

REFERENCES

BOOKS

1. Avery, G. B. (editor): *Neonatology.* Philadelphia: J. B. Lippincott, 1975.
2. Behrman, R. E. (editor): *Neonatal–Perinatal Medicine.* Saint Louis: C. V. Mosby, 1977.
3. Brunner, L. S., and Suddarth, D. S.: *The Lippincott Manual of Nursing Practice* (2nd ed.). Philadelphia: J. B. Lippincott, 1978.
4. Evans. H. E., and Glass, L.: *Perinatal Medicine.* New York: Harper and Row, 1976.
5. Leifer, G.: *Principles and Techniques in Pediatric Nursing* (3rd ed.). Philadelphia: W. B. Saunders, 1977.
6. Marlow, D. R.: *Textbook of Pediatric Nursing* (5th ed.). Philadelphia: W. B. Saunders, 1977.
7. McCracken, G. H., and Nelson, J. D.: *Antimicrobial Therapy for Newborns: Practical Application of Pharmacology to Clinical Use.* New York: Grune and Stratton, 1977.
8. *Pocketbook of Pediatric Antimicrobial Therapy.* Philadelphia: J. B. Lippincott, 1975.
9. Pillitter, A.: *Nursing Care of the Growing Family.* Boston: Little, Brown and Company, 1977.
10. Schaffer, A. J., and Avery, M. D.: *Diseases of the Newborn* (4th ed.). Philadelphia: W. B. Saunders, 1977.
11. Schuberth, K. C., and Zitelli, B. J. (editors): *Harriet Lane Handbook* (8th ed.). Chicago: Year Book Medical Publishers, 1978.
12. Scipien, G. M., et al.: *Comprehensive Pediatric Nursing.* New York: McGraw-Hill Book Company, 1975.
13. Scranton, P. E., Jr.: *Practical Techniques in Venipuncture.* Baltimore: Williams and Wilkins, 1977.
14. Shirkey, H. C.: *Pediatric Drug Handbook.* Philadelphia: W. B. Saunders, 1977.
15. Shirkey, H. C. (editor): *Pediatric Therapy.* St. Louis: C. V. Mosby, 1975.
16. Silver, H. K., et al.: *Handbook of Pediatrics.* Los Altos, CA: Lange Medical Publications, 1977.
17. Vaughan, V. C., and McKay, R. J. (editors): *Nelson's Textbook of Pediatrics* (10th ed.). Philadelphia: W. B. Saunders, 1975.
18. Waechter, E. H., Blake, F. G.: *Nursing Care of Children* (9th ed.). Philadelphia: J. B. Lippincott, 1976.

IMPORTANT NOTE:
Consult Drug Information section in the back of this book or *current* manufacturer's literature for recommended dosages and other information, since changes are constant as research and testing continue.

19. Winters, R. W. (editor): *The Body Fluids in Pediatrics.* Boston: Little, Brown and Company, 1973.

ARTICLES

1. Conway, A., and Williams, T.: Parenteral Alimentation. *American Journal of Nursing,* 76 (4):575-577, April 1976.
2. Evans, M.: Adaption of the Infant at Birth and Intervention Techniques for distressed Neonate. *Journal of Nurse Midwifery,* 20 (4):18-28, Winter 1975.
3. Gruber, D. L.: Helping the Child Accept I. V. Therapy. *American Journal of I. V. Therapy,* 4:50-1, February/March 1977.
4. Hanid, T. K.: Intravenous Injections and Infusions in Infants. *Pediatrics,* 56 (6):1080, December 1975.
5. Luciano, K., and Shumsky, C. J.: Pediatric Procedures. *American Journal of Nursing.* 75 (5):49-52, January 1975.
6. McCalla, J., and Davis, R.: Chemotherapy: Conceptual Basis and Nursing Implications. *APON Newsletter,* 3 (2):7-18, February 1977.
7. McCalla, J., and Davis, R.: Chemotherapy: Conceptual Basis and Nursing Implications. *APON Newsletter,* 3 (4):9-18, August 1977.
8. McCalla, J., and Davis, R.: Classification of Chemotherapeutic Agents. I. V.: Hormones. *APON Newsletter,* 4 (2):21-43, April 1978.
9. Podratz, R.: The Nursing Management of Pediatric Infusion Therapy. *Pediatric Nursing,* 2 (1):13-15, January/February 1976.
10. Robinson, L. A., and Whitacre, N. F.: Intravenous Administration of Antibiotics in Children. *Pediatric Nursing,* 3 (3):21-25, May/June 1977.
11. Ungvarski, P. J.: Parenteral Therapy. *American Journal of Nursing,* 76 (12):1974-77, December 1976.
12. Visintainer, M. A., and Wolfer, J. A.: Psychological Preparation of Surgical Patients: The Effect on Children's and Parents' Stress Responses and Adjustment. *Pediatrics,* 56 (2):187-202, August 1975.

7 Complications of Intravenous Drug Therapy

Although intravenous drug therapy is now a commonplace procedure, it is not an innocuous one. As discussed in Chapter 4, some hazards are associated with the venipuncture itself, particularly when a central vein such as the subclavian or jugular is used. However, the risk of complications certainly does not subside once the cannula is inserted, but persists as long as fluids and medications are given and the cannula remains in place.

Because of the many potential hazards associated with intravenous therapy, from minor to potentially lethal, most nursing functions related to intravenous drug therapy (apart from the activities surrounding drug administration) are directed toward the prevention of complications.

The extent of the staff nurse's responsibility is determined by whether or not the institution has an intravenous therapy team. In the absence of such a team, the staff nurse assumes total responsibility for maintenance of the intravenous system including daily changing of the administration set and care of the cannula. In some institutions, or in special situations within a given institution, the nurse also has responsibility for performing the venipuncture. In hospitals where such functions are assumed by the intravenous therapy team, the primary care nurse must nonetheless share the responsibility for safeguarding the patient against potential complications.

Complications can be either local or systemic, or can start locally and become systemic, such as thrombosis resulting in an embolus, or a local infection developing into septicemia.

There are three general categories of complications, specifically, those associated with: (1) insertion of the cannula, (2) intravenous infusion, and (3) intravenous drug administration. They can be subdivided further as follows:

I. Complications associated with cannula insertion
   A. Peripheral insertion
   B. Central venous insertion
II. Complications associated with intravenous infusion
   A. Interference with accurate delivery of fluid and drugs
   B. Pyrogenic reaction

C. Inflammation and thrombosis
D. Infection
E. Emboli
III. Complications associated with intravenous drug therapy
  A. Hypersensitivity
  B. Toxicity
  C. Other adverse effects, e.g., idiosyncratic reactions

These complications will now be considered in greater depth.

COMPLICATIONS ASSOCIATED WITH VENIPUNCTURE

Peripheral insertion

Complications are generally transient and fairly minor, including:

1. *Penetration of a nerve, ligament or tendon* can occur, resulting in pain (30).
2. *Hematoma* can be caused by piercing of both vein walls or by slipping of the needle out of the vein. This can be serious in individuals with bleeding disorders, as in far advanced liver disease, or with prolonged clotting mechanisms secondary to anticoagulants, or when it occurs in a large vein in which case bleeding can be extensive. Though rare, a massive hematoma can press against an artery and compromise arterial flow.
3. *Collapsed vein* can occur in patients with poor peripheral circulation or if a syringe is used during the insertion process with the exertion of too much negative pressure on the plunger (see Chapter 4).

Central venous insertion

With subclavian vein insertion, complications include:

1. *Pneumothorax*—resulting from puncture of the pleura, allowing air to enter, resulting in lung collapse.
2. *Hemothorax*—due either to laceration of the vein or to arterial puncture.
3. *Hydrothorax*—caused by infiltration of the fluid into the chest cavity.
4. *Air embolism*—when the jugular vein is entered, either directly or via the subclavian, the catheter can be misdirected superiorly. Should any

air enter, it can embolize rapidly to the brain. (See page 104 for further details on air embolism.)

COMPLICATIONS ASSOCIATED WITH INTRAVENOUS INFUSION

Interference with the delivery of fluids and drugs

CLOTTING OF THE CANNULA

Any prolonged cessation of flow will result in clotting of the needle or catheter. Whenever a container empties, or the tubing becomes kinked or otherwise occluded, or the flow rate slows excessively, the venous pressure causes blood to back up into the cannula, and within a matter of minutes, it will clot. An intermittent winged-needle unit (heparin lock) will clot if it is not flushed regularly with heparinized saline. Frequent checking of the total intravenous line is therefore essential to identify the cause of an interrupted flow and to correct it before the cannula becomes clotted.

Preventive measures include: not letting a container run dry; correct taping and positioning of the distal tubing to prevent kinking; maintaining an adequate flow rate, and when extremely slow rates are required (less than 10 ml./hr.), using an infusion pump (see Chapter 5). When intermittent cannulae (heparin locks) are used, they should be flushed with heparinized saline after each dose of drug or at least every 8 hours.

Once the flow has stopped and clotting is suspected, an attempt can be made to restore flow by raising the container, opening the flow control clamp, and milking the tubing. Forceful irrigation when resistance is met should never be done since it can dislodge clots and cause emboli to the lungs (particularly when large gauge cannulae are used), as well as introduce contaminants into the bloodstream (23). If attempts to restore flow are unsuccessful, the cannula should be removed and a new one inserted.

EXTRAVASATION AND INFILTRATION

These terms are often used synonymously to signify leakage of the infused fluid into the tissues. Technically, extravasation refers to an escape of fluid or blood from a blood vessel, and it can result from a leakage of fluid or blood around a venipuncture site while the cannula is still within the vein (30). Infiltration of fluid into the tissues generally occurs when the needle has pulled out of the vein, although occasionally the bevel of a needle may be partially within and partially outside the vein. With either situation, the escape of fluid may represent a minor problem if it involves a small amount of isotonic fluid or a nonirritating drug. However, large volumes of hypertonic fluids, such as 10 percent dextrose, or those that are very acidic or alkaline, can cause tissue irritation and necrosis. As fluid enters the subcutaneous tissues, the skin becomes separated from the fascia, resulting in stretching of the vessels and obstruction of the arterioles, producing cellular death (20). Even small amounts of powerful vasopressors such as levarterenol (Levophed) and highly toxic drugs such as many chemotherapy (antineoplastic) agents, including doxorubicin (Adriamycin), can produce rapid and severe necrosis and sloughing of the tissues if infiltration occurs. If unchecked, severe disfigurement, requiring skin grafting, or even loss of a limb can occur (32).

Guarding against extravasation and infiltration, therefore, represents a major goal in intravenous drug therapy. Prevention is directed toward selecting the most appropriate type of cannula and inserting it into an area which is not subjected to excessive movement. Secure taping of the cannula and tubing as well as use of an armboard provides further protection, particularly when insertion near a joint is unavoidable or if additional security is needed. For patients who are unable or unwilling to cooperate, restraints may be required as discussed in Chapter 2.

The infusion site should be checked frequently, ideally at least hourly and more frequently with toxic drugs. Instruct the patient who is able to immediately report any pain or swelling at the infusion site. Swelling can range from slight puffiness to overt edema. Compare the size of the limb with the opposite one. The degree of pain is related to the extent of infiltration and type of drug or fluid infusing. Inflammation is often absent initially, but is apt to occur with antineoplastic drugs. The area of infiltration is likely to be cooler than the surrounding skin in the initial stages. Vasopressors will cause pronounced blanching of the tissues. In addition to these signs and symptoms, infiltration can be documented by an absence of flashback of blood on lowering the container, along with continued flow of solution when a tourniquet is applied *lightly*, proximal to the tip of the cannula (23).

When infiltration occurs, early detection and removal of the cannula are essential to prevent pain and disability. With highly toxic drugs, treatment measures may need to be instituted by the physician to prevent permanent tissue damage. With levarterenol (Levophed), for example, phentolamine (Regitine) is given subcutaneously throughout the involved area (30). With nonirritating fluid and drugs, elevation of the limb and application of heat to the affected area are measures often used to reduce discomfort and promote reabsorption of fluid. Specific therapies for each drug are described in the drug information section of this book.

RAPID UNCONTROLLED INFUSION (RUNAWAY IV)

Failure to maintain the prescribed flow rate can result in the rapid infusion of dangerously large volumes of fluid and/or high dosages of drugs. The flow rate can suddenly increase if the clamp slips or if the patient tampers with the clamp, perhaps increasing the flow in hopes that the IV will be discontinued once the container has infused. If the flow rate was adjusted while the limb was in a position which caused kinking of the tubing or occlusion of the cannula tip, repositioning of the limb can relieve the obstruction and give rise to a sudden rapid flow.

Another occurrence is the readjustment of flow rate by the nurse in an attempt to infuse the fluid within the initially specified time after it has gotten behind schedule. Because of the sometimes dire consequences mentioned in Chapter 5, such rapid "catching up" must never be done. While small readjustments of rate can sometimes be made, when fluids get significantly behind schedule, particularly at the end of a 24-hour period, it is usually best to discard the unused fluid and initiate a new container, not only to prevent fluid overload, but also for reasons of sterility and drug stability.

Consequences of a rapid infusion may be minimal in a "healthy" adult; however, depending on the type and volume of drug and fluid infused and the age and condition of the patient, the outcome can be serious or even fatal. The major complications are circulatory overload with resultant congestive heart failure and possibly pulmonary edema, and drug toxicity.

1. *Congestive heart failure and pulmonary edema* result when the volume of rapidly infused fluid plus the volume of blood returned to the heart exceeds the volume which can be pumped by the heart through the vascular system. Patients with acute myocardial infarction or a history of congestive failure or renal failure, as well as the elderly, infants and young children, are most prone to develop these problems. For all patients receiving intravenous therapy, but especially for these high-risk individuals, nursing intervention must focus on preventive measures aimed at insuring an accurate flow rate. For all patients, it is essential to monitor the infusion at frequent intervals (at least hourly whenever possible) to insure that the desired rate is being maintained. Some recommend use of double clamps in case one slips (23). When more precise delivery is required, as in the pediatric setting, use of volume control units and other special devices discussed in Chapter 5 are advisable. When the need to control flow rate is critical, an infusion pump or controller should be used. It must be remembered that the nursing responsibilities are not replaced by the infusion pump; there remains a need for close attention to insure proper function of the pump and accurate flow rate.

In spite of all precautions, it is possible that a patient at high risk may develop congestive failure and pulmonary edema. The recognition of early signs and symptoms is essential. These include tachypnea (rapid respirations), dyspnea, orthopnea, tachycardia, agitation, increased blood pressure, moist rales heard on auscultating the lungs, distended neck veins, and elevated central venous pressure (CVP). Unless treatment is instituted immediately, frank pulmonary edema can ensue, as manifested by severe dyspnea, cough productive of frothy, pink sputum, and cyanosis (29). Should any of these signs be present, the infusion should be slowed to its minimum rate and the patient put in a high Fowler's position. Notify the physician immediately and prepare to assist with treatment measures (e.g., morphine, oxygen, digitalis, diuretics, aminophylline, and rotating tourniquets) (12).

2. A second consequence of a rapid uncontrolled intravenous infusion can result from the effect of drugs being infused at such a rapid rate. The administration of a high dosage enables toxic concentrations of the drug to accumulate, and depending on the drug, this can produce a shocklike syndrome with early signs of tachycardia, decreased blood pressure, and progression to syncope, shock and cardiovascular collapse. This is sometimes referred to as "speed shock" (23, 30). Preventive measures are the same as for circulatory overload (pulmonary edema), primarily close monitoring of the infusion to insure that the correct rate is maintained. Should this type of toxic reaction occur, the infusion must be terminated, the physician notified immediately, and the vital signs closely monitored. Treatment is based on the type of drug infused and the severity of symptoms.

Pyrogenic reaction

A pyrogenic reaction is a systemic febrile reaction caused by the introduction of pyrogens into the blood. Pyrogens have been defined by Turco and King as "metabolic products of living organisms or the dead microorganism themselves, causing a specific pyretic response upon injection" (30, p. 31). Pyrogens can gain entrance to intravenous drugs and fluids by means of the chemicals and drugs used during their preparation and through the containers in which they are prepared or stored (30).

Pyrogenic reactions can be prevented by elimination of pyrogens from intravenous fluids and drugs at the time of their manufacture. Pyrogen testing is now a standard part of quality control measures in manufacture and preparation, and thus pyrogenic reactions are infrequent. When one does occur, however, it is characterized by fever of sudden onset, accompanied by chills, malaise and headache. The treatment consists of immediate discontinuation of the intravenous fluid. Some patients may require antipyretic agents to control the fever. Before attributing such a febrile reaction to pyrogens, steps should be taken by the physician to try to rule out infection and toxic drug reactions as possible fever sources.

Inflammation and thrombosis

Thrombosis and phlebitis are interrelated insofar as their causes are concerned. They can occur either singly or in combination.

THROMBOSIS

Thrombosis is a reaction involving a thrombus or clot without any inflammation. It occurs as a result of damage to the inner lining or *intima* of the vein with subsequent deposition of fibrin, clot formation, and occlusion of the vessel lumen (27). The intimal damage can occur as a result of a traumatic venipuncture or irritating drugs and fluids. Another source of thrombus formation is the cannula itself, particularly with certain types of plastic catheters. One study comparing two types of catheters found twice the rate of thrombosis in polypropylene than in Teflon catheters (8). In another study, clots were formed on the surface of all types of catheters used, though the clots were much smaller on catheters made of such materials as silastic. However, these investigators found that such clotting can be eliminated by maintaining a low level of systemic heparinization (21).

Pure thrombosis is generally associated with little or no pain, and so, unless it results in complete cessation of flow, it can go undetected until secondary complications arise. The major hazards associated with thrombosis are infection due to entrapment of bacteria by the clot, and embolism resulting from dislodgement of a portion or all of the thrombus.

Preventive measures include careful avoidance of traumatizing the vein during cannula insertion; use of veins in the upper extremities rather than those in the legs; selection of a large vein when irritating drugs and fluids are given; and choice of a cannula made of materials which have been found to be less thrombogenic (see Chapter 3). For patients who are at greater risk, the physician may institute low-dose heparin therapy for the duration of intravenous therapy. Bleeding, even at the time of cannula removal, is usually not a problem in these patients, since the dosage of heparin used is very low.

Because inflammation and pain are usually absent, recognition may be difficult. Generalized swelling may be present along the involved area or the thrombus itself may be sharply defined and palpable. When thrombosis is confirmed or suspected, treatment measures should be instituted, including removal of the cannula and anticoagulation for deep thrombosis. Avoid further palpation, massaging or trauma to the thrombosed area since it could precipitate disruption and embolization of the clot.

INFUSION PHLEBITIS

Infusion phlebitis is a common occurrence which is felt to be related to both chemical irritation and infection (13, 27). Ranging from simple inflammation of a vein with minimal discomfort to an extremely painful area with a palpable venous cord present, phlebitis frequently subsides spontaneously upon removal of the cannula.

While no single element has been found to cause infusion phlebitis, several predisposing factors have been identified by Maki (13):

1. *Physiochemical Factors*
   a. *Type of Cannula Used.* Steel needles result in less phlebitis than plastic catheters. Catheters constructed of silicone and certain types of Teflon have been found to be less irritating than those made of polyvinyl chloride (PVC) and polyethylene (see Chapter 3) (27).
   b. *Size of Cannula.* It is believed that larger bore cannulae may result in more venous irritation because the blood flow around them is impaired.
   c. *Site of Cannula Insertion.* Leg veins are more prone to development of phlebitis and thrombosis because of the relatively diminished flow. Hand veins have been associated with fewer complications than those in the wrist or forearm (27).
   d. *Location of Cannula Tip.* When the tip of the cannula is within a peripheral vein, more irritation occurs than when it is in a central vein. This, once again, is due to patterns of flow around the cannula, as well as to less rapid dilution of fluids and drugs infused through the cannula.
   e. *Duration of Time Cannula Remains in the Vein.* Venous irritation and phlebitis are directly proportional to the length of time a cannula remains in one location (7). The occurrence of phlebitis is low when the cannula is removed within 48 hours, but rates begin to increase between 48 and 72 hours and are significantly higher after 72 hours.
   f. *Type of Fluid or Drug Infused.* The chemical composition of a fluid or drug, and particularly the pH, influence the occurrence of phlebitis (22). In general, fluids and drugs with a low pH (acid) and hypertonic fluids are more likely to cause venous irritation.

2. *Infection.* Although infusion phlebitis is primarily a physiochemical phenomenon, it can also have an infective component. Organisms can be introduced at the time of cannula placement or subsequently by entering at the cannula insertion point (15).

Infusion phlebitis is technically confined to localized inflammation involving the inner layer (intima) and middle layer (media) of the vein, without thrombus formation. However, when present, *thrombo*phlebitis can result, and the risk of bacteremia or sepsis developing is significantly increased (18-fold) (13).

Prevention is aimed at eliminating contributory causes such as limiting the use of plastic catheters to situations in which a secure line is needed for long-term therapy or when a central venous line is required; when a plastic catheter is necessary, select one composed of a material which has a relatively low incidence of causing phlebitis; and select a cannula that is smaller than the lumen of the peripheral vein. Perhaps the most important preventive measure, along with use of strict aseptic technique during insertion, is changing the cannula every 48 to 72 hours, and should it be necessary to keep a cannula in one location for an extended length of time (such as with a central venous catheter), it is essential that the insertion site be cleaned and redressed daily using sterile technique.

The hallmark of infusion phlebitis is inflammation of the vein in which the cannula is located. An area of erythema or redness may surround the involved vein, or a red streak along the course of the vein may be present. Warmth is common, as well as varying degrees of discomfort ranging from mild tenderness to moderately severe pain. A palpable venous cord is present in only some cases.

The most effective treatment is generally removal of the cannula at the earliest sign of phlebitis. Failure to do so will almost always give rise to thrombophlebitis (27). A percentage of patients will develop systemic infection. Other treatment besides removal of the cannula is rarely required, but symptomatic measures may be used, including application of warm soaks to the area.

THROMBOPHLEBITIS

The same factors that predispose to infusion phlebitis can also give rise to thrombophlebitis.

Once phlebitis has developed, the resultant damage of the lining or intima of the vein can cause the formation of a thrombus or clot. Unless recognized and treated, the thrombosis will be progressive and inflammation will further involve the media (middle layer) and adventitia (outer layer), as well as the surrounding tissues (27).

Aside from the discomfort and interference with administration of needed drugs and fluids, a more serious consequence of thrombophlebitis is the risk of a portion of the clot dislodging and embolizing to the lung. This complication, which is often serious and can prove fatal, is discussed in detail below. Another potential outcome is the development of sepsis with or without suppuration (33).

Prevention of thrombophlebitis involves elimination of predisposing factors. Attention to the measures discussed above, under *Infusion Phlebitis*, will likewise diminish the risk of thrombophlebitis.

Local symptoms similar to phlebitis include pain, redness, warmth and swelling along the involved vein. When it is extensive, motion of the part may be affected (30). Malaise, fever and leukocytosis (increased white blood count) are not uncommon (27). To prevent serious consequences, the cannula should be removed and the physician notified as soon as these signs and symptoms are noted. If reinsertion of a cannula is necessary, it should be done in the opposite limb. Heat and elevation of the extremity are measures often used to decrease swelling and discomfort.

Infection

Infection represents both a common and also a serious hazard of intravenous therapy. It can be introduced at the time of cannula insertion or subsequently through contaminated fluids or equipment. While simple infusion phlebitis sometimes has an infective component, it is felt to have a physiochemical basis more frequently. When localized infection is clearly present, it is often treated conservatively, and only rarely are antibiotics needed.

Two types of intravenous-associated infections have a very serious significance, however: septicemia and suppurative thrombophlebitis.

SEPTICEMIA

Septicemia is a generalized infection throughout the bloodstream resulting from the introduction of organisms (bacteria or fungi) into the circulation (bacteremia or fungemia). Although *sepsis* technically refers to a toxic infection in any part of the body, it is commonly used interchangeably with septicemia. For patients on intravenous therapy, organisms can enter the bloodstream as the result of contamination of virtually any component of the intravenous system. Contamination can be intrinsic, that is, introduced *prior to use* during the manufacturing or storage of the product. Intrinsic contamination of intravenous fluids was responsible for a nationwide epidemic of septicemia in 1970 and 1971. The discovery that the source of contamination was the liner of the screw-cap bottle closure of one manufacturer prompted the recall of all contaminated products and the redesign of the bottle closure (15). Three other outbreaks of sepsis occurring between 1971 and 1973 were also traced to intrinsically contaminated intravenous fluids (15).

Improved manufacturing methods have virtually eliminated such outbreaks. However, extrinsic contamination, which occurs *during* use of fluids and other intravenous equipment, remains an ever present problem. As discussed in previous chapters, contamination can be introduced at the time of cannula insertion or during any manipulation of the intravenous system causing a break in sterility, such as changing of the container or tubing or during preparation or administration of drugs and admixtures.

Clinical data have shown that septicemia occurs with much higher frequency in patients receiving total parenteral nutrition (TPN) (15). This may be accounted for by several factors: patients requiring TPN are usually seriously ill and sometimes immunosuppressed; the cannula, which is generally in a central vein, is likely to remain in place for an extended period of time; the cannula insertion site is often covered with an occlusive dressing which is felt to alter the microbial flora and favor the growth of fungi such as *Candida*. *Candida*, the organism responsible for the majority of cases of septicemia in patients receiving TPN, has been found to proliferate in TPN solutions.

A variety of other organisms has also been associated with infusion septicemia, including *Staphylococcus* and gram-negative bacilli (*Klebsiella, Enterobacter, Serratia,* and *Pseudomonas*). *Bacteremia* can resolve uneventfully after removal of the contaminated fluid or cannula, in some instances, without need for other treatment. However, since the septicemia it may lead to is a severe systemic infec-

tion, it can represent a serious hazard for many patients, particularly if the source of infection is not immediately suspected and detected and the intravenous line is allowed to remain in place. After apparent improvement, secondary complications such as endocarditis and endophthalmitis can occur. In severely debilitated or immunosuppressed patients, sepsis often proves fatal. Because of its potential seriousness, a major effort must be directed toward its prevention.

The following represents an adaptation of the guidelines set forth by the Center for Disease Control (CDC) for preventing infusion-associated sepsis (10):

1. Use winged-needle units (scalp-vein needles) whenever possible. Reserve use of plastic catheters for central venous lines or for very secure lines.
2. If an intravenous line is required only for the intermittent administration of drugs, an intermittent device (heparin lock) should be used.
3. Avoid use of veins in the lower extremities.
4. For cannula insertion, follow strict aseptic technique, including thorough handwashing, and ideally, use of sterile gloves and drapes. Disinfect the skin with tincture of iodine or an iodophor.
5. If aseptic technique cannot be strictly followed, as in an emergency, a new intravenous line should be inserted as soon as possible (18).
6. Anchor the cannula securely to prevent any movement. Apply antiseptic ointment and sterile dressing to the insertion site.
7. Change the cannula at least every 72 hours; preferably every 48 hours. This practice can be promoted by noting the date and time of cannula insertion on the tape as well as on an appropriate part of the patient's record, such as the nursing care plan or intravenous infusion record.
8. Inspect the insertion site daily for signs of local infection, clean the area with an iodophor, and apply antiseptic ointment and a sterile dressing (Fig. 7-1). If any signs of infection are noted, remove the cannula and notify the physician. In some institutions, central venous catheters are removed only by the physician.
9. Examine all fluid containers for cracks or punctures. Do not use any fluid that has turbidity or a precipitate.

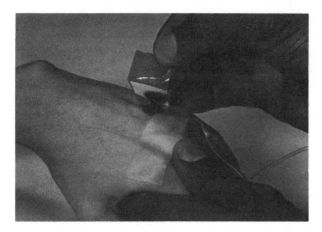

Fig. 7–1. The use of a sterile plastic bandage facilitates daily inspection and redressing of the cannula insertion site. Note the use of iodophor ointment to further minimize the risk of infection.

10. Use the container as soon as possible after opening it. Do not allow any container to run for more than 24 hours. Using small (approximately 250 ml) containers for keep-open IV's helps to insure this practice, while minimizing waste.

11. Consider using a micropore filter, especially with TPN solutions (Fig. 7-2). Avoid touch contamination when adding or changing any adjunctive devices. Maintain a closed system unless changing the tubing. Do not disconnect the tubing to change the patient's gown.

12. Change the administration set and any adjunctive devices every 24 hours. (More recent data from CDC indicate that contamination rates are no higher when sets are changed every 48 hours than when changed every 24 hours. Aseptic insertion and maintenance of the system are the most important factors [5].)

13. Observe the patient for signs and symptoms of septicemia. These include sudden onset of fever, chills, hypotension, cold sweat; occasionally, there may be nonspecific gastrointestinal symptoms (nausea, vomiting and diarrhea) and neurological symptoms and shock (9).

Since up to half the patients with infusion-related septicemia do not show local signs of phlebitis, other sources of infection such as urinary tract infection or pneumonia may initially be suspected. If treated with antibiotics without removal of the intravenous infusion system, the signs and symptoms will persist, although perhaps somewhat abated. Such refractoriness is a characteristic feature of infusion-associated septicemia (13). An intravenous line, when present, should be regarded as a likely source of septicemia. When suspected, the cannula and all other components of the infusion should be removed immediately and the cannula tip cultured. Cultures should also be done of the infusion fluid and blood, as well as any purulent drainage which may be present at the insertion site or on the cannula tip. The lot number of the suspected fluid should be recorded. If a positive culture is obtained, all fluid of the same lot should be removed from use. Local and federal authorities should be notified to conduct an appropriate epidemiological investigation.

When antimicrobial therapy is required, the final choice of drugs is based on culture and sensitivity results. Until they are available, a combination of drugs effective against both gram-negative bacilli (e.g., an aminoglycoside such as gentamicin or tobramycin) and gram-positive organisms such as *staphylococci* (e.g., a cephalosporin such as cephalothin) should be used (13). Should the likely organism be *Candida albicans,* as in patients receiving TPN, antifungal therapy may be required with a drug such as amphotericin. Follow-up of all patients with infusion-related septicemia is essential to insure total eradication of the infection, and, thus, prevention of secondary complications such as endocarditis.

SUPPURATIVE THROMBOPHLEBITIS

Suppurative thrombophlebitis is one of the most dreaded complications of intravenous drug therapy. Fortunately, the overall incidence is low. Unlike the thrombophlebitis described above, this type is characterized by a pocket of pus within the infected segment of the vein. The purulent material, containing vast numbers of organisms, is carried throughout the blood, producing an overwhelming septicemia.

The organisms most frequently associated with suppurative thrombophlebitis include resistant forms of gram-negative bacilli, such as *Enterobacter* and *Klebsiella,* and coagulase-positive *Staphylococcus aureus* (15).

Unless detected and treated surgically, the condition is generally lethal. One hindrance to early treatment is the absence of local signs of inflammation or infection in as many as 70 percent of cases (15). Consequently, many cases remain undetected until death occurs. The diagnosis can sometimes be established in patients with surgical cutdowns by opening the incision, manually milking the vein, and expressing purulent material. In contrast to simple thrombophlebitis with infection, the infection does *not* clear upon removal of the intravenous cannula. In fact, signs of septicemia may first appear approximately two to ten days *after* the cannula has been removed (26).

As with any intravenous-associated infection, prevention must focus on absolute adherence to aseptic practices from the time of cannula insertion throughout the duration of intravenous therapy. While this is certainly advocated for *all* patients receiving intravenous drugs or fluids, it is mandatory that special attention be directed toward those patients who are known to be the most susceptible to development of suppurative thrombophlebitis. At highest risk are patients with burns (26). Individuals on immunosuppressive therapy or with cancer are also more prone to its occurrence. In patients without burns, suppurative thrombophlebitis almost exclusively involves central veins or veins in the lower extremities. It is generally associated with a plastic catheter remaining in place for an extended period of time, but it has also been reported following cannulation with a scalp-vein needle (14). For high-risk patients, and ideally all patients, the guidelines set forth above, under *Septicemia* should be followed.

Signs and symptoms of suppurative thrombophlebitis are essentially the same as for septicemia, with fever being the major presentation. Blood cultures are usually positive, as are cultures of the catheter tip. Leukocytosis (increased white count) is generally present. When these or other signs lead to suspicion of suppurative thrombophlebitis, exploratory venotomy should be done and appropriate treatment must be instituted immediately. The only definitive treatment is surgical excision of the affected segment of the vein and any involved tributaries (15). Broad coverage antibiotics should be initiated until culture results are available, at which time the antibiotic regimen should be changed as then indicated. Antibiotics and anticoagulants given in the absence of surgical intervention usually fail to eradicate the focus of infection, and death frequently is the consequence.

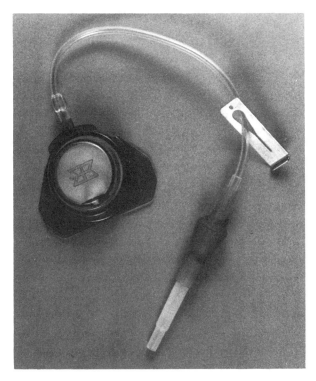

Fig. 7–2. A 0.5 micron filter traps most bacteria as well as air and particulate matter, reducing the likelihood of infection and other complications. (Travenol Laboratories, Inc., Deerfield, Illinois 60015)

Embolism

Embolism refers to the sudden obstruction of a blood vessel by a clot, air or foreign matter carried via the bloodstream from another location. Emboli associated with intravenous therapy, since they originate in the venous system, migrate to a central location, generally reaching a pulmonary arteriole. Those associated with arterial infusions may be carried to various parts of the arterial system in the extremities, brain, kidneys, etc., depending upon the infusion site. The three types of embolism associated with intravenous (and intra-arterial) infusions are thromboembolism, air embolism and catheter embolism.

THROMBOEMBOLISM

Should a thrombus or clot form within a vein, portions may become dislodged and embolize to other areas, primarily the pulmonary arterioles. As discussed above, several factors associated with intravenous therapy can predispose to thrombosis and subsequent embolization:

1. The venipuncture itself and subsequent manipulation of the cannula can traumatize the intima of the vein, thereby stimulating the clotting process.
2. Investigations have shown that a fibrin clot forms around most plastic catheters, but some types have been shown to be associated with a lower incidence of clot formation.
3. Alterations in blood flow can occur when a cannula is inserted into a vein, particularly when the external diameter of the cannula is nearly as large as the lumen of the vein. The relative hemostasis produced can predispose to thrombus formation.
4. A diminished flow may also occur in the lower extremities or in a limb following trauma or surgery, and should a cannula be placed in one of these situations, the risk of thrombosis is heightened.
5. Clotting occurs within a cannula when the flow stops, since the venous pressure causes a backup of blood into the cannula.

Once a thrombus has formed in or around the cannula, subsequent manipulation, particularly flushing to restore flow, can dislodge pieces of the clot, resulting in pulmonary embolism. While such clots may be very tiny, they may serve as a focus for subsequent clot formation.

The severity of the pathophysiological changes accompanying a pulmonary embolism depends on the extent of obstruction of pulmonary arterial blood flow to the lung. Respiratory effects include an area or areas of nonperfusion, which means that blood does not get to those regions and therefore there is no gas exchange. There is gradual loss of alveolar surfactant resulting in some atelectasis occurring after 24 to 48 hours. Infarction (actual death of lung tissue) is believed to be rare, occurring in less than 10 percent of cases (29). While most treated pulmonary thromboemboli can resolve without serious consequences, their occurrence in patients with pre-existing cardiac or pulmonary conditions can be serious or even fatal.

Prevention involves elimination of predisposing situations: carefully inserting the cannula to avoid trauma, using upper extremity veins whenever possible and limiting use of leg veins to situations in which there are no alternative veins available. *Never* forcefully flush the cannula to restore flow.

When it does occur, pulmonary thromboembolism is manifested primarily by tachycardia and dyspnea; pleuritic chest pain and hemoptysis may also be present. If the embolism is massive, additional symptoms can include substernal chest pain, restlessness, hypotension and cyanosis (4). The occurrence of any of these signs and symptoms must be reported to the physician immediately.

Treatment depends on the extent of embolization. Anticoagulation with heparin is routinely performed. Oxygen, analgesics, and fluids and drugs to counteract hypotension and shock are administered as needed. Massive, life-threatening embolism may require emergency surgery (embolectomy). When thrombosis or thrombophlebitis is present at the infusion site, the cannula is removed as discussed above.

AIR EMBOLISM

An air embolism, though rare, represents one of the most serious hazards of intravenous therapy. While strict adherence to details in the insertion and maintenance of the intravenous line make its occurrence unlikely, if an air embolism occurs, the outcome can be rapidly fatal.

Air can enter the vascular system through several routes:

1. The greatest risk of air embolism occurs during insertion of a catheter into a central vein such as the subclavin. During inspiration, the pressure is lower in the central veins than in the peripheral veins. On inspiration, negative pressure can occur, which can draw air into the vascular system (23). The measures discussed in Chapter 4, including having the patient perform a Valsalva maneuver and covering the open end of the needle with a gloved finger until the catheter is inserted, are important to the prevention of air entry during catheter insertion (Fig. 7-3). Air can enter subsequently during changing of the administration tubing or accidental disconnection of the tubing. Grace reports two cases of air embolism due to disconnection of the tubing, each resulting in severe neurological damage (11).
2. Air bubbles can remain in the administration tubing due to inadequate priming or might enter later during administration of a drug or changing of the solution container. Small bubbles, though perhaps innocuous in themselves,

can aggregate to form large air pockets and can be carried into the bloodstream.

3. When a fluid container runs dry, the fluid in the tubing drops to the level of the right atrial (central venous) pressure. Should venous pressure drop below that in the tubing (which is more likely with central vein lines), air can be sucked into the vein.
4. The infusion of two bottles simultaneously via a Y-type administration set or using a piggyback setup with no back-check valve (see Chapter 8) enables introduction of air if the secondary container empties.
5. Using plastic fluid containers in series connections (connecting one bottle to a second at the level of the drip chamber) can enable the residual air (about 15 ml.) from the primary container to be drawn into the tubing before complete infusion of the fluid from the secondary container. As a result, all manufacturers of plastic containers warn against this practice.

Air entering the bloodstream is rapidly transported to the heart where it can cause a fatal airlock or be carried into the pulmonary artery where it can occlude the pulmonary capillaries and likewise result in cardiovascular collapse and death. The lethal volume of air is variable, but is believed to be between 5 and 15 milliliters per kilogram (12).

The primary focus, of course, must be directed toward prevention of air entry by attending to the situations described. Both insertion and maintenance of the intravenous line require attention toward preventing the introduction of air and prompt removal of any air that has gotten into the tubing. To remove any air, clean the lowest injection site with alcohol, pinch or clamp the tubing below the injection site, insert a sterile needle or needle and syringe, and aspirate the air.

When a central venous line is present, additional precautions against air embolism are required because of the added risk involved. All tubing connections, especially the junction between the tubing and cannula, should be securely taped to prevent disconnection. As further protection, the use of a micropore filter is recommended to trap any air passing through.

When air embolism does occur, it is evidenced by sudden onset of pallor, cyanosis, dyspnea, cough, and tachycardia, progressing to syncope

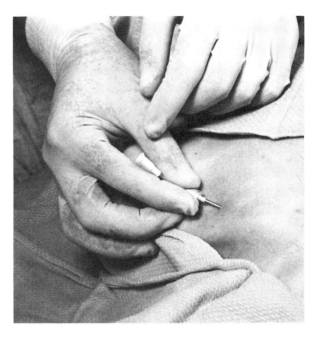

Fig. 7-3. As pictured, failure to cover the catheter hub prior to attachment of the administration tubing during subclavin venipuncture can result in an air embolism.

and shock (12). Unless treatment is instituted immediately, death can rapidly ensue. When these symptoms occur in a patient with an intravenous line, particularly if the container is found to be empty or if the administration set is disconnected, air embolism must be considered as a likely cause. When cardiopulmonary function is still intact, immediate treatment consists of placing the patient on his left side with the head and shoulders lowered. This is done to try to trap the air within the right atrium and prevent advancement into the pulmonary artery. Reconnecting the administration tubing and other measures to prevent entry of more air are of paramount importance. The physician is called immediately, and oxygen is administered. Cardiopulmonary resuscitation measures may be necessary. Definitive treatment by the physician consists of insertion of a cardiac needle (18 or 20 gauge, 3½ inches in length) into the right ventricle to aspirate the air (12). Additional nursing responsibilities consist of remaining with the patient to monitor vital signs and to provide continued psychological support. To enable the rapid institution of treatment, additional nursing personnel should prepare the equipment needed

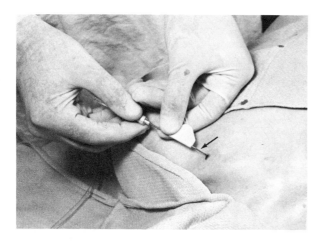

Fig. 7-4. Note the incorrect placement of the needle guard with exposure of the needle tip which can result in severing and embolization of the catheter.

to aspirate the air: intracardiac needle, sterile gloves, drapes, 4 inch by 4 inch gauze sponges, and iodophor solution.

CATHETER EMBOLISM

Reports of intravenous needle fragments and other foreign bodies embolizing and lodging within the venous system have been found in the literature since 1935 (6). With the introduction of the plastic intravenous catheter in 1945, another potential embolic hazard was created (19). The first report of a catheter embolism was in 1954 (31). Since then, as the use of plastic catheters became widespread, hundreds of additional cases have been reported. There are probably many cases occurring which are not reported, so the true incidence of morbidity and mortality is unknown (24).

Early cases of catheter embolism involved inlying catheters which consisted of segments of polyethylene tubing without any hub. A blunt needle was inserted into the end of the tubing and the administration tubing was connected to the needle hub (19). Although the catheter tubing was taped or sutured in place, it could separate from the needle and enter the bloodstream.

With the introduction of intravenous catheters with an attached hub, the problem of separation was eliminated; however, catheter emboli can occur by other means. Catheters introduced through a needle can be sheared off during insertion if an attempt is made to pull back the catheter while the needle is in the vein. Such a practice must

NEVER be done. Once the catheter has been inserted and the needle withdrawn, severing can occur if the needle guard has not been properly placed (Fig. 7-4). Severance and embolization of the catheter have been found to occur in association with emergency insertion of the catheter, particularly if the patient is uncooperative.

Once a catheter fragment has entered the bloodstream, it can lodge anywhere in the venous circulation proximal to the site of origin. The majority of fragments eventually reach the pulmonary artery; others remain in the vena cava, right atrium or right ventricle. Some lodge in a peripheral vein while a few eventually reach the lung periphery (24).

The consequences of catheter embolism vary from minor or no complications to death. Among the nonfatal complications reported are thrombosis, endocarditis, perforation of the ventricle and cardiac arrhythmias. Of course, these complications may be fatal in and of themselves. While the reported mortality rate varies widely among investigators, it has been considerably higher when removal of a fragment was not or could not be attempted. Of 202 cases reviewed by Richardson, the mortality rate for catheter emboli not removed was 24 percent (24). No deaths were reported among patients in whom the catheter fragment was removed. Causes of death included perforation of the heart or great vessels, arrhythmias, endocarditis, pulmonary thrombosis or embolus, and sepsis. The highest incidence of death is associated with fragments embolizing to the right ventricle and pulmonary arteries (24).

Although the occurrence of catheter embolism is quite low in view of the overall frequency of intravenous therapy, its potential for fatal outcome makes prevention imperative. The primary preventive measure is adherence to correct technique during insertion of long intravenous catheters. Ideally, such catheters should be of the type which is encompassed by a short introducer catheter, so that shearing cannot occur during insertion, and since the needle is completely removed from the system, subsequent severing is likewise avoided.

This type of catheter is of particular value in restless or uncooperative patients or in emergency situations when the catheter must be inserted rapidly. When it becomes necessary to utilize a through-the-needle catheter, it is very important that once the catheter has been advanced through the needle, it must NEVER be pulled back. After the needle has been withdrawn from the skin, if it is to remain on the system, the rigid needle guard *must* be properly placed over the tip of the needle. A final security precaution involves using only catheters which are radiopaque, so that if severing and embolization occur, the fragment can be readily located by fluoroscopy or x-ray. These measures are discussed in greater detail in Chapter 4.

Catheter embolization is sometimes readily apparent at the time of placement or removal of the catheter due to absence of a portion of the catheter. In some patients, the embolization is evidenced by signs and symptoms relating to where the fragment has lodged, particularly if it gives rise to a catastrophic complication. Its presence within the heart can produce arrhythmias ranging from minor (isolated premature ventricular contractions, or PVCs) to lethal (ventricular tachycardia and fibrillation). If the fragment punctures the myocardium, signs of cardiac tamponade (leakage of blood from the heart into the pericardial sac causing compression of the heart) may be seen. Embolization to the lung can produce the same symptoms as with a pulmonary thromboembolism.

Other patients remain asymptomatic, and catheter embolism may not be suspected unless signs of later complications occur, such as sepsis, endocarditis, hemorrhage, or thrombosis. In the absence of any secondary complications, the presence of an embolized catheter fragment can remain undetected for years.

If the nurse discovers a severed catheter fragment which can be seen or palpated within a peripheral vein, the following steps should be taken:

1. Lightly apply a tourniquet or an inflated blood pressure cuff in an attempt to prevent further migration of the fragment.
2. Notify the physician immediately.
3. Monitor vital signs, including pulse, respirations and blood pressure, observing particularly for cardiac arrhythmias, respiratory distress or a sudden drop in blood pressure.
4. Prepare the patient to be x-rayed or fluoroscoped for visualization of the catheter fragment.
5. Provide the patient with psychological support and explanation of any required treatment measures.

Because of the potential complications associated with catheter fragments, most clinicians advise their removal, particularly if the fragment has lodged in the right ventricle or pulmonary artery. Prior to 1964, removal of catheters and other foreign bodies involved a surgical procedure: either a cutdown with or without forceps retrieval if lodged in a peripheral vessel, or thoracotomy if the embolus had migrated to a central vein or the heart. In 1964, Thomas reported a percutaneous technique using bronchoscopic forceps to retrieve a broken guide wire from the inferior vena cava (28). In 1967 the first successful percutaneous removal of a catheter fragment from the right atrium and ventricle was achieved by Massumi using a snare (16). Since that time a variety of devices has been employed, including the Fogarty balloon catheter (17), endoscopic forceps (25), gastric biopsy catheter (2), myocardial biopsy catheter (3) and biliary stone basket (1).

The use of snares and other flexible instruments has been shown to be a safe and generally successful means of removing catheter emboli, in most instances requiring only local anesthesia. In situations in which these techniques are unsuccessful, a major surgical procedure such as thoracotomy may be required, but it can often be done without need for cardiopulmonary bypass. However, because of the risk associated with such a major operative procedure, some investigators maintain that patients who are seriously ill from other causes can be managed conservatively by observation, without need for removal of the catheter fragment (24).

COMPLICATIONS ASSOCIATED WITH INTRAVENOUS DRUG THERAPY

The administration of drugs is, in itself, associated with several potential complications. An individual may experience an unpredictable response to a drug, known as an idiosyncratic reaction. Another type of complication known as toxicity results from the administration of a dose that exceeds the therapeutic dose. It can also occur when the dose given is within the normal therapeutic range, but exceeds the individual's ability to metabolize or excrete it, as, for example, in hepatic or renal impairment. Hypersensitivity or allergic reactions represent the most frequently occurring drug-associated complications, and can produce a serious or even fatal outcome.

Drug incompatibilities, particularly therapeutic incompatibilities, can be regarded as a type of complication. These occur when two or more drugs given concurrently result in an undesirable pharmacologic response in the patient. These complications are discussed in detail in Chapter 8.

REFERENCES

1. Aldridge, Harold E., and Lee, Janet: Transvascular Removal of Catheter Fragments from the Great Vessels and Heart. *Canadian Medical Association Journal*, 117(11): 1300–1304, December 3, 1977.

2. Banks, Tazewell, and Yeoh, Hock H.: Removal of Embolized Catheter from the Heart. *Postgraduate Medicine*, 51:116–118, April 1972.

3. Bashour, Tali T., Banks, Tazewell, and Cheng, Tsung O.: Retrieval of Lost Catheters by a Myocardial Biopsy Catheter Device. *Chest*, 66(4):395-6, October 1974.

4. Beeson, Paul, and McDermott, Walsh (editors): *Textbook of Medicine* (14th ed.), Philadelphia: W. B. Saunders Company, 1975.

5. Buxton, Alfred E., Highsmith, Anita K., Garner, Julia S., West, C. Michael, Anderson, Roger L., and McGowan, John E., Jr.: Contamination of Intravenous Fluid: Effects of Changing Administration Sets. Paper presented at Seventeenth Interscience Conference on Antimicrobial Agents and Chemotherapy, New York City: October 12–14, 1977.

6. Fair, George L., Foreign Body in the Heart: Report of a Case with Retention of a Large Needle with Recovery. *New York State Journal of Medicine*, 35:453, 1935.

7. Ferguson, Robert L., Rosett, Walter, Hodges, Glenn R., Barnes, William G.: Complications with Heparin Lock Needles. *Annals of Internal Medicine*, 85:583–586, 1976.

8. Geiger, Elizabeth M., and Jansen, George A.: Complications Associated with the Use of Plastic Catheters. *American Journal of I.V. Therapy*, 3:42–44, 46, October/November 1976.

9. Goldmann, Donald A.: Improving Infection Control in IV Therapy. *American Journal of I.V. Therapy*, 4:27–28; 31–32; 37, February/March 1977.

10. Goldmann, Donald A., Maki, Dennis G., Rhame, Frank S., Kaiser, Allen B., Tenney, James H., and Bennett, John V.: Guidelines for Infection Control in Intravenous Therapy. *Annals of Internal Medicine*, 79:848–850, 1973.

11. Grace, D. M.: Air Embolism with Neurologic Complications: A Potential Hazard of Central Venous Catheters. *Canadian Journal of Surgery*, 20:51–53, January 1977.

12. Hurst, J. Willis, Logue, R. Bruce, Schlant, Robert C., and Wenger, Nanette Kass: *The Heart* (4th ed.), New York: McGraw-Hill Book Company, 1978.

13. Maki, Dennis G.: Preventing Infection in Intravenous Therapy. *Hospital Practice*, 11:95–104, April 1976.

14. Maki, Dennis G., Drinka, Paul J., and Davis, Thomas E.: Suppurative Phlebitis of an Arm Vein from a "Scalp-Vein Needle." *New England Journal of Medicine*, 292:1116–1117, May 22, 1975.

15. Maki, Dennis G., Goldmann, Donald A., and Rhame, Frank S.: Infection Control in Intravenous Therapy. *Annals of Internal Medicine*, 79:867–887, 1973.

16. Massumi, R. A., and Ross, A. M.: Atraumatic Nonsurgical Technic for Removal of Broken Catheters from Cardiac Cavities, *New England Journal of Medicine*, 277(4):195–196, July 27, 1967.

17. Mathur, A. P., Pochaczevsky, R., Levowitz, B. S., and Feraru, F.: Fogarty Balloon Catheter for Removal of Catheter Fragment in Subclavian Vein. *Journal of the American Medical Association*, 217(4):481 (Letter), July 26, 1971.

18. McGowan, John E.: Six Guidelines for Reducing Infections Associated with Intravenous Therapy. *American Surgeon*, 42(9):713–715, September 1976.

19. Meyers, Lawrence: Intravenous Catheterization. *American Journal of Nursing*, 45(11):930–931, November 1945.

20. Mukherjee, G. D., and Guharay, B. N.: Digital Gangrene and Skin Necrosis Following Extravasation of Infusion Fluid. *Journal of the Indian Medical Association*, 68(4):77–79, February 16, 1977.

21. Nejad, M. S., Klaper, M. A., Steggerda, F. R., and Gianturco, C.: Clotting on the Outer Surfaces of Vascular Catheters. *Radiology*, 91:248–250, August 1968.

22. O'Brien, Thomas E., Ashford, Thomas P., Vetter, Thomas G., Wilson, Mary Jane, and Schilling, Barbara A.: Phlebitis from IV Therapy: Prospective Study of an In-line Filter. *Hospital Formulary*, 12:315, 319–320, May 1977.

23. Plumer, Ada Lawrence: *Principles and Practice of Intravenous Therapy* (2nd ed.), Boston: Little, Brown and Company, 1975.

24. Richardson, J. David, Grover, Frederick L., and Trinkle, J. Kent: Intravenous Catheter Emboli. *American Journal of Surgery*, 128(6):722–727, December 1974.

25. Smyth, Nicholas P. D., Boivin, Michael R., and Bacos, James M.: Transjugular Removal of Foreign Body from the Right Atrium by Endoscopic Forceps. *Journal of Thoracic and Cardiovascular Surgery*, 55(4):594–597, April 1968.

26. Stein, John M., and Pruitt, Basil A. Jr.: Suppurative Thrombophlebitis: A Lethal Iatrogenic Disease. *New England Journal of Medicine,* 282(26):1452–1455, June 25, 1970.

27. Thomas, Edward T., Evers William, and Racz, Gabor B.: Postinfusion Phlebitis. *Anesthesia and Analgesia,* 49(1):150–159, January-February 1970.

28. Thomas, John, Sinclair-Smith, Bruce, Bloomfield, Dennis, and Davachi, Asghar: Nonsurgical Retrieval of a Broken Segment of Steel Spring Guide from the Right Atrium and Inferior Vena Cava. *Circulation,* 30:106–108, July 1964.

29. Thorn, George, Adams, Raymond, Braunwald, Eugene, Isselbacher, Kurt, and Petersdorf, Robert (editors): *Harrison's Principles of Internal Medicine* (8th ed.), New York: McGraw-Hill Book Company, 1977.

30. Turco, Salvatore, and King, Robert E.: *Sterile Dosage Forms—Their Preparation and Clinical Application,* Philadelphia: Lea and Febiger, 1974.

31. Turner, David D., and Sommers, Sheldon C.: Accidental Passage of a Polyethylene Catheter from Cubital Vein to Right Atrium. *New England Journal of Medicine:* 251(18):744–745, October 28, 1954.

32. Yosowitz, Philip, Ekland, David A., Shaw, Richard C., and Parsons, Robert W.: Peripheral Intravenous Infiltration Necrosis. *Annals of Surgery,* 182:553–556, November 1975.

33. Zinner, Michael J., Zuidema, George D., and Lowery, Brian D.: Septic Nonsuppurative Thrombophlebitis. *Archives of Surgery,* 111:122–125, February 1976.

8 Principles of Intravenous Drug Administration

Apart from the complications associated with the insertion and maintenance of the intravenous line, the actual intravenous administration of drugs is fraught with numerous potential hazards. To achieve the maximal therapeutic benefit with minimal hazards, the nurse must be familiar with the basic principles of drug action as well as specific considerations associated with the intravenous route. This chapter will also include adverse reactions, including drug allergies, the objectives and techniques of preparation, and the administration of drugs intravenously.

USES OF DRUGS

Drugs in general are given for three reasons: diagnostic, prophylactic, and therapeutic (17). Drugs administered intravenously also fall within these three categories.

Diagnostic agents include those used to assess the function of certain organs or organ systems. Among these are such drugs as sulfobromophthalein, which tests liver function; corticotropin, which is used to assess pituitary function; and so-dium dehydrocholate (Decholin), which is used to determine circulation time. Other agents are used to aide in the diagnosis of specific diseases. Edrophonium chloride (Tensilon) is used to diagnose myasthenia gravis; histamine is used in the diagnosis of pheochromocytoma.

Drugs intended primarily for prophylactic use are generally those used to prevent communicable diseases. These vaccines are not given by the intravenous route. Antibiotics may also be used to prevent infections such as streptococcal infections in susceptible persons. An example is the administration of antibiotics to patients with cardiac valvular lesions prior to dental or genitourinary procedures. However, in these cases the drugs are usually given either orally or intramuscularly. There are a few instances, though, in which intravenous drugs normally used therapeutically are given for prophylactic reasons. In the immediate period following occurrence of a myocardial infarction, a patient may be given lidocaine to prevent ectopic beats even though the cardiac rhythm is normal at that time. Some clinicians add intravenous heparin to infusion bottles in low doses for patients on long-term intravenous therapy to decrease the likelihood of postinfusion phlebitis.

The vast majority of drugs given by the intravenous route are used for therapeutic purposes. The effect may be curative, as in the case of antibiotics, or merely palliative, relieving symptoms or reducing the severity of the condition, such as analgesics or chemotherapeutic agents for advanced cancer. Some drugs serve a supportive role, sustaining the patient while other types of therapy are employed. They may temporarily alter normal processes. Anesthetics and anticoagulants are examples. Replacement therapy, which represents a substitutive function, involves administration of substances such as vitamins, insulin, and electrolytes, which are normally in the body but may be depleted or absent in certain disease states (17).

COURSE OF DRUGS WITHIN THE BODY

To understand why the intravenous route is not only preferable but in certain instances mandatory for some drugs, it is necessary to discuss the course of drug action within the body. The five stages of drug activity include: administration, distribution, drug interaction with the target cell, metabolism, and excretion (27).

Administration

A drug can enter the body through one of many routes, the most common being the oral and parenteral routes. Oral administration requires that the drug survive exposure to gastrointestinal contents and finally be absorbed into the circulation before reaching its site of action. Many drugs are unsuitable for the oral route, since some are inactivated by gastric secretions; others are highly irritating to the gastrointestinal tract; while still others are poorly absorbed from the intestines. Those that are ultimately absorbed into the circulation may require a considerable amount of time for the total process.

Parenteral routes include subcutaneous, intramuscular, and intravenous. The *subcutaneous* route involves injection of drugs into the tissue underlying the skin. While absorption is generally faster than with the oral route, care must be taken to avoid injection of very large volumes or irritating substances which can result in tissue damage (27).

Intramuscular injection is that route in which the medication is injected within a muscle. Absorption is quite rapid when the drug is in solution, while delayed absorption occurs when it is in a suspension. Some drugs, including phenytoin (Dilantin), diazepam (Valium), and tetracycline, are absorbed more slowly by this route than orally due to a relative insolubility in water. Many drugs can be given by this route with a minimum of discomfort; injections of some drugs, such as cephalosporins, are quite painful, particularly when repeated doses are required. Care must be taken to avoid inadvertent puncture of a nerve or entry into a vein.

Like the others, the *intravenous* route offers both advantages and disadvantages. The major advantages include (44):

1. Administration directly into a vein insures almost immediate and total absorption and rapid delivery to the site of action. The therapeutic effects begin almost immediately. This is essential for drugs which must be given in life-threatening situations.
2. Because the total dose is absorbed, precise dosage calculation and flow rates can be achieved. The dose can be titrated to sustain continuous control of the therapeutic response (15). Should an adverse reaction occur during administration, the remainder of the dose can be instantly discontinued.
3. Pain and irritation to the tissues, which can accompany intramuscular and subcutaneous administration, can usually be avoided by the intravenous route if the proper concentration and flow rate are used and the vein selected is large enough to permit adequate dilution.
4. The intravenous route is often selected as an alternative means of delivery of both drugs and fluids to individuals who cannot tolerate them orally. It is also used for drugs which are highly irritating to the gastrointestinal tract or are inactivated by gastric secretions.

Disadvantages of the intravenous route include (27):

1. Once a medication has been given, it cannot be recalled. Since untoward reactions can occur with the same rapidity as the desired response, unexpected effects can be serious and sometimes fatal.

2. Intravenous drug administration presents the risk of additional complications, particularly infection. Aseptic techniques must be faithfully adhered to.

3. Venipuncture requires considerable degree of skill, which limits the group of nurses and other health professionals who can perform it. Even when the medication is to be given into an established intravenous line, limitations on specific drugs, modes of administration, etc. are often established by state laws and institutional policies.

4. Even when performed skillfully, intravenous cannula insertion and drug administration are not without some discomfort. Depending on the patient's age, past experiences, and psychological status, it can be a source of emotional trauma.

Distribution

After being administered, the drug must be delivered to the site of action. As with absorption, distribution times vary due to route of administration and other factors, including protein binding and the blood-brain barrier (22). Drugs given intravenously reach their destination much more rapidly, usually within a few minutes. However, distribution time is also dependent on the circulatory status of the individual. For example, in states of shock, impaired blood flow prevents medications from being delivered as rapidly as desirable; and in cardiac arrest, distribution of life-saving drugs is dependent on the effectiveness of cardiopulmonary resuscitation in maintaining a satisfactory blood flow.

Drug interaction with target cells

Once a drug has been delivered to the site of action, it acts biochemically to produce the desired response. Although all modes of action are not completely understood, it is believed that three general mechanisms operate: drug-receptor interaction, enzymatic effects, and a general action at the cell membrane.

Some drugs interact with the target cells at specific receptor sites (Fig. 8-1). The drug receptors are believed to be molecular-sized structures, most likely making up part of the lipoprotein structure of the cell membrane (37). Somewhat like pieces of a puzzle, the drug and target cell interlock at the receptor sites of the target cell, resulting in some alteration of function of the target cell, thus producing the drug's effect. Drugs such as epinephrine and histamine are believed to act in this way.

Another mechanism of action involves the activation or inhibition of enzymes. Theophylline is thought to inhibit the activity of certain enzyme systems. Some drugs may act as coenzymes, catalyzing or facilitating other reactions (22). Vitamins are one group of drugs believed to be coenzymes.

A third mechanism is a general action on the cell membrane without involvement of receptor sites or enzymes. General anesthetics are believed to act in this manner.

Metabolism

Having produced the desired effects, the drug is metabolized, undergoing chemical alteration or biotransformation, which usually renders it less active or inactive. Some drugs may undergo transformation, which changes them to other pharmacologically active compounds, while others are conjugated, a process which renders them more water-soluble (37). This increased solubility allows certain drugs to be excreted through the kidneys, thus preventing their accumulation and subsequent overdosage or toxicity. Some drugs, particularly those that are strong acids or bases, do not require metabolism to any significant degree (15). Others must be metabolized before they can exert their therapeutic action.

Metabolism is generally accomplished by the liver, through the activation or inhibition of liver microsomal enzymes. Some metabolic transformation is also done by the kidneys, plasma, and intestinal mucosa, likewise through the utilization of enzymes. This must be considered in prescribing drugs to infants and young children, since the degree of maturation of these organ systems will determine the extent to which the drugs will be metabolized. In neonates and premature infants in particular, these enzyme systems are likely to be undeveloped.

Excretion

Eventually, the drug itself, if unaltered, or its metabolic products are excreted from the body. The kidney is the primary organ of excretion, particularly for drugs given intravenously. After being filtered through the glomeruli, part of the drug may be reabsorbed by the tubules. The amount actually excreted is in part affected by the degree of acidity or alkalinity of the urine. Drugs such as gaseous anesthetics are removed from the body by way of the lungs while others are excreted through the gastrointestinal tract in the bile or feces.

RANGE OF RESPONSE

A drug is given with the expectation of achieving a specific response; but, depending on the dose given and other factors, the response may not be therapeutic. Three levels of response are possible.

Ineffective response

If less than the minimum required dose is given or if factors such as competitive antagonism by another drug interfere with its action on the target cells, an ineffective level of response is seen and the desired effect, such as relief of pain or control of a microbial infection, will not occur.

Therapeutic response

With a therapeutic response, the desired effects are produced. For most drugs there is generally a range of doses and blood levels which produce the therapeutic effect. The time required to achieve the therapeutic effect is also variable. With some medications, such as succinylcholine and other muscle relaxants used in surgery, the therapeutic effect is almost instantaneous. With other drugs, including antibiotics, even though they are administered intravenously, the therapeutic response is not seen until adequate blood levels have been reached and maintained for a given period of time. It is essential for the nurse to have some knowledge of the time frame in which a therapeutic response is expected so that the patient can be monitored to determine whether the drug has been effective. To maintain the therapeutic response, the dose administered within a given period of time must not exceed the rate at which it is metabolized and excreted.

Toxic response

Should metabolism and/or excretion be impaired (as occurs in certain types of liver and renal disease) or if an overdose is given, the drug will accumulate in the body, ultimately producing a toxic response. Toxicity may be manifested either by an

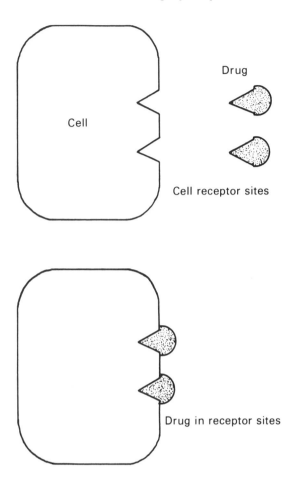

Fig. 8–1. The interaction of a drug with a cell at cell receptor sites. The drug's effect is seen after the interaction.

exaggeration of the usual pharmacologic actions of the drug or by signs and symptoms specific for that drug or class of drugs. Some drugs produce gastrointestinal symptoms such as nausea, vomiting, or diarrhea, while others may cause cardiac arrhythmias or blocks. The drug information section in this book presents signs of toxicity for each drug. When administering drugs intravenously, the nurse should be alert for any of these signs. She should slow down or discontinue the drug if it is being given by continuous infusion, and report the problem to the physician immediately.

The most extreme toxic response, which can occur if a drug is given at a dose or rate far exceeding that recommended, is the *lethal response.* Potassium chloride is a good example of this. If given too rapidly or if administered undiluted as a bolus, it will be fatal.

FACTORS AFFECTING RESPONSE AND THEREFORE DOSAGE GIVEN

Although it is not a nursing responsibility to calculate drug dosage, the nurse must be familiar with the factors involved in determining dosage. While each drug has a minimum and maximum recommended therapeutic dose, the specific dosage required to produce the desired effect in an individual is affected by several factors:

1. Size of the individual
2. Age
3. Sex
4. Genetic factors
5. Presence of other disease processes
6. Route of drug administration
7. Interaction with other drugs given concurrently

Size of the individual

Since the final concentration of a drug in the body is dependent on body mass, a drug dose which is within the therapeutic range for the "average" 70-kilogram (150-pound) adult may be ineffective for a very obese person. Similarly, that dose might be toxic for very lean individuals and lethal for infants and children. In most instances, the adult dosage may be determined according to the kilogram or poundweight of the individual. However, weight alone is not reflective of body mass; so in some instances and, particularly in infants and children, surface area should be used instead of weight to calculate dosage. Surface area can be rapidly calculated by using a standard nomogram (see pp. 543–544, Appendix). (More specific information regarding the determination of drug dosage in infants and children is presented along with other pediatric considerations in Chapter 6.)

Age

Along with body size, age is a determinant of the dose required. There is no doubt that children are more sensitive to drugs than are adults, and thus they require an altered dose. Some methods of calculating pediatric dosages on the basis of age rather than weight, such as Fried's Rule and Young's Rule, have been utilized. However, due to the complexity of factors involved with infants and children, the use of body mass as reflected by surface area is currently recommended as the primary basis for dosage determi-nation. Age should be used as a guideline rather than an absolute determinant of dosage.

Likewise, elderly individuals may require a smaller dosage than young adults. This is most likely due to declining physiological function associated with the aging process.

Sex

Perhaps due to differences in body size and proportion, women are often more susceptible to the actions of some drugs than are men (21). During pregnancy, special consideration must be given to altering doses as recommended by the manufacturer and, whenever possible, to avoid giving drugs unless absolutely necessary, in order to avoid harm to the fetus.

Genetic factors

The response to some drugs, including occurrence of adverse reactions, is influenced by genetic factors. This is felt to be due to genetically determined enzyme activity which affects the body's ability to metabolize the drug (21). Delayed or incomplete metabolism will result in an idiosyncratic response. Since identification of such individuals is essential prior to giving the drug, the physician must consider genetic factors associated with various ethnic and racial groups when determining drug dosage.

Presence of disease processes

Drug dosage will need to be altered when certain disease states are present. As mentioned above, hepatic and renal impairment interferes with the normal metabolism and excretion of many drugs, thus necessitating a lower dosage. The presence of other pathological conditions alters an individual's sensitivity to the effects of a particular drug. A hyperthyroid state makes a person more sensitive to some substances, such as epinephrine; while an asthmatic condition makes an individual hypersensitive to the vasoconstrictor effect of histamine (22). For drugs which require a modified dosage in the presence of renal impairment or other disease, the recommended schedule is included in the drug information section in the back of this book.

Route of administration

The magnitude of response evoked by a drug will be limited by how much is absorbed into the circulatory system and thus distributed to the appropriate sites of action. As mentioned, many oral drugs are only partially absorbed; and with drugs given by the subcutaneous or intramuscular route, absorption rates vary. Absorption decreases in the presence of shock; so if an increased dosage is given at that time, toxic effects can occur later if there is a sudden improvement in the circulatory status.

Since drugs administered intravenously go directly into the circulation, they do not require absorption. As a result, a higher serum level is reached more rapidly, and thus the dosage required is frequently less than with other routes. In some instances the same amount of drug is given but is infused over a specific time interval rather than being given in one discrete dose.

Interaction with other drugs given concurrently

While the dose of a given drug may produce a response within the therapeutic range when it is given alone, the addition of other drugs to the treatment regimen can markedly alter its effects. Drug interactions can be due to interference with any phase of the drug cycle: absorption, particularly from the gastrointestinal tract; distribution; action at the cellular level; metabolism; or excretion. The action of the drug may be intensified or reduced, or other untoward effects can occur.

The two primary types of drug interaction include antagonism and synergism. *Antagonism* is the inhibition of a drug's action by another drug (22). *Synergism* refers to an interaction in which the combined effect of the two drugs is greater than that of either one alone (21). When the combined effect equals the sum of the effects of both drugs, it is sometimes referred to as a *summation* or an additive effect. Two drugs exhibit *potentiation* when their combined effects exceed the sum of their separate actions. One mechanism by which potentiation is believed to occur is through the inhibition of the destruction of one drug by the other (22).

These interactions can occur when the drugs are given concurrently but separately; that is, not as an admixture. Adjustment of both dosage and time of administration can help to achieve the desired therapeutic response while minimizing untoward effects. Additional problems are presented, however, when drugs are administered simultane-

ously as admixtures or are injected in rapid succession into the same intravenous line. This not only presents the potential for untoward therapeutic effects but also creates the risk of physical and chemical incompatibilities. These problems are discussed later in this chapter.

UNTOWARD DRUG RESPONSES

Even when great care is given to prescribe the dose of a drug based on the parameters discussed above, untoward effects, that is, effects which are unexpected and undesired, can occur due to various factors within an individual. These should be distinguished from side effects which, though therapeutically undesirable, are a consequence of the drug's normal action (37), such as loss of potassium from the body when certain diuretics are given and dryness of the mouth associated with atropine.

Untoward responses can occur regardless of the route of administration but are potentially more hazardous when the drug is given intravenously because of the immediacy of response. Untoward responses can be either quantitative or qualitative.

Quantitative responses

TOLERANCE

Tolerance refers to the need for increasing amounts of a drug to produce the same therapeutic response (22). Tolerance develops after a drug has been given repeatedly over a period of time. Though the specific mechanism is not well understood, some investigators maintain that increased production of enzymes involved with metabolism of the drug, or changes within the tissues themselves, are responsible.

Once tolerance to one drug has developed, cross-tolerance can occur when a chemically related drug is administered. An increased dose of that second drug is needed to achieve the desired effect.

TACHYPHYLAXIS

Tachyphylaxis is rapidly developing tolerance to a drug occurring after very few doses have been given. Since it tends to be associated with drugs having a relatively long duration of action, one theory suggests that the first dose is still active at the receptor sites of the target cells; and when the second dose is given, it is unable to gain access to the receptor sites, thus having little or no effect (22).

CUMULATION

Cumulation is the administration of a drug at a faster rate than it can be metabolized and excreted. Thus, with each dose given, more of the drug accumulates; and if administration is continued, toxic effects will result. This must be taken into consideration by the physician when drug dosage is determined. Dosage is frequently based on daily requirements. However, the total metabolism-excretion time for some drugs is greater than 24 hours, and the normal metabolism-excretion time may be prolonged in an individual due to hepatic or renal disease. Examples are digitalis preparations and gentamicin in patients with renal impairments. In these instances, either the dose or the frequency of administration must be adjusted. It is important to remember that drugs with a normally short metabolism-excretion time may also require dosage adjustment in the presence of renal or hepatic impairment. Lidocaine, administered by intravenous drip, is an example.

INTOLERANCE

Intolerance refers to a response which is greater than normal, due to the lowering of the threshold to normal pharmacologic action (37). It is sometimes referred to as hypersusceptibility and requires that a lower than normal dose be given.

Qualitative responses

Qualitative responses are those which are different in type rather than magnitude from the expected effects.

IDIOSYNCRASY

Definitions vary, but idiosyncrasy generally refers to an unpredictable reaction or symptoms which are different in quality from the expected response and which are not due to an allergic reaction. Evidence suggests that such reactions result from an enzyme deficiency interfering with the normal metabolism of the drug. While this is sometimes an individual response, it is believed to be a genetic deficiency of a familial or racial nature. A classic example of this is seen in individuals whose red blood cells lack an enzyme known as glucose 6-phosphate dehydrogenase

(G6PD). When certain drugs such as primaquine are administered to them, a hemolytic anemia results (37).

TOXICITY

As previously mentioned, toxicity refers to adverse effects which result directly from a pharmacologic action of a drug (22). They are generally dose-related, occurring when the dose given exceeds the therapeutic level. Because of a biological variation, which include the above-mentioned factors affecting an individual's response to a drug, toxicity can occur unexpectedly in some persons with therapeutic doses. Digitalis preparations and the aminoglycoside antibiotics (gentamicin, tobramycin, amikacin, etc.) are examples of drugs to which toxicity can occur unless the dosage is altered under certain circumstances. Refer to the toxic effects and modified dosage for specific drugs in part two of this text.

DRUG ALLERGY

Drug allergy is not the most frequent type of adverse reaction, but it is often responsible for some of the most serious and occasionally fatal outcomes. Also referred to as hypersensitivity, drug allergy is a response resulting from an antigen-antibody reaction or cell-mediated immunity. This is a mechanism of the body's immunological system in which the drug or its metabolite, bound to tissue protein, acts as the antigen. Exposure to the drug stimulates the person's immune system to form antibodies. Once the antibodies are present, the individual is said to be sensitized; and on subsequent exposure to the drug, an allergic response is evoked.

Four possible mechanisms have been described, each of which represents different types of allergic responses (11):

TYPE I. The *anaphylactic* or *immediate* type involves a reaction between the antigen and antibodies that are bound to cells. Ultimately, certain chemicals such as histamine are released which act on target organs and tissues, giving rise to the allergic symptoms. The most serious type of reaction in this category is anaphylactic shock, in which symptoms may appear within a few minutes of drug administration. Initial symptoms may include dyspnea, tightness in the chest, pruritus, or nausea and vomiting (41). Classic signs include urticaria (hives), bronchospasm, laryngeal edema, hypotension, and finally shock and circulatory collapse. Unless treatment is initiated immediately, death rapidly ensues. Measures for prevention and treatment of anaphylactic shock are discussed below.

TYPE II. The *cytotoxic* or *cytolytic* type is also called autoimmunity. The antigen-antibody reaction occurs on the cell surface, resulting in cell destruction (37). This mechanism is the one responsible for hemolytic anemia of an allergic basis and other blood cell destruction (decreased platelets, decreased granulocytes, etc.) as well as possible damage to individual organs. Cytotoxic reactions can be induced by such drugs as penicillin, cephalothin, quinidine, chloramphenicol, and the sulfonamides.

TYPE III. The *Arthus* type produces the systemic reaction known as serum sickness, in which antigen-antibody complexes form microprecipitates and circulate in the serum (36). Symptoms, which can be either accelerated or late, range from fever, urticaria, and arthralgia to lymphadenopathy, edema, and neuritis. Serum sickness has been reported from penicillins, sulfonamides, and phenytoin among others (41).

TYPE IV. The *delayed* type is cell-mediated immunity due to lymphocytes which have been sensitized. Contact dermatitis is believed to be due to this type of mechanism; however, this mechanism is responsible for producing other types of allergic responses as well (32).

Drug allergy can produce several clinical manifestations besides the ones discussed above. The most frequent include:

Skin reactions, which are probably the most common type of allergic symptom. Nearly every known type of skin eruption can be produced by drug allergy, ranging from a mild rash or urticaria to potentially lethal exfoliative dermatitis (41).

Fever, which can occur in association with skin reactions or other symptoms or can be an isolated symptom. In drug fever the temperature can rise suddenly, sometimes as high as 105°F (40.6°C) (32).

Hematologic changes, which can include other manifestations in addition to the blood dyscrasias discussed under the cytotoxic mechanism. While a decrease in such blood components as erythrocytes (red cells), platelets, and leukocytes (white cells) can be serious, they generally resolve when the drug is withheld and/or treatment is instituted. However, occasionally bone marrow involvement occurs, resulting in hypoplastic or aplastic anemia, in which the bone marrow is unable to produce adequate number of blood cells. As many as 50 percent of patients with the complication may fail to respond to treatment, with death ultimately resulting. While a relatively infrequent occurrence, it has been seen in association with chloramphenicol and rarely with sulfonamides and tetracyclines (26).

Nursing implications

Virtually any drug has the potential for evoking an allergic response, though some are more frequently associated with systemic reactions and anaphylaxis, even though the overall incidence is relatively low. Among the drugs which can elicit an anaphylactic reaction are penicillin and its synthetic derivatives such as ampicillin; the cephalosporins, such as cephalothin (Keflin); phenytoin (Dilantin); and diagnostic agents, including sulfobromophthalein (BSP), dehydrocholate sodium (Decholin), and iodine-containing contrast media (41). If a person is allergic to one drug, he may be allergic to drugs that are chemically similar. This is known as cross-reactivity or cross-allergenicity. Drug allergies are more likely to occur in adults than in children (41).

One factor influencing the likelihood and speed of onset of an allergic reaction is the route of administration. Serious reactions, including anaphylaxis, are more frequent in parenterally administered, especially intravenous, drugs. Because of the immediate and total absorption and higher concentrations, such reactions occur almost immediately (32). Thus the nurse who is responsible for administering intravenous medications must be able to:

1. Identify patients who are most susceptible to drug allergy
2. Institute appropriate preventive measures
3. Monitor for signs of allergic reaction when administering an intravenous drug
4. Initiate and assist in treatment of allergic reactions that occur

IDENTIFICATION OF SUSCEPTIBLE PATIENTS

All patients should be questioned as to a past history of allergies, both on admission to the hospital and when intravenous drug therapy is initiated. While this information is sought primarily by the physician, the nurse can also play a key role in identifying a history of allergy when obtaining the admission assessment or nursing history. The patient should also be questioned about food or other allergies, such as hay fever or asthma, or symptoms such as urticaria as well as a family history of allergies. Persons with a personal or family history of allergy are more likely to develop allergies to drugs (41).

In infants less than three months old, the mother's allergic history should be obtained, since antibodies can be present in the infant (35).

If a patient states that he is allergic to a drug or drugs, he should be questioned further to determine the type of allergic symptoms which occurred. Some individuals consider any type of reaction, such as pain at an injection site, faintness, or an upset stomach when taking aspirin, to be an allergy. Any questionable allergy should be evaluated further by the physician.

When a patient is too ill or otherwise unable to give a history, the information should be sought from family members and past medical records. With comatose or confused patients, the nurse should check for the presence of a medical identification tag or card.

INSTITUTION OF PREVENTIVE MEASURES

If an allergy is confirmed, certain precautions should be taken:

1. Clearly mark the front of the patient's chart, specifying the drug to which he is allergic. Special eyecatching tape is available for this purpose. The allergy should also be recorded on the nursing care plan and either on the problem list (if the problem-oriented method of charting is employed) or elsewhere in the chart (such as history or progress notes) for a permanent record. Some institutions also find it helpful to record allergies on the medication record as an additional safeguard.
2. If a new allergy has been identified, be sure that the patient (or with a child, the family) is informed of the allergy and is advised or assisted in ordering a medical identification tag.
3. Be aware of related drugs that can produce cross-reactions. An individual who is allergic to penicillin may be allergic to ampicillin or other semi-synthetic penicillins, such as carbenicillin, or to the cephalosporins. Cross-reactivity can also occur among the aminoglycosides (genta-

micin, kanamycin, amikacin, etc.). A person who is allergic to one of them may also develop an allergic response to others (41).

Persons with multiple drug allergies may also be more likely to develop allergic responses to even chemically unrelated drugs.

4. When an intravenous drug, especially penicillin, is ordered, determine whether the patient has previously received the drug. Even with a negative history of allergy, previous exposure could have sensitized the person to it without any overt allergic symptoms. Subsequent doses can elicit an allergic reaction.
5. As a general rule, avoid giving a drug to which a patient is known to be allergic, even if previous reactions have been mild. Successive exposure generally results in increasingly severe reactions. In certain rare instances, such a drug must be given. This is discussed below.

MONITORING FOR SIGNS OF ALLERGIC REACTIONS IN PATIENTS RECEIVING INTRAVENOUS DRUGS

Precautions are necessary for all patients receiving drugs intravenously so that, should allergic symptoms occur, they will be recognized immediately and treatment instituted without delay.

Patients with no allergic history who are receiving drugs rarely associated with allergy are at a fairly low risk of developing an allergic reaction. However, as a safeguard, routine nursing measures should include:

1. Staying with the patient during the first 5 to 15 minutes that the drug is infusing, observing for urticaria (hives), rhinitis (nasal congestion), dyspnea, wheezing, angioneurotic edema (suddenly occurring areas of painless edema, usually on the face), or local reactions around the intravenous site.
2. Instructing the patient, without unduly alarming him, to report any of the above symptoms should they occur. For the bedfast patient, be sure that the call bell is within reach.
3. Checking the patient at 5- to 10-minute intervals until the first dose has infused, particularly if the patient is unable to report symptoms.
4. With subsequent doses, checking the patient frequently during the initial part of the infusion. Once a course of therapy is under way, as long as the drug is given without interrupted

doses, serious reactions including anaphylaxis are unlikely (41).

For patients with a history of allergies to other substances or with drugs that are more likely to be allergenic (such as those referred to above or specified in the drug information section in the back of this text), special precautions required include:

1. Remaining with the patient while the first dose is being administered or for 10 to 20 minutes if the drug is in a large volume infusion. Both for efficiency and to prevent patient apprehension, try to plan his care, or that of a neighboring patient, so that it will be necessary to remain in his room.
2. Keeping emergency medications (as described below) on hand.
3. After the medication has infused, checking the patient every 30 minutes for the next few hours. Reactions which occur later are less likely to be severe, though the nurse must continue to monitor for allergic manifestations. Check the temperature at least every four hours for the first 24 hours or for the duration of therapy to detect the occurrence of drug fever.
4. Instructing the patient to report any of the symptoms mentioned above, particularly breathing difficulties, swelling of the face, or other parts of the body or skin reactions. Be sure that the nurse-call bell is within the patient's reach.
5. At the first appearance of any allergic symptoms, discontinuing the drug and notifying the physician immediately. The intravenous line should be kept open in case any emergency medications are required. If allergic symptoms appear, consideration must be given to any other drugs that the patient is receiving concurrently, particularly parenteral ones (including blood), which may be the source of the reaction.
6. If no allergic manifestations occur, observing the patient for 5 to 10 minutes during the administration of subsequent doses. Observe for late signs, including fever, arthralgia, lymph-node enlargement, skin eruptions (maculopapular type), and neuritis. Changes in the blood, particularly the eosinophil count, are also sometimes seen. Monitoring of the blood count can be helpful.

ADMINISTRATION OF A DRUG TO WHICH A PATIENT IS KNOWN TO BE ALLERGIC

As mentioned, generally a patient should not be given any drug to which he is allergic. However, in rare instances, the benefits of giving a particular drug outweigh the risk of a potentially serious allergic reaction. The major example of this is in the case of bacterial endocarditis or septicemia in which penicillin is the treatment of choice. There is generally no effective substitute which is not cross-allergenic (41). In such cases, the drug can be given if the following procedures are followed.

A skin test using the scratch method is performed on individuals with known or suspected penicillin allergy, employing all possible penicillin antigens to determine the likelihood of an anaphylactic reaction. If the scratch test is negative, an intradermal skin test is done, unless there is a previous history of adverse reaction to penicillin. If the tests are negative, the drug can be given following the precautions discussed above. Should either test be positive, the following measures must be carried out before the penicillin can be given:

1. *Rapid hyposensitization* involves the administration of small increasing doses of drug, by the physician, every 2 to 6 hours. If time and the patient's condition permit, the oral route should be used since the chance of anaphylaxis is much less (41). If the oral route cannot be used or if the therapeutic oral dose has been reached without serious reactions, doses are given intradermally. If no adverse reactions occur, subcutaneous and intramuscular injections are given before the course of intravenous therapy can be instituted. A period of at least 20 minutes should elapse after the intramuscular injection to insure that allergic symptoms will not occur. Parenteral injections should be given in a distal extremity (the calf is recommended) with an uninflated blood pressure cuff applied to the thigh. Should a reaction occur, the cuff is inflated to retard distribution of the drug (26).

   HYPOSENSITIZATION IS ALWAYS CARRIED OUT BY THE PHYSICIAN. If there is sufficient time, it should be started a few days before the drug therapy is started.
2. *Drug suppression* is an alternative measure which utilizes either antihistamines or glucosteroids

to prevent a reaction. A day of pretreatment is recommended, followed by a test dose of the drug. As with hyposensitization, it is conducted by the physician, preferably using a calf muscle with a blood pressure cuff around the thigh. It is essential that equipment needed to treat anaphylaxis be on hand while the test dose is being given. If no reaction occurs, therapy with the drug can be initiated with the glucosteroids being gradually tapered off (26).

When the course of therapy is started, the first dose, and ideally the first several doses, should be administered by the physician. Emergency medications and equipment which must be kept close at hand throughout both the testing and drug therapy include:

- Epinephrine, 1:1,000 and 1:10,000 solutions
- Antihistamines, such as diphenhydramine (Benadryl) for intravenous use
- Glucosteroids, hydrocortisone (Solu-Cortef) and methylprednisolone (Solu-Medrol)
- Calcium preparations in case cardiac arrest should occur
- Vasopressors [dopamine (Intropin), levarterenol (Levophed), isoproterenol (Isuprel)]
- Lidocaine
- Airway and manual resuscitation bag (Puritan, Hope, Ambu, etc.)
- Endotracheal tube and laryngoscope
- Tracheostomy tray, in case laryngeal edema or spasm prevents oral intubation
- Intravenous fluids

TREATMENT OF ALLERGIC REACTIONS

1. *Anaphylactic Shock.* Should anaphylaxis occur in spite of all possible precautions, it is essential that treatment be instituted immediately since death can ensue in a matter of minutes. While specific regimens may vary slightly according to physician preference, essential elements of treatment generally include:
   a) Aqueous epinephrine, 1:10,000, given intravenously by *slow* injection. The initial dose is 2 to 5 milliliters. For milder symptoms such as urticaria, 0.2 to 0.5 milliliters of 1:1,000 strength can be initially given subcutaneously, repeated at three-minute intervals if required (48). A continuous infusion of epinephrine diluted with normal saline or 5 percent dextrose in water may be given.

   b) Establish and/or maintain a patent airway. Endotracheal intubation or emergency tracheostomy may be required if airway obstruction, due to either laryngeal edema or bronchospasm, is present. In these instances, either antihistamines such as diphenhydramine (Benadryl) 50 to 80 milligrams IV or IM, or chlorpheniramine (Chlor-Trimeton), 10 milligrams IV; or aminophylline, 0.25 to 0.50 grams IV (6 milligrams per kilogram over a 20-minute period), may be given as adjunctive measures (26, 48).
   c) Establish a secure, preferably central, intravenous line if the one already present is at risk of dislodgement or infiltration.
   d) Provide intravenous volume expansion with agents, such as dextran, saline, or albumin, and treat acidosis as needed.
   e) If bronchospasm or hypotension persists, corticosteroids may be used (48).
   f) Maintain close nursing observation of the patient for at least 24 hours after the reaction or until stable. Monitoring of vital signs, particularly blood pressure, respiration, and pulse rate, are essential for the assessment of the patient's progress.

Following anaphylactic shock or any significant allergic reaction, it is vital that the patient, or the parent or responsible person when indicated, be informed of the allergy and its significance. With a school-aged child, the parents should be advised to inform the child's teacher or school nurse of the allergy so that the information can be entered into the health record. Another important aspect of the nurse's teaching responsibility includes explaining the value of wearing a medical identification tag and assisting the patient in obtaining one if indicated.

2. *Treatment of Less Severe Allergic Manifestations.* The primary measure is to discontinue the drug. In cases of mild reactions, this is often the only measure required; symptoms subside spontaneously. For more severe reactions, epinephrine may be given. Antihistamines may also be used, both to relieve symptoms and as a prophylaxis against serum sickness. If signs of exfoliative dermatitis appear, steroids are used (41). Drug fever and other isolated symptoms are often treated symptomatically. Nursing intervention in drug allergy includes:

a) Providing psychological support to help allay the patient's anxiety. Asthmatic or other symptoms which interfere with breathing as well as extensive skin reactions are particularly anxiety provoking.

b) Continuing close observation following discontinuation of the drug to be sure that the symptoms are not worsening.

c) Providing symptomatic relief for skin reactions, such as urticaria and rashes, with such measures as tepid baths, use of a bed cradle to prevent pressure and irritation from the bed linen and, unless the skin is broken, application of lotion to relieve itching (8).

RECONSTITUTION OF DRUGS AND PREPARATION OF ADMIXTURES

Since one of the limitations of intravenous administration is that the drug must be in a solution, drugs supplied by the manufacturer in solid form must be reconstituted before use. While it is desirable from the standpoint of the pharmacist and the nurse that a drug be made available in a ready-to-use form, this is not always possible, since potency and stability are often affected once the drug has been reconstituted. To extend the shelf life of intravenous drugs with limited stability, most of them are supplied in a dry powdered form. As a further protection against deterioration, it is often recommended that they be protected from light, moisture, and marked temperature changes during storage. A cool, dry place is acceptable for the storage of most intravenous preparations, but a few require refrigeration before they are reconstituted. (Note specific recommendations for preparation and storage in the drug information section in the back of this text.)

For many years, in most hospitals, the pharmacy dispensed intravenous drugs to the nursing units in an unprepared state. When a dose of the drug was due, the nursing staff, or rarely a physician, was responsible for reconstituting the drug, adding it to a solution if so prescribed, and finally administering it to the patient. During the past 10 to 15 years, there has been a growing trend for the preparation and admixture functions to be assumed by the pharmacy department. This shift in functions has been adopted for a number of reasons.

Safety

Drugs and drug usage represent the specialty area of pharmacists. The pharmacist is more familiar with the drug's mechanism of action, the correct dosage range, potential toxicity, and incompatibilities than the nurse, and, in most instances, the physician. The nurse should have resources available to provide the necessary information to prepare drugs and admixtures safely, but she must also have the necessary time and skill to use them. Should an error in drug dosage or mode of administration, or a compatibility problem, be noted by the nurse and reported to the physician, it may be accepted less readily than if noted by the pharmacist.

The pharmacy, by virtue of its location away from patient areas, is generally a cleaner environment in which to prepare intravenous drugs and solutions which must be kept sterile. While most nursing units have specially designed medication preparation areas, relatively few hospitals are equipped with laminar flow hoods (a device essential in admixture preparation) on each nursing unit. However, each pharmacy should contain such a unit to insure that airborne microorganisms and particulate matter are eliminated from the area in which admixtures are prepared.

Legality

The preparation of admixtures can be regarded as compounding, a function which is within the scope of a pharmacist's practice but is not an accepted function of the nursing profession. Support of this view is found within the Standards of the Joint Commission on Accreditation of Hospitals (1973) which state that when possible, admixtures should be prepared by the pharmacy service (27).

This concept is further upheld by several professional groups, including the American Society of Hospital Pharmacists, which, in a statement issued in 1974, recommended that injectable drugs be reconstituted by pharmacists before being dispensed to the patient unit (6). The National Coordinating Committee on Large Volume Parenterals, a group of professionals from several health disciplines, including nursing, expressed a similar view in a paper published in 1975 (38).

Economy

Preparation of drugs and admixtures in a central area within a hospital by the most highly skilled group of individuals can result in conservation and the most efficient utilization of supplies and equipment. Also, removal of these functions from nurses' daily responsibilities can result in the saving of a significant amount of time, which can be redirected to other patient-care activities.

Nursing implications

The role of the nurse in preparing drugs and admixtures is thus determined by whether the institution utilizes the traditional approach or a centralized pharmacy-based program. In hospitals which have a total pharmacy preparation and admixture service, the nurse's primary responsibilities, in regard to intravenous medications, will be to know the correct dosage, to administer the medications, and to provide follow-up care, including observation for untoward effects. (Techniques of drug administration are discussed later in this chapter.)

In hospitals which do not have a pharmacy admixture program, the responsibility for reconstituting drugs and preparing admixtures remains a nursing function. Whether such tasks are performed by nurses on the intravenous therapy team or by the general nursing staff on the patient units, the same high standards must be adhered to as would be followed in a pharmacy-based program (38).

OBJECTIVES IN PREPARATION OF DRUGS FOR INTRAVENOUS USE

Because the intravenous route is the most dangerous of all routes of administration, several objectives must be met when drugs are prepared for intravenous use to insure their safe and effective administration. These include:

1. Maintenance of sterility
2. Prevention of incompatibilities
3. Insurance of accurate dosage

MAINTENANCE OF STERILITY

The hazards of local and systemic infections have already been discussed in Chapter 7. Since a seemingly minor complication such as phlebitis, can evolve into a potentially fatal infection, such as septicemia or suppurative thrombophlebitis, preventing all intravenous-associated infections remains a primary responsibility of everyone associated with intravenous therapy.

Each component of the intravenous system, from the fluid container to the cannula and including the administration tubing, represents a potential vehicle of infection. Contamination may be intrinsic; that is, having been introduced before use, such as during the manufacturing, delivery, or storage of the product. It can also be extrinsic, occurring during clinical use.

The fluid container and its contents are more subject to intrinsic contamination than other parts of the system. Many types of fluids serve as excellent growth media for bacteria and fungi. Current manufacturing techniques utilize quality controls to insure the sterility of intravenous fluids up to the time of use. However, as can be seen from the intrinsic contamination of intravenous fluids that occurred several years ago on a nationwide basis, such sterility cannot be guaranteed (33). Despite changes in container design that resulted from that epidemic, the potential for contamination of the fluid source still exists.

Thus, at the time of use, each drug and fluid container must be thoroughly inspected for evidence of intrinsic contamination. Unless a careful examination is done, tiny cracks in the bottle or puncture of the bag may go undetected.

Inspection of fluid and drug containers

1. Check glass bottles, vials, or ampuls of medication for obvious cracks, chips, and damaged or missing metal seals. Glass bottles should be slowly rotated in front of a light, to look for a sudden flash of light which signals a hairline crack not otherwise visible.
2. Squeeze plastic containers to detect leaks.
3. Holding the container in front of an illuminated surface, using both black and white background, look for: color changes, precipitates, any particulate matter, or other signs of contamination.
4. Check the expiration date to be sure that the fluid or drug is safe to use.
5. Whenever a defect in the container or intrinsic contamination is noted, do not use the fluid or drug. It should be returned to the pharmacy or department responsible for dispensing such supplies, which in turn should report the defect to the manufacturer.

Adherence to aseptic practices throughout drug preparation

Once the absence of detectable intrinsic contamination has been verified, the introduction of subsequent contamination must be avoided by rigidly adhering to aseptic techniques.

1. The hands must be thoroughly washed before preparing any medication or admixture, using friction and ideally a surgical scrub such as an iodophor preparation. Handwashing facilities should be available in the medication preparation area so that the hands can be rewashed if they become contaminated.
2. Since touch contamination is common and perhaps represents the most frequent break in aseptic practices, it must be avoided (27, 31, 38). Sterile areas that are particularly vulnerable include: the rubber stopper of the fluid bottle or vial, the medication port of the plastic fluid container or administration set, the shaft of the needle, and the plunger of the syringe.
3. When available, prepare drugs and admixtures under a laminar flow hood (Fig. 8-2). The risks of airborne contaminants entering intravenous solutions have been well documented (7).

   Drugs and admixtures prepared in an unsterile environment can become contaminated from airborne microorganisms. Such contamination is likely to occur as a result of turbulent air currents which enable particles and organisms to settle onto objects.

   The laminar flow hood is designed to eliminate airborne contamination from the work area by creating a pattern of flow in a specific direction, usually horizontally from the back of the hood toward the room in front (27). To create the flow, air entering either the lower or upper part of the hood is initially passed through a prefilter to remove gross matter and is then compressed and circulated through a bacterially retentive filter known as a high-efficiency particulate air (HEPA) filter. The purified air, which should be free of virtually all bacteria, is then directed out into the work area of the hood in uniform parallel streams. The direction and velocity of flow prevents nonsterile room air from entering the hood (53).

   While the hood provides a nearly sterile environment for the performance of such tasks as

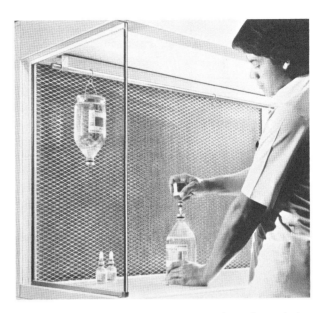

Fig. 8-2. Clean Air Center. Preparation of an admixture under a laminar flow hood reduces the risk of airborne contamination. (Courtesy of Abbott Laboratories, North Chicago, Illinois 60064)

reconstitution of drugs and preparation of admixtures, failure to follow the basic principles of operation will defeat the basic purpose of the hood; and the expected benefits will not be achieved. In institutions in which laminar hoods are available for use by an intravenous therapy team or are located on patients' units, particularly intensive care areas, the nursing staff involved in their operation must be familiar with the basic principles of laminar flow and adhere to certain guidelines:

a) Proper functioning of the hood must be insured by periodic inspection by the hospital's preventive maintenance department or other qualified personnel. Any leaks in the HEPA filter would allow contaminated air to pass through the filter into the work area, thus decreasing operating efficiency (53).

b) Preparation for operation is essential. A 15- to 30-minute warm-up period is required to rid the unit of particulate matter. In pharmacies or units which would use the hood frequently throughout each 24 hour period, it is recommended that the hood run continuously. Clean the hood thoroughly, particularly the work surface, with alcohol or other recommended disinfecting agent (38).

c) Use of the hood:
   (1) While airborne contamination is eliminated, surface contamination of objects placed in the hood is not removed. Therefore, any obvious surface dust or dirt should be wiped off before the object is placed in the hood.
   (2) Hands should be thoroughly scrubbed before the hood is used. Whenever multiple or complex admixtures or drugs are to be prepared, it is recommended that sterile gloves as well as mask and gown be worn (38).
   (3) Placement of objects within the hood should be planned so as to avoid interference with airflow from the filter throughout the work area. Large items should not be placed behind smaller ones lest air turbulences be created or contaminants blown off of the larger objects and settle onto the smaller ones or onto the hands.
   (4) To prevent turbulent air currents from pulling in outside air, work must be carried out at least 6 inches within the hood (27, 38). This principle is often neglected when drug preparations are carried out in haste.
   (5) The work surface should be cleaned whenever anything is spilled and at the end of drug preparation (27).
   (6) When using a laminar flow hood, avoid developing a false sense of security. The hood does not protect against touch contamination; thus strict aseptic technique is mandatory (38).
4. When no laminar flow hood is available, an appropriate clean work area is essential. The medication area should be set apart from heavy traffic flow and be relatively free of air turbulences. It should have a sink and be well lighted. The total work area must be kept clean and dust-free. The counter top used for medication preparation should be cleaned at least once daily with a suitable disinfectant.
5. Always clean the rubber stopper on the top of the fluid bottle and on the medication vials before inserting a needle or administration set. Their sterility is not always guaranteed.
6. For obvious reasons, sneezing and coughing should be avoided during medication preparation and in the drug-preparation area.

Avoiding particulate contamination

While the hazards of microbial contamination are well known to nurses, the dangers associated with particulate matter are not common knowledge. Particulate matter has been defined as "the mobile, undissolved substances unintentionally present in parenteral products" (53, p. 26). It can include rubber, glass, metal, plastic, or almost any substance. As with bacterial contamination, such particles can be introduced into intravenous fluids and drug containers at the time of manufacture or during preparation and use. In a series of studies conducted between 1969 and 1972, Davis and Turco noted large quantities of particulate matter in intravenous fluids from all four major manufacturers (13, 14, 51). However, over that time period, there was a considerable reduction in particle levels in all brands. Masuda and associates found high levels of particulate matter in antibiotics manufactured by one particular technique which did not utilize terminal filtering (34).

Particulate contamination occurring in use is generally derived from two sources: *equipment,* including fluid containers, vials, ampuls, and administration equipment; and *drugs.*

EQUIPMENT

Particles of rubber can be introduced into the fluid bottle when the piercing pin on the administration set is thrust through the rubber stopper. This phenomenon, known as coring, is more likely to occur when the pin is inserted at an angle or with a twisting motion. Manufacturers warn against this practice (3).

Coring can also occur when a needle is introduced either through the latex overseal on vented fluid bottles, into the latex injection port of the administration tubing, or through the rubber stopper of a vial. The sharp needle bevel, whether of a small or large gauge, can cut away fragments of the rubber. With vials, this problem can be minimized by following a suggested technique (53). (Fig. 8-3):

1. Hold the needle bevel up at an angle of 45° to 60°.

2. Maintaining this angle, insert the needle into the rubber stopper.
3. Before the needle tip has fully penetrated the stopper, lift the needle to a 90° angle.
4. Follow the standard technique for the rest of the procedure.

The use of the smallest gauge needle may also help to reduce coring, but any particles created will be difficult to visualize and are likely to pass through the intravenous cannula (44).

Opening a glass ampul and the subsequent withdrawal of medication or diluent can result in the introduction of glass particles which are then transferred into the intravenous setup and ultimately into the patient when the drug is added to the fluid container or administration tubing (52).

DRUGS

Drugs represent another potential source of particulate matter of two varieties:

1. Undissolved drugs occurring as a result of incomplete reconstitution from the powdered form
2. Precipitates produced by the physical incompatibility of admixtures (1)

The greater the number of medications added to a solution, the greater the chance of introducing particles. Solutions such as those used for total parenteral nutrition (TPN) carry a higher risk of particulate contamination for this reason.

While other foreign substances (metal, wood, etc.) may be inadvertently introduced into the intravenous system, their occurrence is less likely than that of the above-mentioned types of particles.

Unless removed, particulate matter in the intravenous line will be carried into the patient's venous circulation and, following the route of venous return, will pass through the right heart and into the pulmonary artery. Whether the particles will pass through the pulmonary capillary bed and into the pulmonary veins, eventually reaching the systemic circulation, or become entrapped within an arteriole, is determined primarily by their size.

It is believed that in general only particles smaller than 5 microns will pass through a pulmonary capillary, though occasionally some particles that exceed that size may pass through. Sub-

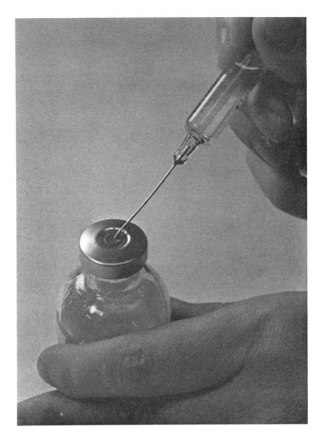

Fig. 8-3. Correct technique for inserting a needle into a vial to prevent coring.

stances of such size are difficult to envision, since a micron is equivalent to about forty millionths of an inch (44). By comparison, the thickness of a human hair is approximately 125 microns.

Particles too large to pass through a pulmonary capillary will become lodged within an arteriole, occluding the blood flow. Consequently, a portion of lung tissue will be deprived of its food and oxygen supply, resulting in an infarction of the involved area unless blood is supplied through collateral channels. Even in the absence of total occlusion, entrapped particles can produce an inflammatory response.

Particles smaller than 5 microns, and larger ones that have somehow passed through the pulmonary capillaries, enter the systemic circulation and can embolize to a vital organ, particularly the brain or kidneys, where an interruption of blood flow can result in profound, permanent consequences.

Eliminating particulate matter

To reduce the hazard that particulate matter presents to patients, efforts must be directed toward two areas: preventing the introduction of particulate matter into the intravenous system and removing any particles that are in the system before they infuse into the patient.

The presence of particulate matter in intravenous solutions and its resultant hazards have been known for many years (49). While the levels have decreased substantially, particles are still known to be present in fluids at the time of manufacture in spite of intensive efforts being directed toward their complete elimination. To achieve this goal, there will be a need not only for stronger standards regulating the level of particulate matter allowed, but also for technological advances to enable the manufacture of particle-free fluids and drugs.

Some recent evidence suggests that particulate matter can be generated from plastic intravenous fluid containers, especially after shaking the bag (10, 39). However, these substances, rather than being true particles, are believed by some to be minute-sized balls of liquid plasticizer, which is a substance added to the plastic to make it more flexible (10). Any one of a number of other substances can be added to the plastic to improve its physical characteristics, and the resultant material may interact with a solution or its additives. In some instances, substances from the plastic are leached; that is, drawn into the solution. Likewise, elements from the solution can be adsorbed by the plastic (53).

PREVENTING THE INTRODUCTION OF PARTICULATE MATTER

A major focus of nurses must be on preventing the introduction of additional particulate matter. This can be done by using care when inserting the piercing pin of the administration set into the fluid bottle and in the insertion of a needle through the rubber stopper of a vial or medication port of the administration set. (Use the technique described on page 124 above.) In addition, reconstitution of drugs and preparation of admixtures must be done according to the recommendations of the manufacturer and following the guidelines discussed later in this chapter. The use of a laminar flow hood can help to reduce particulate contamination.

After preparation, all admixtures should be inspected carefully for the presence of particulate matter. Under adequate lighting, the container should be held against a light background to detect dark-colored particles and against a dark background to visualize lighter particles. If the solution has a hazy appearance or shows evidence of any precipitation or particulate matter, it must not be used.

REMOVING PARTICULATE MATTER THAT IS IN THE SYSTEM

Since the introduction of particles cannot be avoided completely, it is essential to be alert to situations in which they are likely to be present in significant numbers and take measures to remove them. Patients who are most likely to be exposed to a high level of particulate matter are those receiving intravenous fluids containing multiple additives, such as total parenteral nutrition solutions; those receiving large volumes of intravenous fluids; and those at a high risk of a serious reaction from particulate matter, such as patients receiving steroids, which through a modification of the tissue response can cause a localized process to become generalized throughout the lung (53). For such patients, the use of a micropore filter is recommended.

TYPES OF MICROPORE FILTERS

Depth filters consist of beds or mats of asbestos or silicone particles bonded together to provide a tortuous pathway along which particles become trapped. Because they do not contain pores of uniform size, they cannot be given an absolute micron rating (46). They generally filter out particles that are approximately 5 microns and larger. Thus, they are used to filter gross matter such as glass particles from ampuls and cored rubber particles from vials.

Membrane filters, the type most widely used, consist of a discoid-shaped housing with a porous membrane inside. Both the membrane material and pore size determine which substances will pass through and which will be blocked. Many filters are constructed of a material which allows fluid to pass but not air. Any air in the intravenous line containing such a filter would be trapped within the filter, providing a safeguard against air emboli. A disadvantage of this air-blocking type is that careful priming is essential to insure that all air is removed *prior* to wetting the filter. Once wet, any air already trapped, or subsequently entering it, will create a block, thereby interrupting the flow of solution.

This problem is eliminated in filters that contain a material which allows the passage of air. However, should air enter the system, it can readily infuse into the patient. Consequently, this type is not frequently employed.

A third type of membrane filter, which vents the air into the atmosphere, combines the desirable features of the first two while eliminating their disadvantages. Should air enter the system, disruption of flow is prevented, yet the hazard of air embolism is avoided.

FILTER-SIZE POROSITY

Regardless of principle utilized, the versatility of a filter is determined by its porosity or the size of particles that it will allow to pass. The largest pores are approximately 5 microns in size which, in addition to glass and rubber particles, will filter drug crystals and foreign substances of a similar size. Thus, particles smaller than 5 microns will pass through and, upon entering the patient's vascular system, would be small enough to pass through the pulmonary capillaries. While filters of this size reduce the risk of such hazards as pulmonary infarction, the potential for other complications is not eliminated. Furthermore, bacteria will readily pass through since they generally range in size from 0.3 to 0.5 microns (44). Filters with a much smaller pore size, ranging from 1 micron down to 0.22 micron, are available for the removal of bacteria as well as particulate matter.

Perhaps the most versatile filters are those falling within the 0.45 to 0.5-micron range. Capable of filtering gross particulate matter, they also remove many bacteria except for smaller species, specifically pleomorphic *Pseudomonas* (45). They are practical for continuous large volume infusions since they permit the maintenance of acceptable flow rates. They can be used to administer total parenteral nutrition (TPN) solutions as well as dextran, though the flow rates will be slow. Blood and blood products cannot pass through.

The smallest available pore size, 0.22 micron, is sometimes regarded as a sterilizing filter since it is capable of filtering nearly all bacteria and, when used properly, can contribute to a decrease in intravenous-associated infections. The major limita-

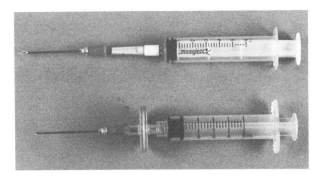

Fig. 8–4. Membrane syringe filters prefilter particulate matter during preparation of drugs and admixtures. (*Top*) MP-5, 5 micron (Travenol Laboratories, Inc., Deerfield, Illinois 60015); (*Bottom*) ADD-MIX, 1.0 micron (Abbott Laboratories, North Chicago, Illinois 60064)

tion of this size filter is the significant reduction in flow rate that can occur, particularly with additives such as antibiotics. In some instances, it may be necessary to use an infusion pump to maintain a satisfactory flow. Since some filter models contain a warning against using with systems producing a specified level of pressure, this parameter should be checked if a pump is to be used. Furthermore, small-pore filters (< 1.0 micron) should not be used with some drugs in suspension, such as amphotericin, since the drug will be filtered out.

CLINICAL USES OF FILTERS

Syringe filters, which are generally in the 1- to 5-micron range, are designed to prefilter substances during preparation of drugs and admixtures (Fig. 8-4). These disposable units are easily connected between a syringe and needle. Since they allow bidirectional flow, they can be used *either* to aspirate medication from an ampul or vial *or* to add the medication to a fluid container or administer it directly into the intravenous line. It is essential that the same filter *never* be used for both aspirating and administering the drug, or the purpose of its use will be defeated. After the solution has been withdrawn from the ampul or vial, any glass, rubber, or other particles will be trapped within the filter. If the same filter were to be used to add the solution to a fluid container, those particles would be ejected into the container. Thus, when the filter is used to withdraw solutions, it must be removed from the syringe prior to adding the solution to the container.

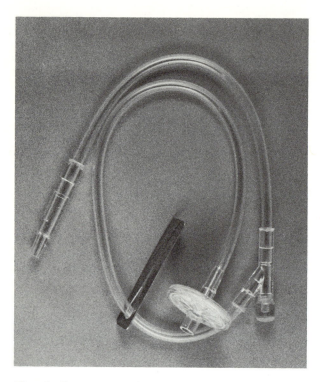

Fig. 8–5. S-A-I-F (Solution Additive Inline Filter). Add-on micropore filters can be attached to any intravenous administration set. (Abbott Laboratories, North Chicago, Illinois 60064)

Additives available in prefilled syringes can be filtered prior to their addition to the fluid or administration into the intravenous line. In these instances, it is essential to remove all air from the syringe before attaching the filter in order to prevent an air lock which will block the flow. The same filter can be reused to add the contents of another syringe containing the same medication as long as great care is taken to preserve the sterility of the filter.

In-line Filters. While syringe filters are of great value in eliminating gross particulate matter during drug reconstitution and admixing, both particulate and bacterial contamination can be introduced at many sites along the intravenous line prior to and during drug administration. Thus, the concept of final filtration has emerged as a means of removing contaminants at the terminal point of the administration tubing. In-line, final filtration devices are usually of the membrane type in the 0.22- to 0.45-micron range to enable removal of both microbial and particulate contamination. Some models are available as add-on

units so they can be used with any type of administration set (Fig. 8-5). Though convenient, this addition of two more connections to the intravenous line creates the potential for contamination either above or downstream from the filter. Thus, in-line filters integrated into the administration set are becoming increasingly popular (Fig. 8-6). Not only can they reduce the risk of touch contamination, but they can save nursing time if used correctly. A disadvantage, however, is that, should the filter develop an air lock or otherwise become blocked, the entire administration tubing must be changed.

Regardless of the type used, the manufacturer's instructions should be strictly followed to insure proper function. The following general guidelines are applicable to most units:

1. With add-on filters, strict aseptic practices must be followed.
2. Thorough priming by inverting the unit and tapping, if necessary, is mandatory to remove all air bubbles.
3. If blood, suspensions, or emulsions are to be given via the same intravenous line, they must be "piggybacked" at the injection site *below* the filter. The slide clamp below the filter must be completely closed to prevent back flow and subsequent occlusion of the filter (1).
4. With filters with very small pore size, particularly the 0.22-micron size, the reduced flow rate produced by the filter can be somewhat compensated for by raising the height of the fluid container (the standard height is about 36 inches above the intravenous site) and by using a large gauge needle.
5. Change the filter at least every 24 hours or sooner if it becomes clogged. When a filter becomes occluded by trapped particles (as opposed to an air lock), this should be regarded as beneficial, a sign that the filter is accomplishing its function, rather than as a nuisance and an excuse for omitting the filter from the intravenous line (12).

The value of filters in the removal of particulate matter has been well documented (50); but despite awareness that bacterial contaminants are also filtered out, study results disagree as to the effectiveness of filters on reducing the incidence of infusion phlebitis. One study of 100 patients found that of 49 who received intravenous fluids

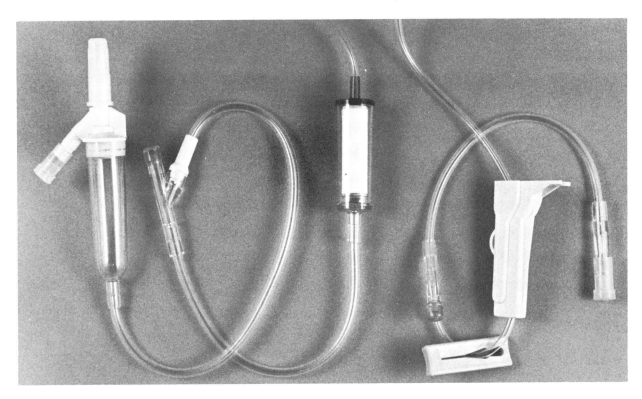

Fig. 8-6. Ivex membrane filter, incorporated into the administration tubing, avoids separate connections. (Abbott Laboratories, North Chicago, Illinois 60064)

without a filter, 22 (44.9 percent) developed phlebitis; while out of the remaining 51 patients, on whom filters were used, only one (1.9 percent) developed phlebitis (47).

However, differing results were obtained by other investigators. Of 15 patients receiving non-filtered intravenous solutions, 6 (40 percent) developed phlebitis; but out of 33 patients with a filter, 14 (42 percent) developed phlebitis (40). These investigators suggested that the incidence of phlebitis is more strongly influenced by the presence of additives and thus has more of a chemical than an infective basis. With such variable findings, it seems evident that there remains a need for further studies in this area.

PREVENTION OF INCOMPATIBILITIES

With an increasing number of medications being given by the intravenous route, the problem of incompatibilities has become a major concern. The potential for incompatibilities is present not only when several drugs are added to a large volume of fluid to produce an admixture, but also when drugs in separate solutions are administered either concurrently or in close succession via the same intravenous line. An incompatibility can also result when a single drug is reconstituted or diluted with the wrong solution.

The likelihood of incompatibilities is reduced when the responsibility for the preparation of drugs and admixtures is centralized within the pharmacy department. Having access to the most current information available on drugs, the pharmacy team can insure greater accuracy and safety. Should a prescribed admixture contain incompatible components, the pharmacist can consult the physician for a modification of the prescription and thus prevent any harm to the patient.

In those hospitals which have not incorporated parenteral admixture preparation into the pharmacy service, this responsibility will remain with the nursing staff. As with maintenance of sterility, the prevention of incompatibilities is of major concern. A basic understanding of the types of incompatibilities is crucial; but because of the complexity of factors involved, a thorough acquaintance with up-to-date resources and assurance of their accessibility remains the best safeguard against compatability problems.

Incompatibilities are generally classified into three groups: physical, chemical, and therapeutic.

Physical incompatibility

Physical incompatibility refers to any visible change in the solution. This may be evidenced by color changes, haze, turbidity, precipitate or gas formation (53). Such changes can result from a decreased solubility due to the addition of a drug to an inappropriate fluid vehicle. This creates either an incomplete solution or a precipitate; that is, solid particles settling out. In a solution containing multiple additives, two or more ingredients which would be soluble if present alone may interact to form an insoluble product (18). Some examples of physical reactions involving commonly used drugs are:

1. Sodium bicarbonate and epinephrine, combinations of which result in the increased degradation of the epinephrine. Since these drugs are often administered by intravenous injection in rapid succession during cardiopulmonary resuscitation, this effect must be considered. To avoid the incompatibility, the administration tubing should be flushed with solution after either of these drugs is given.
2. Sodium bicarbonate and calcium chloride, which when given together form calcium carbonate, an insoluble precipitate. As with the situation above, these drugs are often given in combination during resuscitation attempts. After either one is given, it is essential to thoroughly flush the intravenous line before the second one is given.
3. Phenytoin (Dilantin) and diazepam (Valium), which when administered in combination form a precipitate. These anticonvulsants may be prescribed together for patients with protracted seizures. They must never be mixed together nor with any other solution. The correct technique is to give each separately via the lowest injection port on the administration set, flushing the line in between or directly into the intravenous cannula (18). (See p. 133.)

Chemical incompatibility

Chemical incompatibility is the reaction of a drug with other drugs or solutions which results in some chemical degradation of the drug. Such a reaction is not visible and can be detected only by laboratory analysis. Of the many factors contributing to incompatibilities, the one most commonly responsible is a change in pH that is, the hydrogen ion (H+) concentration which determines the acid-base environment of the substance or solution. A specific pH or narrow range of pH values is required for the solubility of a drug and for the maintenance of its stability once it has been mixed.

Antibiotics are one drug category whose activity and stability are affected by pH. Penicillin, for example, which is most stable in a slightly acidic environment of 6.5, becomes rapidly inactivated in either a very acidic pH (3.5) or an alkaline one (8.5). A buffering agent added to penicillin enables it to be compatible with standard dextrose and sodium chloride solutions which are moderately acidic by changing the pH of the solution to 6.0. However, the addition of penicillin to other fluids with a high buffering capacity, that is, the ability to resist changes in pH, such as protein hydrolysate solution, would maintain the solution's normal pH range of 5.0 to 6.0 and result in inactivation of the penicillin. Likewise, the addition of other drugs such as ascorbic acid or tetracycline hydrochloride to an otherwise stable solution containing penicillin would lower the pH to a point of inactivating the penicillin (53).

Other factors affecting activity or stability of drugs

NUMBER OF ADDITIVES

The greater the number of drugs in an admixture, the greater the chances of one of them becoming unstable. Thus, the number of drug additives should be kept to a minimum.

ORDER OF ADDING DRUGS

When multiple additives cannot be avoided, as with total parenteral nutrition (TPN) solutions, the order in which the substances are added can determine whether incompatibilities will result. Each substance must be thoroughly mixed before the others are added, to insure complete dilution.

TPN and other complex admixtures, for which order of mixing is crucial, should be prepared by the pharmacy.

DOSE AND CONCENTRATION OF A DRUG

The stability of a drug may be dependent on the dose and/or concentration that is added to a solution. A low dose of a drug such as hydrocortisone, added to a solution to counteract an adverse effect of a second drug, may present no compatibility problems. Yet, should a dose within the therapeutic range be added, an incompatibility may occur (27).

COMPLEXATION

Two drugs administered together can combine to form a chemical complex and thus can become inactivated.

TYPE OF SOLUTION

Properties of a solution other than the pH can affect the stability of drugs added to it. Admixture studies have been conducted by investigators independently and in conjunction with manufacturers of intravenous fluids (16). Such studies present the effects (in terms of changes in pH and solubility) of adding one or two drugs to each of the most common intravenous solutions. Study results, summarized in the form of booklets or compatibility charts, are available to hospital personnel. They will be discussed with other drug resources below.

TIME

Once reconstituted, most drugs will deteriorate over a given period of time, and the addition of a drug to a solution will often hasten the deterioration. It is essential that the drug or solution be used within the safe time period. Such information is either available from the package insert or from the pharmacist. The duration of stability can often be prolonged by refrigeration if other precautions specified by the manufacturer are adhered to.

TEMPERATURE

A drug is generally more stable at lower temperatures. Thus, if a drug is reconstituted or a solution is prepared in advance of use, refrigeration is required to prolong the stability. A drug such as cephalothin (Keflin) once reconstituted remains stable at room temperature only for about 6 hours; however, when refrigerated, it remains stable for up to 48 hours (27).

LIGHT

Exposure to light can result in degradation of certain drugs. Such drugs as atropine sulfate, furosemide (Lasix), and levarterenol (Levophed) are particularly sensitive to light and are usually supplied in brown vials or ampuls. It is recommended that these, and ideally all drugs, be stored in their original package as an added precaution.

Nitroprusside (Nipride) and amphotericin B (Fungizone) are drugs which must be shielded from light after being added to a solution. Some manufacturers supply a metallic foil jacket with which to cover the fluid container; however, aluminum foil or any opaque wrapper, such as a paper bag, can also be used.

Therapeutic incompatibility

Therapeutic incompatibility is an undesirable pharmacologic reaction occurring within a patient as a result of two or more drugs given concurrently. The effect may be one of potentiation (increasing the therapeutic response) or antagonism (negating the desired response). Examples of such incompatibilities are: penicillin and heparin, which result in decreased anticoagulation effects of the heparin; penicillin and tetracycline, which inhibit the bactericidal effect of the penicillin.

A therapeutic incompatibility may initially go undetected until it is noted that the patient has failed to show the expected clinical response to the drugs. If an incompatibility is not suspected, the patient may be given increasingly higher doses of the drug to try to obtain the therapeutic effects. Should the incompatibility then be alleviated by the discontinuation of the other drug which caused it, an overdosage could result.

With many variables contributing to the occurrence of incompatibilities and considering the vast number of potential drug combinations, it is obvious that an individual cannot keep abreast of all the information needed to assess the probability of incompatibility with a given combination of drugs. Therefore, in order to minimize the risk of incompatibilities, it is essential that several guidelines be followed:

1. When reconstituting a drug, be sure that it is thoroughly mixed before administering it or adding it to a solution.
2. Avoid adding two or more additives to a large volume solution whenever possible since the risk of incompatibility increases markedly as more drugs are added.
3. When two or more drugs, particularly antibiotics, are prescribed for intermittent infusion, devise a staggered time schedule so that each can be infused individually. As a rule, more than one antibiotic should not be given at a time (28).
4. When preparing a drug, follow all instructions and note all precautions given by the manufacturer. This information is included in the drug information section in the back of this book as well as in the package insert.
5. Be alert for admixtures involving drugs with a very high or very low pH. Such information is not readily available but may be obtained from admixture charts or from the pharmacist. Most drugs are moderately acidic, with tetracycline being one of the most acidic (2.5). A few drugs, however, have a high pH, putting them in the alkaline range. Sodium bicarbonate (7.3), ampicillin sodium (8.75), and sodium thiopental (Pentothal) (10.45) are a few of these (16). Before adding such drugs to a solution, compatibility charts and the compatibility information contained in the drug information section in the back of this text should be checked to avoid incompatibility (27).
6. Calcium and magnesium salts frequently cause precipitation when added to other basic salts. Thus, the mixing of calcium and magnesium preparations with other substances should be done only after checking compatibility references (30).
7. Do not mix any additives with blood or blood products (27, 53).
8. Whenever possible, prepare drugs and admixtures immediately before administration. If they must be prepared in advance, follow manufacturers' direction regarding type of storage and length of time the solution remains stable. Never allow one solution to infuse for longer than 24 hours. With keep-open containers, discard any remaining solution and prepare a new container at least once every 24 hours (53).
9. Never mix in a syringe two drugs which will be administered intravenously. While this practice is generally used for drugs given intramuscularly to avoid multiple injection sites, it could conceivably be used to administer two drugs by intravenous injection or "IV push." Because of the increased likelihood of incompatibility resulting from the mixing of drugs which are highly concentrated, this practice must always be avoided. Administer drugs separately; and as a further precaution, the intravenous tubing should be flushed between drugs.
10. If the compatibility of drugs cannot be determined from the available resources, avoid mixing them (28).
11. Be familiar with compatibility references and know how to interpret the data.

COMPATIBILITY CHARTS

Compatibility charts are available from each of the major manufactures of intravenous fluids. Using a graphic format, most charts are of value in determing the physical incompatibility between two drugs. While certainly quite helpful, they do not provide a complete picture of potential incompatibilities e.g., when multiple drugs are mixed or when different solutions are used.

Because a particular intravenous fluid may be available in a fairly wide range of pH values (depending on the manufacturer), it is best that each institution use the charts designed for the brand of fluids used. While charts available from other sources can also be helpful, it should be remembered that their data may not always be applicable to other products.

ADMIXTURE GUIDES

Some guides currently available provide more detailed information about compatibility. The *Guide to Parenteral Admixtures* from Cutter Laboratories (29) is a reference which includes duration of time that an admixture remains compatible as well as chemical and physical incompatibilities. To insure that the material is kept up to date, supplements are continually being issued.

The *Admixture Studies for Fluids in Viaflex Plastic Containers* is available from Travenol Laboratories (16). This study presents incompatibility data based on 33 common additives, singly and in combination, when mixed with each of 19 of the

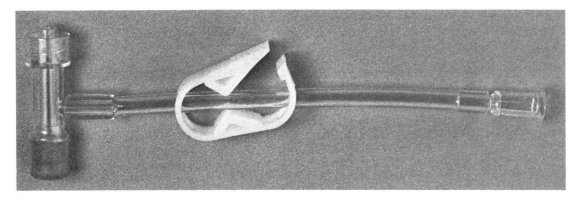

Fig. 8-7. "T" Port. By providing an injection site directly above the cannula hub, devices such as this minimize the likelihood of incompatibilities. (Deseret Company, Sandy, Utah 84070)

most frequently used intravenous solutions. The pH of each admixture is given along with any physical incompatibility (in terms of changes in color or clarity and presence of particles) noted at specified intervals from immediately after mixing up to 48 hours thereafter. The information in the study is not intended to provide a final judgment on the compatibility of specific drugs and solutions. If major changes in the pH or physical appearance have been found, the drugs should not be combined. Absence of such changes does not guarantee that the substances are compatible. Check other references; and if there are any doubts, consult the pharmacist before preparing the solution.

Compatibility of drugs given via the injection port of the administration tubing

As is discussed at the end of this chapter, drugs administered by intravenous injection are generally given via the injection port on the lower end of the administration tubing. This necessitates that the drug mix with the primary solution in the distal portion of tubing. While this represents only a short segment of tubing, the volume of drug being injected is generally quite small, and the resulting mixing of the solution and drug have been shown in one study to occur in about a one-to-one ratio (5). Therefore, drugs which are highly incompatible when added to large volume solutions would also be incompatible when injected into the injection port of the tubing. Of the drugs studied by these investigators, three that were found to produce such incompatibilities were:

phenytoin sodium (Dilantin), diazepam (Valium), and methylprednisolone sodium succinate (Solu-Medrol). For these and other drugs which the manufacturer advises not to inject into the medication port (see drug section at the back of this text), the drug may be injected into the latex sleeve or flashbulb site at the distal end of the administration set. For sets that do not have a latex bulb or sleeve, a new T-shaped adaptor, known as the "T" Port is available (Fig. 8-7). Resembling an intermittent adaptor plug, it consists of a latex injection site with a Luer-lock connection for attachment to the cannula hub. In addition, it has a 4-inch side tubing enabling connection to a standard administration set. A pinch clamp on the side tubing is designed to prevent mixing of the primary fluid with any drug that is administered via the injection site. In the absence of such a device, the only alternative method of administration is direct injection into the cannula. A suggested procedure for this is as follows:

1. Loosen the connection between the administration tubing and cannula.
2. Disconnect the needle and its protective cap from the syringe with the drug, taking care to avoid contamination of all exposed sites.
3. Quickly attach the syringe to the hub of the cannula, and place the capped needle onto the end of the administration tubing to keep it sterile.
4. Inject the medication at the recommended rate.
5. Maintaining sterility, detach the needle from the administration tubing and syringe from the

cannula, and reconnect the tubing to the cannula.

INSURANCE OF ACCURATE DOSAGE

Accuracy in dosage is important for medications given by any route, but it is of particular concern for intravenous medications, since even minor alterations in dosage can be reflected in marked variations in the therapeutic response.

When drugs are prepared by the pharmacy service and supplied to the nursing unit, either in the form of an admixture or in a prefilled syringe, the nurse has only to check the label on the container or syringe to verify the contents and dosage and compare it with the physician's prescription, being certain that the prescribed dose is within the normal range.

If the nurse must assume responsibility for preparing drugs and admixtures, as much attention must be given to calculation of a correct dose as to maintaining sterility and avoiding incompatibilities. The major requirements for this are a clear understanding of fundamental mathematics and knowledge of the normal dose range of drugs. While basic mathematical calculations are well known to most if not all nurses, anyone who is uncomfortable with calculations would do well to refer to a basic nursing pharmacology textbook to review the essential material.

Even though a nurse may have a thorough knowledge of how to calculate dosages, errors can occur unless other factors are attended to:

1. Drug preparation must be done in a quiet place without interruption. Frequent distractions can result in the omission or duplication of steps in the preparation process. Unless the drug or admixture is for emergency use, the calculation and preparation process must not be done hurriedly.
2. Always verify the prescribed drug and dose by checking the physician's order sheet. If unclear, obtain clarification from the physician. When in doubt about the correctness of a dosage, mode of administration, or potential for incompatibility, consult an appropriate written resource (such as the drug information section in this book). If there is a discrepancy between information from different sources, consult the

pharmacist. In situations where a pharmacist may not be immediately available, such as during the night in a small community hospital, the safest reference to rely on is the *Physicians' Desk Reference* (43), which contains the recommendations of the drug manufacturers. Though rare, occasions may arise in which the nurse is requested to administer a drug in a dose which is outside the usual recommended range or via a mode which is not recommended by the manufacturer. Therefore, to avoid not only possible adverse effects on the patient but legal consequences as well, the nurse should inform the physician why she cannot administer it. If the physician still wants the drug to be given, the nurse might provide the drugs and supplies to the physician, who then assumes full responsibility for the preparation and administration of the drug and any consequences. Such a course of action has been suggested by some pharmacists and intravenous therapy nurses (30).

3. As emphasized above, always check for a history of allergies before preparing and administering an intravenous drug.
4. Be sure that the drug form used is for intravenous use. Some drugs are available in a different form for intramuscular use, which, because of some additives, cannot be given intravenously. Check the label carefully.
5. Check the expiration date to be sure that the drug is not outdated. Though the pharmacy and nursing service generally have routine procedures to eliminate outdated drugs from stock, it is always safest to double-check.
6. When reconstituting a drug from powder form, follow the manufacturer's recommendations regarding quantity of diluent to add. These recommendations are found in the drug information section in the back of this text.
7. With multidose vials, label the bottle with the concentration of the reconstituted solution along with the date and time of mixing and initials of the person preparing it.
8. If only a fraction of the total dose is to be used, the amount needed can be initially computed mentally but should be verified with a written calculation to avoid the chance of error.
9. When doing calculations, consider the system of weights and measures used and be consistent throughout. The dosages of most drugs

are expressed in the metric system with grams and milligrams as the units of weight and liters and milliliters the units of volume. However, drugs such as electrolytes which ionize (split into electrically charged particles) when dissolved in water are expressed in milliequivalents. The electrolyte most commonly added to large volume infusions is potassium chloride. A few drugs are measured in units, either "international units" or "USP units." Heparin and insulin are two such drugs. The apothecary system is not used for drugs given intravenously.

TECHNIQUE FOR PREPARATION OF DRUGS

Drugs in liquid form

Some drugs are supplied in a liquid form so they do not need reconstitution. They may, however, require further dilution before administration. Drugs in liquid form may be supplied in ampuls which provide a single dose or in vials which contain either single or multiple doses. If no further dilution is required, the correct amount of the drug is withdrawn, using sterile technique, at the time the drug is to be administered. If any unused portion remains in the vial, label with the date and time and initial. Store in the recommended manner.

Single doses of drugs, particularly those administered by injection, are sometimes available in prefilled syringes. Some prefilled units come preassembled and ready to use; with others, the drug is in a glass cartridge which must be threaded into a plastic barrel with attached needle. Still others come in disposable cartridges which are inserted into reusable metal holders (Fig. 8-8). Not only are prefilled syringes convenient and timesaving, but they reduce the chance of dosage error and minimize the likelihood of contamination.

Drugs in dry powder form

Drugs supplied in powdered form to extend their stability are generally made available in vials for either single or multiple use. To reconstitute the drug, the following procedure is followed:

1. After determining the dose and concentration required, withdraw the appropriate volume of

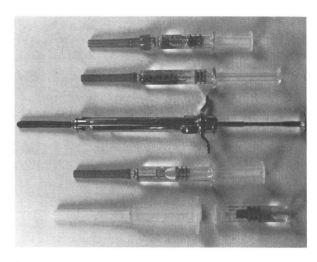

Fig. 8-8. Prefilled syringes offer both convenience and safety in the administration of injectable drugs.

recommended diluent aseptically into a syringe. When special diluents are required they are generally supplied with the drug in a separate ampul.

2. Cleanse the rubber stopper with alcohol, insert the needle, and inject the diluent into the vial. Coring of the rubber stopper can be minimized by holding the needle bevel up at a 45° to 60° angle before inserting it into the vial (as described earlier in this chapter).

3. Mix the contents *thoroughly* until the drug is completely dissolved. Be sure that there is no haze or visible particles.

4. Withdraw the desired volume of solution from the vial. If sterility has been maintained, the same syringe can be used.

5. If additional doses remain in the vial, label it with the following information: date and time the drug was reconstituted; concentration (e.g., 1 ml. = 50 mg.); and initials of the person who prepared the drug.

Store the drug as recommended by the manufacturer and in the drug section in the back of this book. In most cases refrigeration will be required. Follow recommendations regarding length of time the reconstituted drug remains stable, and discard any unused portion as soon as it expires.

Correct labeling and storage are essential to insure that when subsequent doses are given, the dose will be correct and the drug will still be stable. Any drug found unlabeled in the refrigerator

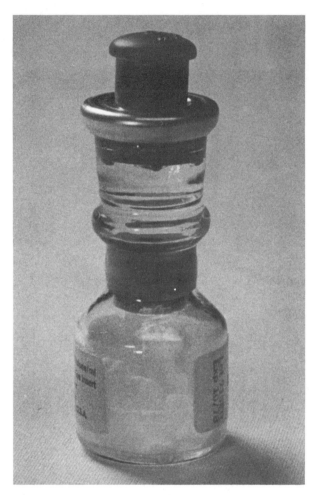

Fig. 8–9. Mix-O-Vial. Double-compartment vials allow rapid reconstitution of a drug without the need of a syringe and needle. (The Upjohn Company, Kalamazoo, Michigan 49001)

or outside of the refrigerator for an undetermined period of time must be discarded.

Reconstituting drugs in special types of vials

DOUBLE-COMPARTMENT VIALS

Occasionally, drugs which require a special diluent are packaged in a double-chambered vial with the powdered drug in the lower chamber and the liquid diluent in the upper chamber (Fig. 8-9). The two compartments are separated by a rubber plug. When pressure is applied to the rubber stopper on top of the vial, the plug inside the vial is dislocated, allowing the diluent to enter the lower chamber. Once this has occurred, mix as with any vial, insuring that the powder is completely dissolved before withdrawing the drug.

PUMP-ACTION VIALS

These are vials with a rubber extension on the top, connected to a plastic spike or piercing pin. Such vials are used for medications which are added to large volume infusions. The advantage is that the drug can be reconstituted by using the solution from the infusion bottle as diluent. Since no other vial or syringe and needle are required, the likelihood of contamination is reduced. Steps include (27):

1. Cleanse the rubber stopper or latex disc on the infusion bottle with alcohol or other agent.
2. Remove the cover from the plastic spike and insert the spike into the stopper site of the infusion bottle.
3. Invert the solution bottle and pump the vial to allow some solution to enter the vial.
4. Carefully agitate the vial until the powder is completely dissolved.
5. Turn the infusion bottle upright again and pump the vial to eject the drug into the infusion bottle. (Steps 3 through 5 can be repeated to insure removal of all the drug.)
6. Label the infusion bottle as described below.

ADDITIVE PIGGYBACK VIALS

A few drugs, primarily antibiotics administered by intermittent infusion, are supplied in vials which can be attached to administration tubing and used to infuse the drug, piggybacked into the main intravenous line (Fig. 8-10). To reconstitute the drug, the same technique can be used as for any standard vial.

After thorough mixing, the secondary administration tubing is inserted through the rubber stopper of the vial. While inserting it, avoid angling or twisting in order to prevent coring. Attach a needle to the end of the tubing. If the administration set does not contain an air inlet, a needle will have to be inserted through the rubber stopper of the vial. The vial is suspended from the intravenous pole by means of either a plastic hanger affixed to the bottom of the vial or by a plastic bag into which the bottle is set.

An alternative reconstitution technique for additive piggyback vials is the backfill method which involves using the fluid from the primary container as the diluent. It is essential that the primary fluid and any additives be compatible with the drug. To use the backfill technique (2):

1. Attach the secondary administration set to the medication container as just described and close the clamp.
2. After cleansing the injection site on the primary tubing with alcohol or other recommended disinfectant, insert the needle from the end of the secondary tubing into the injection site.
3. Lower the medication vial well below the level of the primary container.
4. Open the clamp to allow the recommended amount of fluid to enter the medication vial.
5. Mix thoroughly until the drug is completely dissolved.
6. Close the clamp and hang the secondary container on the IV pole at a level of 6 to 8 inches above the primary container. (The primary container can be lowered by using an extension hook.)
7. Label the bottle as described below.
8. Adjust the flow-control clamp to attain the desired flow rate.

Technique for preparation of admixtures

An admixture is an intravenous fluid to which one or more drugs have been added. Admixture preparation requires strict attention to the three factors discussed above: maintenance of sterility, prevention of incompatibilities, and insurance of accurate dosage.

Once compatibility has been ascertained and the drug additives are prepared, the drugs are aseptically added to the infusion container following one of the techniques described here.

ADDING DRUGS TO GLASS INFUSION BOTTLES (VENTED AND NONVENTED)

1. Using a Syringe and Needle
   a) With the bottle in an upright position, cleanse the rubber stopper (for nonvented bottles) or latex disc (for vented bottles) with alcohol or other recommended agent.
   b) Insert the needle through the rubber stopper (center in nonvented bottles; administration set site in vented bottles).
   c) Inject the medication.

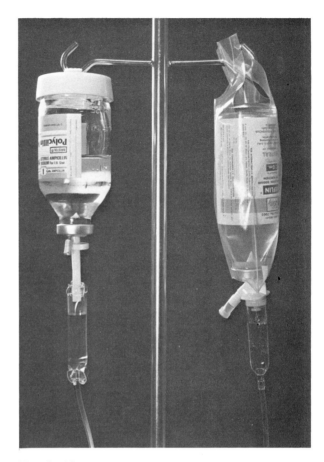

Fig. 8–10. Additive piggyback vials, after reconstitution, are attached directly to the administration tubing, preventing the need for transfer of the drug. (*Left:* Bristol Laboratories, Syracuse, New York 13201; *right:* Eli Lilly and Company, Indianapolis, Indiana 46206)

   d) Invert the bottle to insure thorough mixing.
   e) If an additional drug is to be added, repeat Steps a through d. Always thoroughly mix one drug before adding another one.
   f) Under adequate light with both a black and white background, check the admixture for cloudiness or particulate matter.
   g) Label the bottle in accordance with the recommendations of the National Coordinating Committee on Large Volume Parenterals (38):
      (1) Patient's name, hospital identification number, and room number
      (2) Primary solution
      (3) Additives, including strength and amount
      (4) Preparation date and time

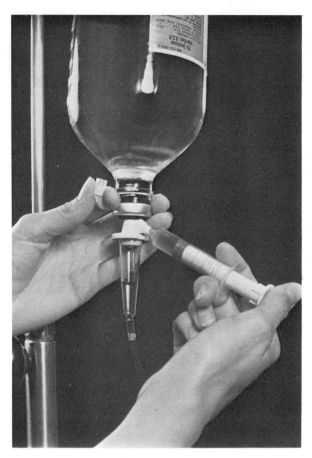

Fig. 8–11. Addition of a drug to a nonvented container while it is infusing. Thorough mixing *must* follow.

(5) Bottle number or pharmacy preparation number

(6) Flow rate, expressed in milliliters per hour and drops per minute

(7) Time bottle starts infusing and time it should be completed

(8) Name of person preparing the admixture (and of the person hanging the infusion container if a different individual)

(9) Expiration date and time if the admixture is prepared in advance

(10) Any special precautions required

Items (9) and (10) are generally included only when the admixture is prepared in the pharmacy.

To insure that all essential information is included, yet to save time when admixtures are prepared by the nursing staff, printed labels can be obtained with spaces designated for all required

information. Some labels can later be removed from the bottle and incorporated into the patient's chart as a permanent record of fluids and drugs administered.

ADDITION OF DRUGS TO BOTTLES THAT ARE INFUSING

Ideally, drugs should be added to the container before it has started to infuse. In certain situations, such as an unexpected change in the patient's condition, a drug may be ordered to be added to the currently infusing bottle. This can be done as long as there is a sufficient volume left in the bottle to insure adequate dilution (e.g., 40 milliequivalents of potassium chloride should not be added to less than 500 milliliters of fluid). To prevent contamination, the administration set should not be removed from the container once it has been attached. Each type of fluid system incorporates a site for subsequent addition of medications.

1. *Nonvented Bottles* (Abbott*, Cutter†)
   a) Medications can be added with the bottle in either the upright or inverted (infusing) position (Fig. 8-11). The inverted position allows an uninterrupted flow but may create the potential for the infusion of a bolus of the drug unless thoroughly mixed.
   b) Remove air filter from the administration set (above the drip chamber), being careful to maintain its sterility.
   c) Disconnect the syringe from the needle and insert syringe into the air inlet.
   d) Inject the medication.
   e) Replace the air filter. *Failure to do so will allow unfiltered air to enter the bottle and contaminate the system.*
   f) Mix thoroughly by rotating the bottle from the inverted to an upright position several times.
   g) Relabel bottle as necessary including name and dose of drug added.
2. *Vented Bottles* (Travenol**, McGaw‡)
   a) The bottle can be in either an upright or inverted position but preferably upright.
   b) Cleanse the medication site (target area) on

---

*Abbott Laboratories, North Chicago, Illinois 60064
†Cutter Laboratories, Berkeley, California 94710
**Travenol Laboratories, Deerfield, Illinois 60015
‡McGaw Laboratories, Division of American Hospital Supply Corporation, Irvine, California 92714

rubber stopper with alcohol or other recommended disinfectant.

c) Insert the needle through the medication site and inject the medication.

d) Withdraw needle and mix thoroughly by rotating bottle from upright to inverted position several times.

e) Relabel bottle as necessary including name and dose of drug added.

ADDING MEDICATIONS DIRECTLY FROM THE VIAL WITH A DOUBLE NEEDLE

Among the timesaving methods available is the direct transfer of a medication from a vial to the infusion bottle using a double needle. Considerable time is saved by eliminating the need to withdraw the contents into a syringe. However, with drugs in powdered form, reconstitution must be done first. Other limitations of the double-needle technique are:

1. It can only be used with fluid containers in which a vacuum is present, so it cannot be used once a bottle is infusing.
2. This method does not allow for use of a syringe filter to remove any particulate matter that may be in a vial.
3. The entire contents of the vial must be added since the amount entering the bottle cannot be measured or controlled (27).

To use the double-needle method (Fig. 8-12):

1. Cleanse the rubber stoppers on the medication vial and infusion bottle (latex seal on vented bottles) with alcohol or other recommended disinfectant.
2. Remove the double needle from the package. Holding the plastic or metal centerpiece, insert the exposed (shorter) end into the vial, using the same technique as with a regular needle to avoid coring (see p. 124). The needle must *never* be inserted into the infusion bottle first, or the vacuum will escape; and the transfer will not be successful.
3. Holding the centerpiece of the needle, remove the protective needle cover. Avoiding contamination of the needle is essential.
4. Insert the needle into the rubber stopper of the infusion bottle. Allow the medication to be drawn into the bottle by the vacuum.

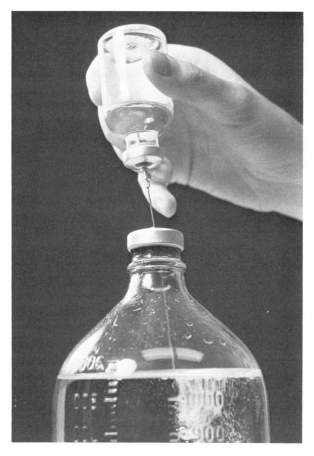

Fig. 8-12. Double-needle technique for transfer of a drug from the vial to an infusion bottle.

5. Remove the needle and vial and mix medication thoroughly.
6. Label the bottle as described above.

USING AN ADDITIVE VIAL WITH A TRANSFER SPIKE (Fig. 8-13)

These vials are constructed with a piercing pin, similar to those of some administration sets, on top of the rubber stopper. They can be used with any container in which the vacuum is intact. Thus, with vented bottles, the latex disc must be kept in place; and like the double-needle technique, it cannot be used once a bottle is infusing. The suggested procedure is:

1. Place the bottle in the upright position.
2. Cleanse the rubber stopper (or latex disc on vented bottles) with alcohol or other recommended disinfectant.

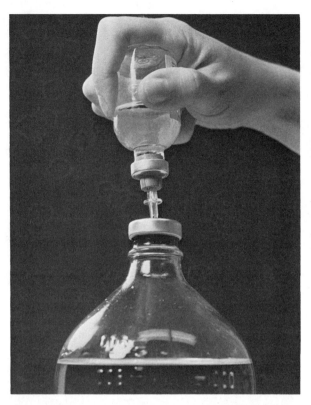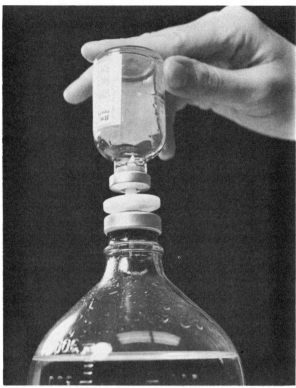

Fig. 8–13. Transfer of a drug to a glass container using a vial with a transfer spike. (*Left*) Inserting the piercing pin through the rubber stopper of the bottle. (*Right*) As pressure is applied, the pin punctures the stopper inside the vial, allowing the drug to be drawn into the bottle.

3. Remove the protective cap from the piercing pin.
4. Invert the vial with the piercing pin centered over the rubber stopper (over administration set site for vented bottles).
5. Using a firm, downward motion, thrust the pin through the rubber stopper. Avoid twisting or angling as it can create cored particles. The pin inside the vial stopper will simultaneously puncture a seal, allowing the medication to flow into the infusion bottle.
6. Remove the vial and mix thoroughly.
7. Label the bottle as described above.

If the vacuum has been lost or only part of the medication dose is required, these vials can be adapted to use with a syringe:

1. Remove the piercing pin from the vial by grasping the top. As long as the rubber stopper is not touched, sterility will be maintained.
2. Insert needle through the well in the center of the stopper and withdraw desired dose as with any vial.

USING A PUMP-ACTION VIAL

As described above, the pump-action vial is used for certain drugs supplied in a powdered form. It allows reconstitution using solution from the infusion bottle and does not depend on a vacuum. For use of this type of vial, follow the steps described on page 136.

ADDING DRUGS TO FLEXIBLE PLASTIC FLUID CONTAINERS (ABBOTT*, TRAVENOL†)

The two types of flexible plastic containers currently available have separate medication ports for the addition of drugs. In one brand (Travenol Viaflex), the medication port is at the end of the bag adjacent to the administration set port. With

---

*Abbott Laboratories, North Chicago, Illinois 60064
†Travenol Laboratories, Deerfield, Illinois 60015

the other type (Abbott LifeCare), the medication port is on the side.

While one manufacturer states that medications can be added either before use with the bag lying flat or during infusion with the bag hanging, the latter practice is not recommended. A study has shown that when drugs are added to a plastic container in the infusion position, poor mixing can result unless the solution is thoroughly mixed by *inverting* and *agitating* the container (9). Failure to do so can result in the patient's receiving a bolus of the additive. Instances of this occurring with potassium chloride have been reported, with the patients experiencing seizure activity as a result (54). Thus, to eliminate this possibility, drugs should always be added with the bag lying on a flat surface or in the upright position, though the flexibility of the bag makes the latter position somewhat awkward.

1. Using a Syringe and Needle (Fig. 8-14)
    a) Cleanse the rubber medication port with alcohol or other recommended disinfectant.
    b) Stabilize the medication port by grasping the tubing (with Viaflex container) or protective collar (with LifeCare).
    c) Using a 21 or 22 gauge (1¼ to 1½ inch) needle, puncture the center of the entry port until the needle is almost fully inserted. The depth of the LifeCare additive port prevents puncturing of the bag.
    d) Inject the medication and withdraw the needle.
    e) Squeeze the medication port to evacuate all of the medication.
    f) Mix thoroughly by inverting and agitating the bag several times.
    g) Label the container as described above (p. 137).
2. Using a Universal Additive Syringe (Abbott). This is a prefilled syringe with a plastic hood or shield extending about one-half inch around the needle (Fig. 8-15). The protective hood surrounding the needle helps to minimize touch contamination, and the design enables it to be used with any type of container: vented and nonvented glass bottles, and plastic containers. No vacuum is required. The technique used is basically the same as with any syringe and needle.
3. Adding Medications Directly from a Vial Using a Double Needle. Since plastic containers have

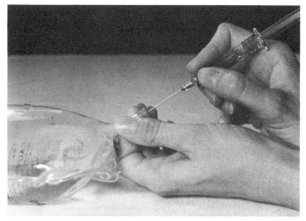
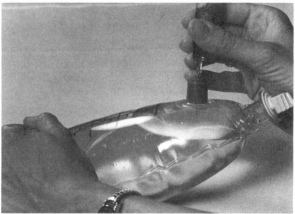

Fig. 8-14. Addition of a medication to a flexible plastic fluid container. (*Top*) Viaflex (Travenol Laboratories, Inc., Deerfield, Illinois 60015). (*Bottom*) LifeCare (Abbott Laboratories, North Chicago, Illinois 60064)

no vacuum, the use of a double needle or similar technique requires a special device to create a vacuum within the bag. Such devices are available for both the Viaflex (Travenol) and LifeCare (Abbott) containers. While the specific steps vary somewhat between the two brands, the general procedure for adding medications is as follows:
    a) Place the bag inside the vacuum unit allowing the medication port to protrude through the designated opening.
    b) Turn on the vacuum pump to allow the vacuum to be created.
    c) Cleanse the top of the vial and the medication port of container with alcohol or other recommended agent.
    d) Remove the double needle from its package and insert the exposed end into the vial.

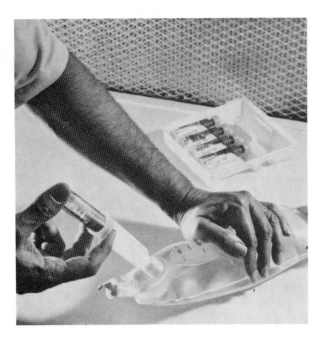

Fig. 8–15. Using a Universal Additive Syringe to transfer a drug to a fluid container. (Courtesy of Abbott Laboratories, North Chicago, Illinois 60064).

e) Remove the protective cover from the other end of the needle and, once the vacuum has been created, insert the needle into the medication port and allow solution to be drawn into bag (Fig. 8-16).

f) Allow the vacuum to be released (in accordance with the manufacturer's specific directions), and remove the needle and vial. After removing the bag from the vacuum unit, invert and agitate the bag to mix thoroughly and inspect for particulate matter.

g) Label the container as described above (p. 137).

One type of unit (Viavac, Travenol) allows both reconstitution and transfer of a drug using the double-needle technique. The vacuum is present while the unit is in a vertical position but is released when the unit is horizontal. Thus, once the needle has been inserted into the medication port, the unit is placed in the horizontal position (Fig. 8-17). This allows solution to flow from the fluid container into the vial. With gentle agitation, the solution is mixed until the drug is dissolved. The unit is then returned to the upright position

recreating a vacuum, thus drawing the drug from the vial into the bag. All other steps remain the same as described above.

In most institutions, such vacuum units are probably limited to the pharmacy or to patient units where large numbers of admixtures are prepared.

ADDING DRUGS TO SEMIRIGID PLASTIC CONTAINERS

A semirigid plastic container has recently become available (Accumed, McGaw*). As described in Chapter 3, this type of container is similar in

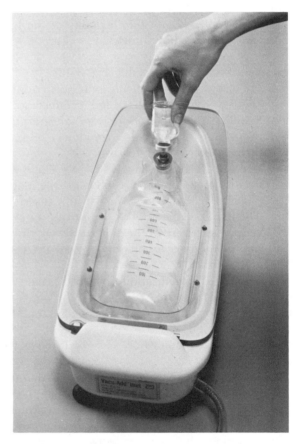

Fig. 8–16. Vacu-Add unit enables the direct transfer of a drug from a vial to a LifeCare flexible fluid container. (Courtesy of Abbott Laboratories, North Chicago, Illinois 60064)

*McGaw Laboratories. Division of American Hospital Supply Corporation; Irvine, California 92714.

some respects to other plastic containers (light-weight and unbreakable), yet shares some properties with glass bottles (more accurate calibrations, impermeable to moisture).

A medication port is provided adjacent to the administration set port. To add medications to these containers, the same basic steps are followed as for glass containers, using a syringe and needle. Since there is no vacuum present, medications cannot be added using a double needle or additive vial with spike.

MODES OF INTRAVENOUS ADMINISTRATION

Having discussed the preparation of drugs and admixtures, we shall now describe their actual administration. The intravenous route of drug administration encompasses three distinct modes which determine the concentration and rate at which a drug will actually be delivered to the patient. With many drugs a particular mode is required, either for efficacy (to achieve the desired pharmacologic effects) or for safety (to prevent adverse reactions). The three modes of administration are:

1. Continuous infusion
2. Intermittent infusion
3. Direct injection

Continuous infusion

This mode involves giving the drug in a relatively large volume of fluid (250 to 1000 milliliters) and infusing it continuously over a period of several hours or days. This mode is employed with:

1. Drugs which must be highly diluted, such as potassium chloride, dopamine (Intropin), and amphotericin B (Fungizone).
2. Drugs which require maintenance of steady blood levels, such as oxytocin (Pitocin) and nitroprusside (Nipride).
3. Replacement of large volumes of fluids and electrolytes.
4. Total parenteral nutrition, the provision of all nutrients intravenously for individuals who cannot ingest or digest food via the gastrointestinal system.

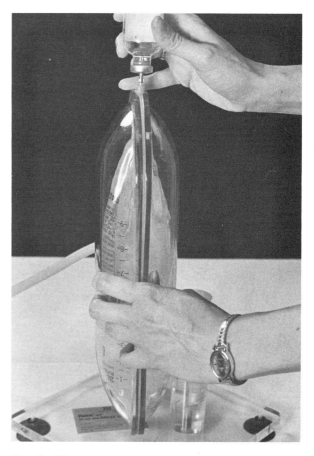

Fig. 8-17. Viavac unit allows both reconstitution and transfer of a drug to a Viaflex container using a double-needle technique. (Travenol Laboratories, Inc., Deerfield, Illinois 60015)

This mode is unsuitable for drugs that are incompatible with other drugs and solutions or for drugs that require a peak blood level to be effective.

Drugs commonly administered by continuous infusion, such as electrolytes, vitamins, and albumin, which do not present a high risk of adverse effects, can be given as the primary infusion. Once the specified dose of medication has been added to the container (as described above), the administration set is attached and then connected to the hub of the cannula or needle in the usual manner, taking care to preserve sterility of all components. After initial adjustment of the flow rate, the infusion should be checked several times during the first hour to insure that the correct rate is being maintained.

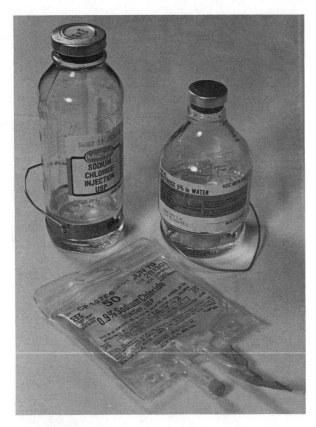

Fig. 8–18. Partially filled fluid containers for piggyback administration of drugs. (*Clockwise from upper left:* McGaw Laboratories, Division of American Hospital Supply Corporation, Irvine, California 92714; Abbott Laboratories, North Chicago, Illinois 60064; Travenol Laboratories, Inc., Deerfield, Illinois 60015)

An alternate method is recommended for drugs associated with rapid changes in vital signs, cardiac arrhythmias, or other untoward physiological responses. These include drugs such as potent vasopressors, antihypertensives, and antiarrhythmics such as lidocaine. Such drugs should be delivered via a secondary fluid source and administration tubing connected to the injection port of the primary tubing (piggybacked). This allows the medication in the secondary bottle either to infuse alone, with the primary fluid on standby in case adverse effects occur and the medication has to be discontinued immediately, or to infuse simultaneously with the primary fluid.

Simultaneous infusion of the medication and the primary fluid can be accomplished by using either a Y-type administration set (one administration tubing which is used with two containers simultaneously) or a standard set with a Y-injection site. With the latter, it is important that the administration set *not* have a check valve, or else the valve will shut off the flow of primary fluid while the medication is infusing. With either type of setup, the two bottles should be hanging at the same height. However, the potential hazard of this type of setup is that should one of the bottles run dry, air can be drawn into the tubing and ultimately into the patient. Thus, close observation is required when this type of system is used.

Intermittent infusion

Some drugs are most effective when a specific dose is given one time or is repeated at fixed intervals around the clock. Each dose is added to a relatively small volume of fluid, varying from 50 to 200 milliliters, depending primarily on the properties of the drug itself as well as on the age and fluid requirements of the patient. The medication is infused over a period of from 20 minutes to 2 hours, initially producing a peak blood level which tapers off before the next dose is given. Drugs such as antibiotics are able to exert their therapeutic activity while the drug level is at its peak; yet it is speculated that the likelihood of the organism developing resistance to the drug is reduced when the drug level diminishes between doses (20).

Two basic techniques are available to administer drugs by intermittent infusion: the piggyback method and volume control units.

PIGGYBACK METHOD

For the majority of drugs given by intermittent infusion, 50 or 100 milliliters of fluid is recommended to dilute the drug. Partially filled glass bottles and plastic containers are available with those volumes of the fluids most commonly used for dilution. There is sufficient space in these containers to allow the addition and mixing of the drug (Fig. 8-18). Except for their small size, these containers are like the standard-sized bottles and bags insofar as adding the drug and attaching the administration set.

The preferred piggyback technique involves the use of a primary administration set which incorporates a check valve just above the Y-type injection port. The check valve allows automatic shutoff of the primary fluid while the medication is infusing and resumption of the primary fluid once the medication has completely infused. To administer a dose of medication, the following procedure is followed (2). (Fig. 8-19):

1. Using aseptic technique, attach a secondary administration set to the container with the medication, and attach a needle to the end of the set.
2. Suspend the secondary container 6 to 8 inches above the primary container. (It may be easier to lower the primary container by means of an extension hook.)
3. After clearing the tubing of air, cleanse the injection site of the primary tubing with alcohol, and insert the needle.
4. Adjust the flow rate of the secondary bottle (medication) by means of the single flow clamp located below the injection site.

As the secondary container begins infusing, pressure exerted against the check valve closes it, shutting off the flow from the primary container. Once the secondary container has infused, the pressure between the two sets equalizes, opening the check valve and re-establishing the flow from the primary bottle. This eliminates the need for the nurse to be present when the secondary container finishes infusing since automatic resumption in flow prevents air from entering the primary tubing and clotting of the cannula. However, since there is only one flow control clamp, the primary fluid will resume at the flow rate set for the medication. Thus, when the nurse returns following the infusion to check for adverse reactions, a flow-rate adjustment may be needed.

The residual medication remaining in the secondary tubing can be infused by temporarily pinching off the primary tubing above the check valve and releasing it when the fluid reaches the end of the secondary tubing near the needle. Care must be taken to prevent air from entering the primary line.

Once a dose has been administered, the secondary container and tubing can be discarded; or if it is to be used for subsequent doses, it is kept attached to the secondary bottle. When the next dose is due:

1. Reprime the secondary tubing by closing the flow control clamp and lowering the empty secondary container, allowing fluid from the primary container to fill the tubing and proceed halfway up the drip chamber.
2. Prepare the container with the next dose of medication.

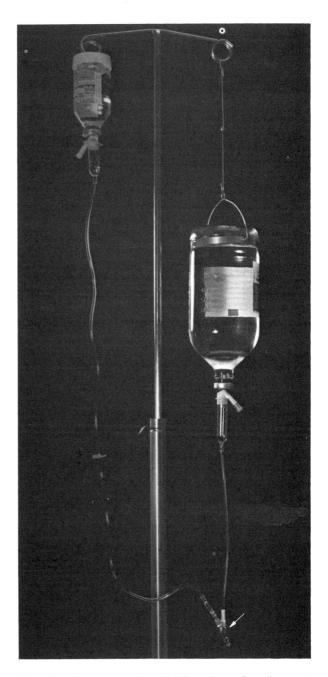

Fig. 8-19. Piggyback administration of a drug. A check-valve at the Y-injection site prevents backflow of medication into the primary container and allows the primary fluid to resume flow after the medication has infused.

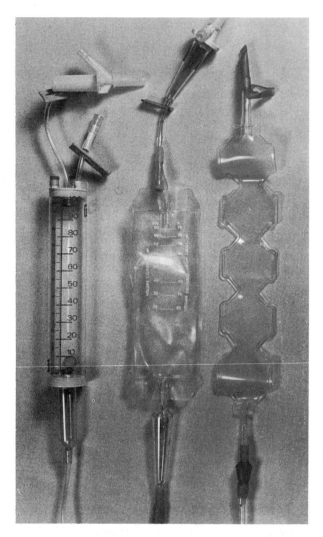

Fig. 8-20. Several types of volume-control sets, (*From left*: Soluset, Abbott Laboratories, North Chicago, Illinois 60064; Volu-Trole-A, Cutter Laboratories, Inc., Berkeley, California 94710; Pedatrol, Travenol Laboratories, Inc., Deerfield, Illinois 60015)

3. Using aseptic technique, remove the piercing pin from the empty container and insert into the new secondary container.
4. Suspend the secondary bottle and open the flow clamp to establish flow of the medication.

An alternative method involves the use of an administration set which does not have a check valve. The system is set up in essentially the same manner, but the primary fluid does not automatically shut off. Either the two solutions can infuse simultaneously, which increases the risk of incompatibilities; or the primary fluid can be manually shut off by closing the clamp above the injection site. In the latter instance, the nurse must return to the patient almost immediately after the medication has infused to prevent air from entering the line as well as clotting of the cannula.

While the "automatic" piggyback technique using the administration set with the check valve does not replace the need for the nurse to monitor the patient who is receiving intravenous medications, it does allow flexibility by eliminating the need to return at a precise time.

Since the piggyback method uses a separate fluid container for each dose of medication, it is somewhat more expensive; but the risk of contamination is reduced.

VOLUME-CONTROL SETS

Another means of delivering drugs intermittently is with a calibrated chamber or burette. This device, which generally consists of a semirigid plastic cylinder with a capacity of 100 to 250 milliliters, is most useful when the volume of fluids and medications must be precisely monitored. Thus, this type of set is frequently used with infants and children. Models are available to deliver 10 drops per milliliter or 60 drops per milliliter (Fig. 8-20).

The burette chamber is connected to a fluid container from which the chamber is filled as required. That fluid may serve as the primary line and provide a continuous flow to keep the vein open between doses of medication. In other instances, the burette chamber and fluid source may represent a secondary line which is piggybacked into the injection site of the primary administration set and is utilized only when doses of the medication are administered. To administer a first dose of drug:

1. Attach the volume control set to the fluid container in the same manner as with any administration set, closing the flow clamp first.
2. Partially fill the burette chamber by opening the clamp above the chamber; then open the main flow control clamp to flush air from the tubing.
3. Fill the burette chamber with the recommended volume of fluid needed to dilute the drug.
4. Cleanse the latex injection port at the top of

the burette with alcohol or other recommended disinfectant.

5. Add the medication, which has already been reconstituted and drawn up in a syringe, by inserting the needle through the injection port and injecting into the burette chamber (Fig. 8-21). In units such as Volu-Trole-A (Cutter), in which the injection site enters the *tubing* above the burette chamber rather than the burette itself, it is necessary to flush the tubing with a small amount of fluid to insure that the full dose of drug has entered the chamber (19).

6. Gently agitate the burette chamber to thoroughly mix the drug.

7. Attach a needle to the end of the tubing below the burette chamber; and after cleansing the injection site of the primary tubing, insert the needle into the injection port.

8. Adjust the flow control clamp below the burette chamber to establish the desired flow rate.

9. After the dose of medication has infused, in many models the flow will automatically shut off due to a rubber diaphragm or a membrane filter at the bottom of the burette chamber. This prevents air from entering the line.

10. The residual medication in the chamber and tubing can be removed by flushing with a small amount of fluid from the secondary bottle.

If the burette chamber is attached to the primary fluid container, it is necessary for the keep-open flow to be re-established as soon as the medication has infused. This is accomplished by closing the air-filter clamp (on top of the chamber) and opening the clamp between the fluid container and burette chamber. The desired flow rate is maintained by adjusting the flow control clamp *below* the burette chamber. To prevent automatic shutoff, approximately 25 milliliters of fluid should be maintained within the chamber (4).

If the volume-control set is used as a secondary line, it can be piggybacked into either a standard administration set or an administration set with a check valve as described above. When combined with the piggyback method, the volume-control chamber can be used with one fluid container for several doses. One set can be used for the *separate* administration of more than one drug, provided

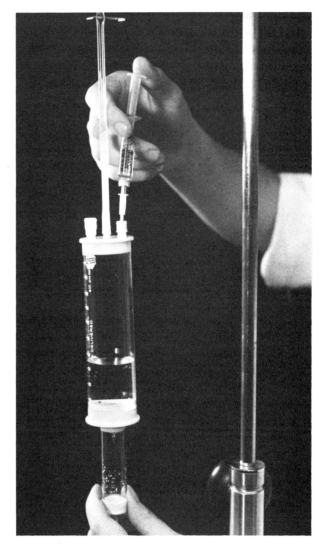

Fig. 8-21. Volu-Trole-B. Intermittent administration of a drug using a volume control set. (Cutter Laboratories, Inc., Berkeley, California 94710)

that the fluid used is compatible with each drug and that the chamber and tubing are flushed with fluid after each dose.

The major advantages of the volume-control unit are the decreased cost to the patient and reduced nursing time (42) However, because of the increased number of manipulations required, there exists a greater potential for contamination.

One group of investigators cite studies which attributed medication errors to the use of volume-control sets (25). The errors cited ranged from omitted or incomplete doses to incompatibilities. It would seem that most of these errors resulted from practices and procedures utilized rather than from the volume-control units themselves. However, because of the increased potential for problems, particularly contamination, the routine use of volume-control sets for the intermittent administration of medications has been discouraged by the National Coordinating Committee on Large Volume Parenterals (38).

Nonetheless, situations remain in which volume-control sets are of value, particularly in the pediatric setting as mentioned above. Such sets provide a means of monitoring the volume of medications and fluids more precisely than with standard containers. Use of a set which is calibrated to deliver 60 drops per milliliter enables the maintenance of very slow flow rates; and should the rate inadvertently increase, the size of the chamber limits the volume that can rapidly be infused.

In pediatrics and other settings in which volume-control sets are used, their safety can be greatly increased by rigorous attention to the manufacturer's recommendations and strict adherence to infection-control measures, including changing of the set and fluid container every 24 hours.

An alternative to the burette chamber type of volume-control set is a device called Pedatrol. Used primarily for the precise control of fluid volumes administered to infants and children, this device consists of five vertically arranged collapsible chambers, each holding 10 milliliters of fluid. The device is used with a standard nonvented administration set (Fig. 8-20). A clamp placed between two of the chambers (determined by the total volume to be administered) creates a closed system, thus preventing air entry after the chambers have emptied. (44)

Direct injection

The third mode of intravenous administration involves injecting by means of a syringe and needle a small volume of a drug directly into the intravenous tubing or cannula or occasionally directly into the vein.

The injection may be instantaneous, taking only the time required to push the plunger of the syringe. Such a rapid injection is referred to as a *bolus* and is used with drugs which must be delivered to the vital organs, primarily the heart and brain, in maximal concentrations. Examples include diazoxide (Hyperstat), a potent, rapidly acting antihypertensive agent, and lidocaine (Xylocaine), an antiarrhythmic.

Most drugs given by intravenous injection, however, cannot be administered as a bolus because the rapid serum concentrations achieved can result in adverse reactions, including seizures, shock, and cardiac arrest. These drugs are given by slow injection, commonly referred to as "IV push." The dose of the drug is administered gradually over a 1- to 2-minute period.

Because of the greater risk of adverse effects, this mode of administration is usually limited to the physician. Exceptions include nurses in critical care areas who, after attainment of a certain level of skill, are generally authorized to administer specific drugs by injection under certain emergency situations. Nurses assigned to oncology units or clinics often give cancer chemotherapy agents by injection (23). It is essential that each hospital establish a written policy for intravenous injections by nurses, including areas where it is allowed, a roster of nurses who have been authorized to give intravenous injections, and a list of drugs allowed in each area.

For nurses who do administer direct intravenous injections, these guidelines are suggested:

1. Injections are usually administered into the injection site of an established intravenous line. Before injecting the drug, it is imperative to confirm the presence of the cannula within the vein, particularly for drugs which cause tissue necrosis.
2. Cleanse the injection site with alcohol or other recommended disinfectant.
3. Insert the needle and syringe containing the drug.
4. Pinch off the tubing above the injection site and attempt to aspirate blood.
5. When a flashback of blood occurs, inject the drug at the appropriate rate. (The drug information section in the back of this text includes recommended rates for each drug.) If presence of the cannula within the vein cannot be confirmed, insert an intravenous line elsewhere or notify the physician in accordance with hospital policy.
6. If an incompatibility exists between the drug and the primary fluid, it is necessary to flush the lower tubing with a compatible solution

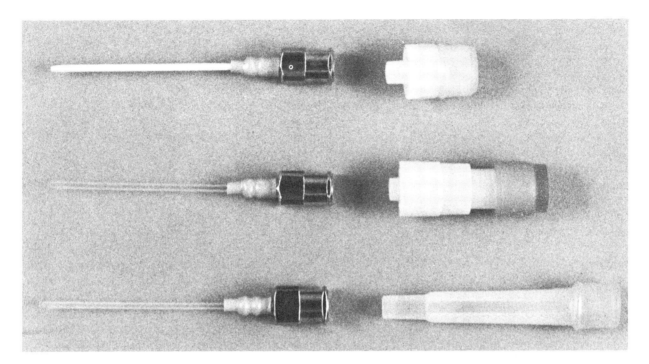

Fig. 8-22. Several types of adaptor plugs which convert a standard over-the-needle cannula into a heparin lock.

both before and after administering the drug. An alternate method is to inject the drug directly into the cannula as described on page 133.

7. When incompatibility is *not* a problem, the primary solution should be run at a rapid rate for a few seconds after the drug is given to insure that the total dose has been delivered.

If no intravenous line is present, a drug may be injected directly into a vein using a syringe and needle. This method is sometimes used for single or isolated doses of drugs, particularly in emergency situations, such as 50 percent dextrose given to patients in hypoglycemic shock or diazepam (Valium) given to patients experiencing seizures. Once venipuncture is performed in the standard manner and the presence of the needle within the vein is assured, the drug is injected at the prescribed rate. Unless the patient is able to cooperate and remain still during the injection, there is a considerable risk of infiltration due to the rigidity of the needle. Thus, drugs which produce necrosis of the subcutaneous tissues should not be given in this manner. For this reason cancer chemotherapy agents which are usually given in isolated doses require the insertion of a winged-needle unit (scalp-vein needle) to insure their safe administration.

Heparin locks

Repeated doses of an intravenous drug such as heparin or antibiotics may be required for a patient who does not need an intravenous line for the continuous infusion of either fluids or drugs. For such patients, the insertion of an intermittent infusion device, known as a heparin lock, is desirable. The standard heparin lock consists of a winged-infusion needle with a short length of tubing (usually 2 to 3 inches) terminating in a resealable rubber injection port (Fig. 3-7, p. 30). Common sites for insertion are the dorsum of the hand or the forearm, depending on the size of the needle required. The insertion technique is described in Chapter 4.

A standard winged-needle unit (scalp-vein needle) or short, over-the-needle catheter can be converted into a heparin lock by using an adaptor plug which consists of a short male adaptor with a resealable injection cap (Fig. 8-22). After it is securely inserted into the cannula hub, the unit is heparinized (flushed with heparinized saline) and used as a standard heparin lock.

The heparin lock provides several advantages for the patient who needs a patent intravenous line for intermittent delivery of drugs but who does not require continuous infusion of fluids or drugs.

SAFETY

The risk of fluid overload is eliminated, and the chance of electrolyte imbalance is minimized. By eliminating the fluid source and administration set, the likelihood of contamination and subsequent infection is also reduced.

COMFORT

For the ambulatory patient, a heparin lock affords greater freedom of movement and easier performance of normal daily activities. For the bedfast individual, such as the patient with a myocardial infarction whose intravenous line is required as a precautionary measure, the elimination of the fluid container and tubing can reduce anxiety during the initial period in the coronary care unit when he is connected to many other pieces of equipment. Later, as he begins to ambulate and resume other activities, he will not be restricted by an IV pole, yet will have an intravenous line should an arrhythmia or other complication occur.

The heparin lock spares the patient the discomfort of having a separate venipuncture each time a dose of the medication is due or being subjected to unpleasant intramuscular injections when the drug can also be given by that route.

When during the course of therapy frequent blood samples are required, they can be obtained via the heparin lock, thus reducing the need for venipunctures, a procedure which can become increasingly difficult and painful as available veins become scarce. The major concern with obtaining blood samples from a heparin lock is clearing the lock of the heparinized saline before the sample is withdrawn because of the dilutional effect and, in some cases, interference with the test itself. Clearing the lock can be done by inserting a needle and syringe into the lock and aspirating until approximately one half to 1 milliliter of blood is withdrawn. This sample is discarded. Using a new syringe and needle, the

blood sample is then withdrawn. It is also essential to re-heparinize the heparin lock after the blood is withdrawn.

ECONOMY

The heparin lock is considerably more economical for administration of drugs by injection since the fluid container and administration set can be eliminated. For drugs being given by intermittent infusion, the primary fluid container and administration set are saved. Since these items are changed at least every 24 hours, the total savings per patient, per days hospitalized, can be considerable.

The savings in terms of nursing time can also be significant, particularly in institutions which utilize a pharmacy-based admixture program. If the medication is prepared and added to the fluid container in the pharmacy, the nurse's primary responsibility, besides monitoring for adverse reactions, is to attach the set to the heparin lock and return as soon as the medication has infused to re-heparinize the lock. The time required to maintain the total intravenous system, including maintenance of the prescribed flow rate and changing the fluid container and administration set each day, is conserved. These duties are also eliminated in hospitals in which drug preparation remains a nursing function.

INJECTION OF A DRUG VIA THE HEPARIN LOCK

1. Cleanse the rubber injection site with alcohol or other suitable disinfectant.
2. Insert the needle and syringe containing the prepared drug into the injection site. Use as small a gauge needle as possible (22 or 25 gauge) to insure complete resealing after multiple punctures.
3. Verify the presence of the needle within the vein by pulling back slightly on the plunger until a flashback of blood is seen.
4. Inject the medication at the appropriate rate. The drug information section in the back of this text includes recommended rates for each drug.
5. Flush the heparin lock with 0.2 to 0.4 milliliter of heparinized saline. The lowest concentration required to maintain patency is recommended so that the blood clotting status will not be altered. A concentration of 10 units of heparin per milliliter of normal saline has been found

to be effective (24). Several preparations of heparinized saline are available in prefilled syringes, making maintenance of the heparin lock convenient and accurate.

6. If the drug being given is incompatible with heparin or saline, flush the heparin lock both before and after the injection with a compatible solution. (See the drug section in the back for compatibilities.) The heparinized saline is then instilled as usual.

USING THE HEPARIN LOCK FOR INTERMITTENT INFUSION OF A DRUG

1. Prepare the dose of medication and add to either a partially filled fluid container or a volume-control chamber, and set up as described on pages 145–147.
2. Cleanse the rubber injection site on the heparin lock with alcohol or other recommended disinfectant.
3. Insert a syringe and needle into the site and aspirate until a flashback of blood is seen, verifying position of the cannula within the vein.
4. Remove the needle and syringe and insert the needle from the end of the administration set.
5. Adjust the flow-control clamp until the desired rate is maintained.
6. Return to check the infusion periodically to insure that the bottle is not allowed to run completely dry in order to avoid air embolism. With some volume-control sets, a membrane filter or valve is incorporated into the bottom of the burette chamber to prevent infusion of air.
7. Upon infusion of the complete dose of the drug, remove the needle and administration set and flush the heparin lock with heparinized saline as described above.

REFERENCES

1. Abbott Laboratories: How and When to Use I.V. Filters. *I.V. Tips,* North Chicago, Illinois, April 1977.
2. Abbott Laboratories: How to Set Up an Automatic Piggyback I.V. *I.V. Tips,* North Chicago, Illinois, April 1977.
3. Abbott Laboratories: How to Use a Universal I.V. Administration Set. *I.V. Tips,* North Chicago, Illinois, October 1975.
4. Abbott Laboratories: How to Use Soluset Precision Volume I.V. Sets. *I.V. Tips,* North Chicago, Illinois, July 1977.
5. Allen, Loyd V., Jr., Levinson, R. Saul, and Phisutsinthop, Daranee: Compatibility of Various Admixtures with Secondary Additives at Y-Injection Sites of Intravenous Administration Sets. *American Journal of Hospital Pharmacy,* 34:939–943, September 1977.
6. American Society of Hospital Pharmacists Statement on Hospital Drug Control Systems: *American Journal of Hospital Pharmacy,* 31:1198–1207, December 1974.
7. Arnold, Thomas R. and Hepler, Charles D.: Bacterial Contamination of Intravenous Fluids Opened in Unsterile Air. *American Journal of Hospital Pharmacy,* 28:614–619, August 1971.
8. Asperheim, Mary K. and Eisenhauer, Laurel A.: *The Pharmacologic Basis of Patient Care,* (3rd ed.), Philadelphia: W. B. Saunders Company, 1977.
9. Bighley, Lyle D., Wille, James, and Lach, John L.: Mixing of Additives in Glass and Plastic Intravenous Fluid Containers. *American Journal of Hospital Pharmacy,* 31:736–739, August 1974.
10. Darby, Thomas D., and Ausman, Robert K.: Particulate Matter in Polyvinyl Chloride Intravenous Bags (Cont.) (Letter) *The New England Journal of Medicine,* 290:579, March 1974.
11. Davies, D. M. (editor): *Textbook of Adverse Drug Reactions,* Oxford: Oxford University Press, 1977.
12. Davis, Neil M. (editorial): It's a Good Thing When Filters Clog, *Hospital Pharmacy,* 8(5):136, May 1973.
13. Davis, Neil M., and Turco, Salvatore: A Study of Particulate Matter in I.V. Infusion Fluids—Phase 2. *American Journal of Hospital Pharmacy,* 28:620–623, August 1971.
14. Davis, Neil M., Turco, Salvatore, and Sively, Edward: A Study of Particulate Matter in I.V. Infusion Fluids. *American Journal of Hospital Pharmacy,* 27:822–826, October 1970.
15. DiPalma, Joseph R. (editor): *Basic Pharmacology in Medicine,* New York: McGraw Hill Book Company, 1976.
16. Durant, Winston, J., Kenna, F. Regis, Hegarty, John, and Tester, William W.: *Admixture Studies for Fluids in Viaflex Plastic Containers,* Deerfield, Illinois: Travenol Laboratories, Inc., 1977.
17. Falconer, Mary W., Ezell, Annette Schram, Patterson, H. Robert, and Gustafson, Edward A.: *The Drug—The Nurse—The Patient* (5th ed.), Philadelphia: W. B. Saunders Company, 1974.
18. Frenier, Edward: Problems of I.V. Incompatibilities. *American Journal of I.V. Therapy,* 3:21–24, May 1976.
19. Geolot, Denise H., and McKinney, Nancy P.: Ad-

ministering Parenteral Drugs. *American Journal of Nursing*, 75 (5):788–793, May 1975.

20. Godwin, Harold N.: Intermittent and Direct I.V. Push: Rationale and Procedures. *American Journal of I.V. Therapy*, 2:27–30, December–January 1975.

21. Goodman, Louis S., and Gilman, Alfred: *The Pharmacologic Basis of Therapeutics* (5th ed.), New York: Macmillan Publishing Company, Inc. 1975.

22. Goth, Andres: *Medical Pharmacology* (8th ed.), Saint Louis: The C. V. Mosby Company, 1976.

23. Grotting, Michael A., Latiolais, Clifton, and Visconti, James: Putting RNs in the I.V. Push Chemotherapy Picture. *The American Journal of I.V. Therapy*, 3:31–34, October–November 1976.

24. Hanson, Robert L. Grant, Alan M., and Majors, Kenneth R.: Heparin-Lock Maintenance with Ten Units of Sodium Heparin in One Milliliter of Normal Saline Solution. *Surgery, Gynecology and Obstetrics*, 142:373–376, March 1976.

25. Henry, Robert H., and Harrison, Willard L.: Problems in the Use of Volume Control Sets for Intravenous Fluids. *American Journal of Hospital Pharmacy*, 29:485–490, June 1972.

26. Hoeprich, Paul D.: *Infectious Diseases*, Hagerstown, Maryland: Harper and Row, Publishers, 1972.

27. Hunt, Max L., Jr., and Latiolais, Clifton J.: *Training Manual for Central Intravenous Admixture Personnel*, Deerfield, Illinois: Travenol Laboratories, Inc., 1976.

28. Jensen, JoAnne C.: Problems of I.V. Incompatibilities. *The American Journal of I.V. Therapy*, 3:24–26, October–November 1976.

29. King, J. C.: *Guide to Parenteral Admixtures*, Berkeley, California: Cutter Laboratories, 1971.

30. Kozma, Minera T., and Newton, David W.: Nursing Guidelines for In-Syringe Mixtures. *Supervisor Nurse*, 6:26–27, 31, 33, August 1975.

31. Letcher, Kenneth I., Thrupp, Laurie D., Schapiro, David J., and Boersma, Johanna E.: In-Use Contamination of Intravenous Solutions in Flexible Containers. *American Journal of Hospital Pharmacy*, 29:673–677, August 1973.

32. MacFarlane, M. David: Allergic Drug Reactions. *Drug Intelligence and Clinical Pharmacy*, 6:342–348, October 1972.

33. Maki, Dennis G., Rhame, Frank S., Mackel, Donald C., and Bennett, John V.: Nationwide Epidemic of Septicemia Caused by Contaminated Intravenous Products. *The American Journal of Medicine*, 60:471–485, April 1976.

34. Masuda, John Y., and Beckerman, Joseph H.: Particulate Matter in Commercial Antibiotic Injectable Products. *American Journal of Hospital Pharmacy*, 30:72–76, January 1973.

35. Melman, Kenneth L., and Morrelli, Howard F.: *Clinical Pharmacology—Basic Principles in Therapeutics*, New York: The Macmillan Company, 1972.

36. Meyer, L., and Peck, H. M.: *Drug Induced Diseases*, Vol. 4., Amsterdam: Excerpta Medica, 1972.

37. Modell, Walter, Schild, Heinz O., and Wilson, Andrew: *Applied Pharmacology*, Philadelphia: W. B. Saunders Company, 1976.

38. National Coordinating Committee on Large Volume Parenterals: Recommended Methods for Compounding Intravenous Admixtures in Hospitals. *American Journal of Hospital Pharmacy*, 32:261–270, March 1975.

39. Needham, T. E., Jr., and Luzzi, L. A.: Particulate Matter in Polyvinyl Chloride Intravenous Bags. (Letter) *The New England Journal of Medicine*, 289:1256, December 6, 1973.

40. O'Brien, Thomas E., Ashford, Thomas P., Vetter, Thomas G., Wilson, Mary Jane, and Schilling, Barbara A.: Phlebitis from I.V. Therapy: Prospective Study of an In-Line Filter. *Hospital Formulary*, 12:315, 319–320, May 1977.

41. Parker, Charles W.: Drug Allergy (3 parts). *The New England Journal of Medicine*, 292:511–514; 732–736; 957–960, 1975.

42. Paxinos, James, and Samuels, Tom M.: Combined Volume Control Set-Piggyback System for Intermittent Intravenous Therapy. *American Journal of Hospital Pharmacy*, 32 (9):892–897, September 1975.

43. *Physicians' Desk Reference* (32nd ed.), Oradell, New Jersey: Medical Economics Company, 1978.

44. Plumer, Ada Lawrence: *Principles and Practice of Intravenous Therapy* (2nd ed.), Boston: Little, Brown and Company, 1975.

45. Rapp, Robert P., Bivens, Brack, and DeLuca, Patrick: In-Line Filtration of I.V. Fluids and Drugs. *The American Journal of I.V. Therapy*, 2:18–19, 22–23, April–May 1975.

46. Russell, J. H.: Pharmaceutical Applications of Filtration. *The Journal of Hospital Pharmacy*, 28:98–100, 125–126, 1970.

47. Ryan, Patrick B., Rapp, Robert P., DeLuca, Patrick P., Griffen, Ward O., Jr., Clark, Joseph D., and Cloys, Don: In-Line Final Filtration—A Method of Minimizing Contamination in Intravenous Therapy. *Bulletin of The Parenteral Drug Association*, 27(1):1–14, January–February 1973.

48. Thorn, George W., Adams, Raymond, D., Braunwald, Eugene, Isselbacher, Kurt J., and Petersdorf, Robert G.: *Harrison's Principles of Internal Medicine* (8th ed.), New York: McGraw Hill Book Company, 1977.

49. Turco, Salvatore, and Davis, Neil M.: Clinical Significance of Particulate Matter: A Review of the Literature. *Hospital Pharmacy*, 8(5):137–140, May 1973.

50. Turco, Salvatore, and Davis, Neil M.: A Comparison of Commercial Final Filtration Devices, *Hospital Pharmacy*, 8(5):141–146, May 1973.

51. Turco, Salvatore, J., and Davis, Neil M.: Particulate Matter in Intravenous Infusion Fluids—Phase 3. *American Journal of Hospital Pharmacy*. 30:611–613, July 1973.

52. Turco, Salvatore, and Davis, Neil M.: Preventing the Injection of Glass Particles with Furosemide Injection. *Hospital Pharmacy,* 7(12):423–424, 1972.

53. Turco, Salvatore, and King, Robert E.: *Sterile Dosage Forms—Their Preparation and Clinical Application*, Philadelphia: Lea and Febiger, 1974.

54. Williams, R. H. P.: Potassium Overdosage: A Potential Hazard of Nonrigid Parenteral Fluid Containers, *British Medical Journal*, 1:714–715, March 24, 1973.

Part Two

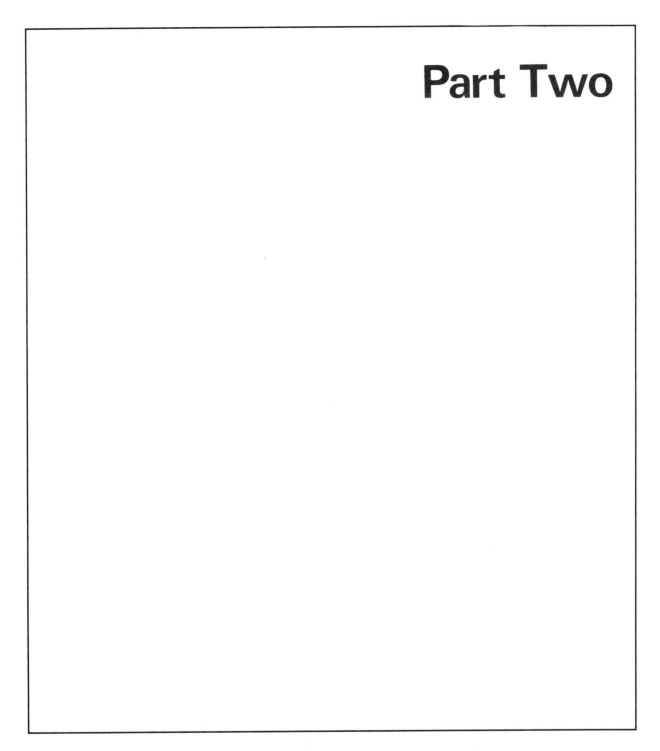

Drug Information

The fact is realized, and discussed in detail in Part One, that an ever increasing number of institutions are preparing to initiate, or are now using, pharmacy-based unit-dose and intravenous admixture programs. We advocate such innovations for the reasons stated in Chapter 8. And, despite the fact that under these systems the nurse does not prepare intravenous drugs, we feel that since she administers them, she must still know all aspects of the drugs as presented in the Drug Information Section. The nurse can be the final checkpoint through which the medication passes before being administered to the patient. This checkpoint can help to insure appropriateness and accuracy. It is an accepted fact that the nurse is the professional closest to the patient to observe for adverse reactions, to administer explanations and comfort measures, and to monitor for drug effectiveness. There have been concerns voiced in the nursing community that unit-dose and admixture programs remove the nurse from her traditional involvement in drug administration. It is our belief that these programs free the nurse from mechanical aspects of drug preparation and allow her to devote more time to professional bedside care: comfort measures, therapeutic intervention, and observation.

The primary source of information is the drug manufacturer. As stated in Chapter 8 of Part One, the current trend is to consider the manufacturer's guidelines as legal standards for the administration of a drug. It behooves the practitioner to use this book coupled with strict adherence to institutional policies and procedures as determined by the pharmacy and therapeutics committee, the director of pharmacy services, a drug information center, hospital pharmacologist, or other pertinent resources. The legal implications of deviations from such standards, policies, and procedures are discussed in Chapter 1.

The drugs listed in this text are those currently available and approved for human clinical intravenous use by the Food and Drug Administration. Agents classified for investigational use only have not been included. All drugs are listed in alphabetical order according to their generic name. The Table of Contents has been cross-indexed to facilitate rapid location of the entry for a drug whether the generic or the trade name is known. The information on each drug is divided into seven major sections in a sequence that follows the order that the information will be needed in preparing to administer a drug. The purpose and the contents of each of the seven sections will be discussed in detail.

ACTIONS/INDICATIONS

The term *actions* in this text refers to the physiologic and pharmacologic effects that the drug produces within the body when it is administered intravenously. The *indications* listed are those clinical situations in which the drug actions can produce a desirable change, such as the relief of pain, or the prevention, diagnosis or treatment of a disease. These indications are those currently recognized by the Food and Drug Administration. A drug may have other uses via alternate routes of administration; these indications are not listed. Besides helping to insure the appropriateness of a drug for a particular patient, knowledge of the actions and indications will facilitate monitoring for drug effectiveness.

DOSAGE

The currently accepted adult and pediatric dosages are given. As with other material, dosages are those recommended by the manufacturer, unless otherwise stated. For some drugs, dosages are given for each indication listed; for the remainder, the one dosage given is for all indications.

Pediatric dosages are given by weight, age and/or body surface area (in square meters). A nomogram for body surface area and a chart for the conversion of pounds to kilograms can be found in the Appendix.

PREPARATION AND STORAGE

As discussed in Chapter 8, each medication has specific preparation requirements in relation to reconstitution, dilution in fluids, protection from environmental factors, and perishability. Strict attention to these details is mandatory for safe and effective drug administration. Alterations can change the actions of the drug in the body.

The volume of diluent added to a drug in its powder form must be precise according to instructions, to produce an accurate concentration (mg./ml.). Accuracy of the concentration of a drug solution will help to guarantee the delivery of an accurate dose to the patient. Similarly, accurate preparation of a drug-fluid solution is also essential to the delivery of an accurate dose.

Conditions under which a prepared solution should not be used, e.g., with the appearance of discoloration, a precipitate, opalescence or a separation, are described.

The stability of prepared drug solutions for stock use and infusion is also listed in this column. The preparer is encouraged to use this information in labeling vials and bottles to prevent the use of a drug after its period of known stability has passed. Special precautions to follow, such as protection of a drug or infusion solution from light, are included.

DRUG INCOMPATIBILITIES

Information in this column was based primarily on information in Lawrence Trissel's *Handbook on Injectable Drugs* from the American Society of Hospital Pharmacists, and data from the drug manufacturer. In most instances, other agents with which the drug *cannot* be mixed are listed. However, the reader is cautioned that for some drugs, the only agents with which the drug *can* be mixed are listed. The warning to avoid mixing certain drugs "in any manner" means that the two agents cannot be combined in a syringe, intravenous tubing, or fluid containers under any circumstances. Caution is advised when mixing drugs, as incompatibility does not always produce a visible change to warn the preparer. Special flushing techniques and intravenous tubing arrangements are required when drugs that are incompatible must be given at the same time. The reader is advised to review the information on this subject in Chapter 8.

MODES OF INTRAVENOUS ADMINISTRATION

Currently, the three methods of intravenous administration of a drug are injection (push), intermittent infusion, and continuous infusion. The mode or modes appropriate for each drug are indicated as "YES." If a drug must not be given by a particular method, it is indicated by a "NO" at the top of the column.

Definitions

Injection: The administration of a relatively small volume of a concentrated solution of a drug directly into the venous system from a syringe via intravenous tubing, a cannula or into the vein itself using a needle. Medications administered in this fashion are given over a short period of time either by rapid injection (bolus) or over several minutes.

Intermittent Infusion: A dose of the drug is added to a small volume of fluid (50 to 100 ml) and the mixture is infused over a period of time ranging from 20 minutes to 2 hours. This technique of delivery is used to produce peaks in the blood level of the drug. Piggyback and volume control units are used.

Continuous Infusion: Administering a medication in a large volume of fluid (250 to 1000 ml.) without interruption, over several hours or days. This method is used to maintain a constant blood level of the medication, or to highly dilute the medication before it enters the body.

Under the *Intermittent Infusion* and *Continuous Infusion* columns the fluids which can be used as vehicles for administration are listed. Use no others. The abbreviations for these solutions are as follows:

D5W	Dextrose 5% in water
D5/NS	Dextrose 5% in normal saline (0.9% sodium chloride)
D5/0.45% Saline	Dextrose 5% in one-half normal saline (0.45% sodium chloride)
NS	Normal saline (0.9% sodium chloride)
0.45% Saline	One-half normal saline (0.45% sodium chloride)
RL	Ringer's Lactate
LR	Lactated Ringer's solution

These abbreviations are used throughout the text.

Appropriate concentrations and injection or infusion times (rates) are given for each medication, and must be observed to avoid adverse reactions.

CONTRAINDICATIONS, WARNINGS, PRECAUTIONS AND ADVERSE REACTIONS

These aspects of the clinical application of the medication are listed and were taken from information given by the manufacturer. Other sources were also used and are so indicated by footnotes. Nursing care is based in large part on this information. Where appropriate, directions for the detection and treatment of drug overdosage are included. Definitions and explanations of these terms are found in Chapter 7.

NURSING IMPLICATIONS

A major component of the nursing intervention involved with drug administration begins after the drug has been given. The suggestions for patient care presented here are based on the information from the preceding six columns of information. Primarily, the nurse must be concerned with monitoring appropriate physiologic parameters to detect desired changes and adverse reactions. How frequently parameters such as heart rate, blood pressure, respiratory rate, arterial blood gases, electrocardiogram, central venous pressure, and urine output should be monitored is stated. Expected changes in these parameters, both desirable and undesirable, are also discussed. Supportive care for minor and major discomforts produced by the drug is described, as are safety precautions and the management of emergencies related to the use of the drug. Suggestions are also made for explanations and patient education where appropriate.

This material was written with all levels of practitioners in mind, from the student to the experienced. Also, keeping in mind that available equipment and institutional policies and procedures vary, the authors have attempted to present the information in a manner that can be applied to all situations.

It must be remembered that the entire entry on each drug has implications for nurses, and that practitioners must not limit themselves to becoming familiar with only the Nursing Implications column. It is the philosophy of the authors that the administration of intravenous medications requires clear, logical thinking, a knowledge of all facets of the drug being administered, and a commitment on the part of the nurse to carry out the procedure with the greatest precision.

Contents

ACETAZOLAMIDE SODIUM (Diamox)

ACTIONS/ INDICATIONS	DOSAGE	PREPARATION AND STORAGE	DRUG INCOMPATIBILITIES	MODES OF IV ADMINISTRATION			CONTRAINDICATIONS; WARNINGS; PRECAUTIONS; ADVERSE REACTIONS
				INJECTION	INTERMITTENT INFUSION	CONTINUOUS INFUSION	
Potent carbonic anhydrase inhibitor.	*Acute closed-angle glaucoma**—250 mg every 4 hrs. May be preceded by an initial dose of 500 mg.	Reconstitute with at least 5 ml of sterile water for injection. Use within 24 hours of preparation. Can be stored for 4 weeks if refrigerated.	Do not mix with any other medications.	YES	YES	YES	CONTRAINDICATIONS
In glaucoma: rapidly decreases the secretion of aqueous humor thus decreasing intraocular pressure; used preoperatively and in acute crisis to lower intraocular pressure.				*Preferred* IV mode. No further dilution needed after reconstitution. Should be given at a rate of 250–500 mg over 5–6 min.	Add to any IV fluid, 50 ml fluid for each 250 mg of drug.	Add to any IV fluid in any volume, at least 50 ml for each 250 mg of drug.	1. In hyponatremic and/or hypokalemic states 2. In cases of marked hepatic or renal dysfunction, or adrenal insufficiency 3. In hypochloremic acidosis 4. Long-term administration in chronic noncongestive angle-closure glaucoma
In convulsive disorders: suppresses abnormal paroxysmal discharge from CNS.	*Convulsive disorders*—children and adults: 8–30 mg/kg/24 hrs in divided doses.						PRECAUTIONS 1. Should not be used in pregnancy, especially the first trimester, unless benefits outweigh potential adverse effects on the fetus. 2. May increase the diuretic effect of other diuretics. 3. Increasing dose does *not* increase diuresis but may increase drowsiness. 4. Monitor CBC throughout therapy.
As a diuretic: produces a renal loss of HCO₃— which carries with it, sodium, water and potassium; used in the reduction of edema due to congestive heart failure, drug induced edema (steroids); seizure disorders, acute angle-closure glaucoma, prior to eye surgery.	*Congestive heart failure**—5 mg/kg, usually 250–375 mg daily on alternate days. Overdosage will decrease diuresis. *Not recommended for pediatric use in this situation.						ADVERSE REACTIONS Rash, renal calculus, casts in the urine, bone marrow depression, thrombocytopenic purpura, pancytopenia, agranulocytosis. Also mild paresthesia, tingling feelings in extremities, anorexia, drowsiness and confusion. Transient myopia (near-sightedness) may be decreased with a lower dose and is reversible with discontinuance of the drug.

NURSING IMPLICATIONS
1. Monitor patient for drug effectiveness:
   a. *Acute glaucoma*—improvement in vision, decreased ocular pain, decreased ocular pressure; disappearance of nausea and vomiting.
   b. *Seizure disorders*—chart frequency, character and duration of all seizures.
   c. *In congestive heart failure* (usually used in mild failure)—weigh all patients daily and record intake and output every 8 hours to document diuresis. Monitor resting heart rate respirations and their changes with exertion. Observe for improvement in peripheral edema (feet, legs and sacrum) and CVP.
2. Examine patient daily for rashes, fever, hematuria and melena.
3. Monitor elderly patients carefully for confusion and take precautions where indicated; e.g., side rails, light restraints, bedside light at night.
4. Instruct patient to drink water as ordered by physician to prevent crys-

taluria, at least 2000–3000 ml/day for adults.
5. Instruct patient about the possibility of myopia (blurred vision).
6. Monitor for signs of mild metabolic acidosis which may be induced in long-term therapy: hyperventilation (also increased depth of respiration), drowsiness, restlessness.
7. Monitor for hypokalemia: muscle weakness, postural hypotension. Administer potassium supplements as prescribed.

SUGGESTED READINGS

Newell, Frank W., and Ernest, J. Terry: *Ophthalmology. Principles and Concepts* (3rd ed.), St. Louis: C.V. Mosby Company, 1974, Chapter 20—Glaucoma.
Condl, E. D.: Ophthalmic Nursing: The Gentle Touch. *Nursing Clinics of North America,* 5:467–476, September 1970.
Seamon, F. W.: Nursing Care of Glaucoma Patients, *Nursing Clinics of North America,* 5:489–496, September 1970.

● ALBUMIN, NORMAL SERUM (HUMAN), 5% (Albuminar-5, Albumisol, Albuspan, Buminate, Pro-Bumin, Proserum-5)

ACTIONS/ INDICATIONS	DOSAGE	PREPARATION AND STORAGE	DRUG INCOMPATIBILITIES	MODES OF IV ADMINISTRATION				CONTRAINDICATIONS: WARNINGS; PRECAUTIONS: ADVERSE REACTIONS
				INJECTION	INTERMITTENT INFUSION	CONTINUOUS INFUSION		
A protein constituent of human plasma, with the following functions: 1. Maintenance of colloid osmotic pressure of the plasma thus its volume. 2. Tissue nourishment. Indicated in: • Shock, regardless of etiology; 5% albumin is the agent of choice because it supplies volume without dehydrating tissues	ADULTS AND CHILDREN: Initially 250–500 ml. Repeated doses must depend on condition and response to initial dose. *Shock*—2–4 ml/min. NEONATES AND INFANTS: 10–20 ml/kg. Rate of administration 5–10 ml/min. Adjust with clinical response	Store at room temperature. Do not use any solution that has been frozen. Do not use if solution is cloudy, discolored or has a sediment. Use containers promptly after opening; discard unused portion. Supplied in 50-ml, 250-ml and 500-ml vials.	Do not add any medications to a solution of albumin.	NO	YES See Dosage column for rates. Administer undiluted into a running IV.	YES May add to IV fluids. See Dosage column for infusion rates. (These rates apply to undiluted albumin.)		CONTRAINDICATIONS 1. Severe anemia 2. Congestive heart failure (not an absolute contraindication) PRECAUTIONS 1. In the presence of dehydration, other fluids must be administered along with albumin. 2. When cardiac and/or circulatory disease are present or threatening, administer 5% albumin at a rate not faster than 5–10 ml/min. Use an infusion pump. Rapid infusion and the resultant increase in blood volume and pressure may cause cardiac decompensation (shock, pulmonary edema). 3. Increased arterial pressure may cause renewed bleeding in the case of trauma, gastrointestinal hemorrhage, etc. Further hemorrhage and shock can follow. 4. This agent does not provide clotting factors to correct clotting defects. 5. Administer with caution in the presence of normal or increased blood volume (this may be present when the patient is receiving albumin for hypoproteinemia).

ALBUMIN, NORMAL SERUM (HUMAN), 5% (Albuminar-5, Albumisol, Albuspan, Buminate, Pro-Bumin, Proserum-5) (Continued)

ACTIONS/ INDICATIONS	DOSAGE	PREPARATION AND STORAGE	DRUG INCOMPATIBILITIES	MODES OF IV ADMINISTRATION			CONTRAINDICATIONS: WARNINGS: PRECAUTIONS: ADVERSE REACTIONS
				INJECTION	INTERMITTENT INFUSION	CONTINUOUS INFUSION	
• Hypoproteinemia and resultant edema Burns, to correct fluid loss through exudation (Threat of hepatitis is minimal because of heat treatment in its preparation.)							6. Whole blood must be given in the presence of anemia secondary to albumin-induced hemodilution (especially in shock). 7. This agent has no oxygen-carrying ability. If the capacity of the blood to carry oxygen is reduced, whole blood or packed red blood cells must be given. ADVERSE REACTIONS 1. Chills 2. Fever 3. Urticaria 4. Congestive heart failure secondary to overexpansion of blood volume

NURSING IMPLICATIONS
1. All patients must have blood pressure monitored frequently, depending on the general clinical condition.
2. Critically ill patients (shock, severe burns, etc.) should have a central circulatory monitoring device in place, i.e., a CVP catheter, or, preferably, a pulmonary artery catheter (Swan-Ganz). This device will allow titration of the infusion rate with the need for volume expansion versus the heart's ability to pump the expanding blood volume. As treatment progresses, there will be a rise in CVP or pulmonary artery pressure (wedge). The physician must set numerical limits of these parameters as goals for albumin administration. Patients with known cardiac disease must be monitored frequently for a rise in CVP or pulmonary artery pressure above desirable levels. (See Precaution No. 2.) Other signs of acute cardiac decompensation secondary to volume overload:
   a. Increased respiratory rate
   b. Orthopnea
   c. Rales
   d. Tachycardia
   e. Onset of a third and/or fourth heart sound
3. Monitor for signs of renewed hemorrhaging after arterial pressures rise.
4. Observe for cyanosis or pallor which may indicate a reduction in the oxygen-carrying capacity of the blood. This can occur with hemodilution produced by the osmotic effect of the protein.
5. Monitor for allergic reactions. Stop infusion on appearance of chills, fever, urticaria. Notify the physician.

ALBUMIN, NORMAL SERUM (HUMAN), 25% (Albuminar-25, Albumisol, Albuspan, Albutein, Buminate, Pro-Bumin, Proserum-25)

ACTIONS/ INDICATIONS	DOSAGE	PREPARATION AND STORAGE	DRUG INCOMPATIBILITIES	MODES OF IV ADMINISTRATION			CONTRAINDICATIONS: WARNINGS: PRECAUTIONS: ADVERSE REACTIONS
				INJECTION	INTERMITTENT INFUSION	CONTINUOUS INFUSION	
A protein constituent of human plasma with the fol-	ADULTS AND CHILDREN OVER 12 YRS:	To prepare an isotonic, isosmotic solution (as compared	Do not mix with Ionosol-DCM or	NO	YES Can be diluted in fluids, D5W	YES Can be diluted in most	CONTRAINDICATIONS 1. Severe anemia 2. Cardiac failure (not an absolute contraindication)

lowing functions:

1. To maintain the colloid osmotic pressure of the plasma, thus its volume.

   This albumin preparation draws 3.5 times its own volume into the blood from the tissues within 15 minutes of infusion, in the normally hydrated patient.[1]

2. Tissue nourishment.

Indications:
- Shock, regardless of etiology, to restore blood volume;
- Burns, to prevent hemoconcentration and to maintain electrolyte-fluid balance;
- Hypoproteinemia with or without edema, to replace plasma protein and blood onconic pressure;
- Prevention and treatment of ce-

Shock—100–200 ml followed by 100 ml as needed to obtain increase in blood pressure and CVP

Burns—100–200 ml of a 5% solution (see Preparation column)

Hypoproteinemia—200–300 ml (do not exceed a rate of 100 ml in 30–45 min). In the presence of congestive heart failure, mix 200 ml 25% albumin in 300 ml D10W at a rate of 100 ml/hr. (Alternate dosage—75 gm/day until desired results are obtained.)

Cerebral edema—60–80 ml infused over 8–10 min.

CHILDREN:
Shock—(1 ml/lb repeated every 15–30 min until desired blood pressure is reached

Burns—1 ml/lb usually

to plasma), add 200 ml albumin to 1000 ml NS or D5W.*

Do not use a solution that is cloudy, discolored or has a precipitate. Store in cool dry area.

Use promptly after opening vial; discard unused portions.

*Albumin is compatible with most IV fluids; see Drug Incompatibilities column.

Ionosol-G with Dextrose 10%.

or NS, or given undiluted. When administered undiluted, infusion rate should not exceed 1 ml/min.

fluids or given undiluted. When administered undiluted, infusion rate should not exceed 1 ml/min.

PRECAUTIONS
1. The effectiveness of an albumin infusion depends on its ability to draw tissue fluid into the bloodstream. In the presence of dehydration, other fluid must be administered with the albumin.
2. Rapid infusion in patients with a decreased cardiac reserve or no albumin deficiency may cause cardiac decompensation (pulmonary edema, cardiogenic shock).
3. The resultant increased arterial pressure produced by this infusion may cause renewed bleeding in the case of trauma, gastrointestinal hemorrhage, etc. Further hemorrhage and shock can occur.
4. This agent does not provide clotting factors to correct clotting defects.
5. Administer whole blood as needed to prevent a secondary anemia due to the hemodilution produced by albumin.
6. This agent has no oxygen-carrying ability. If the capacity of the blood to carry oxygen is reduced, whole blood or packed red blood cells must be given.

ADVERSE REACTIONS
1. Nausea, vomiting
2. Increased salivation
3. Fever and chills
4. Urticaria

169

ALBUMIN, NORMAL SERUM (HUMAN), 25% (Albuminar-25, Albumisol, Albuspan, Albutein, Buminate, Pro-Bumin, Proserum-25) (Continued)

ACTIONS/ INDICATIONS	DOSAGE	PREPARATION AND STORAGE	DRUG INCOMPAT- IBILITIES	MODES OF IV ADMINISTRATION			CONTRAINDICATIONS; WARNINGS; PRECAUTIONS; ADVERSE REACTIONS
				INJECTION	INTERMITTENT INFUSION	CONTINUOUS INFUSION	
rebral ede- ma.	in NS (40 ml albumin in 160 ml NS) Hypoprotein- emia—25 gm daily un- til desired ef- fect is obtained. Cerebral edema— same as adult.						b. Orthopnea c. Rales d. Tachycardia e. Onset of a third and/or fourth heart sound 3. Monitor for signs of renewed hemorrhaging after arterial pressure rises. 4. Observe for cyanosis or pallor which may indicate a reduction in the oxy- gen-carrying capacity of the blood. This can occur with hemodilution pro- duced by the osmotic effect of the protein. 5. Monitor for allergic reactions. Stop infusion on appearance of chills, fever, urticaria. Notify the physician. *REFERENCE* 1. Buchanan, E. C.: Blood and Blood Substitutes for Treating Hemorrhagic Shock. *American Journal of Hospital Pharmacy,* 34:633, June 1977.

NURSING IMPLICATIONS
1. All patients must have blood pressure monitored frequently, depending on the general clinical condition.
2. Critically ill patients (shock, severe burns, etc.) should have a central circu- latory monitoring device in place, e.g., a CVP catheter, or, preferably, a pul- monary artery catheter (Swan-Ganz). This device will allow titration of the infusion rate with the need for volume expansion versus the heart's ability to pump the expanding blood volume. As treatment progresses, there will be a rise in CVP or pulmonary artery pressure (wedge). The physician must set numerical limits of these parameters as goals for albumin administra- tion. Patients with known cardiac disease must be monitored frequently for a rise in CVP or pulmonary artery pressure above desirable levels. (See Pre- caution No. 2.) Other signs of acute cardiac decompensation secondary to volume overload:
   a. Increased respiratory rate

ALPHAPRODINE HYDROCHLORIDE (Nisentil)

ACTIONS/ INDICATIONS	DOSAGE	PREPARATION AND STORAGE	DRUG INCOMPAT- IBILITIES	MODES OF IV ADMINISTRATION			CONTRAINDICATIONS; WARNINGS; PRECAUTIONS; ADVERSE REACTIONS
				INJECTION	INTERMITTENT INFUSION	CONTINUOUS INFUSION	
Narcotic anal- gesic synthet- ic, rapid onset of effects, short duration.	ADULTS: *Range*—0.4 – 0.6 mg/kg. Use the lower dosage initially	Supplied in 1 ml ampuls, 40 mg/ml, and 60 mg/ml.	Do not mix with any med- ication other than: atropine, scopolamine,	YES Administer at a rate no greater than 20 mg/	NO	NO	CONTRAINDICATIONS Known hypersensitivity WARNINGS 1. This drug is a habit-forming narcotic.

Analgesia is comparable to morphine except for duration (30–60 min when given intravenously).

Used when a short duration of analgesia is desirable such as in minor surgery, obstetrics, cystoscopic examinations, or orthopedics.

and evaluate patient response. *Usual adult dose*—30 mg or less.

Do not exceed 240 mg in 24 hrs. May be given with levallorphan tartrate to prevent respiratory depression without abolishing analgesia (especially in obstetric use). When given together, the ratio should be 1 part levallorphan to 50 parts alphaprodine. In obstetrics, if alphaprodine is not administered in this manner, 1–2 mg of levallorphan should be given intravenously 5–10 min prior to delivery. To prevent respiratory depression in the infant, 0.05–0.1 mg of levallorphan should be given into the umbilical vein immediately after delivery.

See page 360 for further information on levallorphan.

CHILDREN:
A dosage for children under 12 years of

min. May be given undiluted.

chlorpromazine, trifluoperazine, prochlorperazine, levallorphan.

This is a Schedule II drug under the Controlled Substances Act of 1970. Maintain hospital or institutional regulations guiding its use.

2. Respiratory depression can occur.
3. The central nervous system depressant effects of alphaprodine are potentiated by barbiturates, general anesthetic agents, and some phenothiazines. Lower dosage of this agent should be used in these circumstances.
4. Use with caution in the presence of increased intracranial pressure, hepatic insufficiency, severe depression of the central nervous system, myxedema, acute alcoholism, delirium tremens, seizure disorders, and Addison's disease.
5. Use with caution if the patient is concomitantly receiving an MAO inhibitor drug because of the possibility of hypotension.
6. Do not use for the relief of chronic pain. The need for frequent administration may make addiction more likely, and frequent injections would be unpleasant for the patient.
7. The safety of the use of this drug in obstetrics has been established. However, its use in early pregnancy has not.

PRECAUTIONS
Respiratory depression is more likely to occur in patients with pre-existing pulmonary disease, postoperative chest surgery, chest trauma, central nervous system depression, and in the elderly and the debilitated.

ADVERSE REACTIONS
1. Respiratory depression (in obstetrics, depression may occur in the mother and infant)
2. Dizziness
3. Drowsiness
4. Diaphoresis
5. Urticaria
6. Nausea and vomiting
7. Restlessness
8. Confusion (rare)

MANAGEMENT OF OVERDOSAGE
Toxic effects of alphaprodine include: coma, shallow respirations, cyanosis, hypotension, and pinpoint pupils. If these signs develop, a narcotic antagonist agent should be administered intravenously, levallorphan tartrate or naloxone (Narcan). (See page 417 for further information on this drug.) Some groups routinely give

ALPHAPRODINE HYDROCHLORIDE (Nisentil) (Continued)

ACTIONS/ INDICATIONS	DOSAGE	PREPARATION AND STORAGE	DRUG INCOMPAT- IBILITIES	MODES OF IV ADMINISTRATION			CONTRAINDICATIONS; WARNINGS: PRECAUTIONS; ADVERSE REACTIONS
				INJECTION	INTERMITTENT INFUSION	CONTINUOUS INFUSION	
	age has not been estab- lished.						naloxone prophylactically when used in obstetrics to prevent respiratory depression in the newborn. Whether or not it is used, the infant should be closely monitored for respiratory depression for the first 4–6 hours of life. In the presence of apnea, artificial ventilation and oxygen should be ad- ministered in addition to the narcotic antagonist. Body warmth and hydra- tion should be maintained and the pa- tient's vital signs and respiratory status monitored carefully for 24 hours (see Nursing Implications, No. 1).

NURSING IMPLICATIONS

1. Onset of action is 1–2 min and lasts for 30–60 min. Monitor the patient continuously for respiratory depression immediately after injection (or im- mediately after delivery of newborn) and for the next hour. Patients with re- nal or hepatic failure should be monitored carefully for at least 2 hours af- ter injection because of delayed metabolism and excretion of the drug. If respiratory rate falls below 8–10/min in an adult or below normal in a child (see chart on page 545 for normal rates), attempt to arouse the pa- tient and to increase the respiratory rate to 12–14/min (or normal rate in a child). Stay with the patient until the effects of the drug have diminished. A narcotic antagonist may be prescribed; keep the agent readily available. If the patient is apneic or unarousable, begin artificial ventilation using an air- way and manual breathing bag. (If this equipment is not immediately avail- able, preceed with mouth-to-mouth breathing.) Maintain respiratory support until a narcotic antagonist can be administered (see above), and spontane- ous respirations of an adequate rate return. If a patient develops respira-

tory depression after a normal dose of this drug, any subsequent doses should be reduced in amount.
2. Patients listed above in Warnings No. 3 and No. 4 must be monitored more closely and for a longer period of time for the development of respiratory depression.
3. If the patient has received an MAO inhibitor agent within the previous 2 weeks, monitor blood pressure carefully for 1 hour after injection; hypoten- sion may develop.
4. Keep the patient supine for at least 15 minutes after an intravenous injec- tion, and then ambulate with caution. (Dizziness can occur.)
5. If the patient is lethargic, drowsy, or in the immediate postoperative period, take precautions to prevent aspiration in the event of nausea and vomiting.

SUGGESTED READING

McCaffery, Margo, and Hart, Linda L.: Undertreatment of Acute Pain with Narcotics, *American Journal of Nursing*, October 1976, pp. 1586–1591.

AMIKACIN SULFATE (Amikin)

ACTIONS/ INDICATIONS	DOSAGE	PREPARATION AND STORAGE	DRUG INCOMPAT- IBILITIES	MODES OF IV ADMINISTRATION			CONTRAINDICATIONS; WARNINGS: PRECAUTIONS; ADVERSE REACTIONS
				INJECTION	INTERMITTENT INFUSION	CONTINUOUS INFUSION	
Antibiotic (semisynthetic) aminogly- coside type, derived from kanamycin.	PRETREAT- MENT WEIGHT MUST BE USED TO DE- TERMINE DOS- AGE.	Available in vials with a concentra- tion of 50 mg/ ml in 2-ml, and in a concentra-	Do not mix with any other medication in any manner.	NO	YES Add dose to 200 ml (smal- ler volumes in children, as tol-	NO	CONTRAINDICATIONS Hypersensitivity to this drug or kanamy- cin. WARNINGS 1. Both auditory (sound perception) and

Used to treat *serious* infections due to gram-negative bacilli, some Proteus species, Pseudomonas, E. Coli, Serratia species, *Staphylococcus aureus* and *epidermis* (especially those strains resistant to other aminoglycosides).

Types of infections to be treated with this drug are: bacteremias (including neonatal sepsis), infections of the genitourinary and respiratory tracts, central nervous system, burns, osteomyelitis, abdominal cavity infections.

Use must be based on susceptibility tests and response of the patient.

tion of 250 mg/ml in 2- and 4-ml vials.

Aqueous solutions may darken without change in potency.

Use prepared solution promptly. Store unopened vials at room temperature.

IN NORMAL RENAL FUNCTION—
ADULTS, CHILDREN AND OLDER INFANTS:
15 mg/kg/day divided into 2-3 equal doses given at evenly spaced intervals. Do not exceed 1.5 gm/day.

NEWBORNS:
Loading dose of 10 mg/kg followed by 7.5 mg/kg every 12 hours.

The usual duration of treatment is 7-10 days; if administration continues beyond this, renal and auditory function must be monitored daily.

IN THE PRESENCE OF RENAL IMPAIRMENT:
1. Monitor serum levels (peaks and valleys); when possible, avoid concentrations over 35 mcg/ml peak.
2. For normally calculated dose (15 mg/kg) at prolonged intervals to allow for excretion of

erated by the patient) of D5W or NS (drug is compatible with most solutions).

Infuse over 30-60 min in adults and older children, and over 1-2 hours in infants.

vestibular (equilibrium) ototoxicity can occur in patients treated with high doses for longer than the recommended duration of therapy. This is secondary to eighth cranial nerve damage. The risk of such damage is increased in the presence of renal failure. High-frequency deafness occurs first and must be detected only by audiometric testing. Vertigo may also appear, indicating vestibular damage. The ototoxicity of this drug in infants is not known; use only when other agents cannot be used and observe closely for signs of damage.

2. This drug can cause renal damage if large doses are given at longer than recommended times. Nephrotoxicity in patients with normal renal function, receiving recommended doses and hydration, is low. Renal impairment may be indicated by proteinuria, casts and cells in the urine, oliguria, decreasing or fixed low specific gravity, rising serum creatinine and BUN, decreasing creatinine clearance. Patients with pre-existing renal impairment may develop further deterioration in renal function.

3. Evidence of drug-induced renal impairment, and auditory and/or vestibular damage requires discontinuation of the drug or reduction in dosage and close monitoring of involved systems. If renal status does not improve with reduction of dosage, the drug should be discontinued.

4. Monitor serum concentrations (peaks and valleys) when possible (see Dosage column).

5. Concurrent and/or sequential administration of topically or systemic neurotoxic or nephrotoxic antibiotics (kanamycin, gentamicin, tobramycin, neomycin, streptomycin, cephaloridine, paromycin, viomycin, polymyxin B, colistin, or vancomycin) should be avoided.

6. Do not give concurrently with potent diuretics (ethacrynic acid, furosemide, meralluride sodium, sodium mercaptomerin or mannitol).

PRECAUTIONS
1. Adequate hydration may reduce chemical irritation to renal tubules, and therefore decrease the likeli-

AMIKACIN SULFATE (Amikin) (Continued)

ACTIONS/INDICATIONS	DOSAGE	PREPARATION AND STORAGE	DRUG INCOMPATIBILITIES	MODES OF IV ADMINISTRATION			CONTRAINDICATIONS; WARNINGS; PRECAUTIONS; ADVERSE REACTIONS
				INJECTION	INTERMITTENT INFUSION	CONTINUOUS INFUSION	
	the drug: 15 mg/kg every (serum creatinine × 9) hours. 3. For lower dosage regimen at fixed time intervals: loading dose of 7.5 mg/kg, maintenance dose determined by: $$\frac{\text{patient's creatinine clearance (ml/min)}}{\text{normal creatinine clearance (ml/min)}} \times \text{calculated loading dose}$$ — every twelve hours 4. Alternative: divide normal dose (15 mg/kg) by the patient's serum creatinine, give at usual intervals. 5. After peritoneal dialysis: 3–4 mg for every 2 liters of dialysate removed.[1] 6. After hemodialysis: 7.5 mg/kg after each dialysis.[2]						hood of renal damage. If urinalysis shows casts, red or white blood cells or albumin, hydration should be increased. If other signs of renal damage appear (see Warning No. 2) a reduction in dosage should be instituted. Further deterioration should prompt discontinuation of the drug. 2. The possibility of neuromuscular blockade and subsequent respiratory paralysis should be monitored for when this drug is given with anesthetic or neuromuscular blocking agents. If blockade occurs, calcium gluconate may reverse the effect. 3. There may be cross-allergenicity with other aminoglycoside drugs (tobramycin, streptomycin, kanamycin, gentamicin, and neomycin). 4. Overgrowth infections due to nonsusceptible organisms may occur. 5. It is not known whether or not this drug may cause fetal abnormalities. Use in pregnant women must be carefully considered and only when absolutely necessary. Nursing should not be continued during therapy with this drug; it is not known whether or not it is excreted in human milk.

ADVERSE REACTIONS
1. Ototoxicity (see Warning No. 1)
2. Nephrotoxicity (see Warning No. 2)
3. Rash
4. Drug fever
5. Headache
6. Paresthesia
7. Muscle tremor
8. Nausea and vomiting
9. Eosinophilia
10. Arthralgia
11. Hypotension during infusion

MANAGEMENT OF OVERDOSAGE AND TOXIC REACTION
Hemo- and peritoneal dialysis can remove this drug from the serum. Monitor

serum concentrations to guide dialysis frequency and duration.

NURSING IMPLICATIONS
1. Weigh the patient prior to treatment to calculate dosage.
2. Obtain urine for creatinine clearance determinations in patients with renal impairment for dosage calculation. Be aware of dosage modifications for patients with renal impairment.
3. Monitor for signs and symptoms of ototoxicity, e.g., high-frequency deafness, in patients on large doses for over 10 days. Arrange for audiometric testing. The patient may complain of ringing or roaring in the ears (this is usually a late symptom). Instruct the patient to report vertigo (vestibular damage), or monitor for signs of dizziness in patients who cannot describe symptoms. Notify the physician.
4. Send urine for urinalysis daily. Be aware of results. Place the patient on intake and output measurements. Notify the physician if the urine output falls below 240 ml/8-hour period (30 ml/hour) in the adult (see chart on page 546 for normal urine output volumes in children). Report fall in specific gravity below 1.020 or the development of a fixed value. Be aware of the patient's serum creatinine and BUN.
5. Keep the patient hydrated via oral or intravenous routes. Monitor for signs of dehydration (concentrated urine, high specific gravity, decreased skin turgor, dry mucous membranes).
6. Patients receiving anesthetic agents or neuromuscular blocking agents while on this drug must be monitored carefully for extension of neuromuscular blockade. These patients may require respiratory support for a longer than normal period following anesthesia.
7. Monitor for signs and symptoms of overgrowth infections:
   a. Fever (take rectal temperature at least every 4–6 hours in all patients)
   b. Increasing malaise
   c. Newly appearing localized signs and symptoms—redness, soreness, pain, swelling, drainage (increased volume or change in character of pre-existing drainage)
   d. Monilial rash in perineal area (reddened areas with itching)
   e. Cough (change in pre-existing cough or sputum production)
   f. Diarrhea

REFERENCES
1. Appel, Gerald B., and Neu, Harold C.: The Nephrotoxicity of Antimicrobial Agents. *New England Journal of Medicine*, 296(3):666, March 31, 1977.
2. Ibid.

● AMINOCAPROIC ACID (Amicar)

ACTIONS/ INDICATIONS	DOSAGE	PREPARATION AND STORAGE	DRUG INCOMPATIBILITIES	MODES OF IV ADMINISTRATION			CONTRAINDICATIONS; WARNINGS; PRECAUTIONS; ADVERSE REACTIONS
				INJECTION	INTERMITTENT INFUSION	CONTINUOUS INFUSION	
Inhibitor of plasminogen activator substances; also has antiplasmin activity. This inhibits fibrinolysis to help control bleeding. Used in the treatment of excessive bleeding which results from systemic hyperfibrinolysis and urinary fibrinolysis.	ADULTS: *Loading dose* —5 gm via infusion. *Maintenance*—1.0–1.25 gm/hr to obtain a plasma level of 0.13 mg/ml or until bleeding has stopped. Maximum 24-hr dose is 30 gm. *In renal failure* —avoid; drug	Available in 20-ml vials with a concentration of 250 mg/ml. After adding desired amount to infusion fluid, discard unused portion of drug vial. Use prepared solutions promptly. Store unopened vials at room temperature.	Do not mix with any other medication in any manner.	NO Direct injection may cause hypotension, bradycardia and other life-threatening arrhythmias.	YES Add loading dose to 100 ml D5W, NS or RL and infuse over 1 hr. Maintenance doses are administered by continuous infusion.	YES Add an 8-hr dose to 1000 ml D5W, NS or RL and infuse at a rate of approximately 1 gm/ hr (or 1/8 of the total dose/hr).	CONTRAINDICATIONS Do not use if there is evidence or suspicion of an intravascular coagulation process. WARNINGS When used in women of childbearing age or in a patient who is pregnant, the potential benefits must be weighed against the possibility of harm to the fetus. PRECAUTIONS 1. Do not infuse rapidly; to do so may result in bradycardia or other arrhythmias or hypotension. 2. Do not administer without a substantiated diagnosis of hyperfibrinolysis (hyperplasminemia). 3. Administer with caution to patients with cardiac, hepatic or renal disease.

AMINOCAPROIC ACID (Amicar) (Continued)

ACTIONS/ INDICATIONS	DOSAGE	PREPARATION AND STORAGE	DRUG INCOMPATIBILITIES	MODES OF IV ADMINISTRATION			CONTRAINDICATIONS; WARNINGS; PRECAUTIONS; ADVERSE REACTIONS
				INJECTION	INTERMITTENT INFUSION	CONTINUOUS INFUSION	
Systemic hyperfibrinolysis can be associated with: • Postsurgical complications following cardiac surgery, portocaval shunts • Hematological disorders such as aplastic anemia • Abruptio placentae • Hepatic cirrhosis • Carcinoma of the prostate, lung, stomach, and cervix • During the administration of thrombolytic drugs i.e., streptokinase and urokinase. Urinary fibrinolysis may be associated with life-threatening complications following severe trauma, anoxia, and shock. This drug is also used to prevent rebleeding associated with intracranial an-	is excreted primarily via the kidneys.[1] CHILDREN: *Loading dose* — 100 mg/kg or 3 gm/M^2 *Maintenance* — 30 mg/kg or 1 gm/M^2 at hourly intervals to obtain a plasma level of .013 mg/ml. Maximum 24-hr dose is 18 gm/M^2.						ADVERSE REACTIONS 1. Nausea 2. Abdominal cramps 3. Diarrhea 4. Dizziness 5. Tinnitus 6. Malaise 7. Nasal stuffiness 8. Headache 9. Rash 10. Thrombophlebitis at infusion site

eurysms by preventing dissolution of the hemostatic clot that occurs because of the normal fibrinolytic mechanism.

NURSING IMPLICATIONS
1. Avoid extravasation; see page 96.
2. Change IV site at the first sign of thrombophlebitis. Apply warm compresses to the area.
3. Monitor heart rate and blood pressure at hourly intervals during the infusion. Notify physician of arrhythmias or hypotension. Strict adherence to infusion rates should prevent complications.
4. Monitor urine output at 4-hour intervals or as patient's condition dictates.

REFERENCE
1. Mullan, S., and Dawley, J.: Antifibrinolytic Therapy for Intracranial Aneurysms. *Journal of Neurosurgery,* 28:21, 1968.

SUGGESTED READING
Guyton, Arthur C.: *Textbook of Medical Physiology* (5th ed.), Philadelphia: W. B. Saunders Company, 1976, Chapter 9, Hemostasis and Blood Coagulation, pp. 99–111.

● AMINOPHYLLINE

ACTIONS/ INDICATIONS	DOSAGE	PREPARATION AND STORAGE	DRUG INCOMPAT- IBILITIES	MODES OF IV ADMINISTRATION			CONTRAINDICATIONS; WARNINGS; PRECAUTIONS: ADVERSE REACTIONS
				INJECTION	INTERMITTENT INFUSION	CONTINUOUS INFUSION	
Bronchodilator. Works directly on spastic bronchial muscles and induces relaxation. Can be used in any condition that produces acute bronchospasm, such as asthma (bronchial or cardiac), status asthmaticus, and pulmonary edema (when accompanied by hypertension.*) Also used as an antispasmotic in biliary colic. *See Contraindications.	ADULTS: *Loading dose* —6 mg/kg given over 20 min followed by 0.9 mg/kg/ hr as a continuous infusion titrated with plasma theophylline levels. (Example: 70-kg patient would receive approximately 420 mg as a loading dose followed by an infusion of 63 mg/hr) Reduce dose by ⅓ in the presence of congestive heart failure and in the elderly.	Available in IV and IM forms; check label carefully.	Do not mix in any manner with: Epinephrine Levarterenol (Levophed) Isoproterenol (Isuprel) Penicillin G potassium Amikacin Cephalothin Cephapirin Clindamycin Erythromycin Nafcillin Oxytetracycline Tetracycline Vancomycin Hydrocortisone Methylprednisolone Insulin (regular) Nitroprusside Vitamin C	YES Only in extreme emergencies. This drug will cause serious tachyarrhythmias, hypotension and seizures when given in concentrated form. DO NOT INJECT AT A RATE GREATER THAN 25 mg (1 ml)/min of the undiluted preparation.	YES Dilute to at least 1 mg in 1 ml of D5W or NS. Total daily dose may be given in 4 divided doses every 6 hrs. DO NOT EXCEED A RATE OF 25 mg/min. Use an infusion pump.	YES *This is the preferred mode of administration.* Prepare a solution concentration that will simplify calculation of drip rate, e.g., 1 mg/ml in D5W or NS. SEE DOSAGE COLUMN FOR HOURLY DOSE Use an infusion pump.	CONTRAINDICATIONS 1. Hypersensitivity to theophylline derivatives 2. In the presence of hypotension 3. In the presence of coronary artery disease or angina when cardiac stimulation could be harmful 4. In peptic ulcer disease WARNINGS 1. Overdosage may lead to circulatory collapse. 2. Rapid injection will produce serious tachyarrhythmias, hypotension and seizures. PRECAUTIONS 1. When the patient is acutely ill and has a history of cardiac problems such as arrhythmias, use with caution and monitor ECG for PVC's, ventricular tachycardia, ventricular fibrillation, or supraventricular tachycardia. 2. Use with caution in patients who have already received epinephrine, or other sympathomimetic drugs (isoproterenol, levarterenol, etc.), who are hypotensive or who have hyperthyroidism. 3. Use extreme caution when adminis-

AMINOPHYLLINE (Continued)

ACTIONS/INDICATIONS	DOSAGE	PREPARATION AND STORAGE	DRUG INCOMPATIBILITIES	MODES OF IV ADMINISTRATION			CONTRAINDICATIONS; WARNINGS; PRECAUTIONS; ADVERSE REACTIONS
				INJECTION	INTERMITTENT INFUSION	CONTINUOUS INFUSION	
	derly. In the presence of liver impairment reduce dose by ½. CHILDREN: *Loading*—5–6 mg/kg or 150 mg/M² given over 20 min. *Maintenance*—0.9 mg/kg/hr by continuous infusion. (Alternative—20 mg/kg/24 hrs, or 600 mg/M²/24 hrs in equally divided doses every 6 hrs. In children and adults, collect blood samples after loading dose or any time during continuous infusion. Optimal plasma level: 10–15 mcg/100 ml.						tering to an infant less than 11 kg (25 lbs). 4. This drug should not be administered concomitantly with other xanthine preparations, such as theophylline, oxtriphylline, dyphylline. ADVERSE REACTIONS 1. Gastrointestinal: anorexia, abdominal cramps, nausea, vomiting, reactivation of a peptic ulcer, and intestinal bleeding. 2. Central nervous system: headache, nervousness, insomnia, anxiety, dizziness, confusion, seizures. 3. Cardiovascular: palpitations, tachy- and bradyarrhythmias, hypotension, chest pain. 4. Fatalities have occurred in overdosage.

NURSING IMPLICATIONS

1. Be aware of hospital policy on the IV administration of aminophylline.
2. Monitor all patients electrocardiographically in an I.C.U. who:
   a. Have a history of arrhythmias
   b. Are acutely ill with pulmonary edema or status asthmaticus
   c. Are hypoxic
   d. Are acidotic
   e. Are receiving other agents that may produce arrhythmias
   Observe for premature ventricular contractions, premature atrial contractions, supraventricular tachycardia and ventricular tachycardia. Slow the infusion rate *immediately* if one of these arrhythmias occurs, or if the sinus rate exceeds 120/min. Notify the physician of the occurrence. Slowing or stopping an infusion will usually control these reactions. However, be prepared to actively treat arrhythmias not controlled in this manner. Keep lidocaine 100 mg at the bedside and administer in accordance with hospital regulations and physician's orders in the event of a ventricular tachyar-

rhythmia. A defibrillator must be readily available.
3. Monitor blood pressure frequently during an infusion (all patients), especially during the first 15 minutes, or if the infusion is being given rapidly for therapeutic reasons. Hypo- and hypertension may occur. (Suggested schedule: Every 2–3 minutes the first 15 minutes of infusion, then every 10 minutes for 1 hour, then every 30 minutes, or as patient's condition dictates.)
4. Observe for drug effectiveness, e.g., decreasing respiratory effort (observable and subjective), decreased wheezing, decreased respiratory rate, decreased cyanosis or pallor. Monitor arterial blood gases for improvement of pCO_2, pO_2, pH and $pHCO_3$, when possible.
5. Monitor for all adverse reactions; all are early warnings of overdosage and toxicity. Slow or stop the infusion at the onset of any one sign. Be aware of the patient's plasma level if obtained (see Dosage column).
6. Initiate seizure precautions.
7. Be prepared to manage vomiting to prevent aspiration.

● AMOBARBITAL SODIUM (Amytal)

ACTIONS/ INDICATIONS	DOSAGE	PREPARATION AND STORAGE	DRUG INCOMPAT-IBILITIES	MODES OF IV ADMINISTRATION			CONTRAINDICATIONS; WARNINGS; PRECAUTIONS; ADVERSE REACTIONS
				INJECTION	INTERMITTENT INFUSION	CONTINUOUS INFUSION	
Barbiturate. Central nervous system depressant, hypnotic, anti-convulsant; moderately long-acting.

Used to control seizures secondary to eclampsia chorea, meningitis, tetanus, drug reactions.

In psychiatry, may be used to control catatonic, negativistic and manic reactions. May also be used for narcoanalysis and narcotherapy. | ADULTS AND CHILDREN OVER 6 YEARS OF AGE: 65–500 mg/ dose (not exceeding 1 gm). Dosage should be determined by patient response.

YOUNGER CHILDREN: 3–5 mg/kg or 125 mg/M^2 per dose. | Available in ampuls of 125, 250 and 500 mg, some accompanied by sterile water for injection, 2.5 ml. To reconstitute from powder, use sterile water for injection in the amounts listed on page 180.

After adding diluent, rotate vial gently; do not shake. Dissolution may take several minutes. Do not use a solution that has not cleared within 5 minutes, or one that contains a precipitate. Use solutions within 30 minutes.

This is a Schedule II drug under the Controlled Substances Act of 1970. Maintain hospital or institutional regulations guiding its use. | Do not mix in any manner with:
Tetracyclines
Metaraminol
Methyldopate
Penicillin
Isoproterenol
Levarterenol
Thiamine
Succinylcholine
Pentazocine
Clindamycin
Chlorpromazine
Propiomazine
Cephalothin
Cephaloridine
Cefazolin
Anileridine
Codeine
Dimenhydrinate
Diphenhydramine
Hydrocortisone
Hydroxyzine
Insulin, regular
Levorphanol
Meperidine
Morphine
Procaine
Vancomycin | YES

Do not exceed a rate of 100 mg/min. for adults or 60 mg/min. for children. | NO

Pharmacologically inappropriate. | NO

Pharmacologically inappropriate. | CONTRAINDICATIONS
1. Impaired liver function
2. Family or patient history of porphyria
3. Hypersensitivity to any barbiturate

WARNINGS
1. May be habit-forming, causing both psychic and physical dependence.
2. The central nervous system depressant effects of this drug may be potentiated by the depressant effects of other similar drugs and alcohol.
3. Safety for use in pregnancy has not been established.
4. This drug may impair the mental and physical abilities to perform potentially hazardous tasks such as ambulating (in the elderly or debilitated), climbing stairs, driving a car.
5. Rapid injection, exceeding recommended rate, or a relative overdosage may cause apnea or hypotension. Respiratory depression may occur if this drug is given concomitantly with other central nervous system depressants.

PRECAUTIONS
1. The liver is the major site of metabolism of this drug. Caution should be observed when administering amobarbital to patients with impaired liver function. Titrate small doses with patient response.
2. Use caution in the dosage and rate of administration of this drug when administering it to patients with hypotension, respiratory disorders, cardiac disease or hypertension.
3. Pulmonary edema may accompany long periods of unconsciousness produced by this drug.

ADVERSE REACTIONS
1. Respiratory depression
2. Drug idiosyncrasy: excitement or "hangover" symptoms
3. Hypersensitivity: asthma, urticaria, angioneurotic edema |

AMOBARBITAL SODIUM (Amytal) (Continued)

ACTIONS/INDICATIONS	DOSAGE	PREPARATION AND STORAGE	DRUG INCOMPATIBILITIES	MODES OF IV ADMINISTRATION			CONTRAINDICATIONS; WARNINGS; PRECAUTIONS; ADVERSE REACTIONS
				INJECTION	INTERMITTENT INFUSION	CONTINUOUS INFUSION	
		Volumes of diluent needed to make specified solution concentrations for each ampul size:[1]					4. Laryngospasm (rarely during normal use or as the result of improper dosage)
							5. Hypotension after rapid injection
							6. Nausea and vomiting

Preparation table:

Concentration (mg/ml)	Volume of Diluent (ml)
125-mg ampul	
10	12.5
25	5.0
50	2.5
100	1.25
200	0.625
250-mg ampul	
10	25.0
25	10.0
50	5.0
100	2.5
200	1.25
500-mg ampul	
10	50.0
25	20.0
50	10.0
100	5.0
200	2.5

MANAGEMENT OF OVERDOSAGE

1. Symptoms: respiratory depression, depression of superficial and deep reflexes, slight pupillary constriction (in severe overdosage pupils may dilate), decreased urine output, fall in body temperature, coma, hypotension.

2. Treatment: administration of fluids; maintenance of blood pressure, body temperature and ventilation. Patients with respiratory depression will require intubation and mechanical ventilation until the drug has been excreted. Hemodialysis can be used to increase the rate of excretion.

NURSING IMPLICATIONS

1. Strictly adhere to maximum injection rate suggestions and maximum dosage limits. Patients with liver impairment should receive smaller doses and should be monitored more closely and for a longer period of time than usual.

2. Keep the patient supine during and after injection. Monitor blood pressure, heart rate and respiratory rate every 5 minutes for 1 hour following an injection. This includes fetal heart rate monitoring. Do not leave the patient unattended.

3. Patients with porphyria are sensitive to barbiturates in that they may experience an acute attack of the disease secondary to the administration of a barbiturate (see Contraindications). The onset of an acute attack is indicated by severe colicky abdominal pain radiating to the back. There is usually severe vomiting, fever and leukocytosis in addition.[2]

the physician. Discontinuation of the injection is usually all that is necessary to prevent further problems. If not, see No. 7 below.

7. Management of acute overdosage:
   a. Continue to stay with the patient and monitor vital signs.
   b. Maintain an open airway and adequate ventilation.
   c. Keep the patient as alert as possible by verbal and physical stimuli. Encourage the patient to breathe at an adequate rate (12–14 breaths/minute for an adult). If necessary, initiate artificial ventilation with a manual breathing bag (Puritan, Hope, Ambu, etc.) or mouth-to-mouth breathing at a rate of 12–14 breaths/minute.
   d. Circulatory support in the form of fluids and drugs may be ordered.

8. The sedation produced by this drug may be preceded by transient changes in mental status, such as feelings of euphoria and confusion. If this occurs, attempt to calm the patient and take measures to prevent injury until the

4. Avoid extravasation; see page 96. Extravascular or intra-arterial injection of this drug can cause tissue necrosis and gangrene of the affected extremity, respectively. Thrombophlebitis can also occur.
5. Take anaphylaxis precautions; see page 118.
6. Monitor for symptoms of acute overdosage (listed in order of progression):
   a. Respiratory depression, i.e., decreased respiratory rate and depth
   b. Peripheral vascular collapse, i.e., fall in blood pressure, pallor diaphoresis, tachycardia
   c. Pulmonary edema (rare)
   d. Decreased or absent reflexes, pupillary constriction
   e. Stupor
   f. Coma
   Stop the injection immediately upon noting one of these symptoms. Notify patient returns to his normal status.
9. If a patient is to be ambulatory following an injection, ambulate with assistance; there may be transient dizziness. Obtain lying, then sitting and standing blood pressures to detect postural hypotension. If this drug has been used for outpatient procedure, a responsible adult should accompany the patient home. The patient should not drive for at least the next 8 hours.

REFERENCES
1. Trissel, Lawrence: Handbook on Injectable Drugs. American Society of Hospital Pharmacists, Washington, D.C., 1977, p. 23.
2. Beeson, Paul B., and McDermott, Walsh (editors): Cecil-Loeb Textbook of Medicine (14th ed.), Philadelphia, W. B. Saunders Company, 1975, p. 1873.

● AMPHOTERICIN B (Fungizone)

ACTIONS/INDICATIONS	DOSAGE	PREPARATION AND STORAGE	DRUG INCOMPATIBILITIES	MODES OF IV ADMINISTRATION			CONTRAINDICATIONS; WARNINGS; PRECAUTIONS; ADVERSE REACTIONS
				INJECTION	INTERMITTENT INFUSION	CONTINUOUS INFUSION	
Antibiotic, antifungal. To be used only in patients with progressive, potentially fatal fungal infections: • Cryptococcosis • Blastomycosis • Disseminated histoplasmosis • Candidiasis • Coccidiomycosis • Disseminated moniliasis • Mucormycosis (phycomycosis) This drug may be helpful in the treatment of American mucocutan-	ADULTS: An initial test dose of 1 mg may be given over 30 min in an infusion. If no adverse reactions occur, full dose may be given. Optimal dose is unknown, but amount given should be gradually increased up to 1 mg/kg/day depending on patient response. Do not exceed 1.5 mg/kg/day. *Usual dose—* 0.25 mg/kg/day. CHILDREN AND NEONATES: Test dose of 0.1 mg/kg	To prepare from powder add 10 ml sterile water for injection* to the 50-mg vial. Shake until solution is clear. The resultant solution is 5 mg/ml. Store powder and reconstituted solution in the refrigerator. Discard reconstituted solutions after 7 days. Use only D5W for infusion vehicle; do not use if solution is not clear. *Do not use diluents containing bacteriostatic agents, or saline.	This drug is incompatible with solutions with a pH less than 6. Use only D5W for infusion. Do not mix with any other medication in any manner. (Heparin and/or hydrocortisone may be added to solution to decrease risk of infusion phlebitis.)	NO Must be highly diluted prior to administration.	YES Preferred mode of administration. Infuse total daily dose over 6 hrs. Use a concentration of 1 mg/ml; use D5W for infusion fluid. In-line filters can be used but the mean pore diameter should not be less than 1.0 micron in order to assure passage of the drug dispersion.	NO	CONTRAINDICATIONS Hypersensitivity, unless administration of this drug is considered to be lifesaving. WARNINGS 1. The possible lifesaving benefits of this drug must be weighed against its untoward and dangerous side effects. 2. Safety for use in pregnancy has not been established. PRECAUTIONS 1. Prolonged therapy is usually necessary. 2. Unpleasant reactions are common; some are dangerous. Therefore, this drug should be used only in potentially fatal forms of susceptible mycotic infections that have been confirmed by culture. 3. Corticosteroids in large doses should not be administered concomitantly unless they are necessary to control drug reactions. 4. May cause renal damage. Serum creatinine and BUN must be monitored at weekly intervals during therapy. If BUN exceeds 40 mg/100 ml or the serum creatinine exceeds 3.0 mg/100 ml, the drug should be discontinued or reduced in dosage until re-

AMPHOTERICIN B (Fungizone) (Continued)

ACTIONS/INDICATIONS	DOSAGE	PREPARATION AND STORAGE	DRUG INCOMPATIBILITIES	MODES OF IV ADMINISTRATION			CONTRAINDICATIONS; WARNINGS; PRECAUTIONS; ADVERSE REACTIONS
				INJECTION	INTERMITTENT INFUSION	CONTINUOUS INFUSION	
eous leishmaniasis, but is not the drug of choice.	over 6 hrs. Increase the dose, if there are no adverse reactions, over the next 4 days. Do not exceed 1 mg/kg/24 hrs (30 mg/m²/24 hrs).						nal function improves. Use with caution in the presence of pre-existing renal failure. 5. Therapy should be discontinued if liver function test results are abnormal, e.g., elevated bromsulphalein, alkaline phosphates and bilirubin. 6. May cause hypokalemia and low serum magnesium. 7. Whenever amphotericin is discontinued for longer than 7 days, therapy should be restarted at test-dose level, and gradually increased to therapeutic levels. 8. Anemia usually occurs with this drug. ADVERSE REACTIONS 1. Intolerance to this drug may be made less severe by administering aspirin, antihistamines and anti-emetics. Administration on alternate days may decrease anorexia and infusion phlebitis. Small doses of intravenous hydrocortisone just prior to or during the infusion may lessen febrile reactions. The smallest possible dosage of the steroid should be employed. 2. Extravasation may cause tissue irritation. 3. Fever (shaking chills) 4. Headache 5. Malaise 6. Diarrhea 7. Muscle and joint pains 8. Normochromic, normocytic anemia 9. Renal function abnormalities: hyperkalemia, azotemia, renal tubular acidosis, nephrocalcinosis. Permanent renal impairment may occur, especially with large doses. Supplemental alkali medication may decrease renal tubular acidosis. 10. Anuria is rare 11. Cardiac toxicity (rare): arrhythmias, cardiac arrest, hypertension, hypotension. 12. Blood dyscrasis: thrombocytopenia, leukopenia or leukocytosis, agranulocytopenia, eosinophilia. 13. Hemorrhagic gastroenteritis

14. Rash
15. Loss of hearing, tinnitus, transient vertigo
16. Blurred vision or diplopia
17. Peripheral neuropathy
18. Convulsions
19. Anaphylaxis
20. Acute liver failure

   f. Hearing loss—notify the physician if any hearing loss, ringing in the ears, or dizziness.
   g. Changes in vision.
3. Administer supplemental medications to prevent or lessen adverse reactions; e.g., antipyretics, antiemetics, analgesics.
4. Notify the physician if jaundice is observed.
5. Avoid extravasation, see page 96. If it occurs, discontinue infusion, apply warm compresses and prevent further damage to the area.
6. Maintain hydration. In the presence of nausea, vomiting and diarrhea parenteral fluids may be indicated. Administer drugs to lessen these effects. Measure intake and output to guide the physician in ordering fluids.
7. Provide emotional support for critically ill patients receiving this drug. Their discomforts and fears will be numerous.

NURSING IMPLICATIONS
1. Take anaphylaxis precautions; see page 118.
2. Monitor for symptoms of toxicity:
   a. Renal damage—measure urinary output every 4 hours; notify the physician if urine output falls below an average of 30 ml/hour; urine for analysis at least every other day to detect abnormalities.
   b. Cardiac arrhythmias—monitor heart rate and rhythm every 2 hours; notify physician of abnormalities. Continuous ECG monitoring is advisable.
   c. Neurologic changes—observe for changes in mental status, numbness of fingers, toes, or face, seizures.
   d. Fever—record temperature every 4 hours (mild elevations are seen in most patients).
   e. Blood disorders—observe for bleeding, petechiae, bruising.

AMPICILLIN, SODIUM (Alpen-N, Amcill-S, Omnipen-N, Pen A/N, Penbritin-S, Pensyn, Principen-N, Polycillin-N, SK-Ampicillin N, Totacillin)

ACTIONS/ INDICATIONS	DOSAGE	PREPARATION AND STORAGE	DRUG INCOMPAT- IBLITIES	MODES OF IV ADMINISTRATION			CONTRAINDICATIONS; WARNINGS; PRECAUTIONS; ADVERSE REACTIONS
				INJECTION	INTERMITTENT INFUSION	CONTINUOUS INFUSION	
Antibiotic, synthetic penicillin, broad spectrum. Bactericidal against penicillin-insusceptible gram-positive and gram-negative organisms. Used to treat infections secondary to susceptible organisms such as streptococci, penicillin-G sensitive staphylococci, gonococci, E. coli, Proteus, H. influenzae and others, for	This drug should not be given in doses larger than those recommended, except where indicated. ADULTS:[1] *Infections of the respiratory tract, skin, and soft tissue—* 250–500 mg every 6 hrs. *Gastrointestinal and urinary tract infections—*500 mg every 6 hrs.	To reconstitute 125-, 250- and 500-mg vials add 5 ml sterile water for injection. For the 1-gm and 2-gm vials add 10 ml sterile water for injection or bacteriostatic water for injection. Use these solutions within 1 hour of reconstitution. For infusion add reconstituted solutions to	Do not add any other medication to ampicillin in IV fluid. Do not mix in an IV line with any other antibiotic.	YES Must be injected over at least 3–5 min for a dose of 125–500 mg. A more rapid injection can result in seizures. Inject into tubing of a running IV.	YES *Preferred route.* Dilute each 500 mg of any fluid listed in the Preparation column. Infuse over 30 min. Do not exceed a 100 mg/min flow rate.	YES Dilute dose in 500–1000 ml of any fluid listed in the table in the Preparation column. Infuse within the time limit specified in that table to insure potency.	CONTRAINDICATIONS Hypersensitivity to any penicillin or ampicillin PRECAUTIONS 1. There may be cross-allergenicity with cephalosporins. Administer with caution to patients with allergy to any cephalosporin. 2. Safety for use in pregnancy has not been established. Potential risk to the fetus must be weighed against benefits to the mother. 3. There is a possibility of secondary (overgrowth) infections due to nonsusceptible mycoses or bacterial pathogens. 4. Monitor renal, hepatic and hematopoietic function before and during therapy. 5. A maculopapular rash and urticaria can occur in a significant percentage of all patients receiving this drug who

183

AMPICILLIN, SODIUM (Alpen-N, Amcill-S, Omnipin-N, Pen A/N, Penbritin-S, Pensyn, Principen-N, Polycillin-N, SK-Ampicillin N, Totacillin) (Continued)

ACTIONS/INDICATIONS	DOSAGE	PREPARATION AND STORAGE	DRUG INCOMPATIBILITIES	INJECTION	INTERMITTENT INFUSION	CONTINUOUS INFUSION	CONTRAINDICATIONS; WARNINGS; PRECAUTIONS; ADVERSE REACTIONS
				MODES OF IV ADMINISTRATION			

infections of the respiratory tract, soft tissue, skin, urinary tract, blood and central nervous system.

DOSAGE:
(Dosage may be higher in severe infections.)

In septicemia and bacterial meningitis— 8–14 gm daily or 150–200 mg/kg/day, in equally divided doses, every 3–4 hours.

Renal impairment (creatinine clearance less than 10 ml/min.)—increase the interval between doses to 8 and 12 hrs, unless a high urine concentration of the drug is needed, then give every 6 hrs.

CHILDREN:
(Children over 40 kg may receive adult dosage.)

Infections of the respiratory tract, skin and soft tissue —25–50 mg/kg/day given in equally divided doses every 6 hrs.

Gastrointestinal and urinary tract infections

PREPARATION AND STORAGE:
any of the IV fluids listed in the table below.

For piggyback units for infusion, use sterile water for injection or NS: to the 1-gm bottle, add 49 ml of diluent, shake well. Resultant solution is 20 mg/ml.

2-gm bottle, add 99 ml of diluent and shake well. The resulting solution is 20 mg/ml.

FLUID USED—INFUSION TIME LIMIT

Solution	Concentration of Infusion (Ampicillin/ml of fluid)	Time Limit for Infusion
NS	up to 30 mg/ml	8 hrs
Sodium lacate		
M/6	up to 30 mg/ml	8 hrs
D5W	10–20 mg/ml	2 hrs
D5W	up to 2 mg/ml	4 hrs
D5/0.45% sodium chloride	up to 2 mg/ml	4 hrs
10% invert sugar	up to 2 mg/ml	4 hrs
R.L.	up to 30 mg/ml	8 hrs

CONTRAINDICATIONS; WARNINGS; PRECAUTIONS; ADVERSE REACTIONS:
have renal dysfunction. This is not thought to be a true penicillin allergic reaction, and is not a contraindication. However, the patient should be monitored closely for other signs of allergy or anaphylaxis.
6. With high urine concentrations, false-positive glucose reactions may occur if Clinitest is used. Clinistix or Tes-Tape should be used.

ADVERSE REACTIONS
1. Allergy: rash, urticaria, anaphylaxis.
2. Gastrointestinal: glossitis (inflammation of tongue), stomatitis (inflammation of mucous membranes of the mouth), nausea, vomiting, diarrhea.
3. Liver: slight rise in SGOT, especially in infants (significance is unknown).
4. Blood cell formation: anemia, thrombocytopenia, leukopenia and agranulocytosis. (These reactions are believed to be due to allergy, and are reversible.)

—50–100 mg/kg/day given in equally divided doses every 6 hrs.

Septicemia and bacterial meningitis—100–400 mg/kg/day via continuous infusion for 3 days followed by intermittent IV or IM doses.

NEONATES (TERM AND PREMATURE):
Less than 1 week of age in life-threatening septicemia and meningitis[2]—100 mg/kg/day in 2 equal doses 12 hrs apart. (Usually given with an aminoglycoside antibiotic).

More than 1 week of age in septicemia and meningitis[3]—200 mg/kg/day in 3 equal doses 8 hrs apart (with an aminoglycoside).

NURSING IMPLICATIONS
1. Take anaphylaxis precautions; see page 118.
2. Monitor for signs and symptoms of overgrowth infections:
   a. Fever (take rectal temperature at least every 4–6 hours in all patients)
   b. Increasing malaise
   c. Newly appearing localized signs and symptoms—redness, soreness, pain, swelling, drainage (increased volume or change in character of pre-existing drainage)
   d. Monilial rash in perineal area (reddened areas with itching)
   e. Cough (change in pre-existing cough or sputum production)
   f. Diarrhea
3. Nausea, vomiting and diarrhea are fairly common side effects with ampicillin. Administer antiemetics or constipating agents as ordered. Maintain hydration. Encourage nutritional intake as allowed by the patient's condition. Record intake and output to guide the physician in ordering parenteral fluids if they are needed.

4. Be aware of the patient's blood cell count. If the white cell count falls below 2000/cu.mm., place the patient in protective (reversed) isolation. Prevent infection by maintaining bodily cleanliness (especially perineal) and avoiding traumatic procedures. Monitor for signs of infection. If the platelet count falls below 100,000/cu.mm., monitor for thrombocytopenic bleeding: gum bleeding, epistaxis, hematemesis, petechiae, hematuria, melena, blood in the stools, vaginal bleeding, ecchymosis.
5. Report all rashes to the physician. They may be prelude to anaphylaxis.
6. Use Clinistix or Tes-Tape for urine glucose determinations.

REFERENCES
1. *American Hospital Formulary Service*, Washington, D.C.: American Society of Hospital Pharmacists. 1977, Section 8:12–16.
2. McCracken, George H., and Nelson, John D.: *Antimicrobial Therapy for Newborns*. New York: Grune and Stratton, 1977, p. 16.
3. Ibid.

● ANILERIDINE PHOSPHATE (Leritine)

ACTIONS/ INDICATIONS	DOSAGE	PREPARATION AND STORAGE	DRUG INCOMPAT- IBILITIES	MODES OF IV ADMINISTRATION				CONTRAINDICATIONS; WARNINGS; PRECAUTIONS; ADVERSE REACTIONS
				INJECTION	INTERMITTENT INFUSION	CONTINUOUS INFUSION		
Narcotic analgesic similar to, but more potent than, meperidine. Used for moderate to severe pain. Has sedative qualities. Can be used as an adjunct to anesthesia or as an analgesic during labor.

Onset of action is in 2–3 min, duration is 25–40 min. | ADULTS AND CHILDREN OVER 12 YEARS OF AGE: *Initially*—5–10 mg by injection followed by an infusion of 0.6 mg/min titrated with patient response

CHILDREN UNDER 12: Not recommended. | Available in 25 mg/ml solutions: 1-ml and 2-ml ampuls and 30-ml multi-dose vials.

Add only to D5W for infusion.

Store at room temperature.

This is a Schedule II drug under the Controlled Substances Act of 1970. Maintain hospital or institutional regulations guiding the use of this drug. | Do not mix in any manner with: Aminophylline Ammonium chloride Any barbiturate Chlorothiazide Heparin Methicillin Novobiocin Phenytoin Sodium bicarbonate Sodium iodide. | YES

ONLY IN GRAVE EMERGENCIES

Dose via this route should not exceed 10 mg.

INJECT SLOWLY OVER 2–3 MIN | YES

Add 50–100 mg to 500 ml D5W. Usual rate is 0.6 mg/min titrated with patient response.

Use an infusion pump. | YES

Same as Intermittent Infusion. | | CONTRAINDICATIONS 1. Respiratory depression 2. Hypersensitivity 3. Patients under 12 years of age

WARNINGS 1. Can cause respiratory depression; occurs more frequently in the elderly, the debilitated or in the presence of pulmonary impairment such as in chronic lung disease, chest trauma, or chest surgery. 2. Can cause circulatory depression. Administer with extreme caution to patients in shock; further decrease in cardiac output and blood pressure may occur. 3. In the presence of deep respiratory and circulatory collapse, nalorphine or levallorphan may counteract the effects. 4. Use with caution in combination with other narcotics, sedatives, phenothiazines, or anesthetics. These drugs may potentiate respiratory and circulatory depressant effects. 5. Rapid injection of a dose greater than 10 mg may result in severe respiratory depression and apnea, hypotension and possibly cardiac arrest. Give via intravenous *injection* ONLY IN EXTREME EMERGENCIES. 6. Safety for use in pregnancy has not been established in regard to the effects on fetal development. Can be used during labor, but precautions must be taken to prevent or to promptly treat respiratory depression in the newborn.

PRECAUTIONS 1. May be habit-forming 2. Use with extreme caution in the presence of hepatic impairment, severe central nervous system depression, patients with head injuries or when intracranial pressure is increased, myxedema, Addison's disease, acute alcoholic intoxication, delirium tremens, seizure disorders, and in patients taking MAO inhibitors |

ADVERSE REACTIONS

1. Respiratory depression (see Warning Nos. 1, 4, and 5)
2. Circulatory depression (see Warning Nos. 2, 4, and 5)
3. Nausea, vomiting, dry mouth
4. Slight transient hypotension and bradycardia
5. Dizziness
6. Diaphoresis
7. Blurred vision
8. Euphoria, restlessness, nervousness and excitement
9. Hypersensitivity: urticaria, rash, anaphylaxis

MANAGEMENT OF OVERDOSAGE

1. Symptoms: Respiratory depression, i.e., decreased respiratory rate possibly leading to apnea, stupor, hypotension.
2. Treatment:
   Adults: Nalorphine intravenously, 5–10 mg repeated at 10- to 15-minute intervals until symptoms of overdosage resolve (or naloxone according to manufacturer's dosage guidelines).
   Newborns: Nalorphine into the umbilical vein (or subcutaneously), 0.2–0.5 mg initially, or 0.2 mg repeated until a 0.5 mg dose has been reached. Oxygen, assisted ventilation, intravenous fluids, blood pressure support and constant attendance are advisable until full respiratory and circulatory functions return and are stabilized.
   In patients who are addicted to narcotics (including newborn of an addicted mother), the use of a narcotic antagonist agent may precipitate an acute withdrawal syndrome. See page 415 for the use of nalorphine.

NURSING IMPLICATIONS

1. Adhere strictly to injection and infusion rate restrictions.
2. Monitor respiratory status during, and for 1 hour after, injection. Count respiratory rate every 2–3 minutes during the first 30 minutes and every 5–10 minutes thereafter. If the patient's respiratory rate (adult) falls below 8–10/minute, attempt to arouse the patient and stimulate a respiratory rate of at least 12–14/minute. If the patient is receiving an infusion of this drug, temporarily stop it. Call for the physician. If the patient cannot be aroused to cooperate, begin assisted ventilation either by mouth-to-mouth breathing or by using a manual breathing bag and airway. Administer oxygen as needed. See Management of Overdosage for the use of a narcotic antagonists. The patient should have complete return of spontaneous respiratory rate, gag, swallow and cough reflexes before being left unattended. (See chart on page 545 for normal newborn respiratory rates.)
3. Monitor blood pressure before, during, and for 1 hour after injection, at 5–10 minute intervals. Report hypotension to the physician. If the patient is receiving an infusion, slow it down to a minimal rate or discontinue. Administer fluids, the narcotic antagonist, and vasopressors as needed. Discontinuation of the drug alone may allow blood pressure to return to normal.
4. Patient situations as listed in Warning No. 4 and Precaution No. 2 should be monitored continuously during and for 2 hours after injection or infusion. These patients are more likely to develop adverse reactions.
5. Be prepared to manage vomiting to prevent aspiration.
6. Monitor patient's response to analgesia to guide infusion rate and/or additional injections.

SUGGESTED READING

McCaffery, Margo, and Hart, Linda L.: Undertreatment of Acute Pain With Narcotics. *American Journal of Nursing*, October 1976, pp. 1586–1591.

187

ANTIHEMOPHILIC FACTOR, HUMAN (Factorate, Humafac, Factor VIII)

ACTIONS/ INDICATIONS	DOSAGE	PREPARATION AND STORAGE	DRUG INCOMPATIBILITIES	MODES OF IV ADMINISTRATION				CONTRAINDICATIONS; WARNINGS; PRECAUTIONS; ADVERSE REACTIONS
				INJECTION	INTERMITTENT INFUSION	CONTINUOUS INFUSION		
A stable lyphilized concentrate of Factor VIII (AHF, AHG), intended for the specific therapy of Hemophilia A., characterized by a deficiency in the production of the antihemophilic factor (Factor VIII).	ADULTS AND CHILDREN: For IV administration only. Dosage must be individualized according to the needs of the patient, by body weight, severity of the hemorrhage, and presence of inhibitors. General dosages:

Overt bleeding—20 units/kg initially, followed by 10 units/kg every 8 hrs for the first 24 hrs and every 12 hrs for 3–4 days.

Muscle hemorrhages—
Minor, in non-vital areas—10 units/kg once a day for 2–3 days.

Massive, in nonvital areas—10 units/kg by infusion for 12 hr intervals for 2 days and then once a day for 2 days.

Near vital organs (neck, throat, subperitoneal)—20 units/kg initially, then | To prepare: warm the drug and diluent provided by the manufacturer, un opened, to room temperature but not above 98°F (37°C).

Use plastic syringes and filter needles provided by the manufacturer. Follow package insert instructions for transfer of diluent. Gently rotate vial to mix; do not shake. This process takes about 5 min. Store drug and diluent at 2–8°C (36–46°F). Do not freeze.

Mix fresh for each administration; discard unused portions. | Do not mix with any other medication. | YES

Use plastic syringes only. Administer at a rate comfortable to the patient, usually 25 ml in 5 min. | YES

Use plastic syringes only and infusion set provided by manufacturer; follow instructions. Use a new set each 24 hrs. Flush set with NS after completion of infusion to insure all medication enters the patient. | YES

Use plastic syringes only. Infuse as directed under "intermittent." Do not mix with large volume of fluids. | | CONTRAINDICATIONS
None known

WARNINGS
There is a possibility, despite manufacturer testing, that viral hepatitis can be transmitted in this drug.

PRECAUTIONS
This drug contains low levels of blood groups A and B isohemagglutinins. When large volumes are given to patients of groups A, B, or AB, the possibility of intravascular hemolysis should be considered.

ADVERSE REACTIONS
There may be mild chills, nausea, or stinging at the infusion site during the administration of this drug. |

10 units/kg every 8 hrs for 2 days, then reduce dose by one-half.

Joint hemor-rhages— 10 units/kg every 8 hrs for 1 day, then twice daily for 1-2 days. If joint aspiration is carried out, 10 units/kg just prior, and 10 units/kg 8 hrs later, and again the next day.

Surgery—30-40 units/kg prior, 20 units/kg every 8 hrs after. Serum antihemo-philic factor should be kept at 40% by lab valves for 10 days postoper-atively.

One unit of AHF will in-crease the cir-culatory AHF by 2%. See dosage charts accompanying the drug.

NURSING IMPLICATIONS
1. Monitor the patient for signs of intravascular hemolysis; e.g., change in urine color to pink, red or brown.
2. All preparations for administration must be carried out *precisely* as manu-facturer directs.
3. Apply comfort measures as indicated for chills and nausea during adminis-tration.
4. All patients and families must be thoroughly educated on the care of the patient with hemophilia. The manufacturers of antihemophilic factor pro-vide useful patient literature.

ANTIVENIN, SNAKE (Crotalidae Species, Polyvalent, Equine Origin)

ACTIONS/ INDICATIONS	DOSAGE	PREPARATION AND STORAGE	DRUG INCOMPAT- IBILITIES	MODES OF IV ADMINISTRATION			CONTRAINDICATIONS; WARNINGS; PRECAUTIONS; ADVERSE REACTIONS
				INJECTION	INTERMITTENT INFUSION	CONTINUOUS INFUSION	
A protective substance against the venom of all rattlesnakes, moccasins, the fer-de-lance and similar species, and the brushmaster.

Used to treat poisoning by crotaline snakes throughout the world.

This serum is of equine origin. | ADULTS AND CHILDREN: *Initial dose*— 15–75 ml: depending on the size of the snake, the time lapsed between time of bite and treatment, and the size and condition of the patient. *The smaller the patient's body*, the larger the amount of initial dose. Besides the initial IV dose, SC and IM injections are usually made at points around the bite, above the level of swelling.

(These injections may consist of half of the initial dose with the remainder being given IV.) Repeated intravenous injections of 15 ml may be given in ½ to 2 hours if pain and active swelling persist. | Reconstitute with diluent provided by the manufacturer; administer in ml doses. Discard unused portions. (Testing material for equine sensitivity also provided.) | Do not mix with any other medication in any manner. | YES

Slowly, directly IV or into the tubing of a running IV. | YES

Add dose to 50–250 ml NS; infuse over 30–45 min. | NO | PRECAUTIONS
1. Sensitivity testing to the horse serum should be carried out before administration (skin and conjunctival).
2. Blood typing should be carried out as soon as possible after injury because the hemolysins present in the venom will alter blood protein structure, preventing accurate cross-matching.
3. Administer antibiotics and tetanus antitoxin.
4. Use barbiturates and opiates in small doses and with caution.

ADVERSE REACTIONS
1. Systemic reactions to this drug begin within 30 minutes of administration: anaphylaxis, itching, urticaria, apprehension, edema of the face, tongue, and throat, cough, dyspnea, cyanosis, vomiting. These symptoms may also be produced by the venom itself.
2. Serum sickness within 6–24 days of administration.
3. Severe accelerated reactions may occur within 2–5 days or in some patients within a few minutes. Future injections may be dangerous, in that they may produce a fatal anaphylaxis. |

NURSING IMPLICATIONS
1. Immediate care of the patient:
   a. Begin monitoring vital signs (blood pressure, heart rate, respiratory rate, and quality); in severe reactions to crotalidae venom, there will be decreasing blood pressure, tachycardia, diaphoresis, and pallor.[1]
   b. The patient is usually anxious and in considerable pain (depending on

and symptoms:
   a. Numbness and tingling of the face
   b. Severe muscle spasms
   c. Alterations in clotting time and resultant bleeding (hematuria and gastrointestinal bleeding)[2]
Monitor for the onset of these signs and symptoms. Notify the physician.

the location of the bite and the amount of venom injected). Analgesia and sedation will be necessary. Explanations of procedures and reassurance are mandatory.

c. Be prepared to manage vomiting to prevent aspiration. Suction equipment should be at the bedside.

d. Tetanus antitoxin will be ordered early in the course of therapy. (Determine if patient has an allergy to this prior to administration.)

e. Respiratory distress is common in severe reactions, secondary to laryngeal edema or chest muscle weakness or paralysis. Monitor respiratory effort, ability to use muscles of respiration, respiratory sounds (stridor or wheezing will be present in the event of airway edema), and patient's color for presence or absence of cyanosis. Be prepared to support ventilation. Keep a manual breathing bag, airways, and oxygen ready for use. Equipment to perform an emergency tracheostomy should be readily available. Treatment must be guided by arterial blood gas determinations.

f. The patient may complain of severe thirst, but should be kept NPO. Fluids and supportive therapy for hypotension will relieve this symptom.

2. Severe systemic reactions to the venom will produce the following signs Such reactions must be treated with antivenin.

3. Assist with obtaining an allergy history and skin-testing procedure if indicated (if patient has a positive history of allergy to horse serum or has other drug allergies) prior to administration of antivenin. After adminstration, monitor for anaphylaxis (see page 118 for precautions and treatment). Keep in mind that the signs of a severe allergic reaction can also be produced by snake venom.

4. Wound care:
a. Protect blebs and necrotic tissue from further damage and from contamination.
b. It is advisable to manage a severe wound as a burn.
c. Monitor the circulatory status of the extremity. Severe edema may cause circulatory embarrassment. Notify the physician in such an event; a fasciotomy may be required.

REFERENCES
1. Beeson, Paul B., and McDermott, Walsh (editors): *Cecil-Loeb Textbook of Medicine* (14th ed.), Philadelphia: W. B. Saunders Company, 1975, p. 90.
2. Ibid., p. 91.

● ANTIVENIN, SPIDER (Black Widow, *Latrodectus mactans*)

ACTIONS/ INDICATIONS	DOSAGE	PREPARATION AND STORAGE	DRUG INCOMPAT- IBILITIES	MODES OF IV ADMINISTRATION			CONTRAINDICATIONS; WARNINGS; PRECAUTIONS; ADVERSE REACTIONS
				INJECTION	INTERMITTENT INFUSION	CONTINUOUS INFUSION	
A protective substance against the venom of the black widow spider. Specific systemic therapy for the bite of the black widow spider. This serum is of equine origin.	ADULTS AND CHILDREN: 2.5 ml (contents of 1 vial) in 10–50 ml of saline over 15 min. IV route is preferred if the patient is under 12 years of age or in shock. One dose is usually sufficient.	Reconstitute by adding 2.5 ml sterile water for injection that accompanies the drug.	Do not mix with any other medication.	YES In 10–50 ml NS; inject over 15 min.	YES In 10–50 ml NS; infuse over 15 min.	NO	PRECAUTIONS 1. Intradermal skin test for hypersensitivity to this drug should be carried out prior to administration. (Use no more than 0.2 ml of the test material.) 2. Evaluate test area in 10 minutes; a positive reaction is indicated by a wheal surrounded by an area of erythema. 3. Sensitivity reactions, serum sickness, and death may occur in sensitive patients. 4. Desensitization should be carried out only if use of this drug is considered essential to the life of the patient. Follow standard desensitization procedures.

NURSING IMPLICATIONS

1. The black widow spider bite can produce the following signs and symptoms:
a. A shock state, hypotension, tachycardia, pallor, diaphoresis
b. Abdominal muscle rigidity
c. Respiratory distress secondary to chest muscle weakness and eventual paralysis
d. Severe reactions can lead to coma[1]

2. Monitor blood pressure and heart rate frequently until stabilization is seen. Supportive care should include fluids and vasopressors.

3. Calcium gluconate, 10 ml of a 10% solution, can be given intravenously to relieve muscle spasms (see page 215 on the administration of calcium gluconate). Muscle relaxants (diazepam) may also be prescribed.

4. Analgesia and sedation will be required to combat pain and anxiety. Reassurance and frequent explanations of procedures are mandatory.

5. Monitor the respiratory status frequently for rate, depth, and effort of respirations. Be prepared to support ventilation in the event of respiratory insufficiency with a manual breathing bag, oxygen, and airways. Intubation may be needed.

6. Antivenin will be required for any patient experiencing the above-listed

ANTIVENIN, SPIDER (Black Widow, *Latrodectus mactans*) (*Continued*)

NURSING IMPLICATIONS (No. 6 continued)
signs and symptoms. Assist with obtaining an allergy history, focusing on allergy to horse serum. If the history is positive or if the patient has multiple allergies, desensitization will be required. Be prepared to manage anaphylaxis; see page 118.

7. Monitor patient response to antivenin injections.

REFERENCE
1. Beeson, Paul B., and McDermott, Walsh (editors): *Cecil-Loeb Textbook of Medicine* (14th ed.), Philadelphia: W. B. Saunders Company, 1975, p. 94.

ARGININE HYDROCHLORIDE 10% (R-Gene 10)

| ACTIONS/ INDICATIONS | DOSAGE | PREPARATION AND STORAGE | DRUG INCOMPAT-IBILITIES | MODES OF IV ADMINISTRATION | | | CONTRAINDICATIONS; WARNINGS; PRECAUTIONS; ADVERSE REACTIONS |
				INJECTION	INTERMITTENT INFUSION	CONTINUOUS INFUSION	
L-arginine is a naturally occurring amino acid, that can induce a pronounced rise in the plasma level of human growth hormone (HGH) in a patient with intact pituitary. Used to stimulate the pituitary to release HGH where the measurement of pituitary reserve can be used to diagnose: panhypopituitarism, pituitary dwarfism, chromophobe adenoma, postsurgical craniopharyngioma, hypophysectomy, pituitary trauma, acromegaly, and giantism. This drug is a diagnostic aid and is not intended for therapeutic use.	ADULTS: 300 ml (30 gm) CHILDREN: 5 ml (0.5 gm)/kg	Store in as cool a place as possible above freezing. Start the infusion within 3 hrs after opening the bottle. Follow instructions in package insert for use of Cutter Saftiflask.	Do not mix with any other medications.	NO	YES Drug is supplied in 300 and 500 ml "Saftiflask" vials. Administer over *exactly* 30 min. See test procedure under "Nursing Implications." Use an infusion pump.	NO	CONTRAINDICATIONS Do not administer to patients with highly allergic tendencies. PRECAUTIONS 1. Administer slowly. For accuracy of the test, infuse dose over 30 min. A more rapid infusion can cause irritation at the infusion site, nausea, vomiting, or flushing. 2. Monitor BUN to evaluate patient's tolerance of the drug's content of metabolizable nitrogen. 3. This drug contains 47.5 mEq of chloride ion per 100 ml. The effect that this amount of chloride could have should be considered prior to infusion. 4. Administer *only* by intravenous infusion because of the solution's hypertonicity.

3. Take anaphylactic precautions; see page 118.

NURSING IMPLICATIONS

1. It is not necessary to warm the solution prior to infusion. Inspect solution for clarity. Discard any flask lacking a vacuum or containing a cloudy solution.

2. Arginine hydrochloride injection is a part of the test for measurement of pituitary reserve of human growth hormone. To prepare the patient for this test and to assure accurate results, the following clinical conditions and procedures should be arranged.
   a. The test should be performed in the morning after a normal night's sleep. The patient should be NPO after midnight and during the test.
   b. The patient should be at rest. Attempt to prevent apprehension and distress 30 minutes prior to the infusion of the drug. This is especially important in children.
   c. Infuse through an indwelling IV cannula in a moderately large vein (antecubital). Blood samples should be taken from the opposite arm.
   d. Blood samples to measure HGH release should be taken 30 minutes prior or to beginning the test, at the time of infusion, and at the following times after the infusion was *started:* 30, 60, 90, 120, and 150 minutes.
   e. The infusion rate should be uniform and must be calculated to infuse the volume in 30 minutes time.
   f. Blood samples should be *promptly* centrifuged and the plasma stored at minus 20 degrees centigrade until assaying.

SUGGESTED READINGS
Spencer, R. T.: *Patient Care in Endocrine Problems,* Philadelphia: W. B. Saunders Company, 1973.
Smith, Dorothy W., and Germain, Carol P. Hanley: *Care of the Adult Patient* (4th ed.), Philadelphia: J. B. Lippincott Company, 1975, Unit Nine.

● ASCORBIC ACID (Calcium Ascorbate [Calscorbate], Sodium Ascorbate [Cenolate], Cevalin, also contained in Multivitamin Infusion [M.V.I.] and Vitamin B Complex Preparations)

ACTIONS/ INDICATIONS	DOSAGE	PREPARATION AND STORAGE	DRUG INCOMPAT- IBILITIES	MODES OF IV ADMINISTRATION			CONTRAINDICATIONS; WARNINGS; PRECAUTIONS; ADVERSE REACTIONS
				INJECTION	INTERMITTENT INFUSION	CONTINUOUS INFUSION	
Vitamin, an antiscorbutic agent. Used by the body in the formation, maintenance and repair of collagen and fibrous tissues, and the metabolism of carbohydrates.	ADULTS: *Therapeutic*— 300–1000 mg/day *Protective*— 70–150 mg/day *Maximum*—6 gm/day CHILDREN: *Therapeutic*— 100–300 mg/ day *Protective*— 30 mg/day PREMATURE AND IMMATURE INFANTS: 75–100 mg/ day	Store at room temperature or as directed by the manufacturer in the original packaging, away from heat and light. Slight darkening of the solution does not affect potency. Can be used in plastic solution bags.	Do not mix in any manner with: Aminophylline Erythromycin Nafcillin Nitrofurantoin Sodium bicarbonate Warfarin Chlordiazepoxide (Librium) Conjugated estrogens Cyanocobalamin Dextran Methicillin Penicillin G potassium Phytonadione	YES Undiluted at a rate no greater than 1 mg/ min. Rapid injection can cause dizziness.	YES Add to any IV fluid in a volume dictated by patient's fluid needs. Infuse at a rate no greater than 1 mg of drug/min.	YES Add to any IV fluid in a volume dictated by patient's fluid needs. Infuse at a rate no greater than 1 mg of drug/min.	CONTRAINDICATIONS None PRECAUTIONS 1. Intravenous ascorbic acid can decrease the activity of all anticoagulants. 2. Avoid extravasation of the calcium ascorbic acid preparations; pain and tissue irritation will result. 3. Calcium preparations have been reported to precipitate cardiac arrhythmias in patients on digitalis; use with caution via slow infusion.
There is an increased need for ascorbic acid in febrile states, chronic illness, and trauma. Indicated in malabsorption states and scurvy. Premature and immature infants require large amounts.							

● **ASCORBIC ACID** (Calcium Ascorbate [Calscorbate], Sodium Ascorbate [Cenolate], Cevalin, also contained in Multivitamin Infusion [M.V.I.] and Vitamin B Complex Preparations) *(Continued)*

NURSING IMPLICATIONS
1. Take precautions to prevent extravasation of calcium preparations of this drug; see page 96.
2. Any patient receiving calcium preparations of ascorbic acid should be monitored closely for cardiac arrhythmias if they are concomitantly receiving a digitalis drug. Stay with the patient during the first 30 minutes of administration. Use only slow infusion technique. Monitor heart rate and rhythm. Obtain an ECG if pulse becomes irregular. Use continuous EKG monitoring if indicated. Premature atrial and ventricular contractions are the arrhythmias most likely to be seen.

● **ATROPINE SULFATE**

ACTIONS/ INDICATIONS	DOSAGE	PREPARATION AND STORAGE	DRUG INCOMPATIBILITIES	MODES OF IV ADMINISTRATION			CONTRAINDICATIONS; WARNINGS; PRECAUTIONS; ADVERSE REACTIONS
				INJECTION	INTERMITTENT INFUSION	CONTINUOUS INFUSION	
Anticholine-sterase that produces the following major effects:	ADULTS: *Antispasmotic, preanesthetic* —0.4–1.0 mg	Store at room temperature. Supplied in ampuls of 0.4 mg in 0.5 ml	Can be combined with most analgesics in a syringe just prior to injection.	YES No dilution required. Inject over 1–2 min.	NO Pharmacologically inappropriate.	NO Pharmacologically inappropriate.	CONTRAINDICATIONS 1. Glaucoma (angle-closure and open-angle types) 2. In the presence of adhesions between the lens and iris of the eye 3. Bronchial asthma 4. Pyloric stenosis
1. Decreases smooth muscle spasm	*Bradycardia, insecticide poisoning*—0.5–2.0 mg		Do *not* mix in any manner with: Sodium bicarbonate Levarterenol Metaraminol Isoproterenol				PRECAUTIONS 1. Use with caution in patients with prostatic hypertrophy; may cause urinary retention.
2. Decreases salivation 3. Decreases the production of respiratory tract secretions	(Do not exceed 2.5 mg in 1 hour; bradycardia may occur.)						2. Use with caution when an excessive increase in heart rate may precipitate cardiac decompensation; e.g., congestive heart failure, acute myocardial infarction.
4. Increases heart rate	CHILDREN: *All indications:* —0.01–0.03 mg/kg repeated as necessary.	Frequently used doses (in mg) and their volumes (in ml) are listed below:					3. May increase intraocular pressure in patients susceptible to angle closure glaucoma or with chronic open-angle glaucoma.
Indications: 1. To treat pyloro-spasm and other spastic conditions of the gastrointestinal tract		Dose	Volume				4. May produce premature ventricular contractions or ventricular tachycardia, especially in patients with pre-existing cardiac problems.
		0.10 mg	0.12 ml				5. This drug may increase the size of an ischemic area of the heart in patients with acute myocardial infarction. Use only in the presence of severe and symptomatic bradycardia (heart rate less than 50/min) in such patients.
		0.15 mg	0.20 ml				
		0.20 mg	0.25 ml				
		0.25 mg	0.30 ml				
2. As a pre-anesthetic medication to decrease		0.30 mg	0.375 ml				ADVERSE REACTIONS Toxic effects from even minimal over-
		0.40 mg	0.50 ml				
		Multidose vials are also available, 0.5 mg/ml. Doses and volumes:					

secretions and prevent vagal stimulation with its possible slowing effect on heart rate

3. To increase heart rate in A-V block and sinus and junctional bradyarrhythmias

4. To relieve symptoms associated with organophosphorus insecticide poisoning

Dose	Volume
0.10 mg	0.20 ml
0.15 mg	0.30 ml
0.20 mg	0.40 ml
0.25 mg	0.50 ml
0.30 mg	0.60 ml
0.50 mg	1.0 ml

dosage are not uncommon, especially in children. These effects are dose-related as follows:

Dosage	Effect
0.5 mg	Dryness of nose and mouth; bradycardia (not always seen)
1.0 mg	Marked dryness of nose and mouth, thirst, acceleration of heart rate, dilation of pupils
2.0 mg	Extreme dryness of nose and mouth; tachycardia with palpitation; dilation of pupils; blurring of near vision; flushed, dry skin
5.0 mg (within 1 hour)	Above symptoms, plus: difficulty speaking and swallowing; headache; hot, dry skin; restlessness
10.0 mg (within 1 hour)	Above symptoms, plus: excitement; disorientation; hallucinations; coma
65 mg (within 1–2 hours)	May be fatal due to apena.

May produce fever in children due to decreased evaporation on the body surface (even in therapeutic doses).

May produce hallucinations and disorientation in the elderly at therapeutic doses.

In atropine overdosage, administer respiratory support and symptomatic treatment until drug can be excreted.

NURSING IMPLICATIONS

1. Monitor all patients for urinary retention, especially those with known prostatic hypertrophy or urethral strictures, and elderly males. Palpate bladder size every 4 hours. Monitor urinary output. Small voidings or sudden cessation of output may indicate retention.

2. Maintain on continuous ECG monitoring all patients receiving this drug for heart block or bradycardia. Observe for: increase in heart rate greater than 110 in adults or rates higher than normal in children (see page 545), premature ventricular contractions, and ventricular tachycardia. Notify physician immediately if these occur. Be prepared to treat premature ventricular contractions and ventricular tachycardia by keeping lidocaine at the bedside. (Follow ICU policy for nurse's administration of this drug.) A defibrillator must be readily available.

3. If sinus tachycardia occurs, monitor for cardiac decompensation (pulmonary edema). Signs: increasing respiratory rate, orthopnea, dyspnea, elevated (engorged) external jugular veins, rales and wheezing, cyanosis, or pallor (elevated or decreased blood pressure). These signs may appear suddenly. Notify physician. Be prepared to: elevate the body from the waist up if possible. Administer oxygen 2–5 L/min, prepare rotating tourniquets, prepare traditional drugs (potent diuretics, such as furosemide or ethacrynate, morphine, aminophylline). Provide emotional support; do not leave the patient alone.

4. Monitor for signs of an acute increase in intraocular pressure: increase in tear production, decreasing vision, severe eye pain, patient seeing rainbows around light, nausea, vomiting.[1] Notify physician at the first sign. (Doses of atropine greater than 1.0 mg may cause blurred vision in the absence of glaucoma.)

5. Be prepared to protect elderly patients from injury if hallucinations and disorientation occur. Use side rails and light restraints as necessary. These changes may last for 24 hours after the last dose. Provide reassurance and close observation.

6. Maintain hydration to prevent drying of bronchial secretions that could lead to respiratory complications. When indicated, treat dry mouth with fluids and mouth care in patients receiving this drug for indications other than

195

ATROPINE SULFATE (Continued)

NURSING IMPLICATIONS (No. 6 continued)
preanesthesia.
7. In the comatose patient, prevent corneal damage due to dryness (decrease in tear production) by using methylcellulose eyedrops or saline and eye dressings as indicated. Corneal damage is evidenced by scleral redness and edema.
8. In patients receiving large doses, be prepared to give respiratory support. Keep the following equipment readily available: airways, suction, oxygen, endotracheal tubes and laryngoscope, manual breathing bag and mask.

REFERENCE
1. Newell, Frank W., and Ernest, J. Terry: *Ophthalmology—Principles and Concepts* (3rd ed.), St. Louis, C. V. Mosby Company, 1974, p. 337.

SUGGESTED READINGS
Scarpa, William J.: The Sick Sinus Syndrome, *American Heart Journal,* 92(5):648–660, November 1976 (complete review article on sick sinus syndrome and the use of atropine in its early management).
Stuckey, John G.: Atropine in Bradycardia in the Coronary-Care Unit and Elsewhere. *Heart and Lung.* 2(5):666–668, September–October 1973.
DeMaria, Anthony N., et al.: Atropine: Current Concepts of its Use in Acute Myocardial Infarction. *Heart and Lung.* 3(1):135–137, January–February 1974 (references).

AZATHIOPRINE SODIUM SALT (Imuran)

ACTIONS/ INDICATIONS	DOSAGE	PREPARATION AND STORAGE	DRUG INCOMPAT- IBILITIES	MODES OF IV ADMINISTRATION			CONTRAINDICATIONS; WARNINGS; PRECAUTIONS; ADVERSE REACTIONS
				INJECTION	INTERMITTENT INFUSION	CONTINUOUS INFUSION	
Immuno-suppressant and antimeta-bolite. Used to prevent organ rejection after transplantation by depressing the antibody-producing response of the lymphoid tissue occurring after the new organ has been placed in the body.	ADULTS AND CHILDREN: *Initial*—3–5 mg/kg/day. *Mainten-ance*—(Usually oral)—1–2 mg/kg/day in 1 or 2 doses, with periodic adjustments to prevent rejection without drug toxicity (bone marrow depression).	To prepare: Add contents of one 10-ml vial of sterile water for injection to azathioprine vial. Swirl gently until mixed. Use immediately, discard unused portions. Store at room temperature away from light (in original box).	Do not mix with any other medication in any manner.	YES Inject slowly, diluted as described in "Preparation" column.	YES Use D5W or NS in any volume.	YES Use D5W or NS in any volume.	CONTRAINDICATIONS Hypersensitivity WARNINGS 1. Can produce severe irreversible bone marrow depression. CBC, including platelet counts, should be done at least daily during the initial phase of therapy and when high doses are used. A fall in leukocyte count should prompt a decrease in or discontinuation of the dosage. 2. In the presence of severe, unremitting organ rejection, it may be better to allow rejection to occur and remove the organ rather than attempt to prevent rejection with very high doses of this drug that will produce toxicity. 3. Infection is a persistent hazard. In this event, appropriate antibacterial, antifungal or antiviral therapy should be initiated and the dose of azathioprine decreased. 4. There have been reports of patients developing lymphomas while receiving immunosuppressive drugs after kidney transplantation. 5. Persistent negative nitrogen balance has been observed when the patient is concomitantly receiving corticosteroids. If this occurs, reduce the dosage of azathioprine. (Signs: weight loss, increased BUN [azotemia], loss of muscle mass.)

6. This drug should probably be withheld if signs of toxic hepatitis or biliary stasis occur (elevated bilirubin, SGOT, jaundice).
7. This drug has potential teratogenic activity (can cause fetal abnormalities).

PRECAUTIONS
1. In the presence of a cadaveric kidney with tubular necrosis and delayed onset of function, use reduced dosage of this drug.
2. Use reduced (1/3 to 1/4) dosage in patients concomitantly on allopurinol.

ADVERSE REACTIONS
1. Bone marrow depression: leukopenia, anemia, thrombocytopenia, bleeding.
2. Allergy: rashes, drug fever.
3. Skin: oral lesions and hair loss.
4. Gastrointestinal: nausea, vomiting, diarrhea (especially in higher doses), pancreatitis (rare).
5. Hepatic: jaundice.

NURSING IMPLICATIONS
1. Be aware of the patient's white cell count during administration period; a fall in leukocytes is the first sign of bone marrow depression. If count falls below 2,000 place the patient in protective (reversed) isolation, hold the next dose and notify the physician.
2. Observe for bleeding from any site; prevent trauma that may lead to bleeding.
3. Monitor temperature at least every 4 hours to detect infection or drug fever. Also observe for drainage, swelling, soreness, redness, signs of local infections. Therapy must be initiated as soon as possible after the onset of these findings.
4. Avoid any unnecessary venipunctures, catheterizations, nasotracheal suctioning and other instrumentation that can increase the chance of infection.
5. Monitor for jaundice of skin and sclera in fair-skinned patients and sclera in dark-skinned patients. Observe for darkening of urine.
6. Examine for oral lesions. Hydrogen peroxide-saline mouthwashes may be prescribed. Order a soft, bland diet and nonirritating oral fluids.

7. Reassure the patient, if hair loss occurs, that the hair will grow back when the drug is discontinued.
8. Be prepared to manage nausea, vomiting and diarrhea. Antiemetics may be used prior to meals.
9. Monitor for early signs of rejection (renal transplantation): decrease urinary output, fever, increasing proteinuria, increasing blood pressure, pain and tenderness near the organ.

SUGGESTED READINGS
Ihar, Sisir K., and Smith, Earl C.: Renal Transplantation. *Heart and Lung* 4(6):897–899, November–December 1975.
Topor, Michele A.: Kidney Transplantation (Especially in Pediatrics). *Nursing Clinics of North America*, 10(3):503–516, September 1975.
Harrington, Joan DeLong, and Brener, Etta Rae: *Patient Care in Renal Failure*, Saunders Monographs in Clinical Nursing–5, Philadelphia, W. B. Saunders Company, 1973, p. 199.

BENZQUINAMIDE HYDROCHLORIDE (Emete-Con)

ACTIONS/ INDICATIONS	DOSAGE	PREPARATION AND STORAGE	DRUG INCOMPAT- IBILITIES	MODES OF IV ADMINISTRATION			CONTRAINDICATIONS: WARNINGS: PRECAUTIONS: ADVERSE REACTIONS
				INJECTION	INTERMITTENT INFUSION	CONTINUOUS INFUSION	
Antiemetic. For use during anesthesia and surgery to depress the che-	ADULTS: 25 mg (0.2– 0.4 mg/kg), repeat in 1 hr, then every 3–	Reconstitute with 2.2 ml of sterile water for injection, or bacteriostatic	Do not mix with any other medication.	YES Slowly, 1 ml/ min, undiluted.	NO	NO	CONTRAINDICATIONS 1. Do not administer IV to patients with any form of acute cardiac disease; sudden hypertensive episodes and arrhythmias have been reported.

BENZQUINAMIDE HYDROCHLORIDE (Emete-Con) (Continued)

ACTIONS/INDICATIONS	DOSAGE	PREPARATION AND STORAGE	DRUG INCOMPATIBILITIES	MODES OF IV ADMINISTRATION			CONTRAINDICATIONS; WARNINGS; PRECAUTIONS; ADVERSE REACTIONS
				INJECTION	INTERMITTENT INFUSION	CONTINUOUS INFUSION	
moreceptor trigger zone and prevent nausea. Prophylactic use should be limited to those patients in whom emesis would be hazardous. Onset of action is 15 minutes following injection.	4 hrs as needed. Use IM route after initial IV dose. Give 15 min prior to patient's awakening from anesthesia. Dosage in the elderly or debilitated should be decreased.	water for injection. This yields a solution volume of 2 ml (25 mg/ml). Store powder and reconstituted solution in light occlusive containers. Reconstituted form is stable for 14 days at room temperature.					2. Safety for use in pregnancy has not been established. 3. Do not use in children under 12 years of age. PRECAUTIONS 1. Arrhythmias (such as atrial and ventricular premature contractions) have been reported after IV injection. 2. As with any antiemetic, this drug may obscure signs of overdosage of other drugs, or the diagnosis of an intracerebral lesion or intestinal obstruction that would normally be present with nausea and vomiting. ADVERSE REACTIONS 1. Most frequent reaction is drowsiness. 2. Allergic reactions will present with a rash and pyrexia. 3. Other reactions include dry mouth, blurred vision, dizziness and insomnia.

NURSING IMPLICATIONS
1. Administer appropriate supportive care to the patient with adverse reactions. Report them to the physician.
2. Maintain continuous ECG monitoring of all patients with past history of cardiac arrhythmias, during and for 2 hours after injection. Be prepared to treat brady- and tachyarrhythmias, premature atrial and ventricular arrhythmias. Keep both lidocaine 100 mg and atropine 1.0 mg at the bedside.
3. Monitor blood pressure. Obtain a resting, pre-injection reading and then subsequent measurements every 2–3 minutes during and for 15 minutes following injection. Obtain readings every 30 minutes for the next 2 hours.
4. In patients undergoing neurologic surgery, who have had recent head trauma, or who may be suspected as having an intracranial lesion, monitor for signs of increased intracranial pressure other than nausea and vomiting, such as neurologic signs: unequal pupillary reaction to light, unequal hand grip, change in mental status.
5. In susceptible patients, monitor for signs of bowel obstruction other than nausea and vomiting, such as increasing abdominal girth, rigid abdomen, abdominal pain, loss of bowel sounds.
6. Take precautions to prevent injury in patients with secondary drowsiness. Ambulate with assistance, use side rails when indicated.

BENZTROPINE MESYLATE (Cogentin)

ACTIONS/INDICATIONS	DOSAGE	PREPARATION AND STORAGE	DRUG INCOMPATIBILITIES	MODES OF IV ADMINISTRATION			CONTRAINDICATIONS; WARNINGS; PRECAUTIONS; ADVERSE REACTIONS
				INJECTION	INTERMITTENT INFUSION	CONTINUOUS INFUSION	
Anticholinergic agent. Used in addition to other drugs for all forms of par-	IM and IV routes produce the same amount of time; IV route is rarely used.	Supplied in 2-ml ampuls, 1 mg/ml. Further dilution prior to injection is not necessary.	No specific incompatibilities known; do not mix unnecessarily with any other medications.	YES Inject slowly over 3 to 5 min undiluted.	NO Pharmacologically inappropriate.	NO Pharmacologically inappropriate.	CONTRAINDICATIONS Children less than three years of age (use with great caution in children up to 13 years of age). WARNINGS 1. Safety for use in pregnancy has not

kinsonism and to control the extrapyramidal effects* of phenothiazines and reserpine.

*Uncontrolled abnormal ocular movements, staggering gait, tremors, etc.

Store at room temperature.

ADULTS:

In parkinsonism—Initial dose is 0.5 to 1.0 mg. Gradually increase the daily dose by 0.5—mg. increments until daily maintenance dose is reached by desired effect. Do not exceed 6 mg/day. Older or thinner patients tolerate lower doses.

In drug-induced extrapyramidal effects—Initial dose and management are the same as in parkinsonism above. Maintenance dose is usually 1.0 to 4.0 mg once or twice a day guided by patient response.

been established.

2. Should probably not be used in the presence of angle-closure glaucoma (acute).

PRECAUTIONS

1. Because of effects on mentation and possibly vision, patients must be cautioned on performing potentially hazardous tasks after an injection; e.g., climbing stairs, taking a bath or shower. In elderly or debilitated patients, ambulation may be hazardous without assistance.

2. This drug has cumulative effects.

3. May produce anhidrosis (loss of sweating).

4. There may be an acute exacerbation of tachycardias (paroxysmal atrial, junctional and ventricular) in patients with active cardiac problems or a history of arrhythmias.

5. There may be urinary retention in patients with prostatic hypertrophy.

6. Large doses can produce weakness in certain muscle groups.

7. Mental confusion and hallucinations can occur and should be closely monitored.

8. In patients with acute or chronic mental disorders, there may be intensification of those mental symptoms. This is especially true of patients on high doses of this drug and other antiparkinsonian drugs.

9. This drug can precipitate acute glaucoma.

ADVERSE REACTIONS

1. Side effects may be anticholinergic or antihistaminic in nature: dry mouth, blurred vision, nausea, nervousness, constipation, listlessness, numbness in fingers.

2. Allergic rashes.

3. All reactions listed above can be controlled by temporary discontinuation of the drug or reduction of dosage.

4. Observe all patients for change in mental status after the injection. Take precautions to prevent injury. Changes such as confusion, agitation, and hallucinations may last for several hours.

While the Patient is on Daily Doses of this Drug:

1. Anhidrosis (loss of the ability to perspire) may decrease the patient's ability to control body temperature by skin evaporation. Temperature elevation may be seen. Monitor oral or rectal temperature every 4–6 hours.

2. With anhidrosis, the sign of diaphoresis will be absent in clinical situations such as shock due to any cause, including hypoglycemia in diabetics. Moni-

NURSING IMPLICATIONS

During and Immediately After Injection:

1. Keep the patient in a supine or semi-Fowler's position.

2. Obtain a preinjection blood pressure.

3. All patients with acute cardiac disorders or a past history of cardiac problems, especially arrhythmias, should be observed for acute arrhythmias via a continuous ECG monitor. Be prepared to treat tachy- and bradyarrhythmias (lidocaine 100 mg and atropine 1.0 mg should be readily available). Observations should continue for at least 4 hours.

BENZTROPINE MESYLATE (Congentin) (Continued)

NURSING IMPLICATIONS (No. 2 continued)
tor for other signs of shock such as pallor, extreme weakness, fall in blood pressure, tachycardia, rapid respirations, cyanosis.

3. Elderly male patients and all male patients with a history of prostatic disorders should be monitored for urinary retention by frequent palpation of bladder size and measurement of urinary output (at least every 4 hours). Encourage adequate fluid intake.

4. Observe for any type of muscle weakness or rigidity. (This frequently occurs in the neck muscles.) Report this sign to the physician; a reduction in dosage will probably be ordered. Reassure the patient of the temporary nature of this side effect.

5. Warn patients and families, when appropriate, of side effects such as nervousness and depression. Dosage reduction can usually relieve the symptoms. Reassurance and support can allay fears and reduce the intensity of the effects.

6. Anticipate an acute intensification of a currently active mental disorder. Reassure the patient of the transient nature of the effects and take protective measures.

7. Monitor patients with a past history of a psychotic problem for an acute exacerbation of symptoms. Reassure the patient of the transient nature of the effects and take protective measures.

8. This drug usually does not affect the intraocular pressure of patients with simple, chronic (wide-angle) glaucoma, usually seen with aging; but it should *not* be administered to patients with known acute, closed (narrow) glaucoma. Because both forms of glaucoma may go undetected in early states, monitor all patients for acute rise in intraocular pressure: severe eye pain, rainbow and blurred vision, nausea, and vomiting. Notify the physician immediately.

9. Assist in preventing the constipation associated with this drug by high fiber diet, fluids, activity, or laxatives.

BICARBONATE, SODIUM

ACTIONS/ INDICATIONS	DOSAGE	PREPARATION AND STORAGE	DRUG INCOMPAT- IBILITIES	MODES OF IV ADMINISTRATION				CONTRAINDICATIONS; WARNINGS; PRECAUTIONS; ADVERSE REACTIONS
				INJECTION	INTERMITTENT INFUSION	CONTINUOUS INFUSION		
Alkalizing sodium salt. Dissociates in solution into sodium and bicarbonate radicals (Na+, HCO₃⁻). The bicarbonate then combines with free hydrogen ions to form H²CO³ a weak acid. This reduces the number of free hydrogen ions and thus increases the serum pH.

Used to treat metabolic acidosis secondary to cardiac arrest, renal failure; as an adjunct in the management of salicylate intoxication in the absence of | ADULTS: *Initially*—1–5 mEq/kg. Subsequent doses must be guided by arterial blood gases.

Cardiac arrest —50 mEq is given every 5– 10 min, with the frequency guided by arterial blood gases.

INFANTS AND CHILDREN: 0.9 mEq/kg diluted 1:1 in sterile water, guided by arterial blood gases. Children over 15 kg can receive the adult dose. | Available in the following forms:

Ampuls and prefilled syringes—50 ml of an 8.4% solution (50.0 mEq, 1 mEq/ml); 50 ml of a 7.5% solution (44.6 mEq)

Bottles—500 ml of a 5% solution (297.5 mEq, 0.6 mEq/ ml); 500 ml of a 1.4% solution (83 mEq, 0.16 mEq/ml). | Do not mix with the following fluids: Alcohol 5% in Ringer's injection, lactated

Ionosol B with invert sugar 10%

Ionosol D with invert sugar 10% modified

Ionosol G with invert sugar 10%

Ringer's injection

Ringer's Lactate

Sodium Lactate

Other medications: Because of the alkalinity of solutions produced by sodium bicarbonate, it is | YES

Using a 7.5 or 8.4% solution, undiluted (except in children, see Dosage column), injection may be rapid. This is the preferable mode for the treatment of cardiac arrest. | YES

This mode is for nonemergency situations. Titrate rate with arterial blood gases.

See Incompatibility column for fluids that cannot be used for sodium bicarbonate solutions, or use 500-ml bottles of prepared 5% or 1.4% sodium bicarbonate. Use an infusion pump. | YES

This mode is for nonemergency situations. Titrate rate with arterial blood gases.

See Incompatibility column for fluids that cannot be used for sodium bicarbonate solutions, or use 500-ml bottles of prepared 5% or 1.4% sodium bicarbonate. Use an infusion pump. | | CONTRAINDICATIONS
Arterial blood pH greater than 7.4

PRECAUTIONS
1. Patients with congestive heart failure may need a diuretic following the administration of sodium bicarbonate to enhance the excretion of the sodium contained in this agent.
2. Dosage must always be guided by arterial blood gases, when possible. Administration should stop when the pulse returns in the management of a cardiac arrest. Further injections must be guided by arterial blood gases.[1]
3. During cardiac arrest, or any severe acidotic situation, effective ventilation must accompany sodium bicarbonate to remove carbon dioxide in the blood.[2]

ADVERSE REACTIONS
Metabolic alkalosis and hyperosmolarity, secondary to excessive unguided dosage. |

respiratory alkalosis, and in ketoacidosis.

advisable not to add any other medication to a solution of sodium bicarbonate for infusion.

When injecting sodium bicarbonate into intravenous tubing containing any one of the following drugs, flush the line with a compatible solution prior to injecting the sodium bicarbonate, or inject directly into the vein or intravenous catheter:

Anileridine
Ascorbic acid
Codeine phosphate
Corticotropin
Hydromorphone
Insulin, regular
Levarterenol
Levorphanol
Magnesium sulfate
Meperdine
Methicillin
Morphine
Any tetracycline
Dopamine
Epinephrine
Pentazocine
Any barbiturate
Penicillin G potassium
Procaine
Promazine
Vancomycin
Vitamin B complex
Calcium preparations
Isoproterenol

BICARBONATE, SODIUM (Continued)

ACTIONS/ INDICATIONS	DOSAGE	PREPARATION AND STORAGE	DRUG INCOMPAT- IBILITIES	MODES OF IV ADMINISTRATION			CONTRAINDICATIONS; WARNINGS; PRECAUTIONS; ADVERSE REACTIONS
				INJECTION	INTERMITTENT INFUSION	CONTINUOUS INFUSION	
			In using any other medica- tions, observe carefully for signs of pre- cipitation or color changes, which denote physical in- compatibility.				spiratory rate, muscle spasms, hyperactive reflexes, tetany seizure, change in mental status.

NURSING IMPLICATIONS
1. This drug is indicated when the arterial blood pH is 7.3 or less.
2. Monitor for signs of excessive sodium and water retention (especially in pa- tients with congestive heart failure or renal impairments); increased weight; dyspnea, increased respiratory rate, orthopnea, rales; increasing resting heart rate; peripheral edema.
3. Be aware of arterial blood gas values during titration of this drug. Monitor for signs of metabolic alkalosis (blood pH greater than 7.45): decreased re-

REFERENCES
1. Standards for Cardiopulmonary Resuscitation (CPR) and Emergency Cardiac Care (ECC). JAMA, 227: Supplement, February 18, 1974, p. 857.
2. Ibid., p. 858.

BIPERIDEN LACTATE (Akineton)

ACTIONS/ INDICATIONS	DOSAGE	PREPARATION AND STORAGE	DRUG INCOMPAT- IBILITIES	MODES OF IV ADMINISTRATION			CONTRAINDICATIONS; WARNINGS; PRECAUTIONS; ADVERSE REACTIONS
				INJECTION	INTERMITTENT INFUSION	CONTINUOUS INFUSION	
Anticholinergic agent. Used to treat extra- pyramidal dis- turbances sec- ondary to re- serpine and phenothiazines (e.g. profuse sweating, mus- cle weakness, agitation, rest- lessness, trem- ors, muscle spasm, muscle rigidity, eye movement dis- turbances). Also used as an adjunct to therapy for	ADULTS: 2 mg, repeat- ed every ½ hr until resolution of symptoms. No more than 4 consecutive doses in 24 hrs.	May be administered undiluted into the vein or IV tubing. Store at room temperature. Discard any un- used portions. Available in 1 ml ampuls, 1 mg/ml.	Do not mix with any other medication.	YES Slowly, over 2 to 3 min. Keep the patient su- pine during in- jection. Rapid IV injection may cause transient pos- tural hypoten- sion and dizzi- ness.	NO Pharmaco- logically inap- propriate	NO Pharmaco- logically inap- propriate	CONTRAINDICATIONS Hypersensitivity to biperiden WARNINGS 1. There may be mental confusion, agita- tion or euphoria. 2. Safety for use in pregnancy has not been established PRECAUTIONS 1. Administer with caution to patients with any form of active glaucoma; there may be further elevation of intraocular pressure. 2. Patients with a history of prostatic hy- pertrophy may develop urinary reten- tion. 3. There may be an acute exacerbation of cardiac arrhythmias in susceptible patients. 4. Mild transient postural hypotension

parkinsonism of postencephalitic, idiopathic and arteriosclerotic types.

can occur after rapid IV injection.

ADVERSE REACTIONS
1. Reactions are anticholinergic in nature, e.g., dry mouth, tachycardia, urinary retention, blurred vision, drowsiness.
2. Overdosage resembles atropine toxicity: CNS depression or stimulation, depressed respirations, fall in blood pressure, hyperthermia. These effects can be treated symptomatically until the drug is excreted. Barbiturates can be used to treat CNS stimulation. Respiratory depression should be treated supportively as needed with tracheal intubation and ventilation. Hypotension can be treated with vasopressor agents. Hyperthermia should be controlled with cool baths or cooling blanket.

NURSING IMPLICATIONS
1. Monitor all patients for changes in mental status and instigate protective measures as needed, e.g., bed rails, light restraints, ambulation with assistance, reassurance.
2. Monitor for signs of increased intraocular pressure in all patients, e.g., severe ocular pain, loss of visual field or acuity, rainbows around lights, dilated pupils, nausea and vomiting.
3. Monitor all elderly male patients and patients with positive histories of prostatic hypertrophy for urinary retention. Initiate intake and output recording. Palpate bladder size every 4 hours.
4. Observe susceptible patients (e.g., those with a past history of arrhythmias or with active arrhythmias), for rhythm disturbances via continuous ECG monitoring, both during and after the injection. Tachy- and brady-arrhythmias are possible. Keep lidocaine 100 mg and atropine 0.5 mg at the bedside. In the event of a serious arrhythmia, administer these drugs according to hospital policy and physician's orders. Notify the physician.
5. Keep the patient supine during and for 1 hour after the injection to prevent postural hypotension. Dangle the patient for at least 3–5 minutes before ambulating. Take lying and standing blood pressure. Report large differences between lying and standing pressures to the physician.
6. Monitor for signs of overdosage:
   a. Central nervous system depression or stimulation
   b. Respiratory depression (count respirations continuously during, and every 5 minutes for 1 hour after, injection)
   c. Hypotension (obtain blood pressure readings every 2–3 minutes during, and for 30 minutes after, injection, and then every 30 minutes for the next hour)
   d. Hyperthermia (take a baseline temperature before the injection and then every 15 minutes for the next hour, followed by hourly temperatures for the next 2 hours)
   See Adverse Reaction section for management of toxicity.
7. Patients who will be placed on chronic oral therapy of this drug should be educated on self care measures.

● BLEOMYCIN SULFATE (Blenoxane)

ACTIONS/ INDICATIONS	DOSAGE	PREPARATION AND STORAGE	DRUG INCOMPAT- IBILITIES	MODES OF IV ADMINISTRATION			CONTRAINDICATIONS; WARNINGS; PRECAUTIONS; ADVERSE REACTIONS
				INJECTION	INTERMITTENT INFUSION	CONTINUOUS INFUSION	
Antineoplastic; antibiotic; impairs correct DNA formation in the cell. In- dicated in the	ADULTS: *In squamous cell carcinoma, testicular car- cinoma, Hodg- kin's disease,*	Available in am- puls containing 15 units. To re- constitute from powder, add 5 ml (or more) of	Do not mix with any other medication in any manner.	YES No need to fur- ther dilute re- constituted so- lution. Inject	YES Add reconsti- tuted solution to 20 ml D5W or NS for ev-	YES For intra- arterial per- fusion of tumor site.	CONTRAINDICATIONS Hypersensitivity WARNINGS 1. This agent can (rarely) cause renal im- pairment at any time during therapy,

203

● **BLEOMYCIN SULFATE** (Blenoxane) (*Continued*)

ACTIONS/ INDICATIONS	DOSAGE	PREPARATION AND STORAGE	DRUG INCOMPAT- IBILITIES	MODES OF IV ADMINISTRATION			CONTRAINDICATIONS; WARNINGS; PRECAUTIONS; ADVERSE REACTIONS
				INJECTION	INTERMITTENT INFUSION	CONTINUOUS INFUSION	
treatment of: • Hodgkin's disease (in combination with other drugs) • Non-Hodgkin's lymph- omas (in combination) • Squamous cell carcin- omas • Testicular carcinoma (in combina- tion) • Malignant pleural and peritoneal effusions	*and lympho- cytic and his- tocytic lym- phoma*[1]— 0.25–0.50 units/kg (10– 20 units/ M²) weekly or twice weekly until a total dose of 400 units has been reached. Re- sponse is usu- ally seen with- in 2 weeks or as a total dos- age of 200 units is reached. *In Hodgkin's disease,* after the above dos- age following a 50% regres- sion of tumor size, begin a dose of 1 unit/ day or 5 units/ week. For regional in- fusion—(intra- arterial) 30– 60 units/day over 1–24 hrs into affected areas. Dosage should be modified in the presence of renal or he- patic failure, usually by 25% (see Pre- cautions for further qualifi- cations for dosage).	D5W or NS. 5 ml of diluent will produce a solu- tion of 3 units/ ml. Discard un- used portion.		over a 10-min period.	ery 15 units of drug adminis- tered. Infuse over 10 min.	Use D5W or NS and in- fuse over 12– 24 hrs.	indicated by rising BUN and creati- nine. Use with extreme caution, if at all, in patients with pre-existing renal impairment. 2. Hepatic toxicity has also been report- ed (rarely) and is indicated by deterio- ration in liver function tests. Use with extreme caution in the presence of hepatic failure. 3. Pulmonary toxicity has been reported to occur in approximately 10% of all patients treated. Patients at greatest risk are those over 70 years of age, those receiving over 400 units or those with an underlying lung dis- ease. First signs of symptoms include cough, dyspnea, and bilateral basilar rales. Chest x-ray will show bilateral basilar and perihilar reticulonodular infiltrates with fibrosis. These chang- es may occur up to 1 month after the drug has been discontinued. Pulmo- nary function tests reveal a decreased vital capacity and a decreased diffu- sion capacity.[2] To monitor for pulmo- nary toxicity, obtain chest x-rays every 1–2 weeks. The drug should be dis- continued when x-ray or other clinical findings are noted and until it is deter- mined if they are drug-related. This toxicity can occur at lower dosages when the drug is used in combination with other agents. 4. Idiosyncratic reactions similar to ana- phylaxis have been reported in 1% of lymphoma patients treated. These re- actions usually occur with the first or second dose, immediately on injec- tion or after several hours of injection. Some groups administer a skin test, or test dose prior to full dosage. 5. Safety for use in pregnancy has not been established. PRECAUTIONS Improvement of Hodgkin's disease and testicular tumors is prompt and can be noted within 2 weeks of initiation of ther- apy. If no improvement is seen by this time, it is unlikely that it will occur. Squa- mous cell cancers respond more slowly, sometimes 3–4 weeks.

Patients with lymphoma are more susceptible to anaphylactic reactions to this drug and should therefore receive a 2- to 5-unit test dose for the first 2 doses. If no acute reaction occurs, a regular dosage schedule can be initiated.

CHILDREN: *All indications—* 10–15 units/M² /week. Do not exceed a total cumulative dose of 400 units.

ADVERSE REACTIONS

As with all antineoplastic agents, adverse reactions are frequent and numerous.
1. Pulmonary toxicity: pneumonitis, fibrosis
2. Skin changes: vesicles, hair loss, hyperpigmentation, hyperemia, hyperkeratosis, rashes, itching, mucous membrane ulceration
3. Renal impairment (rare)
4. Liver impairment (rare)
5. Febrile reactions (seen in 25% of all patients treated)
6. Anaphylaxis and anaphylaxislike idiosyncratic reactions (more frequent in patients with lymphomas)
7. Minimal bone marrow supression
8. Nausea, vomiting and anorexia
9. Pain at tumor site (this can be considered a favorable sign of tumor destruction)

NURSING IMPLICATIONS
1. The patient receiving this medication will be experiencing the emotional and physical effects of the malignancy. Knowledge of the patient's feelings about his disease and its implications will assist in helping him tolerate the chemotherapy. The incidence of uncomfortable side effects and adverse reactions is high. It is within the nurse's role to assist the patient in coping with the discomforts of the disease and its treatment, and to help him work through depression and anger toward acceptance of the disease at his own pace. Despite the unpleasantness this drug may bring, it can be a source of hope for the patient.
2. Take anaphylaxis precautions (see page 118).
3. Monitor for febrile reaction; fever usually begins 1 hour after injection and rises slowly over the next 2–4 hours. Take temperature every hour. Acetaminophen and/or cooling baths can be given for chills and fever. Inform the patient that this is not a hazardous complication.
4. Monitor for signs and symptoms of pulmonary toxicity:
   a. First symptoms are usually dyspnea, mild chest pain, and tachypnea
   b. First signs are x-ray changes (see under Warnings), bilateral basilar rales
   Notify the physician of the onset of any one of these signs or symptoms.
5. Monitor urinary output every 8 hours. Notify physician with the onset of oliguria (less than 240 ml of urine in 8 hours for an adult; see page 546 for normal urine output in children). Weigh the patient daily to detect onset of fluid retention. Be aware of the patient's BUN prior to each dose.
6. Management of hair loss
   a. Use scalp tourniquet during injection, if ordered, to help prevent hair loss. This technique may be ineffective in preventing hair loss because of the prolonged presence of this drug in the blood.
   b. Counsel the patient on the possibility of hair loss to enable him to prepare for this disfigurement.
   c. Reassure him of regrowth of hair following discontinuation of the drug.
   d. Provide privacy and time for the patient to discuss his feelings.
7. Reassure the patient that pain in the tumor site may occur. This can be considered as a favorable sign of drug effectiveness.
8. Management of nausea and vomiting (usually minimal):
   a. Administer antiemetics when appropriate to prevent nausea following injections and/or before meals.
   b. Small frequent meals, timed with periods when the patient feels his best, are advisable. Bland foods may be more easily tolerated. Carbohydrate and protein content should be high.
   c. If the patient is anorexic, encourage high nutrient liquids and water to maintain nutrition and hydration.
   d. Keep accurate measurements of emesis volume and total intake and output to guide the physician in ordering parenteral fluids when necessary.

REFERENCES
1. Shinn, Arthur F., et al.: Dosage Modifications of Cancer Chemotherapeutic Agents in Renal Failure. *Drug Intelligence and Clinical Pharmacy,* 11:141, 1977.
2. Silver, Richard, Lauper, R. David, and Jawroski, Charles I.: *A Synopsis of Cancer Chemotherapy,* The York Medical Group, Dun-Donnelley Publishing Corporation, 1977, p. 75.

BLEOMYCIN SULFATE (Blenoxane) (Continued)

SUGGESTED READINGS

Bolin, Rose Homan, and Auld, Margaret E.: Hodgkin's Disease. *American Journal of Nursing.*74: 1982–1986, November 1974.

Bruya, Margaret Auld, and Madeira, Nancy Powell: Stomatitis After Chemotherapy. *American Journal of Nursing.* 75:1349–1352, August 1975.

Foley, Genevieve and McCarthy, Ann Marie: The Disease (Hodgkin's) and Its Treatment. *American Journal of Nursing.* 76:1109–1114, July 1976, (references).

Giadquinta, Barbara: Helping Families Face the Crisis of Cancer. *American Journal of Nursing,*77: 1583–1586, October 1977.

Gullo, Shirley: Chemotherapy—What To Do About Special Side Effects. *RN,* 40:30–32, April 1977.

Hannan, Jeanne Ferguson: Talking is Treatment, Too. *American Journal of Nursing* 74:1991–1992, November 1974.

LeBlanc, Dona Harris: People With Hodgkin Disease: The Nursing Challenge. *Nursing Clinics of North America,* 13(2):281–300, June 1978.

McMullen, Kathleen: When the Patient is on Bleomycin Therapy. *American Journal of Nursing.* 75:964–966, June 1975.

Vietti, Teresa J., and Valeriote, Frederick: Conceptual Basis for the Use of Chemotherapeutic Agents and Their Pharmacology. *Pediatric Clinics of North America,* 23:67–92, February 1976.

Showfety, Mary Patricia: The Ordeal of Hodgkin's Disease. *American Journal of Nursing,* 74:1987–1991, November 1974.

Sovik, Corinne: The Nursing Care of Lung Cancer Patients. *Nursing Clinics of North America,* 13(3):301–317, June 1978.

BLOOD (Whole) and Packed Red Blood Cells

ACTIONS/ INDICATIONS	DOSAGE	PREPARATION AND STORAGE	DRUG INCOMPAT- IBILITIES	MODES OF IV ADMINISTRATION			CONTRAINDICATIONS; WARNINGS; PRECAUTIONS; ADVERSE REACTIONS
				INJECTION	INTERMITTENT INFUSION	CONTINUOUS INFUSION	
Blood replacement, used in: • Sickle-cell disease • Acute blood loss • Bone marrow failure • Severe anemia • Hemolytic anemia • Coagulation disorders One unit of whole blood or packed cells can raise the hemoglobin about 1 gm/ 100 ml, or the adult hematocrit 3 percentage points. Whole blood is used when volume and all blood components are needed, e.g.,	ADULTS: *Whole blood*— 500 ml. *Packed RBC's* —200 ml. Titrate with blood pressure and/or hematocrit. CHILDREN: *Whole blood*— 100–250 ml. *Packed RBC's* —100 ml. Titrate with blood pressure and/or hematocrit. NEONATES: *Whole blood*— 10 ml/kg. *Packed RBC's* —5 ml/kg. Titrate with blood pressure and/or hematocrit.	Do not mix with IV fluids except as a secondary IV line. Store at 1–10°C (approximately 40°F). Check unit number with cross-match data on the patient. Follow hospital regulations on the administration of blood.	Do not add any medication to blood.	NO	YES Add as a secondary IV to a primary line containing NS (only), at a rate of 5–10 ml/ min or as indicated.	YES Add as a secondary IV to a primary line containing NS (only), at a rate of 5–10 ml/ min or as indicated.	PRECAUTIONS 1. Except in extreme emergencies, blood must be typed and cross-matched with the recipient's blood. In emergencies typed blood or "O" blood or plasma expanders (dextran, saline) can be given until completely typed and cross-matched blood is ready for use. Obtain a cross-matching blood sample before giving emergency typed blood. Avoid using a noncross-matched blood whenever possible. 2. Administer blood only when absolutely necessary. Risks are—allergic reactions, hepatitis, bacterial, malarial and syphilis contaminations. 3. If blood is more than 2–4 hours old, it will be deficient in platelets and other clotting factors. Also erythrocyte oxygen-carrying capacity may be altered. 4. Stored blood may also have a lower pH (6.6) than normal blood; it may be hypercalcemic and hyperkalemic. 5. The patient's normal blood volume can be estimated to assist in determining whole blood replacement dosage: Female body weight in kg × 67 = total blood volume Male body weight in kg × 77 = total blood volume Radioactive iodine can also be used

coagulation factors.

Packed cells are used when keeping volume low is critical, or when the patient cannot tolerate sodium or potassium, and needs a rise in hematocrit (renal, hepatic and cardiac insufficiency). Also used in hemolytic anemia.

to give a more exact volume.

6. Packed RBC's (PRBC's) are safer than whole blood in raising the hematocrit, because they contain less sodium, potassium and other elements, making them safer to use in patients with congestive heart failure or impaired renal or hepatic functioning. There also may be fewer transfusion reactions with PRBC's.

7. If more than 2000 ml of blood must be infused rapidly, administer 10% calcium gluconate solution, 10 ml for each subsequent 1000 ml of blood. Give calcium in a separate IV line.

ADVERSE REACTIONS
The signs and symptoms of a transfusion reaction are similar to other drug reactions or anaphylaxis:

1. Fever (can also result from contamination)

2. Hemolytic reactions (early onset, usually after 50 ml has been infused): throbbing headache, severe lumbar pain, chest pain, dyspnea, anxiety, oozing at venipuncture site or incision, flushed face then cyanosis, slowed pulse followed by tachycardia, all symptoms of shock, bleeding; renal failure may occur several days later.

3. Allergic reactions produce urticaria, pain at infusion site, asthma, shock. Diphenhydramine (Benadryl) 50 mg may be given prior to transfusion to prevent reaction.

4. Bacterial contamination can result in shock and sepsis.

5. Citrate intoxication resembling hypocalcemia can occur but is rare. (Symptoms are minimal until intoxication is severe; then tetany may occur if condition is untreated.) See Precaution No. 7 above.

6. Hyperkalemia produces the following signs and symptoms: lethargy, confusion, diarrhea, arrhythmias (see Precaution No. 4 above).

7. Congestive heart failure. To prevent, use packed cells in susceptible patients; digitalize; use diuretics.

8. Bleeding disorders can occur when stored blood lacking in coagulation factors is used; use fresh blood and plasma when possible. With bleeding disorders, oozing will appear at venipuncture sites, incisions, etc.

9. Noncardiac pulmonary edema —

BLOOD (Whole) and Packed Red Blood Cells (*Continued*)

ACTIONS/ INDICATIONS	DOSAGE	PREPARATION AND STORAGE	DRUG INCOMPATIBILITIES	MODES OF IV ADMINISTRATION			CONTRAINDICATIONS; WARNINGS; PRECAUTIONS; ADVERSE REACTIONS
				INJECTION	INTERMITTENT INFUSION	CONTINUOUS INFUSION	
							thought to be caused by the leukocytes of the donor blood, produces pulmonary infiltration, chills, fever, shortness of breath. This condition clears in 48 hours.

NURSING IMPLICATIONS

1. Check blood unit with cross-match and typing information from the patient.
2. Stay with the patient during the first 15–20 minutes of the infusion, monitor for all types of transfusion reactions (see Adverse Reactions). The first signs of an allergic reaction can be blanching along the vein tract, pain and itching in the extremity, chills, hypotension. These may occur before any of the other reactions described above. In the young child who cannot verbalize symptoms, observe also for restlessness, crying, color changes, and changes in respiratory and heart rates.
3. Stop the infusion *immediately* at the first sign of a reaction and notify the physician. Be prepared to treat anaphylaxis; see page 118.
4. If no reactions occur during the initial observation period, instruct the patient to call immediately if he feels itching, pain in the extremity, chest pain or tightness, dyspnea.

For patients who cannot report symptoms (obtunded or anesthetized) check venipuncture site every 30 minutes for oozing of blood; skin for diaphoresis, urticaria, blanching along vein tract; and other signs of reactions.

5. Administer at slower rates to patients with cardiac failure. Monitor for decompensation: increased heart and respiratory rates, dyspnea, orthopnea, engorged external jugular veins (rising central venous pressure), rales in the lungs, decreasing blood pressure. Notify the physician at the onset of any one of these signs and symptoms.
6. Titrate infusion rate with blood pressure if indicated.
7. Monitor temperature hourly during administration and every 4 hours for the next 24 hours.
8. Monitor urine output every 8 hours for the next 4–5 days to detect the onset of oliguria secondary to a hemolytic reaction.
9. Administer calcium gluconate as ordered; see Precaution No. 7.

BOTULISM ANTITOXIN BIVALENT (Types A and B, Globulin Modified)

ACTIONS/ INDICATIONS	DOSAGE	PREPARATION AND STORAGE	DRUG INCOMPATIBILITIES	MODES OF IV ADMINISTRATION			CONTRAINDICATIONS; WARNINGS; PRECAUTIONS; ADVERSE REACTIONS
				INJECTION	INTERMITTENT INFUSION	CONTINUOUS INFUSION	
An antitoxin serum derived from the plasma of hyperimmunized horses. Used to treat all cases of toxemia due to, or suspected to be due to, *Clostridium botulinum* (whether Type A, B or undetermined). *Cl. botulinum* neurotoxin Type E is a frequent cause of ill-	ADULTS AND CHILDREN: 10,000 units (1 ml) as early as possible after onset of symptoms. Repeat at 4-hr intervals until symptoms of toxicity are alleviated.	Store in refrigerator. May be warmed to body temperature prior to injection (not necessary). Place vial in water bath no warmer than 37°C, or 98.6°F. DO NOT ALLOW SERUM TO BECOME WARMER THAN BODY TEMPERATURE.	Do not mix with any other medication in any manner.	YES Dilute 1 ml of antitoxin in 9 ml of D10W, D5W or NS. Inject over 5 min.	NO	NO	WARNINGS Anaphylaxis can occur due to animal (equine) origin of serum. PRECAUTIONS 1. Allergic reactions (including anaphylaxis) can occur during and after injection. To be prepared for such reactions: a. Obtain a history of allergic disorders, specifically asthma, angioneurotic edema, sensitivity to horse hair, and horse serums. Determine if the patient has received an injection of serum of equine origin within the last 7 days. b. *Skin Testing:* Inject intradermally, 0.1 ml of a 1:10 saline dilution of antitoxin (see Injection column for dilution. 1:100 dilution can be

used in patients with a positive history of allergy to equine serum.) Read the reaction within 10–30 minutes. A positive reaction will produce a wheal surrounded by an area of redness. The size of the positive reaction will not indicate the severity of systemic reaction to the antitoxin. A negative test does not mean that the patient will not react systemically to the antitoxin. The positive reaction does indicate a likely dangerous degree of sensitivity and can constitute a contraindication to the use of the drug. Sensitivity testing should be done only by a physician.

c. A conjunctional test can be used when there is a history of previous serious reaction to horse serums, to avoid a severe systemic reaction to the intradermal test dose. Drop 0.1 ml of a 1:10 dilution of antitoxin in into the lower conjunctival sac. A positive response will produce redness, dilated vessels, edema, itching and tear formation within 10–15 minutes. Terminate the reaction by rinsing the eye with a 1:1000 solution of epinephrine. The meaning of a positive reaction applies as described above.

d. Desensitization can be done in cases where there has been a positive skin or conjunctival test and when administration of the antitoxin is necessary to save the patient's life. Procedure:

1. Using the *subcutaneous* route for initial injections, a small amount of a 1:500 dilution is injected. In 15 minutes a second injection of a larger amount is given. Gradually increase concentration and volume of the antitoxin solution as injections are tolerated.
2. After subcutaneous injections are tolerated, intravenous injections of highly diluted (1:500) solutions may be made.
3. Epinephrine 1:10,000 for intravenous injection should be at the bedside in the event of a highly allergic reaction.

2. Serum sickness may occur 5–13 days after administration of the antitoxin. Signs and symptoms will be urticaria, fever, pruritus. Antihistamines will relieve most symptoms.

ness in man, usually secondary to contaminated fish, and is not affected by the A- and B-type antitoxin. Monovalent antitoxin for Type E and a trivalent antitoxin containing neutralizing agents against types A, B and E are available from the Center for Disease Control in Atlanta, Ga.

BOTULISM ANTITOXIN BIVALENT (Types A and B, Globulin Modified) (Continued)

NURSING IMPLICATIONS

1. Botulism intoxication is not an infection, but rather an illness secondary to neurotoxins ingested in food containing the bacteria. There are three major types found in humans in the United States: A, B and E. Mortality rates are as follows: Type A: 60–70%, Type B: 10–30%, Type E: 30–50%.[1]

2. The neurotoxin blocks conduction in cholinergic nerve fibers and thereby prevents the release of acetylcholine at the neuromuscular junction; paralysis results. Symptoms may be mild to severe and fatal, and begin 12–36 hours after ingestion of the contaminated food. NOTE: Fecal analysis must be done for the presence of botulin toxin.[2]

   Early signs and symptoms in adults and older children: nausea and vomiting (severe in Type E, not always present in A and B), weakness, dizziness, severe dryness of mouth, pharyngeal pain.

   Late signs and symptoms: blurred and/or double vision, difficulty speaking, difficulty swallowing, extreme weakness, respiratory difficulty, abdominal distention, urinary retention, dilated and fixed pupils, patient remains alert.

   Signs and symptoms in infants and young children: generalized weakness, decreased head control, cranial nerve deficits, weak sucking and crying ability, pooling or oral secretions (inability to swallow).

3. Respiratory difficulty can suddenly lead to apnea. Until the patient is intubated and on a respirator, monitor continuously for decreasing respiratory rate and cyanosis. A baseline vital capacity can be helpful in monitoring for respiratory changes. Begin manual breathing if respiratory rate falls below 8–10 in an adult (see chart on page 545 for normal respiratory rates in children). Use oxygen if necessary. The patient should be intubated without delay. Once the patient is on a respirator, he should be managed as would a patient receiving a neuromuscular blocking agent. Initiate the use of respiratory apnea alarms, monitoring of arterial blood gases and constant attendance.

4. Monitor temperature rectally every 2–4 hours to detect the onset of secondary infection. Report elevations to physician.

5. Monitor for urinary retention; bladder catheterization may be advisable.

6. Assist in skin testing prior to the use of the antitoxin. Take anaphylaxis precautions; see page 118. Keep epinephrine 1:10,000 at the bedside.

7. Cleansing enemas may be ordered to remove remaining, unabsorbed toxin in from the colon.

8. Assistance in diagnosis, treatment and in obtaining trivalent (A, B and E) antitoxin can be obtained from the Enteric Disease Branch of the Center for Disease Control in Atlanta, Georgia: Telephone Numbers (404) 633-3311 (daytime) and (404) 634-2561 (nights). If type E intoxication is suspected, there must be no delay in obtaining trivalent serum; do not use bivalent unless a delay is expected.

9. Patients with botulism can be alert despite paralyzing neurologic symptoms. Do not leave the patient alone. Give pertinent information in simple form as to his condition and what is being done to treat it. Explain all procedures prior to their performance. If the patient is able to write, allow this form of communication to help decrease the anxiety of being unable to speak. Sedation, and analgesia should be prescribed by the physician.

10. Recovery can be complete without residual neurologic deficit.

11. Prevention: Exposure of food to moist heat at least 120°C (216°F) for 30 minutes will kill Clostridium botulinum bacteria (all 6 types). When preparing food for canning: to destroy toxin, all food should be boiled for 10 minutes or be exposed to at least 80°C (144°F) heat for 30 minutes. Foods that are contaminated may taste and appear normal.[3]

REFERENCES

1. Beeson, Paul B., and McDermott, Walsh (editors): Cecil-Loeb Textbook of Medicine (14th ed.), Philadelphia, W. B. Saunders Company, 1975, p. 49.
2. Arnon, Stephen S., et al.: Infant Botulism, Epidemiological, Clinical and Laboratory Aspects. JAMA, 237(18):1950, May 2, 1977.
3. USDA Home and Garden Bulletin No. 8: Superintendent of Documents, Washington, D.C. 1973 (Order Number 001-000-03398-9).

SUGGESTED READINGS

Arnon, Stephen S. et al.: Infant Botulism, Epidemiological, Clinical and Laboratory Aspects. JAMA, 237(18):1946–1951, May 2, 1977 (references).
Taylor, Andrew: Botulism and Its Control. American Journal of Nursing, 73:1380–1382, August 1973.
Watson, Kenneth C.: Botulism. Nursing Mirror, 144:14–16, June 30, 1977.

CAFFEINE AND SODIUM BENZOATE INJECTION

ACTIONS/ INDICATIONS	DOSAGE	PREPARATION AND STORAGE	DRUG INCOMPATIBILITIES	MODES OF IV ADMINISTRATION			CONTRAINDICATIONS; WARNINGS; PRECAUTIONS: ADVERSE REACTIONS
				INJECTION	INTERMITTENT INFUSION	CONTINUOUS INFUSION	
Potent central nervous system stimulant. Used as a respiratory stimulant in the treatment of respiratory depression due to alcohol,	ADULTS: 500 mg (maximum 1 gm)	Supplied in 2-ml ampuls of a 250 mg/ml solution. Discard unused portions.	Do not mix in solution with any other medication.	YES Slowly, over 1–2 min, undiluted.	YES Use any IV fluid, 50-100 ml. Titrate drip rate with patient's response.	NO Pharmacologically inappropriate.	CONTRAINDICATIONS Acute myocardial infarction PRECAUTIONS 1. Doses over 1 gm can cause further respiratory depression. 2. Administration to patients on MAO inhibitors (isocarboxazid, etc.) can precipitate a hypertensive crisis. 3. When used to treat respiratory de-

narcotic analgesics (narcotic antagonist is *preferred* agent to combat respiratory depression due to these drugs), barbiturates and electrical shock. Can also be used to relieve the headache caused by spinal tap.

pression secondary to propoxyphene (Darvon) overdose, convulsions may result.

ADVERSE REACTIONS
1. Nausea
2. Insomnia, excitement, restlessness
3. Tinnitus
4. Tachycardia, premature ventricular contractions
5. Diuresis

NURSING IMPLICATIONS
1. Monitor for the effectiveness of this drug when used as a respiratory stimulant: respiratory rate and depth, presence or absence of cyanosis, mental status, arterial blood gases.
2. Support breathing as necessary. Have the following equipment at the bedside: airways, suction, endotracheal tubes and laryngoscope, oxygen, manual breathing bag (Ambu, Hope, Puritan).
3. Monitor for overdose of caffeine: rapid, shallow respirations, tachycardia, restlessness (differentiate from restlessness due to hypoxia), mental excitement, muscle tremor, premature ventricular contractions.
4. Monitor blood pressure continuously during injection, every 15 minutes for the first hour after injection and then hourly for the next 4 hours.

● CALCIUM CHLORIDE

ACTIONS/ INDICATIONS	DOSAGE	PREPARATION AND STORAGE	DRUG INCOMPAT- IBILITIES	MODES OF IV ADMINISTRATION			CONTRAINDICATIONS; WARNINGS; PRECAUTIONS; ADVERSE REACTIONS
				INJECTION	INTERMITTENT INFUSION	CONTINUOUS INFUSION	
Electrolyte, the most potent provider of calcium ions. Calcium is necessary for the proper functioning of cell membranes, nerves, muscles, blood clotting, myocardial conductivity and excitability, maintenance of the skeletal and vascular muscle tone. Used in the treatment of hypocalcemia when prompt	ADULTS: *For indications other than cardiac arrest*— 6.8–13.6 mEq (5–10 ml of a 10% or 1.36 mEq/ml solution). Additional doses must be guided by serum calcium levels. *In cardiac arrest*—2.7–5.4 mEq (2–4 ml of a 1.36 mEq/ml or 10% solution). May also be administered via intracardiac injection.	Store at room temperature. Discard unused portions of vials. Supplied in ampuls of 10 ml, 1.36 mEq/ml (10% solution) and prefilled syringes. To make a 2% solution, add 1 ml of the 10% calcium chloride solution to 4 ml of a suitable diluent (see Infusion columns).	Do not mix with: Sodium bicarbonate Streptomycin Tobramycin Amphotericin Cephalosporins Chlorpheniramine Tetracyclines Epinephrine	YES This mode is appropriate for emergency situations. In cardiac arrest: total dose can be administered within 15–30 seconds. All other situations: Do not exceed a rate of injection greater than 0.7–1.5 mEq/min (approximately 0.5–1.0 ml of a 10% solution).	YES Add dose to D5W, NS, D5/NS, RL in any volume. Infusion rate should not exceed 0.7–1.5 mEq/min.	YES Add dose to D5W, NS, D5/NS. Infusion rate should not exceed 0.7–1.5 mEq/min.	CONTRAINDICATIONS 1. Hypercalcemia 2. Metastatic bone disease when there is a possibility of hypercalcemia PRECAUTIONS 1. Avoid extravasation. Do not use a scalp vein when giving this drug to children. 2. Administer with caution to patients concomitantly receiving digitalis. Myocardial tetany and/or arrhythmias may result. 3. Monitor serum calcium at frequent intervals to guide dosage. 4. Rapid administration can cause tingling sensations in the extremities and cardiac arrhythmias. Follow infusion rate suggestions. 5. Administration of calcium to patients with high serum phosphate levels has resulted in the precipitation of dibasic calcium phosphate in vital organs, lungs, kidneys, arterial walls, thyroid

CALCIUM CHLORIDE (Continued)

ACTIONS/ INDICATIONS	DOSAGE	PREPARATION AND STORAGE	DRUG INCOMPAT- IBILITIES	MODES OF IV ADMINISTRATION			CONTRAINDICATIONS; WARNINGS; PRECAUTIONS; ADVERSE REACTIONS
				INJECTION	INTERMITTENT INFUSION	CONTINUOUS INFUSION	
increase in serum calcium is needed: • Neonatal tetany • Parathyroid deficiency • Vitamin D deficiency • Magnesium sulfate overdose • Sensitivity reactions with urticaria and hypocalcemia • Hypocalcemia in acute renal failure • Electromechanical dissociation of the heart (as a positive inotropic agent) • Maintenance therapy in parenteral nutrition • Treatment of hyperkalemia.	CHILDREN: *Indications other than cardiac arrest*—4 mEq/kg/24 hrs. Use a 2% solution (see Preparation column.) Dosage must be guided by serum calcium levels. *In cardiac arrest*—IV: 1 ml of a 10% solution/kg (maximum); Intracardiac— 1 ml of a 10% solution diluted 1:1 in NS.[1]						gland. Death can result. Monitor serum phosphate levels during calcium therapy. 6. If bradycardia occurs during an injection or infusion, discontinue administration.

NURSING IMPLICATIONS
1. The normal serum calcium is 8.5–10.5 mg/100 ml (higher in children).
2. Signs and symptoms of hypocalcemia:[2]
   a. Neuromuscular excitability, muscle twitching, convulsions
   b. Numbness and tingling of extremities
   c. Emotional lability
   d. Carpopedal spasm (muscle spasms of hands, wrists, feet and ankles). Trousseau's sign—carpopedal spasms of the hands (inability to open the hand) following inflation of blood pressure cuff to a pressure to occlude circulation for at least 3 minutes
   e. Chvostek's sign—facial muscle twitch following tap over the facial nerve just in front of the ear
   f. In infants and small children, hypotonia and abdominal distention may be seen. As the severity of hypocalcemia increases, laryngeal stridor and

5. In the presence of hypocalcemic tetany, protect the patient from injury through the use of padded side rails. Keep the room quiet and reduce stimulation to a minimum until therapy is effective. Monitor the patient frequently for signs of laryngeal spasm and resultant airway obstruction (this rarely occurs).
6. If this preparation is being administered during cardiopulmonary resuscitation, remind the physician if the patient has been digitalized; he may decide to withhold the drug, use another agent, or use the calcium in a lower dosage.
7. Take precautions to prevent extravasation; see page 96. Do not administer via a scalp vein in children.
8. Use an infusion pump to maintain an accurate flow rate.
9. Follow incompatibility guidelines carefully.

tetany may appear.

3. Monitor for signs of hypercalcemia secondary to overdosage of calcium chloride (these signs will appear as the serum calcium reaches 12 mg %):[3,4]

   a. Changes in mental status secondary to central nervous system depression, e.g., lethargy, confusion, sluggish peripheral nerve reflexes, muscular weakness
   b. Decreased Q-T interval and bradycardia on ECG
   c. Anorexia, constipation, nausea and vomiting
   d. Rise in BUN, polyuria

4. Patients who are digitalized must be observed continuously on an ECG monitor for the onset of arrhythmias such as premature atrial or ventricular contractions, sinus bradycardia or ventricular tachycardia. Be prepared to treat such arrhythmias. Atropine and lidocaine should be readily available.

REFERENCES
1. Standards for Cardiopulmonary Resuscitation (CPR) and Emergency Cardiac Care. *JAMA,* 227(7):859, February 18, 1974.
2. Guyton, Arthur C.: *Textbook of Medical Physiology,* (5th ed.), Philadelphia: W. B. Saunders Company, 1976, p. 1056.
3. Ibid., p. 1056.
4. Beeson, Paul, and McDermott, Walsh (editors): *Cecil-Loeb Textbook of Medicine,* (14th ed.), Philadelphia: W. B. Saunders Company, 1975, p. 1810.

SUGGESTED READING
Tripp, Alice: Hyper- and Hypocalcemia. *American Journal of Nursing,* 76(7):1142–1145, July 1976.

CALCIUM DISODIUM EDETATE (EDTA, ENDRATE)

ACTIONS/ INDICATIONS	DOSAGE	PREPARATION AND STORAGE	DRUG INCOMPATIBILITIES	MODES OF IV ADMINISTRATION			CONTRAINDICATIONS; WARNINGS; PRECAUTIONS; ADVERSE REACTIONS
				INJECTION	INTERMITTENT INFUSION	CONTINUOUS INFUSION	
Chelating agent, combines with metallic ions to form nonionized, water-soluble complexes. Mobilizes heavy metals from the body in the urine. Used in acute and chronic lead, cadmium, zinc, manganese, vanadium, gold, plutonium, yttrium, and arsenic poisoning.	ADULTS: 1 gm every 12 hrs for up to 5 days. After initial 5 days, stop dosage for 2 days and then repeat for 5 more days if needed. Do *not* exceed 50 mg/kg/day. CHILDREN: IM route preferred. Do not exceed 75 mg/kg/day in symptomatic cases. *Asymptomatic patients*—50 mg/kg/day. Administer every 8 or 12 hrs for 3–5 days. A second course may be given	Discard unused portion of vials. Supplied in 5 ml (1 gm) ampuls, 200 mg/ml.	Do not add any other medication to IV bottle; do not add to IV lines containing other drugs.	NO	YES — ADULTS: Add 5 ml of a 20% solution (1 gm) to 250–500 ml of D5W or NS. Infusion times of 6–8 hrs. are preferable; however, infuse over at least 1 hour in asymptomatic patients. Infusion time should be no less than 2 hours in symptomatic patients. CHILDREN: Add dose to 50–100 ml D5W or NS and infuse over 6–8 hrs.	NO	CONTRAINDICATIONS Anuria WARNINGS 1. Never exceed recommended dosage. 2. In lead encephalopathy, avoid rapid infusion to prevent a sudden increase in intracranial pressure. 3. Intramuscular administration is preferred in the presence of lead encephalopathy. 4. Use with caution in the presence of active or healed tuberculosis. PRECAUTIONS 1. Urinalysis should be done daily. This drug should be discontinued if signs of significant renal damage appear (presence of large renal epithelial cells, red blood cells, or increasing proteinuria and rising BUN.) 2. Monitor for cardiac arrhythmias during infusions. 3. In the presence of lead encephalopathy with increased intracranial pressure, excess parenteral fluids must be avoided, yet an adequate urine output must be established by giving fluids before the first dose is given. Once an adequate urine output is obtained, ad-

CALCIUM DISODIUM EDETATE (EDTA, ENDRATE) (Continued)

ACTIONS/INDICATIONS	DOSAGE	PREPARATION AND STORAGE	DRUG INCOMPATIBILITIES	MODES OF IV ADMINISTRATION			CONTRAINDICATIONS; WARNINGS; PRECAUTIONS; ADVERSE REACTIONS
				INJECTION	INTERMITTENT INFUSION	CONTINUOUS INFUSION	
	after a 4-day rest.						minister fluids in volumes to only meet basal fluid and electrolyte requirements. 4. Stop drug infusion if urine output stops, to prevent high serum levels of the drug from developing. 5. Monitor serum electrolytes daily during therapy. 6. Safety for use in pregnancy has not been established. ADVERSE REACTIONS 1. Renal tubular necrosis. Associated signs and symptoms: rise in BUN and serum creatinine, proteinuria, red and white blood cells and renal epithelial cells in the urine, oliguria and anuria, nocturia, dysuria, frequency.[1] 2. Thrombophlebitis at injection site 3. Malaise 4. Thirst 5. Fever 6. Muscular pain 7. Symptoms No. 3–6 may herald the onset of renal toxicity[2]

NURSING IMPLICATIONS

1. In the presence of lead encephalopathy, monitor for signs of increasing intracranial pressure:
   a. Decreasing level of consciousness
   b. Changes in pupil size and equality
   c. Increasing systolic blood pressure and possibly decreasing diastolic blood pressure
   d. Decreasing pulse
   e. Irregular and decreasing respiratory rate
   Notify the physician at the onset of any sign.
2. Administer supportive care if increased intracranial pressure occurs:[3]
   a. Maintain airway
   b. Maintain adequate ventilation guided by arterial blood gases
   c. Correct body positioning; i.e., keep patient on his side, prevent neck flexion, elevate head 15–30 degrees, turn hourly
   d. Prevent valsalva maneuver; i.e., use stool softeners, avoid enemas, instruct alert patients to avoid bearing down and breath-holding
   e. Plan nursing-care procedures so that those that might precipitate increased pressure are not performed together
   f. Follow fluid restriction orders carefully; use of an infusion pump may be advisable.
3. Assist in monitoring renal function:
   a. Send urine for urinalysis daily
   b. Monitor urine output every 8 hours or more frequently if patient has documented renal impairment. Notify physician if urine output falls below 240 ml in 8 hours for adult. (See normal urine output for children, page 546, report fall in output below normal levels.) Slow infusion until the physician determines appropriate therapy.
   c. Be aware of serum BUN.
   d. Examine for malaise, thirst, muscular pain in the conscious patient, report symptoms to the physician.

REFERENCES
1. Craven, Philip and Morrelli, Howard: Chelation Therapy. *The Western Journal of Medicine*, 122:277, March 1975.
2. Ibid., p. 278.
3. Mitchell, Pamela, and Mauss, Nancy: Intracranial Pressure: Fact and Fancy. *Nursing '76*, June 1976, p. 56.

CALCIUM GLUCONATE AND CALCIUM GLUCEPTATE (Calcium Glucoheptonate)

ACTIONS/ INDICATIONS	DOSAGE	PREPARATION AND STORAGE	DRUG INCOMPATIBILITIES	MODES OF IV ADMINISTRATION			CONTRAINDICATIONS; WARNINGS; PRECAUTIONS; ADVERSE REACTIONS
				INJECTION	INTERMITTENT INFUSION	CONTINUOUS INFUSION	
Electrolyte, provider of calcium ions. Calcium is necessary for proper functioning of nerves, muscles, blood clotting, myocardial conductivity, maintenance of the skeletal, and vascular muscle tone. Used in the treatment of hypocalcemia when prompt increase in serum calcium is needed: • Neonatal tetany • Parathyroid deficiency • Vitamin D deficiency • Magnesium sulfate overdose • Sensitivity reactions with urticaria and hypocalcemia • Hypocalcemia in acute renal failure • Electro-mechanical dissociation of the heart (as a positive inotropic agent); calcium *chloride* is usually the preferred preparation,	ADULTS: *Cardiac arrest*—10 ml of a 10% solution (4.8 mEq), repeated as necessary. Administer via IV injection or intracardiac injection. *For indications other than cardiac arrest*—Initial dose, 10 ml of a 10% solution (4.8 mEq or 97 mg). Additional doses must be guided by serum calcium levels. CHILDREN: *Cardiac arrest*—1 ml of a 10% solution/kg, maximum dose; intracardiac: 1 ml of a 10% solution diluted in an equal volume of NS.[1] *For indications other than cardiac arrest*—5—10 ml of a 10% solution (500 mg/kg/24 hrs, or 12 g/ M²/24 hrs).	Store at room temperature. Discard unused portions of vials. Supplied in 5-ml ampuls, of a 10% solution, 0.9 mEq/ml.	Do not mix in any manner with: Tobramycin Clindamycin Folic acid Cephradine Cephalothin Cephazolin Fat emulsion Amphotericin-B Sodium bicarbonate Magnesium sulfate Novobiocin Oxytetracycline Prochlorperazine Tetracycline Prednisolone Sodium or potassium phosphate Epinephrine Sodium bicarbonate.	YES This mode is appropriate for emergency situations. In cardiac arrest: total dose can be administered within 15—30 seconds. In all other situations: do *NOT* exceed a rate of injection greater than 0.5—1.0 ml/min (of a 10% solution) or 0.7—1.5 mEq/min.	YES Add dose to D5W, NS, D5/NS, RL. Infusion should be set at a rate no greater than 0.7—1.5 mEq/min., in any convenient volume of fluid.	YES Add dose to D5W, NS, D5/NS, RL or hyperalimentation fluid.	CONTRAINDICATIONS 1. Hypercalcemia 2. Metastatic bone disease PRECAUTIONS 1. Avoid extravasation; do not use a scalp vein when giving this drug to children. 2. Administer with extreme caution to patients concomitantly receiving digitalis. Myocardial tetany and/or arrhythmias may result. 3. Monitor serum calcium levels at frequent intervals to guide dosage. 4. Rapid administration can cause tingling sensations in the extremities and cardiac arrhythmias. Follow infusion rate suggestions. 5. Administration of calcium to patients with high serum phosphate levels has resulted in the precipitation of dibasic calcium phosphate in vital organs. This can produce soft tissue calcification, and possibly nephrotoxicity. Monitor serum phosphate levels during calcium therapy. 6. If bradycardia occurs during an injection or infusion, discontinue administration.

CALCIUM GLUCONATE AND CALCIUM GLUCEPTATE (Calcium Glucoheptonate) (Continued)

ACTIONS/ INDICATIONS	DOSAGE	PREPARATION AND STORAGE	DRUG INCOMPATIBILITIES	MODES OF IV ADMINISTRATION			CONTRAINDICATIONS; WARNINGS; PRECAUTIONS; ADVERSE REACTIONS
				INJECTION	INTERMITTENT INFUSION	CONTINUOUS INFUSION	
but gluconate can be used. • Treatment of hyperkalemia • Maintenance therapy in parenteral nutrition	Dosage must be guided by serum calcium levels.						

NURSING IMPLICATIONS
1. The normal serum calcium is 8.5–10.5 mg/100 ml. Calcium therapy must be guided by frequent serum calcium determinations.
2. Signs and symptoms of hypocalcemia:[2]
   a. Neuromuscular excitability, muscle twitching, convulsions
   b. Numbness and tingling of extremities
   c. Emotional lability
   d. Carpopedal spasm (muscle spasms of hands, wrists, feet and ankles). Trousseau's sign—carpopedal spasms of the hands (inability to open the hand) following inflation of blood pressure cuff to a pressure to occlude circulation for at least 3 minutes
   e. Chvostek's sign—facial muscle twitch following tap over the facial nerve just in front of the ear
   f. In infants and small children, hypotonia and abdominal distention may be seen
   As the severity of hypocalcemia increases, laryngeal stridor and tetany may appear.
3. Monitor for signs of hypercalcemia secondary to overdosage of calcium solutions (these signs will appear as the serum calcium reaches 12 mg %):[3]
   a. Changes in mental status secondary to central nervous system depression, e.g., lethargy, confusion, sluggish peripheral nerve reflexes, muscular weakness
   b. Decreased Q-T interval and bradycardia on ECG
   c. Anorexia, constipation, nausea and vomiting
   d. Rise in BUN, polyuria

4. Patients who are digitalized must be observed continuously on an ECG monitor for the onset of arrhythmias such as premature atrial or ventricular contractions, sinus bradycardia or ventricular tachycardia. Be prepared to treat such arrhythmias.
5. In the presence of tetany, protect the patient from injury through the use of padded side rails. Keep in a quiet room, reduce stimulation to a minimum until therapy with calcium infusion is effective. Monitor the patient frequently for signs of laryngospasm (stridor, increased respiratory effort, cyanosis). Keep a tracheostomy tray available for emergency use in the event of severe laryngospasm and resultant airway obstruction (this is rare).
6. During cardiac resuscitation, inform the physician if the patient has been digitalized.
7. Take precautions to prevent extravasation; see page 96. Do not infuse via a scalp vein in children.
8. Use an infusion pump for infusion to prevent overdosage but ensure adequate dosage.
9. Make special note of incompatibilities.

REFERENCES
1. Standards for Cardiopulmonary Resuscitation (CPR) and Emergency Cardiac Care. *JAMA*, 227(7):859, February 18, 1974.
2. Guyton, Arthur C.: *A Textbook of Medical Physiology* (5th ed.), Philadelphia: W. B. Saunders Company, 1976, p. 1056.
3. Ibid.

CARBENICILLIN DISODIUM (Geopen, Pyopen)

ACTIONS/ INDICATIONS	DOSAGE	PREPARATION AND STORAGE	DRUG INCOMPATIBILITIES	MODES OF IV ADMINISTRATION			CONTRAINDICATIONS; WARNINGS; PRECAUTIONS; ADVERSE REACTIONS
				INJECTION	INTERMITTENT INFUSION	CONTINUOUS INFUSION	
Antibiotic, semisynthetic penicillin. Ef-	ADULTS: *Range*—200–500 mg/kg/	Reconstitute with sterile water for injec-	Do not mix in IV bottle with any other anti-	YES Further dilute	YES Use any IV	YES Use any IV	CONTRAINDICATIONS Hypersensitivity to penicillin

fective against several gram-positive and gram-negative organisms; most frequently used in pseudomonas and proteus infections, but may also be used to treat infections due to other organisms tested to be susceptible.

day in 4–6 divided doses or continuous infusion. Maximum recommended dose is 40 gm/day.

DOSAGE IN RENAL FAILURE—SEE FOLLOWING PAGE.

CHILDREN:
Initial—100 mg/kg followed by 100–500 mg/kg/24 hrs divided into 4–6 doses or continuous infusion.

NEONATES:
Initial—100 mg/kg followed by 75 mg/kg every 8 hrs for infants under 7 days for infants under 2000 gm; or 75 mg/kg every 6 hrs for 3 days for infants over 2000 gm; for all infants, subsequent doses after above regimen are 100 mg/kg every 6 hrs.

tion *only.* SEE TABLES BELOW

Refrigerate reconstituted solution. Discard after 72 hours. (When stored at room temperature, discard after 24 hours.)

biotic or vitamins.

Do not mix in IV tubing with: Sodium bicarbonate Aminophylline Sodium iodide Levarterenol Isoproterenol

the reconstituted solution with sterile water for injection, 20 ml/gm of drug.

Inject at a rate no greater than 200–500 mg/min.

fluid. Dilute to 1 gm/20 ml (100 mg/ml for children)

Infuse over 30–60 min.

fluid. Add 6-, 12- or 24-hour dose to 500–1000 ml depending on fluid needs of patient.

This drug is stable in solution for 24 hours.

Preparation and Storage

PIGGYBACK VIALS

Vial Size (gm)	Vol. Diluent (ml)	Vol. of 1-gm Dose
2	100	50 ml
	50	25 ml
	20	10 ml
5	100	20 ml
	50	10 ml
10	95	10 ml

REGULAR VIALS

Vial Size (gm)	Vol. Diluent (ml)	Vol. of 1-gm Dose
1	2.0	2.5 ml
	2.5	3.0 ml
	3.6	4.0 ml
2	4.0	2.5 ml
	5.0	3.0 ml
	6.6	4.0 ml
5	9.5	2.5 ml
	12.0	3.0 ml
	17.0	4.0 ml

WARNINGS
1. Take anaphylaxis precautions.
2. Blood-clotting abnormalities have been reported in uremic patients on high doses of carbenicillin. Hemorrhagic manifestations disappeared on withdrawal of the drug.
3. Safety for use in pregnancy has not been established.

PRECAUTIONS
1. Avoid intra-arterial injection and extravasation.
2. Monitor hepatic, renal and hematopoietic (blood cell production) systems during therapy.
3. This drug contains 5.3–6.5 mEq of sodium per gram.
4. Emergence of organisms resistent to this antibiotic, such as Klebsiella species and Serratia species, has been reported. These organisms can cause a superinfection.
5. Monitor serum potassium; hypokalemia has been reported.

ADVERSE REACTIONS
1. Thrombophlebitis at injection site
2. Allergic reactions: rash, urticaria, drug fever, anaphylaxis
3. Nausea and unpleasant taste (especially with high doses)
4. Blood dyscrasias: leukopenia, neutropenia, thrombocytopenia, hemolytic anemia
5. Elevation in SGOT and SGPT
6. Convulsions or neuromuscular excitability in patients with impaired renal function where high serum concentration may occur.

CARBENICILLIN DISODIUM (Geopen, Pyopen) (Continued)

ACTIONS/INDICATIONS	DOSAGE	PREPARATION AND STORAGE	DRUG INCOMPATIBILITIES	MODES OF IV ADMINISTRATION			CONTRAINDICATIONS; WARNINGS; PRECAUTIONS; ADVERSE REACTIONS
				INJECTION	INTERMITTENT INFUSION	CONTINUOUS INFUSION	

DOSAGE

ADULTS WITH RENAL IMPAIRMENT [1,2]*

Creatinine Clearance (ml/min)	Dosage	Intervals
80–50	Same as for normal adults	q 4 hrs
50–10	2–4 gm	q 6 hrs
10	2 gm	q 12 hrs
Combined renal and hepatic failure	2 gm	q 24 hrs
With hemodialysis	2 gm	After each dialysis
With peritoneal dialysis	2 gm	q 6–12 hrs[3]

*NEONATES: The mode of administration ordered may depend on the organism being treated. More detailed dosage recommendations in relation to site of injection and organism are available from manufacturer's (Geopen, Roerig, Pyopen, Beecham Labs).

NURSING IMPLICATIONS

1. Take precautions to prevent extravasation; see page 96.
2. Take anaphylaxis precautions, see page 118.
3. Monitor for signs of bleeding, especially in patients with impaired renal function: melena or blood in stools (daily guaiacs are advisable), hematuria, nose bleeding, gum bleeding, ecchymosis with no history of trauma, vaginal bleeding (excessive menstrual flow).
4. Monitor patients with active cardiac disease, history of cardiac disease, and renal dysfunction, for fluid retention by daily weights. Check for peripheral edema at least daily. Place the patient on intake and output and record at least every 8 hours, depending on the patient's general condition.
5. Monitor cardiac patients for signs of cardiac decompensation, i.e., congestive heart failure, in addition to those activities listed in No. 4 above: increasing heart rate; increasing respiratory rate, dyspnea or exertion, orthopnea, rales; elevation of jugular venous pulses, engorgement of external jugular veins.
6. Take seizure precautions in patients with renal impairment.
7. Patients on high-dose infusions may have nausea and vomiting; if so, administer antiemetics as ordered, prior to meals. Instruct the patient as to the origin of the bad taste if it occurs.
8. Monitor for signs of hypokalemia: unusual weakness, increasing lethargy, irritability, abdominal distention, poor feeding in infants, muscle cramps.
9. Monitor for signs and symptoms of overgrowth infections:
   a. Fever (take rectal temperature at least every 4–6 hours in all patients)
   b. Increasing malaise
   c. Newly appearing localized signs and symptoms—redness, soreness, pain, swelling, drainage (increased volume or change in character of preexisting drainage)
   d. Monilial rash in perineal area (reddened areas with itching)
   e. Cough (change in pre-existing cough or sputum production)
   f. Diarrhea

REFERENCES
1. Gardner, Pierce, and Provine, Harriet: *Manual of Acute Bacterial Infections.* Boston: Little, Brown and Company, 1975, p. 241.
2. Kagen, Benjamin M., *Antimicrobial Therapy,* (2nd ed.), Philadelphia: W. B. Saunders Company, 1974, p. 433.
3. Hoffman, Thomas A., et al. Pharmacodynamics of Carbenicillin in Hepatic and Renal Failure. *Annals of Internal Medicine,* 73:173, August, 1970.

SUGGESTED READING
Rodman, Morton J.: Antimicrobial Drugs for Septicemia, *RN,* May 1976, pp. 67–80.

● CARMUSTINE (BCNU, BIS-CHLORETHYL NITROSOUREA, BiCNU)

ACTIONS/ INDICATIONS	DOSAGE	PREPARATION AND STORAGE	DRUG INCOMPAT-IBILITIES	MODES OF IV ADMINISTRATION			CONTRAINDICATIONS; WARNINGS; PRECAUTIONS; ADVERSE REACTIONS
				INJECTION	INTERMITTENT INFUSION	CONTINUOUS INFUSION	
Antineoplastic agent, with alkylation and protein modification actions. Used in the treatment of: • Metastatic brain tumors • Gliomas (brain) • Hodgkin's disease • Non-Hodgkin's lymphomas • Melanoma • Multiple myeloma • Epidermoid lung carcinoma • Breast cancer • Carcinoma of colon and rectum • Head and neck tumors	ADULTS AND CHILDREN: 100 mg/M² for 2 days or 200 mg/M² as a single dose every 6–8 weeks. Alternative schedule: 40 mg/M² daily for 5 consecutive days repeated at 6- to 8-week intervals. Subsequent doses must be adjusted according to bone marrow function. A repeat course of this drug should not be given until circulating blood elements have returned to acceptable levels. Subsequent doses should be adjusted according to the hematologic response to the preceding dose. See chart on page 220.	To reconstitute, add 3 ml of accompanying diluent; then 27 ml of sterile water for injection. Concentration of the solution is 3.3 mg/ml. Powder must be kept at 2–8°C until ready to use. After reconstitution, it is stable for 2–4 hrs. Discard unused portions. Avoid contact with skin; it causes brown staining. If this drug is added to 500 ml. D5W or NS, the solution can be stored in the refrigerator for 48 hours without losing stability. If the powder form is exposed to a temperature above 27°C or 80°F, it will liquify, and should be discarded.	Do not mix with other medications in any manner.	NO	YES Add dose to 100–500 ml D5W or NS. Infuse over 60 min. Use an infusion pump to prevent rapid infusion.	NO	CONTRAINDICATIONS 1. Hypersensitivity 2. Bone marrow depression producing decreased platelets, leukocytes, or erythrocytes WARNINGS Safety for use during pregnancy has not been established. PRECAUTIONS 1. Complete blood counts should be obtained frequently for at least 6 weeks following a course of therapy. 2. Do not repeat doses more frequently than every 6 weeks. 3. Bone marrow toxicity is cumulative. Dosage must be adjusted based on CBC at the time of the prior dose. 4. Monitor liver function tests throughout therapy. ADVERSE REACTIONS 1. Bone marrow depression: occurs 4–6 weeks after administration and is dose-related. The lowest level in the platelet count may occur 4–5 weeks after a single dose; the leukocyte count in 5–6 weeks. Anemia also occurs but is less severe than the thrombocytopenia (decreased platelets) or leukopenia (decreased WBC's). 2. Nausea and vomiting: occur within 2 hours of infusion and may last for 4–6 hours. This may be prevented or diminished with antiemetics. 3. Hepatotoxicity: usually reversible, manifested by elevated SGOT, alkaline phosphatase and bilirubin. 4. Burning at infusion site. 5. Rapid infusion may produce intense flushing of the skin and hyperemia of the conjunctiva within 2 hours and may last for about 4 hours.

219

CARMUSTINE (BCNU, BIS-CHLORETHYL NITROSOUREA, BiCNU) (Continued)

ACTIONS/ INDICATIONS	DOSAGE	PREPARATION AND STORAGE	DRUG INCOMPAT- IBILITIES	MODES OF IV ADMINISTRATION			CONTRAINDICATIONS; WARNINGS; PRECAUTIONS; ADVERSE REACTIONS
				INJECTION	INTERMITTENT INFUSION	CONTINUOUS INFUSION	

MANUFACTURER'S SUGGESTED ADJUSTMENT OF SUBSEQUENT DOSES

Lowest Cell Count After Prior Dose		Percentage of Prior Dose to be Given
WBC's	Platelets	
4000	100,000	100%
3000–3999	75,000–99,999	100%
2000–2999	25,000–74,999	70%
2000		50%

NURSING IMPLICATIONS

1. The patient receiving this medication will be experiencing the emotional and physical effects of the malignancy. Knowledge of the patient's feelings about his disease and its implications will assist in helping him tolerate the chemotherapy. The incidence of uncomfortable side effects and adverse reactions is high. It is within the nurse's role to assist the patient in coping with the discomforts of the disease and its treatment, and to help him work through depression and anger toward acceptance of the disease at his own pace. Despite the unpleasantness this drug may bring, it can be a source of hope for the patient.

2. Management of hematologic effects:
   a. Be aware of the patient's white blood cell and platelet counts prior to each injection.
   b. See Adverse Reaction No. 1; anticipate when blood counts will reach the lowest points.
   c. If the WBC falls to 2000/cu mm, take measures to protect the patient from infection, such as protective (reversed) isolation, avoidance of traumatic procedures, maintenance of bodily (especially perineal) cleanliness, carrying out strict urinary catheter care when appropriate, etc. Monitor for infection by recording temperatures every 4 hours, examining for rashes, swelling, drainage, and pain. Explain these measures to the patient.
   d. If the platelet count falls below 100,000/cu mm, monitor for thrombocytopenic bleeding: petechiae, purpura, hematuria, melena, blood in stools, gum bleeding, vaginal bleeding, epistaxis, hematemesis, etc. Avoid trauma. Transfusions may be ordered.
   e. Instruct the patient and family on the importance of follow-up blood studies if this drug is being administered on an outpatient basis.

3. Management of gastrointestinal effects:
   a. Administer antiemetics with each injection; the nausea and vomiting which occur usually 2–6 hours after the injection can be prevented. Repeat antiemetic in 4–6 hours to cover the duration of the nausea produced by the carmustine (4–6 hours).
   b. If nausea and vomiting are not completely relieved by the antiemetics, attempt to maintain nutrient intake. Small, frequent meals, timed with

periods when the patient feels his best, are advisable. Bland foods may be more easily tolerated. Carbohydrate and protein content should be high.
   c. If the patient is anorexic, encourage high nutrient liquids and water to maintain hydration.
   d. Keep accurate measurements of emesis volume and total intake and output to guide the physician in ordering parenteral fluids when necessary.

4. Maintain recommended infusion rate with an infusion pump. See Adverse Reaction No. 5.

5. Warn the patient that there may be local vein discomfort during the infusion.

SUGGESTED READINGS

Gullo, Shirley: Chemotherapy—What To Do About Special Side Effects, *RN,* 40:30–32, April, 1977.

Giaquinta, Barbara: Helping Families Face the Crisis of Cancer, *American Journal of Nursing,* 77:1583–1588, October, 1977.

Foley, Genevieve, and McCarthy, Ann Marie: The Disease (Hodgkin's) and Its Treatment. *American Journal of Nursing,* 76:1109–1114 (references).

———: The Child With Leukemia In a Special Hematology Clinic. *American Journal of Nursing,* 76:1115–1119, July 1976.

Bolin, Rose Homan, and Auld, Margaret E.: Hodgkin's Disease. *American Journal of Nursing,* 74:1982–1986, November 1974.

Hannan, Jeanne Ferguson: Talking is Treatment Too. *American Journal of Nursing,* 74:1991–1992, November 1974.

Martinson, Ida: The Child With Leukemia: Parents Help Each Other. *American Journal of Nursing,* 76:1120–1122, July 1976.

Showfety, Mary Patricia: The Ordeal of Hodgkin's Disease. *American Journal of Nursing,* 74:1987–1991, November 1974.

LeBlanc, Dona Harris: People With Hodgkin Disease: The Nursing Challenge, *Nursing Clinics of North America,* 13(2):281–300, June, 1978.

Morrow, Mary: Nursing Management of the Adolescent: The Effect of Cancer Chemotherapy on Psychosocial Development, *Nursing Clinics of North America,* 13(2):319–335, June, 1978.

CEFAZOLIN SODIUM (Ancef, Kefzol)

ACTIONS/ INDICATIONS	DOSAGE	PREPARATION AND STORAGE	DRUG INCOMPATIBILITIES	MODES OF IV ADMINISTRATION			CONTRAINDICATIONS; WARNINGS; PRECAUTIONS; ADVERSE REACTIONS
				INJECTION	INTERMITTENT INFUSION	CONTINUOUS INFUSION	
Antibiotic, cephalosporin group, broad-spectrum. Active against *Staph aureus* (penicillin-sensitive and penicillin-resistent); Group A beta-hemolytic streptococcus and others. Indicated for the treatment of serious infections of the respiratory and genitourinary tracts; of skin, soft tissue, bones, and joints; and in septicemia and endocarditis.	ADULTS: *Mild gram-positive infections*—250–500 mg every 8 hrs (750–1500 mg/24 hrs). *Moderate to severe infections*—500–1000 mg every 6–8 hrs (1.5–4 gm/24 hrs). *Serious infections*—up to 6–12 gm/24 hrs. All doses may be given by divided doses or continuous infusions. *In the presence of renal impairment*—see table below. CHILDREN: *Mild to moderate infections* —25–50 mg/ kg/24 hrs divided into 3–4 equal doses. *Severe infections*—up to 100 mg/ kg/24 hrs in 3–4 equal doses. NEONATES: 40 mg/kg/24	Reconstitute from powder as follows: *Vial Size* *Diluent to Be Added* 250 mg 2 ml 500 mg 2 ml 1 gm 2.5 ml Refrigerate reconstituted solution; discard after 90 hrs.	Do not mix in any manner with the following drugs: Calcium preparations Chlortetracycline Erythromycin Kanamycin Oxytetracycline Polymyxin B Tetracycline Barbiturates Amikacin	YES Further dilute reconstituted form with 10 ml of sterile water for injection for every 500 mg of the drug. Inject over 3–5 min. Injection may be into the tubing of a running IV containing any fluid listed under the Continuous Infusion column.	YES Dilute reconstituted form in 100 ml of NS or D5W for every gram of the drug. Infuse over 15–30 min.	YES Add 8-, 12- or 24-hr dosage to 500–1000 ml of fluid depending on the patient's fluid needs. Use any of the following fluids: NS D5W D10W RL D5/½ NS D5/0.45% saline D5/0.2% saline 5% or 10% invert sugar Normosol-M in D5W. Solution will be stable for 24 hrs.	CONTRAINDICATIONS Hypersensitivity to any cephalosporin WARNINGS 1. Administer with caution to patients with an allergy to penicillin; there may be cross-allergenicity. 2. Safety for use in pregnancy has not been established. 3. Safety for use in infants under 1 month of age or in premature infants has not been established, and use is not recommended by the manufacturer. PRECAUTIONS 1. Overgrowth of nonsusceptible organisms can occur with prolonged use. 2. False-positive urine glucose testing may result with the use of Benedicts' or Fehling's solution, or with Clinitest tablets. 3. This drug contains 2 mEq of sodium per gram. ADVERSE REACTIONS 1. Allergic reactions: rash, urticaria, drug fever, anaphylaxis 2. Blood dyscrasias: neutropenia, leukopenia, thrombocytopenia, positive direct and indirect Coombs tests 3. Renal and hepatic changes: transient rise in SGOT, SGPT, BUN, and alkaline phosphotase levels have been seen without evidence of organ damage 4. Gastrointestinal: anorexia, nausea, vomiting, diarrhea, oral candidiasis (oral thrush infection) 5. Thrombophlebitis at injection site 6. Perineal monilial infections

CEFAZOLIN SODIUM (Ancef, Kefzol) (Continued)

ACTIONS/ INDICATIONS	DOSAGE	PREPARATION AND STORAGE	DRUG INCOMPATIBILITIES	MODES OF IV ADMINISTRATION			CONTRAINDICATIONS; WARNINGS; PRECAUTIONS; ADVERSE REACTIONS
				INJECTION	INTERMITTENT INFUSION	CONTINUOUS INFUSION	
	hrs in equally divided doses every 12 hrs.[1]						
	Manufacturer does not recommend use of this drug under 1 month of age.						

ADULT DOSAGE IN THE PRESENCE OF RENAL IMPAIRMENT[2]

Creatinine Clearance (ml/min)	Dosage Frequency
20–50	Loading dose: 500 mg followed by 250 mg every 6 hours or 500 mg every 12 hours.
10–20	Loading dose: 500 mg followed by 250 mg every 12 hours or 500 mg every 24 hours.
less than 10	Loading dose: 500 mg followed by 250 mg every 24–36 hours or 500 mg every 48–72 hours.
On Hemodialysis	500 mg after each treatment.

NURSING IMPLICATIONS
1. Take anaphylaxis precautions; see page 118.
2. Monitor for signs and symptoms of overgrowth infections due to nonsusceptible organisms:
   a. Fever (take rectal temperature at least every 4–6 hours in all patients)
   b. Increasing malaise
   c. Newly appearing signs and symptoms of a localized infection: redness, soreness, pain, swelling, drainage (increased volume, or change in character of pre-existing drainage)
   d. Oral lesions (thrush) or perineal rash (monilia) of, *Candida albicans*
   e. Cough (change in character or volume of pre-existing sputum)
   f. Diarrhea
3. Use Tes-Tape or Keto-Diastix for urine glucose determinations.
4. Monitor for signs and symptoms of cardiac decompensation in patients with congestive heart failure because of the sodium content of this drug:
   a. Weight gain—weigh these patients daily; report a gain over pretreatment values to the physician
   b. Increasing in resting heart rate—take pulse every 4 hours
   c. Increasing respiratory rate, dyspnea, orthopnea, rales
   d. Peripheral edema

REFERENCES
1. McCracken, Harry C.: *Antimicrobial Therapy for Newborns,* New York; Grune and Stratton, 1977, p. 28.
2. Leroy, Annie, et al.: Pharmacokinetics of Cefazolin, a New Cephalosporin Antibiotic, in Normal and Uremic Patients. *Current Therapeutic Research,* 16(9):887, September 1974.

CEPHALORIDINE (Loridine)

ACTIONS/INDICATIONS	DOSAGE	PREPARATION AND STORAGE	DRUG INCOMPATIBILITIES	MODES OF IV ADMINISTRATION			CONTRAINDICATIONS; WARNINGS; PRECAUTIONS; ADVERSE REACTIONS
				INJECTION	INTERMITTENT INFUSION	CONTINUOUS INFUSION	
Antibiotic, cephalosporin group, broad-spectrum. Active against *Staph aureus* (coagulase positive and negative) Group A beta hemolytic Streptococcus, *Streptococcus pneumoniae*, Pneumococcus, Gonococcus, *E. coli*, and others. Indicated for the treatment of serious infections of the respiratory and genitourinary tracts, bones, and soft tissues. Indicated in septicemia secondary to susceptible organisms. Can be used to treat syphilis and gonorrhea when penicillin is contraindicated.	ADULTS: *Very susceptible organisms* —500–1500 mg/24 hrs. *Serious infections*—2–4 gm/24 hours. Give in 4 divided doses or by continuous infusion. Do not exceed 4 gm/24 hours. This drug is not recommended in the presence of renal failure. CHILDREN: *Mild to moderately severe infections*—30–50 mg/kg/24 hrs (15–25 mg/lb) in divided doses. *Severe infections*—100 mg/kg/24 hrs (50 mg/lb) in divided doses. Do not exceed recommended adult doses.	To reconstitute from powder, use sterile water for injection or sodium chloride injection that has been warmed to body temperature in the hands, in the volumes given in the table below. Shake vial until powder is dissolved. Solution will be pale yellow. Store in refrigerator, discard after 96 hours. If recrystallization occurs, redissolve by warming in the hands and shaking vial. Store reconstituted solution in manufacturer's box to protect from light.	Do not mix in any manner with: Chlortetracycline Barbiturates Erythromycin Oxytetracycline Tetracycline Heparin	YES Further dilute reconstituted form with sterile water for injection, 10 ml/ gm of drug. Inject over a 3–4 min period.	YES Dilute reconstituted form in 100 ml of D5W or NS for every gm of drug.	YES Add 8-, 12- or 24-hour dose to 500–1000 ml D5W, NS, D5/Ringer's, Ionosol-B, Normosol-M, RL D5/NS, Invert sugar, Ringer's Injection, Sodium lactate, depending on patient's fluid needs. Solution is stable for 24 hours.	CONTRAINDICATIONS Hypersensitivity to any cephalosporin C group antibiotic WARNINGS 1. Administer with caution to patients with an allergy to penicillin; there may be cross-allergenicity. 2. Safety for use during pregnancy has not been established. 3. Safety for use in any infant under 1 month of age or in premature infants has not been established and is not recommended. 4. This drug can cause renal damage in patients with normal renal function, and further renal damage in patients with underlying renal impairment, especially in high-dose therapy.[1] Renal impairment will be evidenced by rising BUN and serum creatinine, casts and protein in the urine, and a falling urine output. 5. Some azotemic patients have developed positive direct Coombs tests while on this drug, although there has been no definite evidence of hemolytic anemia. 6. Administer with caution when used concurrently with other nephrotoxic drugs. 7. Concurrent use with potent diuretics such as furosemide or ethacrynic acid may increase the risk of renal toxicity. PRECAUTIONS 1. Overgrowth of nonsusceptible organisms can occur with prolonged use. 2. False-positive urine glucose testing may result with the use of Benedict's or Fehling's solution, or with Clinitest tablets. ADVERSE REACTIONS 1. Allergic reactions: rash, urticaria, drug fever anaphylaxis 2. Blood dyscrasias: neutropenia, leukopenia, thrombocytopenia, positive direct and indirect Coombs test 3. Renal: tubular necrosis producing severe acute renal failure, may be fatal (usually seen in the critically ill and

DILUTION TABLE

Diluent Added to 1-gm Ampul	Volume of Solution	Concentration (Approx.)
2.5 ml	3.3 ml	300 mg per ml
10.0 ml	10.8 ml	100 mg per ml

Diluent Added to 500-mg Ampul	Volume of Solution	Concentration (Approx.)
2 ml	2.4 ml	200 mg per ml
5 ml	5.4 ml	100 mg per ml

CEPHALORIDINE (Loridine) (*Continued*)

ACTIONS/ INDICATIONS	DOSAGE	PREPARATION AND STORAGE	DRUG INCOMPAT-IBILITIES	MODES OF IV ADMINISTRATION: INJECTION	INTERMITTENT INFUSION	CONTINUOUS INFUSION	CONTRAINDICATIONS; WARNINGS; PRECAUTIONS; ADVERSE REACTIONS
							with the use of high doses) 4. Hepatic: transient rise in SGOT and SGPT, without organ damage 5. Gastrointestinal: nausea, anorexia, vomiting, diarrhea, oral Candida infection 6. Thrombophlebitis at injection site 7. Perineal monilial infections.

NURSING IMPLICATIONS

1. Take anaphylaxis precautions; see page 118.
2. Monitor for signs and symptoms of overgrowth infections due to nonsusceptible organisms
   a. Fever (take rectal temperature at least every 4–6 hours in all patients)
   b. Increasing malaise
   c. Newly appearing signs and symptoms of a localized infection: redness, soreness, pain, swelling, drainage (increasing volume or change in character of pre-existing drainage)
   d. Rash and itching in the perineal area (monilia) or oral lesions (thrush) due to *Candida albicans*
   e. Cough (change character of pre-existing sputum volume and character)
   f. Diarrhea
3. Use Tes-Tape or Keto-diastix for urine glucose determinations.
4. Monitor renal function:
   a. Intake and output recordings at least every 4 hours depending on the patient's condition, report oliguria (adults: urine output less than 120 ml over 4 hours; for normal urine output in children: see chart on page 546)
   b. Urinalysis daily, for casts and proteinuria
   c. Be aware of the patient's BUN and creatinine.

REFERENCE

1. Appel, Gerald B., and New, Harold C.: The Nephrotoxicity of Antimicrobial Agents. *New England Journal of Medicine,* 296(12):669, March 24, 1977.

CEPHALOTHIN SODIUM (Keflin, Keflin Neutral)

ACTIONS/ INDICATIONS	DOSAGE	PREPARATION AND STORAGE	DRUG INCOMPAT-IBILITIES	MODES OF IV ADMINISTRATION: INJECTION	INTERMITTENT INFUSION	CONTINUOUS INFUSION	CONTRAINDICATIONS; WARNINGS; PRECAUTIONS; ADVERSE REACTIONS
Antibiotic, cephalosporin group, broad spectrum. Active against *Staph. aureus* (coagulase positive and negative), Group A beta hemolytic streptococcus, *Strep. pneumoniae* clostridia, *H.*	ADULTS: *Usual range*—500–1000 mg every 4–6 hrs. Up to 12 gm/24 hours for serious infections. *In the presence of renal impairment* (adults)—see table below.	To reconstitute from powder add 4 ml of sterile water for injection for each gram of drug. If drug does not dissolve completely, add an additional small amount of diluent and warm the vial in the hands.	Many incompatibilities; do not mix with other drugs in any manner, except hydrocortisone.	YES Further dilute reconstituted form with sterile water for injection, 10 ml/gm of drug. Inject over 3–5 min.	YES Dilute reconstituted form in 50 ml D5W or NS. Infuse over 15–20 min. For smaller volumes dilute to 1 gm/10 ml.	YES Add 8-, 12- or 24-hour dose to 500–1000 ml of any IV fluid, depending on patient fluid needs. Solution is stable for 24 hours.	CONTRAINDICATIONS Hypersensitivity to any cephalosporin WARNINGS 1. Administer with caution to patients with an allergy to penicillin; there may be cross-allergenicity. 2. Safety for use during pregnancy has not been established. PRECAUTIONS 1. Monitor renal status during therapy, especially in the seriously ill who are receiving maximal doses. Use suggested dosage modifications in the

influenzae, E. coli; Proteus, and others.

Indicated for the treatment of serious infections of respiratory, genitourinary, and gastrointestinal tracts, soft tissue, skin, bones and joints. Indicated in septicemia and endocarditis. Intraperitoneal administration has been used to treat peritonitis, or to prevent it when the peritoneal cavity has been contaminated.

CHILDREN: Most susceptible infections —40–150 mg/kg/24 hrs; give in divided doses every 4–6 hrs.

Serious infections or in lowered resistance—80–225 mg/kg/24 hrs given in divided doses every 4–6 hrs.

NEONATES: 0–7 days of age—40 mg/kg/24 hrs (20 mg/kg every 12 hrs). Over 7 days of age—60 mg/kg/24 hrs (20 mg/kg every 8 hrs).[1]

Store in refrigerator. Discard after 48 hours.

presence of renal impairment.
2. Thrombophlebitis at injection site can be minimized by adding 10–25 mg of hydrocortisone to continuous infusion preparations.
3. Overgrowth of nonsusceptible organisms can occur with prolonged use.
4. False-positive urine glucose testing may result with the use of Benedicts or Fehling's solution, or with Clinitest tablets.

ADVERSE REACTIONS
1. Allergic reactions: rash, urticaria, drug fever, anaphylaxis
2. Blood dyscrasias: neutropenia, thrombocytopenia, and hemolytic anemia; positive direct and indirect Coomb's test (usually seen in the presence of azotemia)
3. Hepatic: transient rise in SGOT and SGPT, without organ damage
4. Renal:
   a. Rise in BUN and decrease in creatinine clearance, especially in the presence of pre-existing renal impairment.
   b. Rise in BUN without a decrease in creatinine clearance, renal damage is not likely, and BUN will return to normal after discontinuation of therapy. Permanent renal damage rarely occurs.
5. Thrombophlebitis at injection site with continuous infusions of large doses.
6. Gastrointestinal: nausea, anorexia, diarrhea, vomiting, oral Candida infection
7. Perineal: monilial infections

4. Monitor renal function in patients with renal impairment:
   a. Intake and output recordings every 4–8 hours, depending on the patient's condition; report onset or changes in oliguria defined as: adults—urine output less than 240 ml in 8 hours; children—see chart on page 546
   b. Urinalysis as indicated, usually every other day
   c. Be aware of the patient's BUN and creatinine

REFERENCE
1. McCracken, George H. and Nelson, John D.: Antimicrobial Therapy for Newborns: Practical Application of Pharmacology to Clinical Usage. New York: Grune and Stratton, 1977, p. 28.

DOSAGE IN RENAL IMPAIRMENT (ADULTS)

Degree of Impairment	Creatinine Clearance	Dosage and Frequency
Mild	80–85 ml/min	2 gm q 6 hrs
Moderate	50–25 ml/min	1.5 gm q 6 hrs
Severe	25–10 ml/min	1 gm q 6 hrs
Marked	10–2 ml/min	0.5 gm q 6 hrs
No function	>2 ml/min	0.5 gm q 8 hrs

NURSING IMPLICATIONS
1. Take anaphylaxis precautions; see page 118.
2. Monitor for signs and symptoms of overgrowth infections due to nonsusceptible organisms
   a. Fever (take rectal temperature at least every 4–6 hours in all patients)
   b. Increasing malaise
   c. Newly appearing signs and symptoms of a localized infection: redness, soreness, pain, swelling, drainage (increasing volume, or change in character of pre-existing drainage)
   d. Oral lesions (thrush) or perineal rash (monilia) due to Candida albicans
   e. Cough (change in pre-existing cough and sputum production)
   f. Diarrhea
3. Use Tes-Tape or Keto-Diastix for urine glucose determinations.

CEPHAPIRIN SODIUM (Cefadyl)

ACTIONS/INDICATIONS	DOSAGE	PREPARATION AND STORAGE	DRUG INCOMPATIBILITIES	MODES OF IV ADMINISTRATION			CONTRAINDICATIONS; WARNINGS; PRECAUTIONS; ADVERSE REACTIONS
				INJECTION	INTERMITTENT INFUSION	CONTINUOUS INFUSION	
Antibiotic, cephalosporin group, broad-spectrum. Active against susceptible strains of the following organisms for the following clinical situations: *Staph. aureus* (penicillinase producing and nonpenicillinase producing)—skin, soft tissue, respiratory, urinary and bone infections; septicemia, endocarditis. *Group A beta hemolytic streptococcus*—skin, soft tissue, bone and respiratory infections, septicemia. *Alpha Streptococcus viridans*—septicemia endocarditis. *S. pneumoniae*—respiratory infections. *H. influenzae*—respiratory infections (this organism is frequently not sensitive to cephapirin).	ADULTS: 500–1000 mg. every 4–6 hrs depending on the severity of the infection. Life-threatening infections may require doses up to 12 gm daily. In the presence of renal impairment, severe oliguria or steady-state serum creatinine greater than 5 mg/100 ml, a dose of 7.5–15.0 mg/kg every 12 hrs (when appropriate, just prior to dialysis, and every 12 hrs. thereafter). CHILDREN (OVER 3 MONTHS OF AGE): 40–80 mg/kg/24 hrs in 4 divided doses. *Severe infections*—100 mg/kg/24 hrs in 4 divided doses. Therapy for beta hemolytic streptococcal infections should continue for at least 10 days.	To reconstitute from powder add 10 ml of sterile water for injection or Bacteriostatic Water for injection to the 1-gm or 2-gm vials. Dilute piggyback packages with at least 10 ml of the above diluents. Solutions may be light yellow. Store in refrigerator, discard after 10 days. If stored at room temperature, discard after 12 hrs.	Do not mix with: Mannitol Aminoglycoside antibiotics Aminophylline Tetracyclines Phenytoin Barbiturates	YES Further dilute reconstituted form with sterile water for injection 10 ml/gm of drug. Inject over 3–5 min.	YES Further dilute prepared 1- and 2-gm vials with 50 ml NS or D5W. For smaller volumes, dilute to 1 gm/10 ml. Piggyback vials may be infused, as prepared, over 3–5 min. Discontinue other infusions while infusing this drug.	YES Add 8-, 12- or 24-hour dosage to 500–1000 ml of any IV fluid, except sodium bicarbonate, depending on patient fluid needs. Solution is stable for 24 hours.	CONTRAINDICATIONS Hypersensitivity to any cephalosporin. WARNINGS 1. Administer with caution to patients with an allergy to penicillin; there may be partial cross-allergenicity. 2. Safety for use in pregnancy has not been established. 3. Safety for use in infants under 3 months of age or in premature infants has not been established and use is not recommended. PRECAUTIONS 1. Renal status should be evaluated before and during therapy. Renal impairment is rarely produced by this drug.[1] However, renal impairment is an indication for reduced dosage (see Dosage column). 2. Prolonged use of this drug may result in the overgrowth of nonsusceptible organisms; major and minor superinfections may be produced. 3. With high urine concentrations of cephapirin, false-positive glucose reactions may occur with the use of Clinitest, Benedict's solution, or Fehling's solution. Clinistix or Tes-Tape should be used. 4. Each 500 mg of this drug contains 1.18 mEq of sodium. ADVERSE REACTIONS 1. Hypersensitivity: maculopapular rash, urticaria, drug fever, serum-sickness-like reaction, anaphylaxis 2. Blood dyscrasias: neutropenia, leukopenia, anemia (secondary to depression of blood cell formation) are rare. Occasionally, patients with azotemia (increased BUN) have developed a positive direct Coombs test 3. Liver: transient elevation of SGOT and SGPT, alkaline phosphatase, and bilirubin have been reported 4. Kidney: transient elevation of BUN, especially in patients over 50 years of age

E. coli— urinary tract, skin and soft tissue infections; septicemia.

Klebsiella— respiratory, urinary tract and bone infections; septicemia.

Proteus mirabilis— Urinary tract and bone infections.

NEONATES: Not recommended for infants under 3 months of age or in premature infants.

NURSING IMPLICATIONS
1. Take anaphylaxis precautions; see page 118.
2. Use Clinistix or Tes-Tape for urine glucose determinations.
3. Monitor for signs and symptoms of nonsusceptible organism overgrowth infection
   a. Fever (take rectal temperature at least every 4-6 hours)
   b. Increasing malaise
   c. Localized signs and symptoms of newly developing infection: redness, soreness, pain, swelling, drainage (change in volume or character of pre-existing drainage)
   d. Cough (change in character or amount of sputum production)
   e. Diarrhea
4. The incidence of venous irritation is low.

REFERENCE
1. Appel, Gerald B., and Neu, Harold C.: The Nephrotoxicity of Antimicrobial Agents. New England Journal of Medicine, 296(13):722, March 31, 1977.

CEPHRADINE (Velosef)

ACTIONS/ INDICATIONS	DOSAGE	PREPARATION AND STORAGE	DRUG INCOMPATIBILITIES	MODES OF IV ADMINISTRATION			CONTRAINDICATIONS; WARNINGS; PRECAUTIONS; ADVERSE REACTIONS
				INJECTION	INTERMITTENT INFUSION	CONTINUOUS INFUSION	
Antibiotic, of the cephalosporin type. Indicated in the treatment of the following infections when caused by susceptible strains of the designated organisms: Respiratory tract— Group A beta hemolytic streptococci, Strep.	ADULTS: 500-1000 mg every 6 hrs; do not exceed 8 gm/ day. ADULTS WITH IMPAIRED RENAL FUNCTION: Each patient must be considered individually. Loading dose —750 mg.	To reconstitute from powder add the following amounts of sterile water for infection, D5W or NS: Vial Size / Volume 250 mg 5 ml 500 mg 5 ml 1 gm 10 ml 2 gm 20 ml 2 gm piggyback 40 ml	Do not mix with any other antibiotics in IV bottle, do not mix in any manner with: Epinephrine Lidocaine Aminoglycoside antibiotics Calcium preparations	YES Directly into the vein or into the tubing of a running IV when the intravenous solution is compatible with the drug. Inject over 3-5 min.	YES Add reconstituted solution to enough D5W or NS to make a 30 mg/ml concentration. Infuse over 30-60 min. If infused at the same time as other infusions, these other fluids must be com-	YES Add reconstituted solution to any of the following IV solutions in an amount determined by fluid and electrolyte needs of the patient: D5W D10W NS Sodium Lactate 1/6 molar D5/NS	CONTRAINDICATIONS Hypersensitivity to any cephalosporin. WARNINGS 1. Administer with caution to patients with an allergy to penicillin; there may be partial cross-allergenicity. 2. Safety for use in pregnancy has not been established. 3. This drug is secreted in breast milk during lactation. 4. Use with caution in premature infants or infants under one year of age. PRECAUTIONS 1. Prolonged use may promote the overgrowth of nonsusceptible organ-

CEPHRADINE (Velosef) (Continued)

ACTIONS/INDICATIONS	DOSAGE	PREPARATION AND STORAGE	DRUG INCOMPATIBILITIES	MODES OF IV ADMINISTRATION — INJECTION	MODES OF IV ADMINISTRATION — INTERMITTENT INFUSION	MODES OF IV ADMINISTRATION — CONTINUOUS INFUSION	CONTRAINDICATIONS; WARNINGS; PRECAUTIONS; ADVERSE REACTIONS
pneumoniae. Otis media— Group A beta hemolytic streptococci, Strep. pneumoniae, H. influenzae, Staphylococci. Skin and soft tissue—staphylococci and group A B-H. Strep. Urinary tract— E. coli, Proteus mirabilis, Klebsiella species. Bone infections— Staph. aureus (penicillin-susceptible and resistant). Septicemia— Strep. pneumoniae, Staph. aureus, P. mirabilis, and E. coli. Sensitivity testing should be carried out prior to therapy.	Maintenance dose—500 mg at the following intervals: Creatinine Clearance (ml/min.) — Time Interval >20 — 6–12 hrs 15–19 — 12–24 hrs 10–14 — 24–40 hrs 5–9 — 40–50 hrs <5 — 50–70 hrs On chronic hemodialysis— 250 mg at start, 250 mg at 12 hrs after start and then 250 mg 36–48 hrs after start. CHILDREN AND INFANTS: 50–100 mg/kg/day in equally divided doses every 6 hrs, regulated by age of the patient and severity of the infection. Maximum dose should not exceed 8 gm/day.	Vial Size — Volume (Continued) 4 gm piggyback — 80 ml Use within 2 hours or if stored in refrigerator discard after 48 hours. Protect solutions from direct sunlight.			patible with cephradine, or be stopped during administration of this drug. Piggyback preparations may be infused as prepared under Preparation and Storage column.	D5/.45% sodium chloride 10% invert sugar Normosol-R Ionosol-B Use *no* other IV solutions. Infuse at a rate to assist in meeting fluid and electrolyte needs. Prepare fresh solution every 10 hrs.	isms. 2. Monitor renal function and adjust dosage accordingly. Renal failure is rarely caused by this drug. 3. False-positive urine glucose reactions may occur if Clinitest tablets, Benedict's solution or Fehling's solution is used. 4. Positive direct Coombs test has been reported to occur during therapy with this drug. 5. This drug will accumulate in the serum and tissues of patients with renal impairment. ADVERSE REACTIONS 1. Gastrointestinal: glossitis (inflammation of the tongue), nausea, vomiting, diarrhea, abdominal pain, tenesmus (spasmotic contraction of anal or bladder sphincter, accompanied by pain and desire to empty bowel or bladder) 2. Hypersensitivity: maculopapular rash, urticaria, erythema, joint pains, drug fever, anaphylaxis 3. Blood dyscrasias: mild transient eosinophilia, leukopenia, and neutropenia 4. Liver: transient elevations in SGOT or SGPT, total bilirubin, alkaline phosphatase and LDH. These values return to normal after discontinuation of therapy. 5. Renal: mild elevations in BUN, more frequently in patients over 50 years or under 3 years of age. 6. Headache 7. Dizziness 8. Paresthesia 9. Candidal overgrowth 10. Thrombophlebitis at injection site

Safety for use in premature infants and infants under 1 year has not been established.

NURSING IMPLICATIONS
1. Take anaphylaxis precautions; see page 118.
2. Use Clinistix or Tes-Tape for urine glucose determinations.
3. Monitor for signs and symptoms of nonsusceptible organism overgrowth infection
   a. Fever (take rectal temperature at least every 4–6 hours)
   b. Increasing malaise
   c. Localized signs and symptoms of newly developing infection: redness, soreness, pain, swelling, drainage (change in volume or character of pre-exisiting drainage)
   d. Cough (change in character or amount of sputum production)
   e. Diarrhea
4. Monitor for the onset of inflammation of the tongue (glossitis). The patient will complain of soreness, and the tongue will be reddened and inflamed. Report this to the physician. Provide a soft diet, analgesics and mouthwashes as ordered. Maintain hydration.
5. Administer antiemetics and/or constipating agents as ordered if gastrointestinal disturbances occur. Maintain hydration and nutritional intake. Record urine output and emesis to assist the physician in ordering fluids if necessary.
6. Examine for thrombophlebitis at the infusion site. Discontinue the IV if this occurs. Apply warm compresses, elevate the extremity, and avoid trauma to the area. Venipunctures should not be performed on that extremity until the inflammation resolves.

CHLORAMPHENICOL SODIUM SUCCINATE (Chloromycetin)

ACTIONS/ INDICATIONS	DOSAGE	PREPARATION AND STORAGE	DRUG INCOMPAT- IBILITIES	MODES OF IV ADMINISTRATION			CONTRAINDICATIONS; WARNINGS; PRECAUTIONS; ADVERSE REACTIONS
				INJECTION	INTERMITTENT INFUSION	CONTINUOUS INFUSION	
Antibiotic, intended for use in serious infections only when less toxic drugs are ineffective or contraindicated. Examples: • Acute infections caused by *Salmonella typhi* (not carrier state) • Serious infections caused by susceptible strains of: a. Salmonella species b. *H. influenzae* (meningeal)	ADULTS: 50 mg/kg/24 hrs in divided doses at 6-hr intervals. Some resistant infections may require up to 100 mg/ kg/24 hrs. Dosage should be reduced in patients with impaired hepatic or renal function. CHILDREN: 50 mg/kg/24 hrs in divided doses at 6-hr intervals. When adequate cerebrospinal fluid concentra-	To reconstitute from powder, add 10 ml of sterile water for injection or D5W. The resulting solution will be 100 mg/ml. Do not use cloudy solutions. Store at room temperature; discard after 30 days.	Do not mix in IV bottle with: Methicillin Gentamicin Nitrofurantoin. Do not mix in any manner with: Chlorpromazine Hydroxyzine Novobiocin Oxytetracycline Polymyxin-B Prochlorperazine Promethazine Sulfadiazine Tetracycline Vancomycin Carbenicillin Erythromycin	YES Use a 10% solution (100 mg/ml). See Preparation column. Inject over at least 1 min. May be injected into the tubing of a running IV.	YES Add dose to 50–100 ml of D5W. Infuse over 15–30 min.	YES Add 6-, 12-, or 24-hr dose to 1000 ml of any IV fluid except protein hydrolysate, depending on the patient's fluid needs. Solution is stable for 24 hrs.	CONTRAINDICATIONS 1. History of hypersensitivity or toxic reaction to chloramphenicol 2. Use as a prophylactic agent to prevent bacterial infections WARNINGS 1. Serious and potentially fatal blood dyscrasias, such as aplastic anemia, hypoplastic anemia, thrombocytopenia and granulocytopenia, have occurred following administration of this drug. Aplastic anemia attributed to this drug has terminated in leukemia. These blood dyscrasias have occurred following short- and long-term therapy. 2. Dose-related bone marrow depression, which is reversible, has also been reported. This type of blood dyscrasia is characterized by vacuolization (development of clear air or fluid-filled spaces in a cell) of the erythroid cells, by reduction of reticulocytes, and leukopenia (decreased white blood cells). These changes disappear with discontin-

CHLORAMPHENICOL SODIUM SUCCINATE (Chloromycetin) (Continued)

ACTIONS/INDICATIONS	DOSAGE	PREPARATION AND STORAGE	DRUG INCOMPATIBILITIES	MODES OF IV ADMINISTRATION			CONTRAINDICATIONS; WARNINGS; PRECAUTIONS; ADVERSE REACTIONS
				INJECTION	INTERMITTENT INFUSION	CONTINUOUS INFUSION	
c. Rickettsia d. Lymphogranuloma-psittacosis group e. Gramnegative organisms causing bacteremia and meningitis f. Other susceptible organisms which have been demonstrated to be resistant to all other appropriate drugs • Cystic fibrosis regimens This drug can be used to initiate antibiotic therapy if one of the above conditions is suspected. It should be discontinued if a less toxic agent will be effective as indicated by sensitivity tests.	tions are needed: 100 mg/kg/24 hrs. Dosage should be reduced as soon as possible. Dosage should be reduced in the presence of impaired hepatic or renal function. NEONATES AND PREMATURE INFANTS (LESS THAN 2 WEEKS OF AGE): 10–25 mg/kg/24 hrs in 3–4 equally divided doses or 6 mg/kg/dose every 6 hrs. Dosage should be reduced in the presence of impaired hepatic or renal function. FULL-TERM INFANTS OLDER THAN 2 WEEKS: 50 mg/kg/24 hrs in 3–4 equally divided doses or 12 mg/kg/dose every 6 hrs.						uation of the drug. 3. This drug should not be used in the treatment of trivial infections such as colds, influenza, sore throats, etc. PRECAUTIONS 1. Blood cell production must be monitored at least every 2 days throughout therapy. 2. Such studies cannot be relied upon to detect irreversible bone marrow depression that occurs prior to development of aplastic anemia. 3. Discontinue this drug with the appearance of reticulocytopenia, leukopenia, thrombocytopenia, or anemia. 4. Avoid repeated courses of this drug. Treatment should not be continued longer than required to produce a cure and to prevent relapse. 5. Avoid concurrent use of other bone marrow depressing agents. 6. Excessive blood levels of this drug will develop in patients with impaired liver or kidney function, including the immature function of these organs in premature or young infants. 7. Safety for use in pregnancy has not been established. This drug crosses the placental barrier and can produce the gray-baby syndrome in the infant: (see Adverse Reaction No. 5). 8. Use with extreme caution in premature and full-term infants; high serum drug levels can produce toxic effects. See Adverse Reaction No. 5 on the gray-baby syndrome. 9. Overgrowth of nonsusceptible organisms may occur. 10. Each gram of this drug contains approximately 2.25 mEq of sodium. ADVERSE REACTIONS 1. Blood dycrasias: a. Idiosyncratic irreversible and potentially fatal bone marrow depression producing aplastic

anemia, hypoplastic anemia, thrombocytopenia, and granulocytopenia

b. Reversible, dose-related bone marrow depression

c. Paroxysmal, nocturnal hemoglobinuria

2. Gastrointestinal:
   a. Nausea, vomiting, diarrhea
   b. Glossitis (inflammation of the tongue) and stomatitis (inflammation of oral mucous membranes)
   c. Enterocolitis (rare)

3. Neurotoxic:
   a. Headache
   b. Mild depression, mental confusion
   c. Optic and peripheral neuritis (usually in long-term therapy; if this occurs, the drug should be discontinued)

4. Rash, angioedema, urticaria, anaphylaxis, herxheimer reaction in typhoid patients

5. Gray-baby syndrome: Seen in premature and full-term newborns receiving this drug or when the mother has received it during labor. This syndrome occurs most frequently when the drug has been used during the first 48 hours after delivery. Symptoms appear after 3–4 days of continued therapy with high doses in the following order:
   a. Abdominal distention with or without vomiting
   b. Progressive, pallid cyanosis
   c. Poor feeding, refusal to suck
   d. Circulatory collapse
   e. Irregular respirations
   f. Flaccidity.
   Infants become gravely ill within 24 hours. Death can occur within the next 12 hours unless the drug is discontinued. The process can frequently be reversed with discontinuation of therapy.

6. Overgrowth infection secondary to organisms not susceptible to chloramphenicol.

NURSING IMPLICATIONS
1. Take anaphylactic precautions; see page 118.
2. Assist the physician in monitoring for the onset of blood dyscrasias:
   a. Complete blood counts should be done every 2 days during therapy (see Precautions No. 1–3).
   b. Be aware of blood count results prior to each dose of the drug.
   c. Monitor for bleeding if the platelet count falls below 100,000/cu mm.
   d. If the white blood cell count falls below 2000, place the patient in protective (reversed) isolation and monitor for signs and symptoms of infection. Avoid traumatic procedures and maintain bodily (especially perineal) cleanliness.
   e. Monitor for nocturnal hematuria.
3. Care of the infant on chloramphenicol:
   a. Monitor for signs of the gray-baby syndrome (see adverse reaction No.

231

CHLORAMPHENICOL SODIUM SUCCINATE (Chloromycetin) (Continued)

NURSING IMPLICATIONS (No. 3 continued)

5). Notify the physician immediately on suspision of the onset of this syndrome. Hold the next dose of the drug until a medical decision is made.

   b. Administer supportive care as needed, e.g., prevention of aspiration, provision respiratory support.

4. Examine the patient daily for the onset of oral lesions (glossitis or stomatitis). Report the occurrence to the physician. Order a soft, bland diet and nonirritating fluids. Administer mouthwashes as ordered (usually half saline, half hydrogen peroxide).

5. Monitor for depression and/or mental confusion. Reassure the patient as to the origin of these problems. Take precautions to prevent patient injury when indicated (e.g., side rails, soft restraints).

6. Observe for signs and symptoms of optic neuritis:

   a. loss of visual acuity
   b. central scotoma (loss of an area of the center of the visual field)
   c. pain on eye movement
   d. tenderness around the eye[1]

   Notify the physician at the onset of these findings; the drug should be discontinued.

7. Observe for signs and symptoms of peripheral neuritis:

   a. Localized neurologic pain
   b. Pain on motion of hands, fingers, feet, toes

   c. Tingling, numbness
   d. Weakness of extremities

   Notify the physician at the onset of these findings; the drug should be discontinued. Reassure the patient as to the origin of the symptoms and their transient nature.

8. If gastrointestinal disturbances occur, notify the physician. If such symptoms are pronounced, the drug will probably be discontinued. Antiemetics, antacids, and a constipating agent can be ordered. Monitor intake and output to assist the physician in planning for parenteral fluid replacement. Maintain hydration orally when possible.

9. Monitor for signs and symptoms of overgrowth infections:

   a. Fever (take rectal temperature at least every 4–6 hours in all patients)
   b. Increasing malaise
   c. Newly appearing localized signs and symptoms: redness, soreness, pain, swelling, drainage (increased volume or change in character of pre-existing drainage)
   d. Monilial rash in perineal area (reddened areas with itching)
   e. Cough (change in pre-existing cough or sputum production)
   f. Diarrhea

REFERENCE
1. Newell, Frank W., and Ernest J. Terry: *Ophthalmology—Principles and Concepts*, (3rd ed.), St. Louis, C. V. Mosby Company, 1974, p. 307.

CHLORDIAZEPOXIDE HYDROCHLORIDE (Librium)

ACTIONS/ INDICATIONS	DOSAGE	PREPARATION AND STORAGE	DRUG INCOMPAT- IBILITIES	MODES OF IV ADMINISTRATION			CONTRAINDICATIONS; WARNINGS; PRECAUTIONS; ADVERSE REACTIONS
				INJECTION	INTERMITTENT INFUSION	CONTINUOUS INFUSION	
Central nervous system depressant; acts on the limbic system involved in emotional reactions. Also depresses the brain stem reticular formation, the cerebral cortex, and the reflex arcs of the spinal cord. Used to control agitation, tremor,	ADULTS *Alcoholism* —50–100 mg initially repeated in 2–4 hrs as necessary. *Acute anxiety* —50–100 mg initially, followed by 24–50 mg, 3–4 times daily. Do not exceed 300 mg in 24 hrs. Lower doses are recommended for el-	Prepared from powder by adding 5 ml NS or sterile water for injection. DO NOT USE DILUENT PROVIDED FOR IM SOLUTION PREPARATION. Inject diluent slowly into the vial. Agitate gently until powder is completely dissolved. Do not use the solution if it is hazy or opalescent. Mix again using oth-	Do not mix with any other medication.	YES Slowly, over 1 min. Do not mix with fluids.	NO This drug is unstable in solution and ineffective.	NO This drug is unstable in solution and ineffective.	CONTRAINDICATIONS Known hypersensitivity WARNINGS 1. Withdrawal symptoms have been reported following discontinuation of this drug. Symptoms may include convulsions. 2. Use during pregnancy, lactation, or in women of childbearing age requires that the potential benefit of the drug be weighed against the possible hazards to the mother and child. 3. The signs and symptoms of overdosage include stupor, confusion, coma, decreased reflexes. PRECAUTIONS 1. Any patient receiving intravenous chlordiazepoxide should be kept un-

der close observation and at bedrest during administration and for 3 hours after the dose.

2. Use of other psychotropic agents during therapy with this drug is not recommended.

3. *Caution should be exercised* when administering to patients with hepatic or renal insufficiency; toxic or adverse effects may be more pronounced.

4. Paradoxical reactions such as increased agitation, excitement, and acute rage have occurred in psychiatric patients, hyperactive children, and the elderly.

5. Variable effects on blood coagulation have been reported in patients concomitantly receiving oral anticoagulants.

6. Should not be given to patients in shock or comatose states.

ADVERSE REACTIONS
1. Mental confusion, syncope, hypotension, tachycardia, skin eruptions, nausea, extrapyramidal symptoms, and blurred vision have been observed. These situations are usually controlled by a reduction in dosage.

2. Blood dycrasias, including agranulocytosis, and hepatic dysfunction have been reported.

er recommended diluent. Use solution *immediately*; discard unused portion. Store dry form in refrigerator.

CHILDREN: 5 mg, 2–4 times a day. Lowest dose should be used initially, increasing as necessary. *Use of this drug in children less than 12 years of age is not recommended.*

derly or debilitated patients.

impending or active delirium tremens resulting from alcohol withdrawal, and for the general relief of anxiety.

patients, hyperactive children, or in the elderly.

3. Monitor for signs of overdose: extreme lethargy, stupor, confusion, decreasing reflexes, eventually, coma. If any one of these signs appears, notify the physician and initiate frequent monitoring of vital signs. Be prepared to manage vomiting to prevent aspiration; keep suction at the bedside. Maintain an open airway and adequate ventilation.

NURSING IMPLICATIONS
1. Keep the patient at rest during the administration of this drug and for 2 hours after the last dose, and then ambulate with assistance. While the patient is on bedrest take precautions to prevent injury, e.g. side rails and restraints as indicated.
2. Be prepared to manage agitation, excitement, or acute rage in psychiatric

● CHLOROTHIAZIDE SODIUM (Diuril)

ACTIONS/ INDICATIONS	DOSAGE	PREPARATION AND STORAGE	DRUG INCOMPAT- IBILITIES	MODES OF IV ADMINISTRATION			CONTRAINDICATIONS; WARNINGS; PRECAUTIONS; ADVERSE REACTIONS
				INJECTION	INTERMITTENT INFUSION	CONTINUOUS INFUSION	
Thiazide diuretic and antihypertensive. Used in the treatment of edema in congestive heart	ADULTS: *For diuresis*— 0.5–1.0 gm once or twice a day. This drug is sometimes more ef-	To reconstitute from powder, add 18 ml (no less) to the 0.5-gm vial. Concentration of this solution	Do not mix in any manner with: Anileridine phosphate Codeine phosphate	YES Slowly, at a rate of 0.1 gm in 1 min.	YES Use D5W or NS as infusion fluid, 50–100 ml.	YES Pharmacologic effectiveness may be compromised by addition to	CONTRAINDICATIONS 1. Anuria 2. Hypersensitivity to this or any sulfonamide-derived drug 3. In *healthy* pregnant women with or without edema

CHLOROTHIAZIDE SODIUM (Diuril) (Continued)

ACTIONS/INDICATIONS	DOSAGE	PREPARATION AND STORAGE	DRUG INCOMPATIBILITIES	MODES OF IV ADMINISTRATION			CONTRAINDICATIONS; WARNINGS; PRECAUTIONS; ADVERSE REACTIONS
				INJECTION	INTERMITTENT INFUSION	CONTINUOUS INFUSION	
failure, cirrhosis, steroid therapy, and renal dysfunction. Also as an adjunct to therapy of hypertension This drug increases the excretion of sodium and chloride. The natriuresis causes a secondary loss of water, potassium and bicarbonate. Onset of action occurs in 15 minutes after IV injection.	fective when given on alternate days *For hypertension*—0.5 gm once a day up to 2.0 gm daily in divided doses. It is recommended that the smallest dose required to achieve the desired effect be used. CHILDREN: Intravenous use in children and infants is not recommended by the manufacturer. When used, the dose is 20–22 mg/kg/24 hrs or 600 mg/M²/24 hrs in 2 divided doses. INFANTS: (not usually recommended) up to 6 months of age: 33 mg/kg/24 hrs.	will be 25 mg/ml. Unused portions may be stored at room temperature; discard after 24 hours.	Regular insulin Levarterenol bitartrate Levorphanol tartate Morphine Prochlorperazine Promazine hydrochloride Promethazine hydrochloride Tetracycline Triflupromazine Vancomycin Avoid concomitant administration with blood or its derivatives			large volumes of fluid. Can be added to all commonly used fluids, except: All Ionosol preparations; all Normosol-M and R solutions; Protein hydrolysate	WARNINGS 1. Use in infants and children is not generally recommended. 2. Use with caution in the presence of severe renal disease. This drug may increase the severity of azotemia. Adverse reactions may develop more easily in patients with renal insufficiency. 3. Use with caution in patients with hepatic failure where alterations in electrolyte balance may precipitate hepatic coma. 4. This drug may potentiate the effects of ganglionic or peripheral adrenergic blocking drugs on blood pressure, i.e., hypotension. 5. Activation or exacerbation of septemic lupus erythematosus has been reported. 6. This drug should not be used concomitantly with lithium because it reduces its renal clearance and increases the likelihood of lithium toxicity. 7. This drug crosses the placental barrier. Adverse reactions have occurred in neonates following administration to the mother (see Adverse Reactions). 8. Thiazides are secreted in breast milk. If therapy is essential, the mother should stop nursing. 9. It is not recommended that this drug be used to reduce mechanically induced edema during pregnancy. It can be used to treat the pathologic states listed under Indications. 10. Extravasation must be avoided. PRECAUTIONS 1. Electrolyte imbalance can occur with therapy; frequent serum electrolyte determinations should be carried out to monitor for hyponatremia (decreased serum sodium), hypochloremic alkalosis and hypokalemia (decreased serum potassium). 2. Hypokalemia is especially likely to develop in rapid diuresis, in the presence of cirrhosis or during the con-

comitant use of corticosteroids or ACTH. Digitalis toxicity is more likely to occur in the presence of low serum potassium. Potassium supplement must be used and guided by serum potassium levels.

3. Insulin requirements in diabetics may be increased, decreased or unchanged. Latent diabetes may become active.

4. If the patient's renal function deteriorates, this drug should be discontinued.

5. Thiazides can increase serum calcium levels; do not use in the presence of hypercalcemia.

6. Hyperuricemia may occur or frank gout may be precipitated in certain patients.

7. May increase the responsiveness to tubocurarine.

ADVERSE REACTIONS
1. Gastrointestinal—anorexia, nausea, vomiting, diarrhea, pancreatitis.
2. Central nervous system—dizziness, paresthesias, headache, xanthopsia
3. Hematologic—leukopenia, agranulocytosis, thrombocytopenia, aplastic anemia.
4. Cardiovascular—postural hypotension, hypokalemia.
5. Hepatic—intrahepatic cholestatic jaundice.

When any of these reactions occur, therapy should be reduced or discontinued, whichever is appropriate.

NURSING IMPLICATIONS
1. Monitor for drug effectiveness:
   a. Urinary output (and fluid intake) at least every 8 hours, depending on the patient's condition
   b. Body weight, daily
   c. When given in an antihypertension regimen, monitor blood pressure every 4–6 hours
   d. In conditions associated with peripheral edema, examine for edema in the legs and sacrum at least every 8 hours
   e. In cirrhosis, measure abdominal girth, daily
2. In patients with renal failure, monitor for deterioration in renal status:
   a. Urinary output (and fluid intake) every 4–8 hours—anticipate a decrease in output
   b. If appropriate, specific gravity every 8 hours
   c. Be aware of the patient's BUN and serum creatinine
3. Monitor for signs and symptoms of hypokalemia: weakness, lethargy, irritability, abdominal distention, muscle cramps.
4. Monitor for signs of hyponatremia: headache, nausea, abdominal cramps, confusion, stupor.
5. Observe for signs of dehydration: dry mucous membranes, extreme weight loss, oliguria, decreased skin turgor, weakness, fall in blood pressure.
6. Take all precautions to avoid extravasation, see page 96. If it occurs, discontinue the infusion or injection immediately. Apply warm compresses and avoid further trauma. Monitor for tissue damage.
7. Monitor for the onset of symptoms of acute gout, e.g., severe joint pain, usually in the feet and ankles. Notify the physician if they occur.

235

CHLORPHENIRAMINE MALEATE (Chlor-Trimeton)

ACTIONS/ INDICATIONS	DOSAGE	PREPARATION AND STORAGE	DRUG INCOMPATIBILITIES	MODES OF IV ADMINISTRATION			CONTRAINDICATIONS; WARNINGS; PRECAUTIONS; ADVERSE REACTIONS
				INJECTION	INTERMITTENT INFUSION	CONTINUOUS INFUSION	
Antihistamine used to prevent allergic reactions to blood or plasma; as an adjunct to the treatment of anaphylaxis; and to treat other allergic conditions when the oral form cannot be used.	ADULTS AND CHILDREN: 5–20 mg/ dose. Maximum adult daily dose is 40 mg.	Use *only* the 10 mg/ml solution for IV use (100 mg/ml solution is for intramuscular injection). Store vials in manufacturer's carton to protect from light.	Do not add to blood container for the prevention of a tranfusion reaction. Do not mix in syringe with: Calcium chloride Kanamycin Levarterenol (Levophed)	YES Aspirate 5–10 ml of the patient's blood into the syringe before injecting. Administer at a rate of 10 mg/ min. Do not inject into IV tubing, inject directly into the vein.	NO	NO	CONTRAINDICATIONS 1. Premature or newborn infants 2. In nursing mothers 3. In acute asthmatic attack or lower respiratory infection 4. Hypersensitivity 5. In patients receiving MAO inhibitors 6. See Adverse Reaction No. 1 WARNINGS 1. This drug has an atropinelike action; therefore, administer with caution in patients with: a. Narrow-angle glaucoma—there may be an exacerbation of the condition with further elevation in intraocular pressure. b. Potential or actual gastrointestinal mechanical obstruction (stenosing peptic ulcer, pyloroduodenal obstruction)—this drug can cause an increase in the severity of the obstruction. c. Prostatic hypertrophy or bladder neck obstruction—urinary retention may result. 2. Hypotension and/or dizziness may occur in the elderly or in debilitated patients. PRECAUTIONS 1. May cause further elevation in blood pressure in patients with hypertension. 2. This drug can decrease the anticoagulant activity of heparin. ADVERSE REACTIONS 1. Transient hypotension accompanied by sweating and pallor; usually subsides within an hour of administration of the drug. If this occurs, the patient should not receive the drug again. 2. Convulsions. 3. Transient dry mouth, dizziness, nausea, headache.

NURSING IMPLICATIONS
1. Monitor for signs and symptoms of increasing intraocular pressure in patients with narrow angle glaucoma (confirm diagnosis with physician): ocular pain (in and around the eye), blurring of vision, rainbows seen around lights, dilated pupils, nausea and vomiting. Notify the physician at onset of

a. Palpate bladder size every 4 hours
b. Measure urine output every 8 hours (also fluid intake)
c. Question patient as to the presence or absence of hesitancy, urgency, dribbling
4. Monitor blood pressure before and immediately after injection, and then

signs or symptoms.
2. Monitor for signs and symptoms of intestinal obstruction in vulnerable patients (see Warning No. 1.b.): vomiting, abdominal distention.[1] Administer supportive care and notify the physician.
3. Monitor for signs and symptoms of urinary retention in elderly males and patients with histories of prostatic hypertrophy or bladder neck obstruction:

every 10–15 minutes for 1 hour. Keep all patients supine for the first hour after injection and ambulate with caution thereafter.

REFERENCE
1. Beeson, Paul B., and McDermott, Walsh (editors): *Cecil-Loeb Textbook of Medicine* (14th ed.), Philadelphia: W. B. Saunders Company, 1975, p. 1211.

● CHLORPROMAZINE HYDROCHLORIDE (Thorazine)

ACTIONS/ INDICATIONS	DOSAGE	PREPARATION AND STORAGE	DRUG INCOMPATIBILITIES	MODES OF IV ADMINISTRATION			CONTRAINDICATIONS; WARNINGS; PRECAUTIONS; ADVERSE REACTIONS
				INJECTION	INTERMITTENT INFUSION	CONTINUOUS INFUSION	
Phenothiazine derivative with psychotropic, sedative and antiemetic activity. Major indications of IV use are: • Intractable hiccups • Nausea and vomiting during surgery • Seizures due to tetanus	ADULTS: Adjust dosage to individual needs and relief of symptoms. Dose should be given in 2-mg increments at 2-min intervals until symptoms are controlled. *Intractable hiccups*—25–50 mg if symptoms are unresponsive to oral administration. Do not exceed 50 mg. (See Continuous Infusion column.) *Tetanus*—25–50 mg, 3–4 times daily. Do not exceed 50 mg/dose. (See Injection and Intermittent Infusion columns.) *Nausea and vomiting during surgery*—	Dilute for injection or infusion in NS *only.* Protect vials from light. Slight yellowing does not alter potency. Discard if undiluted solution is dark yellow or brown.	Do not mix with any other medication in any manner.	YES For tetanus and nausea/ vomiting during surgery, in children and adults. Dilute in at least each 1 mg of drug in 1 ml of NS. Administration rate: *Adults:* 1 mg/min. *Children:* 0.5 mg/min.	YES For tetanus and nausea/ vomiting during surgery, in children and adults. Dilute in at least each 1 mg of drug in 1 ml of NS. Administration rate: *Adults:* 1 mg/ min. *Children:* 0.5 mg/min.	YES For intractable hiccups in adults add 25–50 mg to 500 to 1000 ml NS. Infuse slowly. An infusion pump may be advisable.	CONTRAINDICATIONS 1. Comatose states 2. Concomitant use of other CNS depressants 3. Bone marrow depression WARNINGS 1. Use with caution if there is a history of hypersensitivity to any phenothiazine. 2. Chlorpromazine may counteract the antihypertensive effect of guanethidine or related compounds. 3. Safety for use in pregnancy has not been established. 4. The extrapyramidal symptoms which can occur secondary to chlorpromazine may be confused with the central nervous system signs of an undiagnosed primary disease responsible for vomiting: e.g. Reye's syndrome or other encephalopathy. The use of this drug should be avoided in children and adolescents suspected of having Reye's syndrome. PRECAUTIONS 1. Administer with caution to patients with cardiovascular or hepatic disease (see Adverse Reactions). 2. Use with caution in the presence of chronic respiratory disease, especially in children, because this drug can suppress the cough reflex. With this, there is also an increased likelihood of aspiration of vomitus. 3. Chlorpromazine prolongs and intensifies the action of central nervous system depressants such as anesthet-

237

CHLORPROMAZINE HYDROCHLORIDE (Thorazine) (Continued)

ACTIONS/ INDICATIONS	DOSAGE	PREPARATION AND STORAGE	DRUG INCOMPAT- IBILITIES	MODES OF IV ADMINISTRATION			CONTRAINDICATIONS; WARNINGS; PRECAUTIONS; ADVERSE REACTIONS
				INJECTION	INTERMITTENT INFUSION	CONTINUOUS INFUSION	
	up to 25 mg per dose. CHILDREN: Administer in 1-mg increments at 2-min intervals until symptoms are controlled. (See Injection and Intermittent Infusion columns.) *Tetanus*— ¼ mg/lb every 6 to 8 hrs. Do not exceed 40 mg/day in children up to 50 lbs, or 75 mg/day in children 50 to 100 lbs. *Nausea and vomiting during surgery*— ⅛ mg/lb.						ics, barbiturates and narcotics. The dose of these agents should be decreased in the presence of chlorpromazine. 4. Because of its antiemetic effect, this drug may mask the nausea and vomiting associated with overdosage of toxic drugs, intestinal obstruction, or increased intracranial pressure. ADVERSE REACTIONS SEEN IN SHORT-TERM INTRAVENOUS USE 1. Neurologic: a. Sedation, drowsiness and deep sleep b. Blurred vision c. Extrapyramidal reactions such as motor restlessness resembling Parkinson's disease, drooling, tremors, muscle spasms, shuffling gait, dystonias (involuntary movements), difficulty swallowing d. Agitation and nervousness If these occur, dosage must be reduced or the drug discontinued. Symptoms will subside in 24–48 hours. 2. Rashes usually due to hypersensitivity 3. Hypotension (especially immediately after injection) may be postural type; see Nursing Implications for management 4. Palpitations, especially immediately after an injection 5. Alterations in liver function producing jaundice (cholestatic hepatitis); this is reversible with discontinuation of the drug 6. Anticholinergic reactions such as dryness of the mouth, tachycardia, blurred vision, increased salivation, nasal congestion 7. Exacerbation of seizure disorders 8. This drug is also known to cause (rarely) sudden cardiac arrest after rapid, direct intravenous injection

NURSING IMPLICATIONS
1. Monitor for neurologic disturbances following an injection, or during an infusion; see Adverse Reaction No. 1. Report any of these reactions to the physician immediately. If the patient experiences difficulty in swallowing, sion is significant, report the fact to the physician and keep the patient at rest. As postural effects decrease over time, begin to ambulate the patient if desirable; do so cautiously to prevent injury. Warn the patient not to stand up suddenly until the effects of the drug have disappeared. Ambulate

discontinue an infusion immediately, and remain with the patient until the severity of the reaction is determined; maintain an open airway. The patient may need parenteral hydration and nutrition until swallowing returns.

2. Examine for rashes; report them to the physician.
3. Keep the patient supine during injection or infusion.
4. Monitor blood pressure before, during and after injection or infusion. If hypotension occurs during an infusion, discontinue administration and continue to take the blood pressure until stabilization occurs. Hypotension can usually be avoided with slow injection. If a patient is to be ambulated after an injection, obtain lying and standing blood pressure. If postural hypoten-

the patient with caution if he is experiencing sedation or blurred vision. Initiate safety precautions, such as side rails, to prevent injury.

5. Monitor for jaundice, notify the physician.
6. The patient may experience anticholinergic side effects (see Adverse Reaction No. 6). Inform him of the origin of the symptom and its transient nature.
7. Initiate seizure precautions if not already in effect.
8. This drug can cause the urine to darken or turn orange for 24 hours after administration. Inform the patient of the harmlessness of this effect.

CHLORTETRACYCLINE HYDROCHLORIDE (Aureomycin)

ACTIONS/ INDICATIONS	DOSAGE	PREPARATION AND STORAGE	DRUG INCOMPAT- IBILITIES	MODES OF IV ADMINISTRATION			CONTRAINDICATIONS; WARNINGS; PRECAUTIONS; ADVERSE REACTIONS
				INJECTION	INTERMITTENT INFUSION	CONTINUOUS INFUSION	
Antibiotic, indicated in infections caused by the following micro-organisms: • Rickettsiae • *Mycoplasma pneumoniae* • Agents of psittacosis and ornithosis • Agents of lymphogranuloma venereum • Spirochetal agent of relapsing fever • Gram-negative organisms: *Haemophilus ducreyi, Pasteurella pestis, Pasteurella tularensis, Bartonella bacilliformis* • Bacteriodes • *Vibrio comma* • *Vibria fetus* • Brucella species	ADULTS: 500 mg at 12-hr intervals. Maximum of 500 mg every 6 hrs. CHILDREN: *Older infants and children*—10–15 mg/ kg/24 hrs in 2 equally divided doses. *Children over 40 Kg*—10–20 mg/kg/24 hrs in 2 equally divided doses. Generally not recommended in pediatrics except when another drug is not suitable. See Warning No. 5. Not recommended for neonates or premature infants.	To reconstitute from powder, add 50 ml sterile water for injection, NS, D5W, or D5/ NS. Shake vigorously. Solution contains 10 mg/ml. Use immediately; discard unused portions.	Do not mix with any solution or drug containing calcium, cephalothin, cephaloridine, cefazolin, ammonium chloride, dextran, fructose, polymyxin B, or promazine.	YES Dilute each 100 mg in at least 10 ml sterile water for injection, NS, or D5W. Inject over at least 5 min for each 100 mg.	YES Add to NS or D5W, 10 ml/ 100 mg of drug. Complete the infusion within 1 hr, but no more rapidly than 100 mg/5 min.	YES Add to NS or D5/NS D5W only, 10 ml/ 100 mg of drug. Infuse no more rapidly than 20 mg/ min.	CONTRAINDICATIONS Hypersensitivity to any tetracycline WARNINGS 1. In the presence of renal failure, particularly during pregnancy, intravenous doses exceeding 1 gm/day have been associated with deaths due to hepatic failure. 2. This drug should be avoided in patients with renal insufficiency. Accumulation of the drug in the presence of decreased excretion can cause further renal damage, a catabolic state with acidosis, increasing azotemia and death. If the patient requires a tetracycline, doxycycline may be used with safety.[1] 3. When therapeutic needs outweigh the dangers (during pregnancy, renal or hepatic dysfunction), hepatic and renal function tests should be carried out before, during and after therapy. Monitor serum phosphate, BUN, and chlortetracycline levels. 4. A photoallergic reaction may occur if the patient is exposed to natural or artificial sunlight. If this occurs, the drug should be discontinued. 5. This drug crosses the placental barrier and has been related to retardation of skeletal development. Tetracyclines are also secreted in breast milk and may cause permanent discoloration of the infant's teeth. Use of the drug during the last trimester of pregnancy, neonatal period and early childhood

239

CHLORTETRACYCLINE HYDROCHLORIDE (Aureomycin) (Continued)

ACTIONS/ INDICATIONS	DOSAGE	PREPARATION AND STORAGE	DRUG INCOMPAT- IBILITIES	MODES OF IV ADMINISTRATION			CONTRAINDICATIONS; WARNINGS: PRECAUTIONS; ADVERSE REACTIONS
				INJECTION	INTERMITTENT INFUSION	CONTINUOUS INFUSION	
This drug is also effective against certain gram-positive and other gram-negative organisms. Sensitivity tests are required.							can cause discoloration. 6. The use of this drug may cause increased intracranial pressure. PRECAUTIONS 1. There may be overgrowth of non-susceptible organisms leading to a superinfection. 2. Tetracyclines depress plasma prothrombin activity, thus decreasing dosage requirements in concomitant anticoagulation therapy. 3. In long-term therapy, hematopoietic, renal and hepatic studies should be performed. 4. The use of tetracyclines can decrease the activity of penicillin and should be avoided when penicillin is strongly indicated. ADVERSE REACTIONS SEEN IN INTRAVENOUS THERAPY 1. Gastrointestinal: nausea, vomiting, diarrhea, enterocolitis, glossitis 2. Inflammatory lesions, with monilial growth in the perineal area 3. Skin: rashes, both maculopapular and erythematous 4. Renal toxicity is usually dose-related; see Warning No. 1, 2, and 3 5. Hypersensitivity reactions include urticaria, angioneurotic edema, anaphylaxis, pericarditis, and exacerbation of lupus erythematosus 6. Bulging fontanels have been reported in infants receiving doses in the therapeutic range. This disappeared after the drug is discontinued 7. Hematologic changes: thrombocytopenia, hemolytic anemia, neutropenia, and eosinophilia

NURSING IMPLICATIONS
1. Take anaphylaxis precautions; see page 118.
2. If gastrointestinal disturbances occur, notify the physician. If disturbances such as nausea, vomiting and diarrhea are pronounced, the drug will probably be discontinued. Antiemetics, antacids, and constipating agents can be ordered to control symptoms. Monitor intake and output to assist the physician in planning for parenteral fluid replacement. Maintain hydration orally when possible.
3. If the patient will be taking the oral form of this drug as an outpatient, in-

    e. Cough (change in pre-existing cough or sputum production)
    f. Diarrhea
7. Report the onset of any rash to the physician. If a rash occurs, keep the patient's environment comfortably cool and the skin clean. Diphenhydramine (Benadryl) may be ordered to relieve itching.
8. Report the onset of jaundice to the physician.
9. Report the onset of bulging fontanels, and other signs of increasing intracranial pressure, to the physician.
10. Be aware of this drug's relationship with renal function. Tetracyclines are

struct him/her on the possibility of photosensitivity and the advisability of avoiding exposure to the sun (sun-block lotions may be of help if exposure cannot be avoided).

4. Women of childbearing age and potential, and mothers of children who may receive this drug, should be informed of Warnings No. 1 and 5 by the physician. Assist in the interpretation of these warnings to the patient.

5. Even though blood dyscrasias are infrequently caused by this agent, be aware of the patient's complete blood cell count during therapy. If the platelet count begins to fall, the drug will probably be discontinued. Bleeding secondary to a low platelet count usually begins only after the count falls below 100,000/cu mm.

6. Monitor for signs and symptoms of overgrowth infections:
   a. Fever (take rectal temperature at least every 4–6 hours in all patients)
   b. Increasing malaise
   c. Newly appearing localized signs and symptoms: redness, soreness, pain, swelling, drainage (increased volume or change in character of pre-existing drainage)
   d. Monilial rash in perineal area (reddened areas with itching)

usually not given to patients with renal impairment because:
   a. The drug accumulates in the body because of decreased excretion in renal function
   b. The presence of the drug may cause further deterioration in renal function
   c. It may cause a catabolic state with metabolic acidosis, increasing BUN, and possibly death due to uremia[2]

Know what the patient's pretreatment BUN and creatinine levels are. Monitor for change in these values with initiation of treatment. Monitor urine output in renal patients receiving this drug. Report increasing oliguria to the physician. Send urine for analysis at least every other day.

REFERENCES
1. Barza, Michael, and Schiefe, Richard T.: Antimicrobial Spectrum, Pharmacology and Therapeutic Use of Antibiotics. Part I: Tetracyclines, *American Journal of Hospital Pharmacy*, 34:51, January 1977.
2. Ibid.

CIMETIDINE HYDROCHLORIDE (Tagamet)

ACTIONS/ INDICATIONS	DOSAGE	PREPARATION AND STORAGE	DRUG INCOMPATIBILITIES	MODES OF IV ADMINISTRATION			CONTRAINDICATIONS; WARNINGS; PRECAUTIONS; ADVERSE REACTIONS
				INJECTION	INTERMITTENT INFUSION	CONTINUOUS INFUSION	
Histamine H_2 receptor antagonist, suppresses gastric acid secretion. Promotes healing and relieves pain of peptic ulcers. Used for short-term (less than 8 weeks) treatment of peptic ulcer, and hypersecretory conditions: systemic mastocytosis, multiple endocrine adenomas, and Zollinger-Ellison syndrome (tumor of the non-beta cells of the pancreas	ADULTS: 300 mg. every 6 hrs. If patient requires an increased dosage, increase the frequency of the 300-mg dose. Do not exceed 2400 mg/day. *In the presence of renal failure*—300 mg every 8–12 hrs. Administer at the end of dialysis. CHILDREN: Use for children under 16 years of age is not recommended (see Precaution no. 3).	Supplied in single-dose vials of 300 mg in 2 ml (150 mg/ml). Discard unused portions. When mixed with fluid, the drug is stable for 48 hours at room temperature.	No data available; do not mix with other drugs.	YES Dilute in 20 ml of any IV fluid and inject over 1–2 min.	YES Dilute dose in 100 ml of D5W, NS, or RL and infuse over 15–20 min.	YES Use an appropriate volume of D5W, NS, or RL and add an 8-, 12-, or 24-hour dose or infuse at a rate of 1–4 mg/kg/hr.	CONTRAINDICATIONS None currently known. PRECAUTIONS 1. This drug crosses the placental barrier and should not be used in pregnant women unless in the judgment of the physician, benefits outweigh risks. 2. This drug is excreted in human milk. Nursing should be discontinued while the patient is on therapy. 3. This drug is not recommended for children under 16 years of age unless potential benefits outweigh potential risks. In limited experience, doses of 20–40 mg/kg/day have been used. 4. Antacids should be given concomitantly. 5. This drug can interact with warfarin-type anticoagulants to further prolong prothrombin time. ADVERSE REACTIONS 1. Mild, transient diarrhea 2. Muscular pain (transient) 3. Dizziness (usually transient) 4. Rash 5. Mild gynecomastia (not associated

ACTIONS/ INDICATIONS	DOSAGE	PREPARATION AND STORAGE	DRUG INCOMPATIBILITIES	MODES OF IV ADMINISTRATION			CONTRAINDICATIONS; WARNINGS; PRECAUTIONS; ADVERSE REACTIONS
				INJECTION	INTERMITTENT INFUSION	CONTINUOUS INFUSION	
which stimulates hypersecretion of gastric acid).							with alterations in endocrine function) 6. Neutropenia 7. Slight increase in plasma creatinine (disappears when drug is discontinued) 8. Elevation in SGOT (transient) 9. Confusion, mostly seen in the elderly, seriously ill, patients with renal insufficiency (this may be related to overdosage); this is usually transient.

NURSING IMPLICATIONS
1. Reassure the patient as to the transient nature of diarrhea, muscular pain, dizziness, and gynecomastia, if they occur.
2. Take precautions to prevent patient injury if dizziness or confusion are present.
3. Emotional tension, particularly repressed anger, frustration, and aggression has been cited as predisposing to peptic ulcers. Increased emotional stress is known to aggravate pre-existing peptic ulcer.[1] When possible, assist the patient in identifying factors which produce emotional tension in his/her life. Recognition of the existence of tension or stress may lead the patient to constructive management of the problem, which will subsequently assist in healing and preventing recurrence of a peptic ulcer. Assist in referrals to appropriate supportive agencies as needed.

REFERENCE
1. Smith, Dorothy W., and Germain, Carol P. Hanley: Care of the Adult Patient (4th ed.), Philadelphia, J. B. Lippincott Company, 1977, p. 737.

ACTIONS/ INDICATIONS	DOSAGE	PREPARATION AND STORAGE	DRUG INCOMPATIBILITIES	MODES OF IV ADMINISTRATION			CONTRAINDICATIONS; WARNINGS; PRECAUTIONS; ADVERSE REACTIONS
				INJECTION	INTERMITTENT INFUSION	CONTINUOUS INFUSION	
Antibiotic, indicated in the treatment of serious infections caused by susceptible anaerobic bacteria, susceptible strains of streptococci, pneumococci and staphylococci. Used for penicillin-allergic patients.	ADULTS: *Serious infections*—600–1200 mg/day in divided doses. *More severe infections*—1200–2700 mg/day in divided doses. *Life-threatening infections*—4.8 gm/day. The first dose may be given	Add to any IV fluid. Store unopened vials at room temperature. Discard unused portions.	May be mixed in-line with most other medications and vitamins except: Ampicillin Phenytoin Barbiturates Aminophylline Calcium gluconate Magnesium sulfate	NO Must be diluted; cardiac arrest has been reported associated with this mode.	YES Dilute 300 mg in at *least* 50 ml of any fluid. Infuse over 10 min. Dilute 600 mg in 100 ml, infuse over 20 min. Add 1.2 gm to 200 ml and give over 45 min. Administration of more than 1.2 gm in a single 1-hr in-	YES Do not exceed a rate greater than 1200 mg/ hr. Discard unused portion after 24 hrs.	CONTRAINDICATIONS Hypersensitivity to clindamycin or lincomycin. WARNINGS 1. May cause a possibly fatal colitis. Reserve this drug for cases where less toxic agents are inappropriate. Discontinue use if diarrhea occurs. Antiperistaltic agents such as opiates or diphenoxylate (Lomotil) may prolong or worsen the condition. Onset varies during therapy to several weeks after. Simple cases may respond to discontinuation of the drug. Severe cases may respond to corticosteroids (systemic and/or enemas). 2. Do not use for nonbacterial infections. 3. Safe use in pregnancy has not been

fusion is not recommended.

as a single rapid infusion, followed by a continuous infusion.

CHILDREN OVER ONE MONTH OF AGE:
Serious infections— 15–25 mg/kg/day in 3–4 equal doses.

More severe infections— 25–40 mg/kg/day in 3–4 doses. (Also square meters of body surface may be used: 350 mg/M²/day for serious infections, 450 mg/M²/day for more severe.)

In severe infections, it is advised that the child be given no less than 300 mg/day regardless of body weight.

Not usually recommended for use in newborn infants.

established.
4. Administer with caution to newborns and infants less than 1 month of age. Monitor renal and hepatic function. Observe for the onset of colitis; discontinue if this occurs.
5. This drug is secreted in breast milk. The mother should be advised to stop nursing.
6. Clindamycin does not diffuse adequately enough into the cerebrospinal fluid to be used in the treatment of meningitis.
7. Do not administer concurrently with erythromycin.

PRECAUTIONS
1. Use with caution in patients with active or past history of gastrointestinal disease.
2. Use with caution in patients with numerous allergies, asthma, hayfever, etc.
3. Monitor renal and hepatic function; reduced dosage may be indicated. Hemo- and peritoneal dialysis do not remove the drug from the blood. Monitor serum drug levels if possible.
4. Monitor for overgrowth infections due to nonsusceptible organisms, especially yeasts.
5. This drug has neuromuscular blocking properties that may potentiate neuromuscular blocking agents such as decamethonium, succinylchloine, d-tubocurarine.
6. Monitor carefully for onset of diarrhea, especially the elderly or seriously ill.

ADVERSE REACTIONS
1. Gastrointestinal: nausea, vomiting, diarrhea, abdominal pain, colitis (see Warning No. 1)
2. Hypersensitivity: maculopapular rash and urticaria have been reported; anaphylaxis; rarely, erythema multiforme
3. Hepatic: jaundice and alteration of liver function tests; manufacturer gives no advice as to discontinuation of the drug in this event
4. Hematopoietic: leukopenia and eosinophilia have been observed, as have agranulocytosis and thrombocytopenia
5. Thrombophlebitis can occur after prolonged infusion
6. Polyarthritis (rare)

CLINDAMYCIN PHOSPHATE (Cleocin) (Continued)

NURSING IMPLICATIONS

1. Monitor for the onset of colitis, from the beginning of therapy through 1 month after termination, i.e., abdominal pain, nausea, vomiting and diarrhea. Constipating drugs are not to be given. Notify physician at the first suspicion of this complication. Administer corticosteroids as ordered. Maintain hydration orally when possible. Monitor intake and output to assist the physician in planning parenteral fluid replacement. Observe for symptoms of hypokalemia (secondary to diarrhea), e.g., weakness and muscle cramps. Potassium replacement may be necessary (parenterally).

2. Take anaphylaxis precautions; see page 118.

3. Patients receiving this drug and a neuromuscular blocking agent (see Precaution No. 5) may require respiratory support longer than usual following administration of the neuromuscular blocking agent (see Nursing Implications under individual drugs).

4. Monitor for signs and symptoms of nonsusceptible organism overgrowth infection:
   a. Fever (take rectal temperatures at least every 4–6 hours)
   b. Increasing malaise
   c. Localized signs and symptoms of a newly developing infection: redness, soreness, pain, swelling, drainage (increased volume or change in char-

   acter of pre-existing drainage)
   d. Cough (change in sputum production)
   e. Diarrhea

5. Notify the physician at the onset of jaundice.

6. Complete blood counts should be performed during therapy. If the platelet count begins to fall, the drug will probably be discontinued. Bleeding secondary to a low platelet count usually begins if the count falls below 100,000/cu mm. If this occurs, monitor for bleeding and avoid traumatic procedures.
   If the white blood cell count decreases, the drug may be discontinued. Infections secondary to a low white count usually occur only if the count reaches 2000/cu mm or less. If this occurs (it rarely does), place the patient in protective (reverse) isolation, monitor for infection, avoid traumatic procedures and maintain bodily (especially perineal) cleanliness.

7. Monitor for signs and symptoms of thrombophlebitis at the infusion site, e.g., redness, swelling and pain along the vein tract. If these appear, discontinue the infusion and use another vein. Apply warm compresses and elevate the extremity until symptoms subside. Do not use this extremity for venipunctures until the phlebitis resolves.

COLCHICINE

ACTIONS/ INDICATIONS	DOSAGE	PREPARATION AND STORAGE	DRUG INCOMPAT- IBILITIES	MODES OF IV ADMINISTRATION			CONTRAINDICATIONS; WARNINGS; PRECAUTIONS; ADVERSE REACTIONS
				INJECTION	INTERMITTENT INFUSION	CONTINUOUS INFUSION	
The exact action of this agent in the presence of gout is unknown. It is theorized that it decreases lactic acid production by the leukocytes and thereby decreases urate crystal deposition and inflammatory response.

Intravenous form is used in the treatment of acute gouty arthritis, when a rapid re- | ADULTS 2 mg (4ml), followed by 0.5 mg (1ml) every 6 hrs. until pain has subsided. Do not exceed 4 mg in 24 hrs. | Discard unused portions of vials. | Do not mix in syringe with any other medication. | YES

Dilute in 10– 20 ml NS; inject over 1–2 min. | NO | NO | PRECAUTIONS
1. Use with caution in elderly or debilitated patients; they are more prone to develop adverse effects.
2. Use with caution in the presence of renal, gastrointestinal or heart disease.
3. Reduce dosage if weakness, anorexia, nausea, vomiting or diarrhea occurs; these are symptoms of toxicity (see Management of Acute Overdosage).

ADVERSE REACTIONS
1. Gastrointestinal disturbances are less likely to occur in intravenous administration, but may if recommended dosage is exceeded: nausea, vomiting, diarrhea.
2. Chronic administration may depress bone marrow function and cause agranulocytosis, thrombocytopenia and aplastic anemia.
3. Peripheral neuritis and hair loss have been reported. |

sponse is desired or when the oral form cannot be taken.

ACUTE OVERDOSAGE
1. Deaths have been reported with as small a dose as 8 mg, although higher doses have been taken without fatal results.
2. First symptoms: nausea, vomiting, abdominal pain, diarrhea. Diarrhea may be severe and bloody, secondary to hemorrhagic enteritis. Burning in the throat, stomach and skin may also occur.
3. Extensive vascular damage may ensue, resulting in shock.
4. Renal damage may be evidenced by hematuria and oliguria.
5. There may be marked muscular weakness, with ascending paralysis of the central nervous system. The patient usually remains conscious; however, delirium and seizures may occur.
6. Death may result from respiratory paralysis.
7. Management:
   a. Discontinue the drug at the first sign of toxicity.
   b. Monitor patient carefully for the next 24 hours for progressing symptoms as described above.
   c. Vasopressors and fluids can combat shock.
   d. Atropine and morphine can relieve abdominal pain and diarrhea.
   e. Antiemetics can be used to relieve vomiting.
   f. Provide respiratory support as indicated.

NURSING IMPLICATIONS
1. Monitor closely for signs of acute overdosage; see above.

2. Patients with acute overdosage may require intensive care.

COLISTIMETHATE SODIUM (Coly-Mycin M)

ACTIONS/ INDICATIONS	DOSAGE	PREPARATION AND STORAGE	DRUG INCOMPATIBILITIES	MODES OF IV ADMINISTRATION			CONTRAINDICATIONS; WARNINGS; PRECAUTIONS; ADVERSE REACTIONS
				INJECTION	INTERMITTENT INFUSION	CONTINUOUS INFUSION	
Antibiotic. Has bactericidal activity against sensitive strains of the following gram-negative	ADULTS AND CHILDREN WITH NORMAL RENAL FUNCTION: 2.5–5.0 mg/ kg/24 hrs or,	To prepare 20 mg vial, add 2.2 ml sterile water for injection. Add 2.0 ml to 150-mg vial. Swirl gent-	Do not mix in any manner with: Cephalothin Cephaloridine	YES Further dilute reconstituted solution with 20 ml	YES Add ½ of total daily dose to 50– 100 ml D5W or NS and	YES Add remaining ½ daily dose to 250–1000 ml of fluid	CONTRAINDICATIONS Hypersensitivity to colistimethate sodium. WARNINGS 1. Do not exceed a dosage of 5 mg/kg/ day in the presence of normal renal

245

COLISTIMETHATE SODIUM (Coly-Mycin M) (Continued)

ACTIONS/ INDICATIONS	DOSAGE	PREPARATION AND STORAGE	DRUG INCOMPAT- IBILITIES	MODES OF IV ADMINISTRATION			CONTRAINDICATIONS; WARNINGS; PRECAUTIONS; ADVERSE REACTIONS
				INJECTION	INTERMITTENT INFUSION	CONTINUOUS INFUSION	
bacilli: *Enterobacter aerogenes, E. coli, Klebsiella pneumoniae, Pseudomonas aeruginosa* (most common enteric organisms).	75–150 mg/ M²/24 hrs in 2–4 divided doses. Do not exceed 5 mg/kg/24 hrs in the presence of normal renal function. ADULTS WITH IMPAIRED RENAL FUNCTION: See table below.	ly to mix and avoid frothing. Because of the large difference in the amount of drug in the two sizes of vials, the manufacturer has color-coded them; the 20-mg vial has a green cap, the 150 mg vial a red cap. Refrigerate reconstituted solution; discard after 7 days.	Cefazolin Chlortet-racycline Erythromycin Hydrocortisone Sodium succinate Kanamycin Carbenicillin	sterile water for injection. Inject over 3–5 min. One half of the total daily dose may be given via this mode followed in 1–2 hrs by a continuous infusion (see Continuous Infusion column).	infuse over 30–60 min. Remaining ½ dose can then be administered 1–2 hrs later by continuous infusion (see Continuous Infusion column).	(D5W, NS, D5/NS, D5/ 0.45% sodium chloride, RL or 10% invert sugar) and infuse at a rate of 5–6 mg/ hr (2–3 mg/hr in the presence of renal impairment). Prepare fresh infusions every 24-hrs.	function. 2. Transient neurological disturbances may occur at normal dosage levels: circumoral paresthesias or numbness, ataxia, tingling in the extremities, weakness, vertigo, irritability, slurring of speech, blurred vision. Reduction of dosage may alleviate these symptoms. 3. Safety for use in pregnancy has not been established. 4. Overdosage can cause renal damage indicated by rising BUN, oliguria, proteinuria, casts in the urine, and can cause muscle weakness and apnea. PRECAUTIONS 1. Administer with caution to patients with renal impairment (this drug is excreted mainly via the kidneys). Dosage should be reduced according to the manufacturer's modified dosage schedule (see Dosage column) using serum creatinine levels and urea clearance values. Accumulation of the drug secondary to renal impairment can lead to further renal damage. With renal failure, drug levels in the body can reach toxic levels, precipitating neuromuscular dysfunction and subsequent respiratory failure (apnea). Discontinue therapy if BUN begins to rise and/or urine output falls. 2. Do not administer concomitantly with kanamycin, streptomycin, dihydrostreptomycin, any other polymyxin, or neomycin. In combination the two agents can produce neuromuscular blockade and subsequent respiratory failure (apnea). 3. Drugs which have neuromuscular blocking properties (ether, tubocurarine, succinylcholine, gallamine, decamethonium and sodium citrate) can potentiate these effects in colistimethate sodium and should be used with extreme caution, be prepared to support ventilation for a longer than normal period of time. 4. Calcium chloride can be used as an antidote in the event of respiratory

failure, along with mechanical respiratory support.

ADVERSE REACTIONS
1. Renal damage
2. Neuromuscular blockade at high serum levels (see Precaution No. 1)
3. Neurotoxicity (see Warning No. 2)
4. Drug fever
5. Overgrowth of nonsusceptible organisms
6. Nausea, vomiting, diarrhea

SUGGESTED MODIFICATION OF DOSAGE SCHEDULES OF COLISTIMETHATE SODIUM FOR ADULTS WITH IMPAIRED RENAL FUNCTION (Manufacturers: Warner-Chilcott)

RENAL FUNCTION	DEGREE OF IMPAIRMENT			
	Normal	Mild	Moderate	Considerable
Plasma creatinine (mg/100 ml)	0.7–1.2	1.3–1.5	1.6–2.5	2.6–4.0
Urea clearance % of normal	80–100	40–70	25–40	10–25
	DOSAGE			
Unit dose of Coly-Mycin M, mg	100–150	75–115	66–150	100–150
Frequency, times per day	4 or 2	2	2 or 1	every 36 hrs
Total daily dosage, mg	300	150–230	133–150	100
Approximate daily dose, mg/kg/day	5.0	2.5–3.8	2.5	1.5

eventual paralysis of chest muscles and the diaphragm. Begin ventilating for the patient if respirations fall below 8/minute. Endotracheal intubation will probably be required until serum levels of this drug fall below normal limits. Calcium chloride may be ordered to counteract respiratory depression.
5. Patients who are receiving general anesthetics and/or neuromuscular blocking agents will require respiratory support for a longer than normal period of time following administration of these agents. (Review the Nursing Implications for these drugs.)
6. Take anaphylaxis precautions; see page 118.
7. Monitor for signs and symptoms of nonsusceptible organism overgrowth infection
   a. Fever (take rectal temperature at least every 4–6 hours)
   b. Increasing malaise
   c. Localized signs and symptoms of a new infection: redness, soreness, pain, swelling, drainage (increasing volume, or change in character of pre-existing drainage)
   d. Cough (change in character of the cough or change in sputum production)
   e. Diarrhea

NURSING IMPLICATIONS
1. Monitor renal function (oliguria is a sign of renal damage produced by this drug):
   a. Urinary output (and fluid intake) at least every 8 hours or more frequently as patient's condition indicates. Notify the physician if the output falls below an average of 30 ml/hour for any 8-hour period for adults (see chart on page 546 for normal output values for children).
   b. Urine should be sent for analysis at least every other day to detect the appearance of protein or casts.
   c. Be aware of the patient's BUN during therapy.
2. Be aware of the need for reduced dosage levels in patients with renal impairment.
3. If the patient is able to cooperate, instruct him to report signs of neurotoxicity (see Warning No. 2). Observe ambulatory patients for ataxia and weakness. Infants and small children may become more irritable in the presence of neurotoxicity.
4. Be prepared to support ventilation in patients with myasthenia gravis or renal failure. Keep an oral airway, oxygen, suction equipment and a manual breathing bag at the bedside. Monitor respiratory rate and depth. Respiratory failure associated with this drug will be secondary to weakness and

CORTICOTROPIN (Adrenocorticotropic Hormone, A.C.T.H., Acthar)

ACTIONS/ INDICATIONS	DOSAGE	PREPARATION AND STORAGE	DRUG INCOMPATIBILITIES	MODES OF IV ADMINISTRATION			CONTRAINDICATIONS; WARNINGS; PRECAUTIONS; ADVERSE REACTIONS
				INJECTION	INTERMITTENT INFUSION	CONTINUOUS INFUSION	
Anterior pituitary hormone; stimulates the functioning adrenal cortex to produce and secrete the adrenalcortical hormone: cortisol (the major glucocorticoid) and aldosterone (the mineralocorticoid).	ADULTS: _Diagnostic_— 10–25 units (1 unit is contained in 1 mg. of the International Standard Preparation) infused over 8 hrs. See Nursing Implications section for interpretation of test results.	Available in vials containing 25 or 40 units of the drug. Reconstitute by adding sterile water for injection or NS in the following amounts: 25-unit vial: 1 ml. 40-unit vial: 2 ml. (1 unit is contained in 1 mg. of the International Standard Preparation.) Refrigerate reconstituted solution and use within 24 hours.	Do not mix in any manner with: Aminophylline, Novobiocin, Sodium bicarbonate.	NO Maximum diagnostic and therapeutic effects are only obtained via continuous infusion.	NO Maximum diagnostic and therapeutic effects are only obtained via continuous infusion.	YES Add dose to 500–1000 ml D5W; infuse over 8 hrs. (May also use NS for infusion.)	CONTRAINDICATIONS 1. Scleroderma 2. Osteoporosis 3. Systemic fungal infections 4. Ocular herpes simplex 5. Recent surgery 6. History or presence of peptic ulcer 7. Congestive heart failure 8. Hypertension 9. Sensitivity to pork, beef or equine products (check the origin of the preparation used)
Intravenous mode is used in the diagnostic testing of adrenocortical function. Also can be used as cortisone in disease states where the adrenal glands are functioning (e.g., the drug is ineffective in Addison's disease) such as collagen disease, arthritis, lupus, allergic states, acute inflammations, ulcerative colitis, nephrotic syndrome, periarteritis, dermatologic diseases, palliative treatment of lymphomas and leukemias.	_Therapeutic_— (IM route preferred.) Range: 20–200 units/24 hrs. Dosage varies greatly, depending on the patient's ability to respond. Suggested dosage schedule: 10–12.5 units qid; if there is no effect in 72–96 hrs, increase the dose to 15 units qid; if no effect in 48–72 hrs, increase dose to 20 units qid. Adverse reactions are more common when doses are greater than 25 units qid. Such doses may be neces-	BE CERTAIN THAT BRAND AND PREPARATION BEING USED ARE FOR INTRAVENOUS USE ONLY; DO _NOT_ USE REPOSITORY GEL.					WARNINGS 1. Adrenal responsiveness should be verified by the diagnostic procedure in the Dosage column, before this drug is administered therapeutically. 2. This drug may mask some signs of infection, and new infections including those of the eye due to fungi or viruses. There may be decreased resistance and inability to localize infection. Latent tuberculosis can be reactivated: use chemoprophylaxis. If any infection is present, use anti-infective therapy. 3. Safety for use in pregnancy has not been established; may cause fetal abnormalities. 4. Can cause retention of sodium and water and an increased excretion of potassium and calcium. 5. The usual difficulties encountered with steroid therapy do not apply when this drug is used for diagnostic purposes, except for those effects listed above. PRECAUTIONS 1. Perform a skin test with this drug prior to administration to patients with suspected hypersensitivity to pork, beef or equine products, depending on preparation used. 2. Observe all patients for allergic reactions. 3. There is an exhanced effect of this drug in patients with hypothyroidism and in those with cirrhosis.

sary, however, to produce an adequate clinical response. When remission is reached, begin reducing dosage by 5–10 units over several days.[1]

CHILDREN:
Follow adult guidelines; younger children may require larger doses to produce remission.

ADVERSE REACTIONS IN SHORT-TERM INTRAVENOUS THERAPY
1. Hypersensitivity: dizziness, nausea, vomiting, shock, skin reactions
2. Fluid and electrolyte disturbances, e.g., sodium retention, water retention, potassium loss, calcium loss
3. Musculoskeletal: weakness
4. Gastrointestinal: peptic ulcer, ulcerative esophagitis
5. Skin: impaired wound healing, suppression of skin tests (TB, etc.)
6. Cardiac: precipitation of congestive heart failure due to sodium and fluid retention
7. Endocrine: rise in blood glucose, increased requirement for insulin or oral hypoglycemic agents
8. Metabolic: negative nitrogen balance due to protein catabolism
9. Neurologic:
   a. Increased intracranial pressure
   b. Seizures (increasing frequency in patients with pre-existing seizure disorder)
   c. Vertigo
   d. Headaches
   e. Mental confusion, euphoria, exacerbation of psychosis
10. Eye: Increased intraocular pressure

NURSING IMPLICATIONS
When This Drug Is Used as a Diagnostic Agent:
1. Perform skin testing on all individuals suspected of pork, beef or equine allergy.
2. Monitor for signs of allergic reaction; take anaphylaxis precautions (see page 118).
3. When used as a diagnostic agent, adrenal responsiveness to this drug will produce a rise in urinary and plasma corticosteroid levels. Obtain a 24-hour urine for 17-ketosteroids and 17-hydroxyketosteroids before and after testing period. Normal response is 3–5 times an increase on the first day of the test infusion, and further increases on successive days if testing is continued.

When This Drug Is Used as a Therapeutic Agent:
4. Take precautions to prevent infections in wounds by using strict aseptic technique in dressing changes, etc. Avoid traumatic procedures such as catheterizations. The skin may become more fragile because of the steroid therapy. Patients on bed rest and those with general body weakening secondary to an acute illness should be turned hourly (except during sleep, then every 2–3 hours) to prevent skin breakdown. Initiate the use of supportive measures such as flotation pads, water mattresses, etc. Administer scrupulous skin care to prevent infection.
5. Monitor blood pressure every 2–4 hours, or as the patient's condition dictates. Monitor blood pressure before, during and immediately after intravenous infusion; hypotension can occur.
6. Weigh the patient daily to detect water and sodium retention. Dietary restriction in sodium may be prescribed by the physician. Examine daily for peripheral edema. In susceptible patients, monitor for signs of congestive heart failure, e.g., edema, shortness of breath, rales, dyspnea on exertion, increasing resting heart rate.
7. There may be delayed healing of wounds; take precautions to prevent dehiscence. Sutures may be left in longer than usual for this reason.
8. Monitor urine glucose in patients on high-dose therapy and with diabetes. Diabetic individuals may require a larger dosage of insulin or oral agent.
9. Administer antacid therapy as ordered to assist in preventing peptic ulcer. Monitor for signs of the development of an ulcer and/or acute intestinal bleeding: melena, positive stool guaiac, hematemesis, epigastric pain and/or distention, anemia or falling hematocrit.
10. Monitor for signs and symptoms of hypokalemia:[2] weakness, irritability, abdominal distention, poor feeding in infants, muscle cramps. Dietary or pharmacologic potassium supplements may be ordered, guided by serum potassium levels.
11. Monitor for signs and symptoms of hypocalcemia:[3] (serum calcium less than 6 mg %): irritability, change in mental status, seizures, nausea, vomiting, diarrhea, muscle cramps, late effects—cardiac arrhythmias, laryngeal spasm and apnea. Dietary or pharmacologic supplements may be ordered, guided by serum calcium levels.
12. Patients with a history of seizure activity may have an increasing number of seizures while on steroid therapy. Apply appropriate safety precautions.
13. Monitor for behavioral changes, which may range from simple euphoria to depression and psychosis. Apply appropriate safety precautions. A change in dosage may relieve such symptoms.
14. Tuberculin testing should be carried out prior to initiation of steroid therapy if possible. The patient's reactivity to the tuberculin is altered by the drug, giving a false result.
15. Ambulate the patient with caution if vertigo occurs, and initiate the use of

NURSING IMPLICATIONS (No. 15 continued)
side rails to prevent patient injury. Report the onset to the physician.
16. Be alert to the signs of increasing intraocular pressure:[4] eye pain, rainbow vision, blurred vision, nausea and vomiting. Notify the physician immediately.

REFERENCES
1. Society of Hospital Pharmacists: *American Hospital Formulary Service,* Washington, DC, 1977, Section 68:28.
2. Beeson, Paul, and McDermott, Walsh (editors): *Cecil-Loeb Textbook of Medicine* (14th ed.), Philadelphia: W. B. Saunders Company, 1975, p. 1587.
3. Ibid., p. 1815.
4. Newell, Frank W., and Ernest, J. Terry: *Ophthalmology—Principles and Concepts* (3rd ed.), St. Louis: C. V. Mosby Company, 1974, p. 329.

SUGGESTED READINGS
Glasser, Ronald J.: How the Body Works Against Itself: Autoimmune Diseases. *Nursing '77,* September 1977, pp. 34–38.
Hamdi, M. E.: Nursing Intervention for Patients Receiving Corticosteroid Therapy. In *Advanced Concepts in Clinical Nursing.* K. D. Kintzel, ed., Philadelphia: J. B. Lippincott Company, 1971.
Newton, David W., Nichols, Arlene, and Newton, Marion: You Can Minimize the Hazards of Corticosteroids. *Nursing '77* June 1977, pp. 26–33.
Reichgott, Michael J., and Melmon, Kenneth L.: The Role of Corticosteroids in Shock. In *Steroid Therapy,* Daniel Azarnoff, ed., Philadelphia, W. B. Saunders Company, 1975, pp. 118–133.

● **COSYNTROPIN** (Cortrosyn)

ACTIONS/INDICATIONS	DOSAGE	PREPARATION AND STORAGE	DRUG INCOMPATIBILITIES	MODES OF IV ADMINISTRATION			CONTRAINDICATIONS; WARNINGS; PRECAUTIONS; ADVERSE REACTIONS
				INJECTION	INTERMITTENT INFUSION	CONTINUOUS INFUSION	
A diagnostic agent, synthetic subunit of ACTH. Acts as a corticosteroid stimulating agent in the same manner as ACTH. Used to diagnose patients with primary adrenocortical insufficiency. Can be used to perform a 30-min test where cosyntropin is injected and plasma cortisol levels are determined as response. To be used solely for diagnosis.	Usual test dose for adults and children over 2 years: 0.25–0.75 mg. CHILDREN UNDER 2 YEARS: 0.125 mg The most convenient test method is as follows: 1. Control blood sample taken for basal cortisol level 2. The above doses of the drug are infused intravenously at a rate of 40 mcg/hour.	Reconstitute using diluent provided by the manufacturer. Concentration of resulting solution is 0.25 mg/ml. Store at room temperature. Discard after 48 hours. Cosyntropin 0.25 mg is equivalent to 25 U.S.P. units of corticotropin.	Do not add to blood or plasma.	NO	YES Use D5W or NS. Infuse at a rate of 40 mcg/hour. Use any desired volume. Plasma cortisol levels are taken before and immediately after infusion.	NO	CONTRAINDICATIONS History of previous adverse reaction to this drug PRECAUTIONS 1. Patients receiving cortisone, hydrocortisone or spironolactone should omit their pretest doses on the day of testing. 2. In patients with raised bilirubin or with free hemoglobin in the plasma, falsely high fluorescence measurements will result. 3. Hypersensitivity reactions can occur in susceptible patients. ADVERSE REACTIONS Adverse reactions have rarely been reported; those known have been hypersensitivity reactions in patients with known pre-existing allergic disease and/or a previous reaction to natural ACTH.

3. In exactly 30 min a second blood sample is taken and both are refrigerated. (Some sources advocate that the second blood sample be taken after 60 min.

The normal cortisol response is:
1. Control cortisol level is greater than 5 mcg/100 ml.
2. 30-min level should then be at least 7 mcg/100 ml greater than control, and exceed 18 mcg/100 ml. A response in cortisol levels less than this can indicate adrenocortical insufficiency. This test can be performed any time of day as long as the 30-min technique is used.

NURSING IMPLICATIONS
1. Assist in obtaining an accurate allergy history.
2. Determine if the patient and/or parents fully understand the purpose and technique of the test; supplement information as necessary.
3. Monitor patients closely during the injection and for at least 1 hour following. Make note of any sign of allergic reaction from erythema around the injection site to overt manifestations of hypersensitivity, e.g., urticaria, itching, cough, tightness in the chest, wheezing, hypotension.
4. Be prepared with drugs and respiratory support equipment to treat an allergic reaction. (See chapter 8 on the management of allergic reactions).
5. Assist in interpretation of the test results and their significance to the patient and/or parents.

CYANOCOBALAMIN (Vitamin B$_{12}$)

ACTIONS/ INDICATIONS	DOSAGE	PREPARATION AND STORAGE	DRUG INCOMPAT- IBILITIES	MODES OF IV ADMINISTRATION			CONTRAINDICATIONS; WARNINGS; PRECAUTIONS; ADVERSE REACTIONS
				INJECTION	INTERMITTENT INFUSION	CONTINUOUS INFUSION	
Vitamin, essential in erythrocyte maturation, nucleoprotein and myelin synthesis, and the metabolic processes. Used to treat diseases caused by B$_{12}$ deficiency: • Pernicious anemia • Malabsorption of vitamin B • Macrocytic or megaloblastic anemias • Hemorrhage • Blind loop syndrome Also, in chronic liver disease complicated by vitamin B$_{12}$ deficiency, malignancy, thyrotoxicosis, and renal diseases where there is B$_{12}$ deficiency.	The IV route has no advantage over IM or SC. ADULTS: *Pernicious anemia*—100 mcg once or twice a week until hemoglobin is normal. In severe cases, 100 mcg/day (especially when neurologic changes are present). In pernicious anemia, administration will continue for life. *Nutritional megaloblastic anemia*—15 mcg repeated as necessary. CHILDREN: Dosages vary with age of the child and clinical condition.	Protect from light by storing in manufacturer's package.	Compatible with other vitamins and most IV fluids. May be infused in plastic containers.	YES May be given undiluted. Inject over 1–2 min.	YES In any IV fluid; in any convenient volume	YES In any IV fluid; in any convenient volume	CONTRAINDICATIONS Hypersensitivity to B$_{12}$ or cobalt WARNINGS Patients with inherited congenital atrophy of the optic nerve (Leber's disease) or those predisposed to optic nerve atrophy may develop severe and sudden atrophy when given this drug. PRECAUTIONS 1. Diagnose the need for vitamin B$_{12}$ with caution when the patient is receiving an antibiotic, methotrexate, or pyrimethamine. These drugs may alter blood assay. 2. Colchicine, para-aminosalicylic acid or excessive alcohol intake for more than 2 weeks may produce a malabsorption of vitamin B$_{12}$. 3. Hypokalemia may occur at the beginning of therapy in severe megaloblastic conditions; monitor serum potassium. ADVERSE REACTIONS No evidence of toxicity; allergy only rarely seen. See Warnings.

NURSING IMPLICATIONS
1. Monitor for allergic reactions.
2. Observe for signs of hypokalemia (see Precaution No. 3 above): weakness, muscle cramps, postural hypotension, irritability, abdominal distention.
3. Patients with nutritionally based anemias will need diet counseling and follow-up.

CYCLOPHOSPHAMIDE (Cytoxan, Endoxan)

ACTIONS/INDICATIONS	DOSAGE	PREPARATION AND STORAGE	DRUG INCOMPATIBILITIES	MODES OF IV ADMINISTRATION			CONTRAINDICATIONS; WARNINGS; PRECAUTIONS; ADVERSE REACTIONS
				INJECTION	INTERMITTENT INFUSION	CONTINUOUS INFUSION	
Antineoplastic agent, interferes with growth of neoplastic cells; the mechanism of action is unknown.	ADULTS AND CHILDREN: *Induction*— 40–50 mg/kg usually given in divided doses over 2–5 days.	To reconstitute powder, use sterile water for injection or bacteriostatic water for injection (paraben preserved only), in the following amounts:	Do not mix with any other medication in any manner.	YES A solution of 20 mg/ml can be given without further dilution.	YES Add dose to 100–500 ml D5W or NS and infuse over 1 hr.	NO	WARNINGS 1. In patients who are postadrenalectomy, adjustment of the doses of both replacement steroids and cyclophosphamide may be necessary to prevent toxicity due to the cyclophosphamide.
Indicated in: • Malignant lymphomas, primary drug in induction and maintenance therapy. (Stages III and IV Hodgkin's lymphosarcomas, histiocytic lymphoma, etc.)	Patients with bone marrow depression due to drugs, x-ray therapy, or tumor infiltration should have a dose reduced by $1/3$ to $1/2$.	100-mg vial: 5 ml 200-mg vial: 10 ml 500-mg vial: 25 ml					2. The rate of metabolism and the leukopenic activity of this drug are increased by chronic administration of phenobarbital. Combined drug actions may occur with other agents. 3. This drug may interfere with normal wound healing.
• Multiple myeloma • Chronic and acute leukemias (to induce and maintain remissions)	*Maintenance* —A variety of schedules have been suggested: 10–15 mg/kg every 7–10 days or 3–5 mg/kg twice weekly or 50 mg/kg every 3–4 weeks.	Resulting solution contains 20 mg/ml. Do not heat to promote dissolution. Discard reconstituted solution after 24 hours if unrefrigerated, or 6 days if stored in the refrigerator.					4. Do not use in pregnancy unless the benefits outweigh the potential risks to the fetus. This drug can cause fetal abnormalities. Cyclophosphamide is excreted in breast milk, making it mandatory to terminate nursing prior to instituting therapy. 5. Both male and female patients capable of conception must be warned of the possibility of the drug producing mutations in germinal cells. Contraception is advisable during therapy.
• Mycosis fungoides • Some solid tumors (disseminated neuroblastoma, adenocarcinoma of the ovary, retinoblastoma, oat cell lung carcinoma)	The largest dose tolerated by the patient is usually given. Children may tolerate larger doses than adults. The total leukocyte count can be used to guide dosage. A suppression of the WBC to 3000–4000 cells/cu mm can be tolerat-						6. This drug suppresses lymphocyte formation and this is a powerful immunosuppressant. This fact contraindicates concomitant, though not subsequent, immunotherapy.[1] PRECAUTIONS 1. Administer with caution in the presence of a. Pre-existing leukopenia b. Thrombocytopenia c. Bone marrow infiltration by tumor cells d. Previous x-ray therapy e. Previous therapy with other cytotoxic agents f. Impaired hepatic function g. Impaired renal function These patients will require reduction in dosage to prevent oversuppression of the bone marrow. 2. Cyclophosphamide suppresses immunologic responses to infection. Dosage must be modified in the event of bacterial, fungal or viral infections.

● CYCLOPHOSPHAMIDE (Cytoxan, Endoxan) (Continued)

ACTIONS/ INDICATIONS	DOSAGE	PREPARATION AND STORAGE	DRUG INCOMPAT- IBILITIES	MODES OF IV ADMINISTRATION			CONTRAINDICATIONS; WARNINGS; PRECAUTIONS; ADVERSE REACTIONS
				INJECTION	INTERMITTENT INFUSION	CONTINUOUS INFUSION	
	ed by most pa-tients. (See Ad-verse Reac-tions, No. 1.)						This is especially true in patients with concomitant or recent steroid therapy.

ADVERSE REACTIONS
1. Hematopoietic: Leukopenia is expected due to bone marrow sup-pression, and can be used as a guide to dosage. Leukocyte count should be kept between 3000–5000. Low WBC usually occurs 9–14 days after the first dose and returns to normal 7–14 days after cessation of therapy. Thrombocytopenia and anemia may also occur. These effects are revers-ible when therapy is discontinued.[2] Hemolytic anemia (negative Coombs' test) has been reported.
2. Gastrointestinal: Anorexia, nausea, vomiting are common and dose-relat-ed. Hemorrhagic colitis, oral mucosal ulceration, and jaundice have also been reported. Hepatitis may occur and is indicated by hyperbiliru-binemia.
3. Genitourinary: Sterile hemorrhagic cystitis can occur and has been fatal. Nonhemorrhagic cystitis has also been reported. Both forms can be pre-vented with ample fluid intake to flush the bladder of drug metabolites. If either occur, therapy should be interrupted. Hematuria may disappear from 2 days to several months after cessation of therapy. Blood replace-ment or iron therapy may be neces-sary.
   Nephrotoxicity as indicated by ris-ing BUN and creatinine has been seen. There may be water excretion impairment and subsequent fluid re-tention. Irreversible amenorrhea and absence of sperm production have been reported. Cyclophosphamide af-fects prepuberal gonads. Adult fe-males may have false-positive Pap tests.
4. Skin and soft tissue: Hair loss (50% of patients on IV therapy)[3] darkening of skin and fingernails and nonspecific dermatitis have been seen.
5. Pulmonary: Interstitial fibrosis can be

seen in cases where high doses are administered over a long period of time. This may be irreversible.[4]

6. Secondary malignancies have been reported in association with cyclophosphamide (bladder, myeloproliferative and lymphoproliferative).

7. Cardiotoxicity: With doses greater than 50 mg/kg, congestive heart failure has been seen. This drug may also potentiate the cardiotoxicity of daunomycin and doxorubicin. If the agents are administered concomitantly with cyclophosphamide, their total dose should not exceed 450 mg/M². Impaired water excretion may also precipitate acute congestive heart failure in susceptible patients.[5,6]

the patient.

c. If the platelet count falls below 100,000/cu mm, monitor for thrombocytopenic bleeding: petechiae, purpura, hematuria, melena, blood in stools, gum bleeding, vaginal bleeding, epistaxis, hematemesis, etc. Avoid trauma. Transfusions may be ordered.

d. Instruct the patient and family on the importance of follow-up blood studies if the drug is being administered on an outpatient basis.

e. Patients who develop anemia are often given iron and B vitamin supplements. Decreased exercise tolerance and fatigue are frequently seen in cancer patients, as is anemia (not secondary to drugs). This can be depressing. Assist the patient in developing a daily plan of rest and activity, encourage adequate diet, and allow time for him to discuss frustration.

5. Thrombophlebitis can occur at the injection site. Notify the physician at onset. Apply warm compresses as ordered; elevate the extremity. Protect the area from trauma. Avoid extravasation; if it occurs, apply warm compresses until symptoms (burning pain) subside. Monitor the area for tissue sloughing.

6. Management of hair loss:
a. Use scalp tourniquet during injection if ordered to help prevent hair loss.
b. Counsel the patient on the possibility of hair loss to enable him to prepare for this disfigurement.
c. Reassure him of regrowth of hair following discontinuation of the drug.
d. Provide privacy and time for the patient to discuss his feelings.

7. Management of stomatitis:
a. Administer preventive oral care every 4 hours and/or after meals.
b. For preventive care use a very soft toothbrush (child's) and toothpaste; avoid trauma to tissues.
c. Examine oral membranes at least daily (instruct patient and/or family) to detect the onset of inflammation or ulceration.
d. If stomatitis occurs, notify the physician and begin therapeutic oral care:[7]
   (1) Mild Inflammation: Remove dentures; use a soft toothbrush and a hydrogen peroxide solution (1 part peroxide and 4 parts saline). Do not use toothpaste. Rinse with the peroxide solution and then water. Replace dentures. This procedure should be carried out every 4 hours and/or after meals.
   (2) Severe Inflammation: Remove dentures; use soft gauze pads rather than a toothbrush. Use the peroxide solution as described above.

NURSING IMPLICATIONS

1. The patient receiving this medication will be experiencing the emotional and physical effects of the malignancy. Knowledge of the patient's feelings about his disease and its implications will assist in helping him tolerate the chemotherapy. The incidence of uncomfortable side effects and adverse reactions is high. It is within the nurse's role to assist the patient in coping with the discomforts of the disease and its treatment, and to help him work through depression and anger toward acceptance of the disease at his own pace. Despite the unpleasantness this drug may bring, it can be a source of hope for the patient.

2. Many patients experience fewer injection side effects when they are placed in a prone or reclining position during the administration of this drug.

3. Management of nausea and vomiting:
a. Usually occurs 1–3 hours after injection. Vomiting may subside after 8 hours, but nausea can persist for 24 hours.
b. Administer this drug at night if possible to correlate with normal sleep pattern, accompanied by sedation and an antiemetic drug to combat these side effects.
c. To be effective, antiemetics should be administered 1 hour prior to the injection of the drug.
d. Small frequent meals, timed with periods when the patient feels his best, are advisable. Bland foods are usually tolerated. Carbohydrate and protein content should be high.
e. If the patient is anorexic, encourage high nutrient liquids and water to maintain hydration.
f. Keep accurate measurements of emesis volume and total intake and output to guide the physician in ordering parenteral fluids when necessary.
g. Administer antacids as ordered. Monitor for onset of diarrhea and gastrointestinal bleeding.

4. Management of hematologic effects:
a. Be aware of the patient's white blood cell and platelet counts prior to each injection.
b. If the WBC falls to 2000/cu mm, take measures to protect the patient from infection such as protective (reversed) isolation, avoidance of traumatic procedures, maintenance of bodily (especially perineal) cleanliness, carrying out strict urinary catheter care when appropriate, etc. Monitor for infection by recording temperatures every 4 hours, examining for rashes, swellings, drainage and pain. Explain these measures to

● CYCLOPHOSPHAMIDE (Cytoxan, Endoxan) (Continued)

NURSING IMPLICATIONS (No. 7 continued)
Rinse with water using an asepto syringe and gentle suction until returns are clear. Do not replace dentures. It may be necessary to give this care every 2–4 hours.

e. Order a mechanical soft, bland diet for patients with mild inflammation. If the stomatitis is severe, the patient may be placed on a liquid diet or NPO status by the physician.

f. For patients who can tolerate oral intake, administer Xylocaine Viscous or acetaminophen elixir as a mouthwash prior to meals to decrease pain (do not use aspirin rinses), as ordered by the physician. Patients with severe stomatitis may require parenteral analgesia.

g. Monitor for jaundice; notify the physician at onset.

8. See Adverse Reaction No. 7, cardiotoxicity. If the patient is receiving a dose greater than 50 mg/kg or has pre-existing heart disease, monitor for the onset of congestive heart failure: decreased exercise tolerance, fatigue, shortness of breath, dyspnea, increased respiratory rate, rales, increased resting heart rate, peripheral pitting edema. Notify the physician of these findings when they are noted.

10. Assist in preventing cystitis by ensuring a high fluid intake (preferably water), to keep the bladder flushed of drug metabolites. For the anorexic or vomiting patient, administer antiemetics as described in Adverse Reaction No. 3. Intravenous infusions may be necessary for the patient who cannot maintain a high fluid intake. Encourage voiding every 2–3 hours to keep the bladder empty. Inform the patient as to the rationale for this intervention. The symptoms of chemically induced cystitis include frequency, urgency, pain on urination and hematuria.

11. Pulmonary fibrosis can occur in patients receiving long-term or high dose therapy. The time of onset varies but can be long after the drug has been discontinued. Symptoms include cough, shortness of breath and changes in the chest x-ray. Report the onset of any one of these to the physician. Instruct the patient and/or family to do the same if the patient is at home.

REFERENCES
1. Marsh, John C., and Mitchell, Malcom S.: Chemotherapy of Cancer, Il.: Drugs in Current use. In *Drug Therapy*, (Hospital Edition), October 1976, p. 43.
2. Silver, Richard T., Lauper, R. David, and Jarwoski, Charles: *A Synopsis of Cancer Chemotherapy*, The York Medical Group, New York, Dun-Donnelly Publishing Company, 1977, p. 17.
3. Ibid.
4. Rosenow, E. C.: The Spectrum of Drug-Induced Pulmonary Disease. *Annals of Internal Medicine*, 77(6):978, December 1972.
5. Chabner, Bruce A., et al.: The Clinical Pharmacology of Antineoplastic Agents. *New England Journal of Medicine*, 292(22):1167, May 29, 1975.
6. Marsh and Mitchell, p. 43.
7. Bruya, Margaret Auld, and Madeira, Nancy Powell: Stomatitis After Chemotherapy. *American Journal of Nursing*, 75:1351, August 1975.

SUGGESTED READINGS
Bolin, Rose Homan, and Auld, Margaret E.: Hodgkin's Disease. *American Journal of Nursing* 74(11):1982–1986, November 1974.
Bruya, Margaret Auld, and Madeira, Nancy Powell: Stomatitis After Chemotherapy. *American Journal of Nursing*, 75(8):1349–1352, August 1975 (references).
Donely, Diana L.: Nursing the Patient Who is Immunosuppressed. *American Journal of Nursing*, 76(10):1619–1625, October 1976 (references).
Laatsch, Nancy: Nursing the Woman Receiving Adjuvant Chemotherapy of Breast Cancer. *Nursing Clinics of North America*, 13(2):337–349, June 1978.
LeBlanc, Donna Harris: People with Hodgkin Disease: The Nursing Challenge. *Nursing Clinics of North America*, 13(2):281–300, June 1978.
Schumann, Delores, and Patterson, Phyllis: Multiple Myeloma. *American Journal of Nursing*, 75(1):78–81, January 1975 (references).
Showfety, Mary Patricia: The Ordeal of Hodgkin's Disease. *American Journal of Nursing*, 74(11):1987–1991, November 1974.
Sovik, Corinne: The Nursing Care of Lung Cancer Patients (Emphasizing Chemotherapy). *Nursing Clinics of North America*, 13(2):301–317, June 1978.

● CYTARABINE (Cytosine Arabinoside, Ara-C, Cytosar U)

ACTIONS/ INDICATIONS	DOSAGE	PREPARATION AND STORAGE	DRUG INCOMPAT- IBILITIES	MODES OF IV ADMINISTRATION				CONTRAINDICATIONS: WARNINGS: PRECAUTIONS: ADVERSE REACTIONS
				INJECTION	INTERMITTENT INFUSION	CONTINUOUS INFUSION		
Antineoplastic agent of the antimetabolite (cell-cycle specific) type with cytotoxic effects limited to those tissues with high rates of cellular proliferation, e.g., bone marrow.	ADULTS AND CHILDREN: *Initial Rapid injection*—2 mg/kg/day for 10 days. Continue until blood count shows antileukemic effect or toxicity (see Adverse	To reconstitute from powder add *bacteriostatic water for injection* in the following amounts: 100-mg vial: 5 ml diluent (resulting solution is 20 mg/ml).	Do not mix with any other medication in any manner.	YES Reconstituted solutions can be injected without further dilution. Inject over 2–3 min. See Dosage column. Flush vein with	YES 1-hr infusions are most convenient means of administration. Use D5W or NS in any convenient volume.	YES Add 24-hr dose to 1000 ml D5W or NS and infuse over 24 hours. Flush vein with NS (10–20 ml) after infusion.		CONTRAINDICATIONS Pre-existing drug-induced bone marrow depression WARNINGS 1. This drug is a potent bone marrow suppressant. Leukocyte and platelet counts should be monitored closely during therapy. 2. Cytarabine is known to be teratogenic in some animal species.

Currently used in the treatment of acute and chronic leukemias, myeloblastic and lymphoblastic forms. Some response has also been seen in patients with lymphomas and Hodgkin's disease.

Reactions). If after 10 days there is no effect, increase dose to 4 mg/kg/day, maintain until antileukemic or toxic effect is seen.

Alternate Method of administration:
Infusion—.5–1.0 mg/kg/day in 1-, 4-, 12- or 24-hour infusions. Continue for 10 days. If no response, increase to 2.0 mg/kg/day and treat until toxicity or remission is evident.

Maintenance—
All remissions must be maintained with periodic injections—1 mg/kg weekly or semiweekly. (This drug is sometimes combined with thioguanine or daunomycin HCl.)

See Precaution No. 1.

Safety for use in infants has not been established.

500-mg vial: 10 ml diluent (resulting solution is 50 mg/ml).

Store at room temperature and discard after 48 hours or if solution develops a haze.

NS (10–20 ml) after injection.

NS (10–20 ml) after infusion.

PRECAUTIONS
1. Therapy should be suspended, or modified, when drug-induced marrow depression results in a platelet count under 50,000/cu mm or a white cell count under 1000/cu mm. Cell counts may continue to fall and will reach lowest level 5–7 days after discontinuation. Restart therapy when there are signs of marrow recovery and above cell counts are reached and exceeded. Do not wait for cell counts to return to normal.
2. Nausea and vomiting may be less severe if infusion mode is used. If nausea and vomiting occur, they usually persist for several hours postinjection.
3. Use with caution and at reduced dosage in the presence of hepatic impairment. (This drug is detoxified by the liver.) May cause further hepatic impairment. If liver enzyme levels are significantly elevated, the drug should be discontinued.
4. Monitor renal function during therapy.
5. Safety for use in infants has not been established.
6. Hyperuricemia may occur with the lysis of neoplastic cells.

ADVERSE REACTIONS
1. Blood dyscrasias secondary to bone marrow suppression:
   a. Leukopenia (primarily granulocyte depression; normal lymphoid elements are only minimally affected); lowest white count may not reach a nadir until 5–7 days after treatment
   b. Thrombocytopenia
   c. Anemia
   d. Reduced reticulocytes
   e. Megaloblastosis
2. Mucosal ulceration: oral membranes, eosphagus
3. Nausea and vomiting (incidence is higher when rapid injections are made; very common in children)
4. Hepatotoxicity: elevated liver enzymes
5. Thrombophlebitis at injection site
6. Hair loss

NURSING IMPLICATIONS
1. The patient receiving this medication will be experiencing the emotional and physical effects of the malignancy. Knowledge of the patient's feelings about his disease and its implications will assist in helping him tolerate the chemotherapy. The incidence of uncomfortable side effects and adverse reactions is high. It is within the nurse's role to assist the patient in coping with the discomforts of the disease and its treatment, and to help him work through depression and anger toward acceptance of the disease at his own pace. Despite the unpleasantness this drug may bring, it can be a source of hope for the patient.
2. Take all precautions to prevent extravasation; see page 96.
3. Management of nausea and vomiting:

257

● CYTARABINE (Cytosine Arabinoside, Ara-C, Cytosar U) (Continued)

NURSING IMPLICATIONS (No. 3 continued)

a. Administer this drug by slow (1–8 hours or continuous) infusion to decrease these side effects, unless this method is deemed undesirable by the physician.

b. If nausea and vomiting occur, administer antiemetics at frequency ordered and time doses for 1 hour prior to meals.

c. Small frequent meals, timed with periods when the patient feels his best, are advisable. Bland foods are usually tolerated more readily by a patient who is anorexic or nauseated. Carbohydrate and protein content should be high.

d. If the patient is totally anorexic, encourage high nutrient liquids and water to maintain hydration, to avoid complications of hyperuricemia.

e. Keep accurate measurements of emesis volume and total intake and output to guide the physician in ordering parenteral fluids when necessary.

4. Management of hematologic effects:

a. See Precaution No. 1.

b. Be aware of the patient's white blood cell and platelet count prior to each injection.

c. If WBC falls to 2000/cu mm, take measures to protect the patient from infection such as protective isolation (reversed), avoid traumatic procedures, maintain bodily (especially perineal) cleanliness, carry out strict urinary catheter care when appropriate. Monitor for infection by recording temperatures every 4 hours, examining for rashes, swellings, drainage and pain. Explain these measures to the patient.

d. If platelet count falls below 100,000/cu mm, monitor for thrombocytopenic bleeding: petechiae, purpura, hematuria, melena, blood in stools, gum bleeding, oozing from an incision, vaginal bleeding, epistaxis, hematemesis, etc. Avoid trauma. Transfusions may be ordered.

e. Instruct patient and family of importance of follow-up blood work and the reporting of the signs and symptoms listed above in "b" and "c" if the drug is being administered on an outpatient basis.

5. Thrombophlebitis can occur at the injection site. Notify the physician at onset; apply warm compresses as ordered and elevate the extremity. Protect the area from trauma.

6. Management of hair loss:

a. Use a scalp tourniquet during rapid injection or short-term infusion, if ordered, to help prevent hair loss.

b. Counsel the patient on the possibility of hair loss to enable him to prepare for this disfigurement.

c. Reassure him as to the possibility of regrowth of hair following discontinuation of the drug.

d. Provide privacy and time for the patient to discuss his feelings.

7. Management of stomatitis and eosphagitis:

a. Monitor for symptoms of eosphagitis, e.g., burning chest pain, pain in the throat, pain on swallowing. Administer antacids as ordered. A bland, mechanical soft diet is advisable. Avoid irritating liquids such as fruit juice.

b. Administer preventive oral care every 4 hours and after meals.

c. For preventive care use a soft toothbrush (child's) and toothpaste; avoid trauma to tissues.

d. Examine oral membranes at least daily (instruct family) to detect onset of inflammation and erythema.

e. If stomatitis occurs, notify the physician and carry out therapeutic oral care:[1]

(1) Mild Inflammation: Remove dentures, use soft toothbrush and hydrogen peroxide solution (1 part peroxide and 4 parts saline). Do *not* use toothpaste. Rinse with peroxide solution and then water. Replace dentures. This procedure should be carried out every 4 hours and/or after meals.

(2) Severe Inflammation: Remove dentures, use soft gauze pads rather than a toothbrush. Use peroxide solution as described above. Rinse with water using an asepto syringe and gentle suction until returns are clear. Do not replace dentures. It may be necessary to give this care every 2–4 hours.

f. For stomatitis, order a bland, mechanical soft diet. If inflammation is severe and accompanied by ulceration of oral membranes, the patient may be placed on NPO status by the physician.

g. For patients who can tolerate oral intake, administer Xylocaine Viscous or acetaminophen elixir as a mouthwash prior to meals to decrease pain (do not use aspirin rinses), as ordered by the physician.

h. Patients with severe stomatitis may require parenteral analgesia.

REFERENCE

1. Bruya, Margaret Auld, and Madeira, Nancy Powell: Stomatitis After Cl. therapy. *American Journal of Nursing*, 75(8):1351, August 1975.

SUGGESTED READINGS

Bolin, Rose Homan, and Auld, Margaret E.: Hodgkin's Disease. *American Journal of Nursing*, November 1974, pp. 1982–1986.

Bruya, Margaret Auld, and Madeira, Nancy Powell: Stomatitis After Chemotherapy. *American Journal of Nursing*, 75(8):1349–1352, August 1975.

Foley, Genevieve V., and McCarthy, Ann Marie: The Child with Leukemia in a Special Hematology Clinic. *American Journal of Nursing*, July 1976, pp. 1115–1119.

——— The Disease (Hodgkin's) and Its Treatment, *American Journal of Nursing*, July 1976, pp. 1109–1114 (references).

Giadquinta, Barbara: Helping Families Face the Crisis of Cancer. *American Journal of Nursing*, October 1977, pp. 1583–1588.

Gullo, Shirley: Chemotherapy—What To Do About Special Side Effects. *RN*, April 1977, pp. 30–32.

Hannan, Jeanne Ferguson: Talking is Treatment, Too. *American Journal of Nursing*, November 1974, pp. 1991–1992.

Martinson, Ida: The Child With Leukemia: Parents Help Each Other. *American Journal of Nursing*, July 1976, pp. 1120–1121.

Showfety, Mary Patricia: The Ordeal of Hodgkin's Disease. *American Journal of Nursing*, November 1974, pp. 1987–1991.

DACARBAZINE (DTIC-Dome, Imidazole Carboxamide)

ACTIONS/ INDICATIONS	DOSAGE	PREPARATION AND STORAGE	DRUG INCOMPATIBILITIES	MODES OF IV ADMINISTRATION			CONTRAINDICATIONS; WARNINGS; PRECAUTIONS; ADVERSE REACTIONS
				INJECTION	INTERMITTENT INFUSION	CONTINUOUS INFUSION	
Antineoplastic agent, acts as an alkylating agent. Indicated primarily in the treatment of malignant melanoma (20% response rate), in Hodgkin's disease with other drugs, Kaposi's sarcoma and other soft-tissue sarcomas in combination with other drugs.	ADULTS: 2.0–4.5 mg/ kg/day for 10 days repeated every 4 weeks or 250 mg/M²/ day for 5 days repeated every 2–3 weeks. (Dosage should be reduced in the presence of renal impairment.)	Reconstitute from powder with sterile water for injection or NS in the following amounts: 100-mg vial: 9.9 ml 200-mg vial: 19.7 ml The resulting solutions contain 10 mg/ml. Store in refrigerator and discard 72 hours after opening.	Do not mix with any other medication.	YES Prepared solution (see Preparation column) may be injected without further dilution, over 1 min.	YES Add dose to 50–100 ml D5W and infuse over 30 min.	NO	CONTRAINDICATIONS Hypersensitivity to dacarbazine WARNINGS This drug causes bone marrow suppression that results primarily in reduction in leukocytes and platelets, although mild anemia may also occur. Suppression may be serious enough to cause death. PRECAUTIONS 1. The hemopoietic system must be closely monitored during therapy. 2. Extravasation of this drug into the tissues may cause local tissue damage. ADVERSE REACTIONS 1. Bone marrow suppression: leukopenia usually occurs 10 days after the first injection, and thrombocytopenia 10–15 days after. These may continue 2–4 weeks after the last dose 2. Nausea and vomiting: most patients experience these to some degree, usually within 1 hour of administration, persisting for up to 12 hours. These effects may decrease after 1–2 days of therapy. Phenobarbital and/or prochlorperazine may relieve these symptoms. Intractable nausea and vomiting may necessitate discontinuation of the drug. 3. Diarrhea: restricting oral intake 4–6 hours prior to an injection may help to avoid this problem, which usually subsides 1–2 days after cessation of therapy 4. Flulike syndrome: fever, muscle aches, malaise occur usually 7 days after an injection, and may persist for 7–21 days. This may recur with successive courses of the drug 5. Elevated liver enzymes (transient and rarely seen) 6. Hair loss 7. Facial flushing 8. Mental depression (rare)

NURSING IMPLICATIONS
1. The patient receiving this medication will be experiencing the emotional and physical effects of the malignancy. Knowledge of the patient's feelings about his disease and its implications will assist in helping him tolerate the chemotherapy. The incidence of uncomfortable side effects and adverse reactions is high. It is within the nurse's role to assist the patient in coping with the discomforts of the disease and its treatment, and to help him work through depression and anger toward acceptance of the disease at his own

259

● DACARBAZINE (DTIC-Dome, Imidazole Carboxamide) (Continued)

NURSING IMPLICATIONS (No. 1 continued)
pace. Despite the unpleasantness this drug may bring, it can be a source of hope for the patient.

2. Be aware of the patient's WBC (leukocyte count). If it falls below 2000/cu mm, the drug may be discontinued. Protective (reversed) isolation may be advisable at this time to help prevent infection. Avoid procedures that produce breaks in the skin or mucous membranes, such as intramuscular injections, catheterizations, etc. These could be a source of infection. Monitor for signs and symptoms of infection until white cell count returns to normal.

3. Be aware of the patient's platelet count. Bleeding may occur if the count falls below 50,000/cu mm (normal is 200,000 to 400,000/cu mm). Examine for purpura (purple blotches in the skin that do not blanch on pressure). Monitor for all other signs of bleeding, e.g. melena, hematemesis, hematuria, oozing from an incision, epistaxis, and notify the physician of these lesions or other signs. The patient will probably be given transfusions of fresh whole blood or platelets to alleviate the thrombocytopenia. The drug is usually withheld if the platelet count reaches 50,000/cu mm, and restarted when the level returns to a normal range.

4. Antiemetics can be given prior to the injection of the drug to help control nausea and vomiting (phenobarbital, prochlorperazine, or chlorpromazine). These agents are not effective in some patients. Antiemetics can also be given prior to meals if necessary. Assist in maintaining adequate fluid intake orally if possible, or intravenously if oral intake is limited. The drug is

usually discontinued if vomiting is uncontrollable. In some patients, nausea and vomiting improve after several doses of dacarbazine.

5. If diarrhea occurs following the injection, restrict oral intake for 4–6 hours prior to the next infusion. Lomotil may be used if necessary. Maintain hydration with oral or intravenous fluids. Hypokalemia may occur if diarrhea is severe. This side effect may also subside after 1–2 days of therapy.

6. Prevent extravasation; see page 96. If it occurs, apply warm compresses for 2 hours initially, and for 20–30 minutes every 4 hours until pain and redness subside. Protect the tissue from damage. Necrosis and sloughing may occur.

7. Management of hair loss:
   a. Use scalp tourniquet during injection, if ordered, to help prevent hair loss.
   b. Counsel the patient on the possibility of hair loss to enable him to prepare for this disfigurement.
   c. Reassure him of regrowth of hair following discontinuation of the drug.
   d. Provide privacy and time for the patient to discuss his feelings.

SUGGESTED READINGS
Donley, Diana L: Nursing the Patient Who Is Immunosuppressed. *American Journal of Nursing,* 76(10):1619–1625, October 1976 (references).
Schumann, Delores: Multiple Myeloma. *American Journal of Nursing,* 75(1):78–81, January 1975 (references).

● DACTINOMYCIN (Cosmegen, ACT-D, Actinomycin-D, DACT)

ACTIONS/ INDICATIONS	DOSAGE	PREPARATION AND STORAGE	DRUG INCOMPAT- IBILITIES	MODES OF IV ADMINISTRATION			CONTRAINDICATIONS; WARNINGS; PRECAUTIONS; ADVERSE REACTIONS
				INJECTION	INTERMITTENT INFUSION	CONTINUOUS INFUSION	
An actinomycin antibiotic, antineoplastic agent, cell-cycle specific.	ADULTS: 0.3–0.5 mg daily (15 mcg/ kg/day) for maximum of 5 days. Dosage may vary when drug is used in combination with other agents.	Reconstitute by adding 1.1 ml of sterile water for injection (use no other diluent). This yields a solution of 500 mcg/ml.	Do not mix with any other medication in syringe or IV line.	YES No further dilution needed. Inject into the tubing of a running IV.	YES Use D5W or NS, 100–200 ml, infuse over 30–60 min.	NO	CONTRAINDICATIONS If administered at the time of infection with chickenpox, a severe generalized disease may occur, which may result in death. WARNINGS Use for other than treatment of the conditions listed under Actions/Indications is experimental. PRECAUTIONS 1. This is a toxic drug, and frequent observation of the patient is essential. 2. Anaphylaxis may occur. 3. Abnormalities in renal, hepatic and bone marrow function have been produced by this drug; all three systems should be closely monitored. 4. When administered concomitantly with radiation therapy, there may be
Recommended *only* in the treatment of hospitalized patients with Wilms' tumor (a malignant tumor of the kidney region with metastases to the lungs and lymph), rhabdomyosarcoma, carcinoma	CHILDREN: 15 mcg/kg daily for 5 days, or a total of 2.4 mg/ square meter of body surface over 1 week, usually,	Discard reconstituted solution after 24 hours. Solution is normally yellowgold.					

of the testes and uterus, Ewing's sarcoma in adults, choriocarcinoma that is methotrexate-resistant, Kaposi's sarcoma, and other soft tissue sarcomas.

but dose may vary with patient, tumor and other agents used in combination.

In children and adults a second course may be given after 2 weeks provided all signs of toxicity have passed. May also be used for isolation perfusion (intra-arterial infusion).

an increased incidence of gastrointestinal toxicity and bone marrow suppression.
5. This drug is known to produce abnormalities in fetal development in animals, and the possibility exists in humans.
6. Use of this drug in infants under 6 months of age is not recommended.
7. Extravasation will cause severe tissue damage.

ADVERSE REACTIONS
1. Gastrointestinal: nausea and vomiting 2–4 days after discontinuation of the drug, (reaches maximal intensity in 1–2 weeks), diarrhea, abdominal pain, proctitis, dysphagia secondary to esophagitis, stomatitis
2. Malaise and fever
3. Blood: bone marrow depression producing anemia, aplastic anemia, agranulocytosis, leukopenia, thrombocytopenia
4. Hair loss

d. Instruct the patient and family on the importance of follow-up blood studies if the drug is being administered on an outpatient basis. Also instruct on the importance of reporting possible infections or unusual bleeding.
6. Management of hair loss:
a. Use the scalp tourniquet during injection, if ordered, to help prevent hair loss. This may be ineffective in preventing hair loss because of the prolonged presence of this drug in the blood.
b. Counsel the patient on the possibility of hair loss to enable him to prepare for this disfigurement.
c. Reassure him of the possibility of regrowth of hair following discontinuation of the drug.
d. Provide privacy and time for the patient to discuss his feelings.
7. Management of stomatitis:
a. Administer preventive oral care every 4 hours and/or after meals.
b. For preventive care, use a very soft toothbrush (child's) and toothpaste; avoid trauma to the tissues.
c. Examine oral membranes at least daily (instruct patient and/or family) to detect the onset of inflammation or ulceration.
d. If stomatitis occurs, notify the physician and begin therapeutic oral care:[1]
(1) *Mild Inflammation:* Remove dentures, use a soft toothbrush and a hydrogen peroxide solution (1 part peroxide and 4 parts saline). Do not use toothpaste. Rinse with the peroxide solution and then water. Replace dentures. This procedure should be carried out every 4 hours and/or after meals.
(2) *Severe Inflammation:* Remove dentures, use soft gauze pads rather than a toothbrush. Use the peroxide solution as described above. Rinse with water using an asepto syringe and gentle suction until returns are clear. Do not replace dentures. It may be necessary to give this care every 2–4 hours.
e. Order a bland, mechanical soft diet for patients with mild inflammation. If the stomatitis is severe, the patient may be placed on NPO status by the physician.

NURSING IMPLICATIONS
1. The patient receiving this medication will be experiencing the emotional and physical effects of the malignancy. Knowledge of the patient's feelings about his disease and its implications will assist in helping him tolerate the chemotherapy. The incidence of uncomfortable side effects and adverse reactions is high. It is within the nurse's role to assist the patient in coping with the discomforts of the disease and its treatment, and to help him work through depression and anger toward acceptance of the disease at his own pace. Despite the unpleasantness this drug may bring, it can be a source of hope for the patient.
2. Assist in obtaining an accurate history for recent exposure to chickenpox.
3. Take all precautions to avoid extravasation; see page 96.
4. Management of nausea, vomiting and diarrhea:
a. See Adverse Reaction No. 1.
b. It is likely that the patient will experience these effects while at home. Instruct the patient and/or family on the timing of antiemetic agents, the maintenance of hydration and nutrition, and the signs and symptoms of dehydration, proctitis and esophagitis, and what to do if they occur.
5. Management of hematologic effects:
a. Be aware of the patient's complete blood count and platelet count prior to each injection. Anemia, leukopenia and thrombocytopenia are the dose-limiting side effects.
b. If the white blood count falls to 2000/cu mm, take measures to protect the patient from infection, such as protective (reversed) isolation, avoidance of traumatic procedures, maintaining bodily (especially perineal) cleanliness, carry out strict urinary catheter care when appropriate, etc. Monitor for infection by recording temperature every 4 hours, examining for rashes, swellings, drainage and pain. Explain these measures to the patient.
c. If the platelet count falls below 100,000/cu mm, monitor for thrombocytopenic bleeding: petechiae, purpura, hematuria, melena, blood in stools, gum bleeding, vaginal bleeding, epistaxis, hematemesis, etc. Avoid trauma. Transfusions may be ordered.

● **DACTINOMYCIN (Cosmegen, ACT-D, Actinomycin-D, DACT) (Continued)**

NURSING IMPLICATIONS (No. 7 continued)

f. For patients who can tolerate oral intake, administer Xylocaine Viscous or acetaminophen elixer as a mouthwash prior to meals to decrease pain (do not use aspirin rinses), as ordered by the physician.

g. Patients with severe stomatitis may require parenteral analgesia.

8. Monitor for fever every 4–6 hours. This reaction is usually treated symptomatically with antipyretics.

REFERENCE

1. Bruya, Margaret Auld, and Madeira, Nancy Powell: Stomatitis After Chemotherapy. *American Journal of Nursing,* 75(8):1351, August 1975.

SUGGESTED READINGS

Bruya, Margaret Auld, and Madeira, Nancy Powell: Stomatitis After Chemotherapy. *American Journal of Nursing,* 75(8):1349–1352, August 1975.

Giadquinta, Barbara: Helping Families Face the Crisis of Cancer. *American Journal of Nursing,* 77:1583–1588, October 1977.

Vietti, Teresa J., and Valeriote, Frederick: Conceptual Basis for the Use of Chemotherapeutic Agents and Their Pharmacology. *Pediatric Clinics of North America,* 23:67–92, February 1976.

● **DECAMETHONIUM BROMIDE (Syncurine)**

ACTIONS/ INDICATIONS	DOSAGE	PREPARATION AND STORAGE	DRUG INCOMPAT- IBILITIES	MODES OF IV ADMINISTRATION			CONTRAINDICATIONS; WARNINGS; PRECAUTIONS; ADVERSE REACTIONS
				INJECTION	INTERMITTENT INFUSION	CONTINUOUS INFUSION	
Potent, short-acting skeletal muscle relaxant of the depolarizing type. Produces acceptable muscle relaxation for 4–8 minutes after injection. Muscle activity returns to normal in 20 minutes. Used as an adjunct to general anesthesia and in electroconvulsive therapy to reduce trauma. Can also be used to facilitate endotracheal intubation.	ADULTS: *Electroconvulsive therapy—* 1.50–1.75 mg. Shock should be given at the height of relaxation in 3–5 min after injection. *Anesthesia or Respiratory Control—*initially 2.0–2.5 mg. Additional doses of 0.5–1.0 mg can be given at intervals of 10–30 min as needed. Adult maximum dose is 10 mg. CHILDREN: 0.05–0.08 mg/kg; repeat in 1 to 30 min as needed to	Dilution prior to injection unnecessary. Store at room temperature.	Do not mix with any other medication in any manner.	YES Administer undiluted at 1 mg/min. May be injected into tubing of a running IV.	NO Pharmacologically inappropriate.	NO Pharmacologically inappropriate.	CONTRAINDICATIONS Hypersensitivity to this drug or other bromides WARNINGS 1. Causes respiratory depression secondary to muscle paralysis. Respiratory support equipment must be immediately available. Anticholinesterase agents such as neostigmine are *not* effective antidotes, and manual ventilation must be administered until spontaneous breathing and the swallow, cough, and gag reflexes return. 2. Safety for use in pregnancy has not been established. Benefits to the mother must be weighed against potential risk to the fetus. 3. Use with caution in the presence of other muscle relaxants. 4. Some antibiotics may potentiate the action of this drug, e.g., gentamicin, kanamycin, tobramycin, polymyxins. PRECAUTIONS 1. Administer with caution to the very young and very old. 2. Administer with caution to patients undergoing surgery in the Trendelenburg or lithotomy position; such positions may precipitate significant hypotension. 3. Impaired renal function may cause

maintain effects.

sustained muscular paralysis secondary to delayed excretion of this drug.
4. Administer with caution to patients with severe burns; serious hyperkalemia may occur.
5. Recently digitalized patients or those with digitalis toxicity may have serious cardiac arrhythmias. Cardiac arrest has been reported. Avoid use in these patients.
6. Administer with extreme caution to patients with fractures or neuromuscular disorders; the muscle twitching produced by this drug may cause additional trauma.

ADVERSE REACTIONS
1. Cardiac: bradycardia, tachycardia, and other arrhythmias, hypertension, and hypotension have been reported.
2. Respiratory: respiratory depression and apnea occur secondary to muscle paralysis (see Warning No. 1).
3. After prolonged administration, this agent can take on properties of a nonpolarizing neuromuscular blocking agent. If this occurs, the block can be reversed by neostigmine, edrophonium.

not occur.
7. Be aware of elements which may *prolong* the effects of this drug:
   a. Decreased circulation time, e.g., as in the presence of congestive heart failure or shock
   b. Decreased body temperature
   c. Dehydration
   d. Disturbances in blood pH[2]
   e. Renal insufficiency
   f. Concomitant use of aminoglycoside antibiotics, polymyxin B, or bacitracin
   g. Other drugs, e.g., diazepam, halothane, quinidine
   h. Age, e.g., the elderly
   Patients under the influence of any one of these elements will require prolonged monitoring as described in Nursing Implications No. 5 and prolonged respiratory support.
8. Monitor for changes in vital signs, heart rate and blood pressure; this drug can cause elevation or reduction in both parameters.

Maintenance Care for Ventilatory Control:
1. This drug is usually administered on a PRN basis for controlling ventilation. The criteria for when to administer the drug (by the anesthesiologist, qualified physician, or registered nurse) are determined by the physician. The criteria will include:
   a. A respiratory rate greater than target rate to be set by the physician.
   b. When the patient's respiratory effort is out of phase with the respirator
   c. When the patient is struggling against the respirator
   d. When positive end-expiratory pressure (PEEP) is in use
   Monitor for the onset of any of the criteria and administer (or have administered) the prescribed amount of the drug.

NURSING IMPLICATIONS
Postanesthesia Care:
1. Equipment that should be readily available: suction, manual breathing bag, endotracheal tubes and laryngoscope, oxygen.
2. Patients receiving this agent are usually intubated to assist in maintaining an adequate airway and ventilation (exception: electroconvulsive therapy). Monitor for adequacy of ventilation by presence or absence of cyanosis, and by arterial blood gases.
3. Be aware of the onset and duration of action of this drug (see Actions/Indications column), and when the patient received the last dose.
4. Be aware of the sequence of progression of the paralytic effects, as they will occur after an injection of this drug:
   a. Loss of eye movement
   b. Eyelid droop
   c. Stiffness of jaw muscles
   d. Fasiculations of upper trunk muscles spreading to lower trunk and then extremities
   e. Paralysis of pharyngeal muscles (tongue, swallowing, etc.)
   f. Respiratory paralysis
5. Recovery will be a complete reverse of this sequence.[1] Discharge from the recovery room will depend on the following criteria:
   a. Grip strength
   b. Ability to lift the head
   c. Ability to open the eyes
   d. Respiratory status: e.g., vital capacity and tidal volume. (These values should be obtained preoperatively for comparison.)
6. Reversal agents (anticholinesterase drugs) will not reverse the effects of this drug. Recovery from the paralytic effects occurs over time as the drug is metabolized. Monitor for full recovery as described above. Rebound does

NURSING IMPLICATIONS (No. 1 continued)
2. Make certain that the endotracheal tube is securely and correctly inserted. Check the connection between the tube and the respirator, it must be tight. *Keep respirator alarm systems functioning at all times.*
3. This drug paralyzes skeletal muscles; it does not alter consciousness or relieve pain and anxiety. Therefore, the patient must be adequately sedated to enable him to tolerate the paralyzed state and relieve his anxiety. Analgesics must be given to those patients with wounds, fractures, etc. on a reasonable schedule to insure adequate pain relief. The patient will not be able to make his needs known to those caring for him; they must be anticipated. Many institutions assign one or more RNs to stay in constant attendance with these patients.
4. Monitor vital signs before administration and every 5 minutes after until stabilization is seen, then every 15–30 minutes. Repeat the cycle with each dose. This drug can cause either an elevation or reduction in blood pressure and/or heart rate.
5. Because decamethonium produces muscle paralysis, handle the patient with care to prevent trauma to joints and muscles during turning and positioning.
6. When this drug is discontinued, proceed with the nursing management as described under Postanesthesia Care.

REFERENCES
1. Wylie, W. O., and Churchill-Davidson, H. C. (eds.): *A Practice of Anesthesia,* (3rd ed.). Chicago: Yearbook Medical Publishers, 1972, p. 816.
2. Ibid., p. 833.

● **DEFEROXAMINE MESYLATE** (Desferal Mesylate)

ACTIONS/ INDICATIONS	DOSAGE	PREPARATION AND STORAGE	DRUG INCOMPAT- IBILITIES	MODES OF IV ADMINISTRATION			CONTRAINDICATIONS; WARNINGS; PRECAUTIONS; ADVERSE REACTIONS
				INJECTION	INTERMITTENT INFUSION	CONTINUOUS INFUSION	
Used to facilitate the removal of iron from the body in the treatment of acute iron intoxication. Is an adjunct to, not substitute for, standard measures used to treat acute iron intoxication. Also used to promote iron excretion in patients with secondary iron overload from multiple transfusions. This drug is usually not used in children under 3 years of age. Theoretically, 100 parts by	IV route must only be used for patients in a state of cardiovascular collapse (all others should receive the drug intramuscularly). ADULTS: 1 gm at a rate not to exceed 15 mg/kg/hr. This may be followed by 0.5 gm every 4 hours for 2 doses. Subsequent 0.5-gm doses may also be given if therapeutically indicated. Do not exceed 6 gm in 24 hours.	Reconstitute by adding 2 ml of sterile water for injection to each ampule. Dissolve completely. Add only to NS, D5W or RL for infusion. Discard after 7 days. Store at room temperature.	Do not mix with any other medication.	NO	NO	YES This drug should only be administered by slow IV drip. Rate of infusion must not exceed 15 mg/kg/hr. Use an infusion pump. Use NS, D5W or RL.	CONTRAINDICATIONS Severe renal disease and anuria because the drug is excreted primarily by the kidney. WARNINGS 1. Prolonged treatment has been related to the development of cataracts. This has not been seen in short-term administration. 2. Use in pregnancy is not recommended because of fetal abnormalities seen in animals. Benefits to the mother must outweigh the potential hazards to the fetus. PRECAUTIONS 1. Shock has occurred during rapid IV injection. 2. This drug is not indicated for the treatment of primary hemochromatosis. ADVERSE REACTIONS 1. Pain and induration at injection site have been reported. 2. In patients being treated for acute iron intoxication urticaria, generalized erythema, and hypotension have been seen following rapid IV injection.

weight of this drug is capable of binding approximately 8.5 parts by weight of ferric iron.

CHILDREN:
Initial—20 mg/kg or 600 mg/M². Repeat 10 mg/kg every 4 hrs, times depending on response.[1]

Chronic iron overload (secondary to multiple transfusions)—2 gm with each unit of blood transfused. Infuse at a rate no greater than 15 mg/kg/hour.

3. In long-term therapy, allergic reactions, blurring of vision, abdominal pain, diarrhea, tachycardia, and fever have been reported. These may also be seen in acute therapy.
4. Anaphylaxis has been reported.

NURSING IMPLICATIONS
1. Infusion must be strictly controlled to prevent hypotension; use an infusion pump if available. See Infusion column.
2. Administer other appropriate measures used to treat acute iron intoxication:
   a. Induction of vomiting with syrup of ipecac if the patient is alert
   b. Gastric lavage
   c. Suction and maintenance of airway
   d. Prevention of aspiration
   e. Control of shock with fluids, blood, oxygen, vasopressors
   f. Correction of acidosis.
3. Monitor vital signs frequently until acute crisis has passed and blood pressure, pulse, and respirations are stable.
4. Take anaphylaxis precautions, see page 118.
5. Monitor for adverse reactions, see No. 3 above. Report the onset of any one of these to the physician.

REFERENCE
1. Shirkey, Harry C.: *Pediatric Dosage Handbook,* American Pharmaceutical Association, 1973, p. 53.

DEHYDROCHOLATE, SODIUM (Decholin Sodium)

ACTIONS/INDICATIONS	DOSAGE	PREPARATION AND STORAGE	DRUG INCOMPATIBILITIES	MODES OF IV ADMINISTRATION			CONTRAINDICATIONS; WARNINGS; PRECAUTIONS; ADVERSE REACTIONS
				INJECTION	INTERMITTENT INFUSION	CONTINUOUS INFUSION	
Diagnostic agent: When injected into the venous system, this drug will cause a bitter taste to appear on the tongue when the drug containing blood passes through the	FOR CIRCULATION TIME: 3–5 ml. (See Nursing Implications for test procedure.) FOR HYDRO-CHOLERETIC EFFECT (FOR RADIOGRAPHIC STUDY AND	Store at room temperature; discard unused portions of opened vials. Supplied as a 20% solution in 5-ml ampuls.	Do not mix with any other medication.	YES FOR CIRCULATION TIME: Inject rapidly, within 1–2 seconds. FOR THERAPEUTIC EFFECT: Inject slowly, over 1–3 min.	NO Therapeutically inappropriate.	No Therapeutically inappropriate.	CONTRAINDICATIONS 1. Hypersensitivity 2. Biliary tract obstruction 3. Acute hepatitis 4. History of adverse reactions to the drug PRECAUTIONS 1. Use with caution if the patient has a history of allergy; skin testing prior to administration is advisable. 2. Extravasation may cause a moderate local reaction; i.e., inflammation, pain,

DEHYDROCHOLATE, SODIUM (Decholin Sodium) (Continued)

ACTIONS/ INDICATIONS	DOSAGE	PREPARATION AND STORAGE	DRUG INCOMPATIBILITIES	MODES OF IV ADMINISTRATION			CONTRAINDICATIONS; WARNINGS; PRECAUTIONS; ADVERSE REACTIONS
				INJECTION	INTERMITTENT INFUSION	CONTINUOUS INFUSION	
circulatory system of the tongue.

Hydrocholeretic agent: Increases the volume of the bile produced by the liver, by increasing the water content of the bile. Volume may be increased by 100–200 percent.

Uses
- To determine arm-to-tongue circulation time
- To increase bile flow in cholecystography
- To produce a flushing action in the biliary system for adjunctive treatment of functional and organic disorders of the biliary tract (biliary dyskinesia, postcholecystectomy syndrome, chronic noncalculous (non-stone-forming) cholecystitis and recurrent | THERAPEUTIC USES): 5–10 ml for first dose; 10 ml for second and third. | | | Administer *undiluted.* | | | swelling, lasting several days.
3. This drug should not be used to improve liver function by increasing bile output.
4. Use with caution in patients with acute yellow atrophy of the liver, in children under 6 years of age, and in the elderly. These patients may have a decreased ability to excrete the drug into the bile and may be more likely to develop adverse reactions.
5. Rarely, patients who have been chronic smokers or who have oral sensory impairment may not be able to detect the bitter taste for circulation time determination.

ADVERSE REACTIONS
1. Deaths have occurred following rapid intravenous injection for circulation time determinations in patients with severe congestive heart failure.
2. Anaphylaxis, even after negative skin testing (rare).
3. Gastrointestinal: nausea, vomiting, diarrhea, abdominal discomfort.
4. Cardiovascular: tachycardia, hypotension, faintness, dyspnea, diaphoresis.
5. Allergy (other than anaphylaxis): chills, fever, erythema, pruritus, urticaria. |

nonob-
structive
cholangitis.

NURSING IMPLICATIONS

1. Circulation time procedure:
   a. If a series of determinations are to be done over several days' time, each test should be performed in the same manner as the others.
   b. Keep the patient recumbent for 30 minutes prior to the test.
   c. Keep the patient NPO (except fluids) for 3 hours prior to the test.
   d. Explain the test thoroughly in a manner easily understood by the patient. All efforts should be made to allay his fears. Instruct him to say "now" the moment he experiences the bitter taste.
   e. During the injection, the patient should be lying down and comfortable. One arm should be resting on a pillow to place the antecubital fossa at the level of the right atrium (midchest). If the patient is orthopneic allow him to sit upright.
   f. The sodium dehydrocholate should be injected into a vein without dilution. If a pre-existing intravenous site is being used, remove the system tubing and inject directly into the vein. If a new venipuncture is to be made, use an 18–19 gauge needle (scalp vein needle apparatus is the most convenient).
   g. Attach a syringe containing 3–5 ml of the drug (6–10 ml if two injections are to be given) to the needle. Apply a tourniquet. Insert the needle in the usual manner, making sure that the tip is within the lumen of the vein.
   h. Release the tourniquet, wait 15 seconds, start a stop watch and begin the injection at the same time. Inject the entire dose within 1–2 seconds.
   i. Stop the watch when the patient says "now." A circulation time over 16 seconds is abnormal.

2. Circulation time is usually increased (prolonged) in congestive heart failure, myxedema, polycythemia vera, in some cases of complete atrioventricular heart block, chronic constrictive pericarditis, pericardial effusion with tamponade, and shock. As cardiac compensation is restored toward normal with correction of defect, digitalis, diuretics, etc., circulation time will decrease.
   The time is usually decreased (shortened) in hyperthyroidism, beri-beri, anemia, congenital cardiac anomalies (right-to-left shunts) and reversed blood flow in abnormalities of the great vessels (truncus arteriosus or patent ductus arteriosus). Although this drug is not used to determine circulation time, when it is used the nurse should assist in interpreting the findings to the patient.

3. Take anaphylaxis precautions; see page 118.

4. This drug has a mild diuretic effect. Monitor for urinary retention in patients who have a history of prostatic hypertrophy, bladder neck obstruction, or urinary stricture. Palpate bladder size every 2–4 hours for 8 hours following injection.

● DESLANOSIDE (Cedilanid-D)

ACTIONS/ INDICATIONS	DOSAGE	PREPARATION AND STORAGE	DRUG INCOMPAT- IBILITIES	MODES OF IV ADMINISTRATION			CONTRAINDICATIONS; WARNINGS; PRECAUTIONS; ADVERSE REACTIONS
				INJECTION	INTERMITTENT INFUSION	CONTINUOUS INFUSION	
A digitalis cardiac glycoside, which: • Increases the force of myocardial contraction (positive iotropic effect) • Slows the discharge rate of the sinus node • Slows conduction through the A-V node to decrease the ventricular rate	ADULTS: IV route used only when rapid digitalization is urgent. This can be obtained in 12 hrs by giving 1.6 mg in one dose. PREMATURE AND FULL-TERM NEW-BORNS, AND INFANTS WITH RE-DUCED RENAL FUNCTION OR MYOCARD-ITIS:	Store at room temperature. Discard unused portions of vials. Supplied in 2 ml vials (0.2 mg/ml). Do not add to IV fluids; this drug is unstable when diluted.	Do not add to an IV line containing: Any calcium preparation Protein hydro-lysate	YES At a rate of 0.2 mg/min. Should be given as close to cannula as possible, either into the cannula hub or through the lowest Y injection site, to avoid mixing the drug with IV fluid.	NO Do not dilute in solution.	NO Do not dilute in solution.	CONTRAINDICATIONS 1. Digitalis toxicity. 2. In the presence of ventricular tachycardia unless congestive heart failure occurs after a protracted episode itself not caused by digitalis 3. Ventricular fibrillation 4. Hypersensitivity WARNINGS 1. The arrhythmias that digitalis preparations are indicated for can also be those caused by digitalis toxicity. Digitalis toxicity should be ruled out before administering this drug. 2. Patients in congestive heart failure may complain of nausea, anorexia, and vomiting. These symptoms can also be associated with digitalis toxicity, which should be ruled out prior to administration of the drug.

267

DESLANOSIDE (Cedilanid-D) (Continued)

ACTIONS/ INDICATIONS	DOSAGE	PREPARATION AND STORAGE	DRUG INCOMPAT-IBILITIES	MODES OF IV ADMINISTRATION			CONTRAINDICATIONS; WARNINGS: PRECAUTIONS; ADVERSE REACTIONS
				INJECTION	INTERMITTENT INFUSION	CONTINUOUS INFUSION	

ACTIONS/INDICATIONS

Onset of action is 5 minutes after IV injection, peaks in 2–4 hours, lasts 2–5 days.

Used:
• To treat congestive heart failure of all degrees
• To slow the ventricular rate in atrial fibrillation
• To convert atrial flutter to normal sinus rhythm
• To control paroxysmal atrial tachycardia

In cardiogenic shock, the value of digitalis has not been established, but the drug is frequently used, especially when the condition is accompanied by pulmonary edema.

DOSAGE

For digitalization—
0.022 mg/kg (0.3 mg/M²) in 2–3 doses[1]

CHILDREN 2 WEEKS TO 3 YEARS:
0.025 mg/kg (0.75 mg/M²) in 2–3 doses.

CHILDREN 3 YEARS AND OLDER:
0.0225 mg/kg (0.75 mg/M²) in 2–3 doses.

Oral digitalization can be cautiously carried out with digoxin, 12–24 hrs. after the last dose of deslanoside has been given.

CONTRAINDICATIONS; WARNINGS: PRECAUTIONS; ADVERSE REACTIONS

PRECAUTIONS
1. Toxicity can develop in the presence of hypokalemia, even at usual dosage. Hypokalemia also reduces the positive inotropic effect of the drug. Patients on diuretics, hemodialysis, corticosteroid therapy, or with diarrhea are prone to hypokalemia. Monitor and correct serum potassium levels when indicated.
2. Concomitant conditions may sensitize the myocardium to the effects of digitalis and to toxicity:
   a. Acute myocardial infarction
   b. Advanced congestive heart failure
   c. Fibrotic heart diseases
   d. Severe pulmonary diseases
3. Calcium preparations can produce serious arrhythmias in patients receiving digitalis.
4. Patients with myxedema require lower dosage of this drug.
5. Administer with caution in the presence of any degree of A-V block. Because of its effects on A-V conduction, digitalis may increase the degree of block, slowly.
6. Patients with chronic constrictive pericarditis will react unfavorably to digitalis.
7. This drug, or any digitalis preparation, is usually not given to patients with idiopathic hypertrophic subaortic stenosis.
8. Renal impairment delays excretion of this drug and requires modification of maintenance dosage of digitalis preparations.
9. Electrical conversion of arrhythmias may require adjustment of dosage.

OVERDOSAGE, TOXIC EFFECTS
1. Early symptoms of toxicity are anorexia, nausea, vomiting, and diarrhea in adults, but are rarely present in infants. There may also be weakness, and visual disturbances, such as yellow vision, and headache.
2. Arrhythmias of all types can be seen in toxicity. Premature ventricular contractions are most common except in infants and young children. Junc-

tional rhythms and paroxysmal atrial rhythms are also common.
3. Slowing of the sinus rate and increasing A-V block are advanced signs of toxicity.
4. Treatment must include discontinuing the drug until all signs of toxicity have passed. Potassium may be administered as indicated. Monitor for hyperkalemia. (Do not use in the presence of advanced heart block.)[2] EDTA may also be used to bind serum calcium and counteract arrhythmias. Other antiarrhythmic agents may also be used: phenytoin (drug of choice), quinidine, procainamide, and propranolol. (If propranolol is used, monitor atrioventricular conduction; this drug may increase heart block.) Atropine can be used to treat bradyarrhythmias. See entries for each drug for further details on their use.
5. If profound bradycardia and/or complete A-V block occur, transvenous temporary pacing may be necessary until toxicity resolves.

f. Increased exercise tolerance
Note that worsening congestive failure despite digitalis administration may be a sign of digitalis toxicity.
5. Be aware of the patient's serum potassium. Administer potassium supplements as ordered. These may produce nausea and vomiting (liquid preparations especially) usually soon after administration. The nurse's observations will be needed to differentiate between potassium-induced nausea and vomiting and that due to digitalis toxicity. (Normal serum potassium: 3.5–5.5 mEq/liter.) Potassium supplements, both oral and intravenous, can produce hyperkalemia—monitor serum potassium for elevations. The signs and symptoms of hyperkalemia are: (a) peaked T-waves on ECG, (b) muscular weakness, (c) nausea, abdominal pains, diarrhea, (d) paresthesias of hands, feet, and face.
6. Rarely, elderly patients experience hallucinations, anxiety, and delusions secondary to toxic levels of digitalis preparations. Monitor for onset of this complication, notify the physician, and initiate safety measures, e.g., side rails, restraints as indicated, close observation, reassurance.
7. Patients who will require a digitalis preparation on a chronic basis must be instructed on safe self-administration. Points that must be presented are:
a. The actions of the drug, what it can and cannot do for the patient
b. Correct daily dosage
c. Pulse-taking (if possible, not absolutely required), and actions to take with changes in rate and rhythm
d. Signs and symptoms of toxicity and what to do if they appear
e. Need for follow-up care
f. Potassium intake
g. Diet, activity, etc., necessary for general care of congestive heart failure
The patient and/or family should be able to demonstrate and verbalize knowledge of these areas.

REFERENCES
1. Shirkey, Harry C.: Pediatric Drug Handbook. Philadelphia: W. B. Saunders

NURSING IMPLICATIONS
1. Patients receiving this medication intravenously should, in most instances, be observed for arrhythmias via continuous ECG monitoring. Observe for improvement if the drug is given to treat an arrhythmia, and observe for arrhythmias which may be produced by the drug. Some of the more common arrhythmias produced by toxic levels of deslanoside are : sinus bradycardia, premature ventricular and atrial contractions, atrioventricular block of all degrees, paroxysmal atrial tachycardia. Notify the physician of improvement in arrhythmia being treated, and document with an ECG tracing. If arrhythmias of toxicity appear, notify the physician, document with an ECG tracing, and hold the next dose of deslanoside until the physician decides what course of action is appropriate.
2. Be prepared to administer immediate care in the event of arrhythmias due to toxicity. (See Overdosage, No. 4, above.) Atropine 0.5–1.0 mg can be given for a heart rate less than 50–60/minute. (In units where registered nurses are expected to administer drugs in such an event, the unit physician should decide at what heart rate the atropine should be administered and in what amount.) See page 194 for details on atropine.
   For premature ventricular tachycardia, lidocaine 50–100 mg can be given by intravenous injection. Again, unit policy should dictate when and how much drug is given. See page 365 for details on lidocaine.
3. Observe for noncardiac symptoms of digitalis toxicity: anorexia; nausea; vomiting and diarrhea; visual disturbances, e.g., rainbow vision or yellow vision (rare); in children, poor feeding and irritability; headache (rare); confusion; severe fatigue.[3]
4. Monitor for signs of improvement if the patient is being treated for congestive heart failure:
a. Reduction in weight (weigh the patient daily)
b. Reduction in peripheral edema
c. Increased urine output (measure every 8 hours)
d. Decreased resting heart rate to normal limits (record every 4–8 hours)
e. Decreased respiratory rate, disappearance of rales

- **DESLANOSIDE (Cedilanid-D)** (Continued)

REFERENCES (No. 1 continued)
Company, 1977, p. 133.
2. Davis, Richard H., and Risch, Charles: Potassium and Arrhythmias. *Geriatrics,* November 1970, p. 110.
3. Lely, A. H., and van Enter, C. H. J.: Noncardiac Symptoms of Digitalis Intoxication. *American Heart Journal,* 83(2):150, February 1972.

SUGGESTED READINGS
Amsterdam, Ezra A., et al.: Systemic Approach to the Management of Cardiac Arrhythmias. *Heart and Lung,* 2(5):747–753, September–October 1973 (references).
Arbeit, Sidney, et al.: Recognizing Digitalis Toxicity. *American Journal of Nursing,* 77(12):1936–1945, December 1977 (references).
James, Frederick W., and Love, Ervena: Congestive Heart Failure in Infants. *Heart and Lung,* 3(3):396–400, May–June, 1974 (references).
Lely, A. H., and van Enter, C. H. J.: Noncardiac Symptoms of Digitalis Intoxication. *American Heart Journal,* 83(2):149–152, February 1972.
Rosen, Michael R., Wit, Andrew, and Hoffman, Brian F.: Electrophysiology and Pharmacology of Cardiac Arrhythmias. IV Cardiac Antiarrhythmic and Toxic Effects of Digitalis. *American Heart Journal,* 89(3):391–399, March 1975 Pages 391–399 (references).
———: Treatment of Cardiac Arrhythmias. *Medical Letter on Drugs and Therapeutics,* 16(25):101–108, December 6, 1974.

- **DEXAMETHASONE SODIUM PHOSPHATE** (Decadron Phosphate, Dexacen-4, Hexadrol Phosphate)

ACTIONS/ INDICATIONS	DOSAGE	PREPARATION AND STORAGE	DRUG INCOMPATIBILITIES	MODES OF IV ADMINISTRATION				CONTRAINDICATIONS; WARNINGS; PRECAUTIONS; ADVERSE REACTIONS
				INJECTION	INTERMITTENT INFUSION	CONTINUOUS INFUSION		
Adrenocorticosteroid, synthetic. Used in: • Endocrine disorders, especially adrenocortical sufficiency • Rheumatic disorders with inflammation • Collagen diseases • Dermatologic diseases • Allergy • Ophthalmic disorders with inflammation • Gastrointestinal diseases • Respiratory diseases • Hematologic diseases • Neoplastic diseases • Nephrotic syndrome	ADULTS AND CHILDREN: Dosage requirements are variable and must be individualized according to the disease, the condition of the patient and the response produced by the initial doses. Dosage may vary from day to day. Use the lowest dose possible. *Initial dose—* 0.5–20 mg/ day, given in divided doses every 12 hrs. Do not exceed 80 mg/day. (In shock, dosage may reach 3–6 mg/kg/day.)	Store at room temperature.	Infusions completed within 12 hours are stable with vitamins B and C, sodium bicarbonate, heparin, metraminol and tetracycline. Consider all other medications incompatible.	YES Inject over at least 30 seconds. No further dilution required. Rapid injection can produce premature ventricular contractions.	YES Use D5W or NS in any volume.	YES Use D5W or NS in any volume. Use this mode when constant maximal effect is desired.		CONTRAINDICATIONS 1. Hypersensitivity 2. Systemic fungal infections WARNINGS 1. Dosage should be increased prior to any unusual stress (surgery) and for a short time following. 2. Steroids mask some signs of infection. There may also be decreased resistance and inability to localize infection. 3. Average and large doses cause elevation of blood pressure, salt and water retention, and increased excretion of potassium and calcium. Appropriate diuretic and dietary therapy should be initiated. 4. Immunization procedures should not be carried out, especially for smallpox. 5. Latent tuberculosis may be reactivated, chemoprophylaxis should be ordered. 6. Anaphylaxis has occurred. 7. Use in pregnancy and lactation requires that benefits to the mother be weighed against risks to the fetus or nursing infant. 8. Patients with a stressed myocardium should be observed carefully and the drug administered slowly since premature ventricular contractions may occur with rapid administration.

• Cerebral edema
• Shock

Adrenocortical steroids have anti-inflammatory effects and affect electrolyte balance.

Maintenance—Initial dosage can be maintained if a favorable response is seen in a reasonable amount of time. After a response is obtained, the dosage should be decreased in small decrements until the lowest dosage is reached that produces the desired results.

PRECAUTIONS

1. There is an enhanced effect of corticosteroids in patients with hypothyroidism and cirrhosis; these patients will require lower dosage.
2. Psychic derangements may appear, ranging from euphoria, insomnia, personality changes, depression, to psychosis. Pre-existing problems may be aggravated.
3. Use aspirin with caution when a patient is on corticosteroids, to avoid gastric ulceration. Aspirin should also be used with caution with corticosteroids when the patient has hypoprothrombinemia.
4. Any antiulcer regimen including full theraputic dosage antacid therapy should be instituted.
5. This drug can decrease the number and motility of spermatozoa.
6. There may be an increase in diphenylhydantoin dosage requirements in patients concomitantly receiving that drug and steroids.
7. Steroids should be used with caution in nonspecific ulcerative colitis if there is a possibility of impending perforation or abscess, diverticulitis, fresh intestinal anastomoses, active or latent peptic ulcer, renal insufficiency, hypertension, osteoporosis, and myasthenia gravis.

ADVERSE REACTIONS SEEN IN SHORT-TERM INTRAVENOUS THERAPY

1. Fluid and electrolyte imbalances: sodium and water retention with possible secondary hypertension, hypokalemia, hypocalcemia.
2. Gastrointestinal: peptic ulcer with possible perforation, pancreatitis, ulcerative eosophagitis.
3. Dermatologic: impaired wound healing.
4. Neurologic: increased intracranial pressure, seizures (increasing frequency in patients with pre-existing seizure disorder), vertigo, headaches, mental confusion, euphoria, excerbation of psychosis.
5. Endocrine: decreased glucose tolerance, increased hypoglycemic agent and insulin requirements in diabetics.
6. Eye: increased intraocular pressure.
7. Metabolic: negative nitrogen balance secondary to rapid muscle catabolism.

● **DEXAMETHASONE SODIUM PHOSPHATE** (Decadron Phosphate, Dexacen-4, Hexadrol Phosphate) (*Continued*)

NURSING IMPLICATIONS

1. Take precautions to prevent infections in wounds by using strict aseptic technique in dressing changes, etc. Avoid traumatic procedures such as catheterizations. The skin may become more fragile because of the steroid therapy. Patients on bed rest and those with general body weakening secondary to an acute illness should be turned hourly (except during sleep, then every 2–3 hours) to prevent skin breakdown. Initiate the use of supportive measures such as flotation pads, water mattress, etc. Administer skin care to prevent infection.

2. Monitor blood pressure every 2–4 hours, or as the patient's condition dictates. Monitor blood pressure before, during and immediately after intravenous injection; hypotension can occur. In patients with cardiac disorders, monitor for premature ventricular contractions during and after injection. See Warning No. 8.

3. Weigh the patient daily to detect for water and sodium retention. Dietary restriction in sodium may be prescribed by the physician. Examine daily for peripheral edema.

4. There may be delayed healing of wounds; take precautions to prevent dehiscence. Sutures may be left in longer than usual for this reason.

5. Monitor urine glucose in patients on high-dose therapy and with diabetes. Diabetic individuals may require a larger dosage of insulin or oral agent.

6. Administer antacid therapy as ordered to assist in preventing peptic ulcer. Monitor for signs of the development of an ulcer and/or acute intestinal bleeding: melena, positive stool, hematemesis, epigastric pain and/or distention, anemia or falling hematocrit.

7. Monitor for signs and symptoms of hypokalemia:[1] weakness, irritability, abdominal distention, poor feeding in infants, muscle cramps. Dietary or pharmocologic potassium supplements may be ordered, guided by serum potassium levels.

8. Monitor for signs and symptoms of hypocalcemia (serum calcium less than 6 mg %):[2] irritability, change in mental status, seizures, nausea, vomiting, diarrhea, muscle cramps, late effects—cardiac arrhythmias, laryngeal spasm and apnea. Dietary or pharmacologic supplements may be ordered, guided by serum calcium levels.

9. Patients with a history of seizure activity may have an increasing number of seizures while on steroid therapy. Apply appropriate safety precautions.

10. Monitor for behavioral changes, which may range from simple euphoria to depression and phychosis. Apply appropriate safety precautions. A change in dosage may relieve such symptoms.

11. Tuberculin testing should be carried out prior to initiation of steroid therapy, if possible. The patient's reactivity to the tuberculin is altered by the drug, giving a false result.

12. Ambulate the patient with caution if vertigo occurs, and initiate the use of side rails to prevent patient injury. Report the onset to the physician.

13. Be alert to the signs of increasing intraocular pressure:[3] eye pain, rainbow vision, blurred vision, nausea and vomiting. Notify the physician immediately.

REFERENCES

1. Beeson, Paul, and McDermott, Walsh (editors): *Cecil-Loeb Textbook of Medicine* (14th ed.), Philadelphia: W. B. Saunders Company, 1975, p. 1587.
2. Ibid., p. 1815.
3. Newell, Frank W., and Ernest, J. Terry: *Opthalmology—Principles and Concepts* (3rd ed.), St. Louis: C. V. Mosby Company, 1974, p. 329.

SUGGESTED READINGS

Glasser, Ronald J.: How the Body Works Against Itself: Autoimmune Diseases. *Nursing '77*, September 1977, pp. 34–38.

Melick, Mary Evans: Nursing Intervention for Patients Receiving Corticosteroid Therapy. In *Advanced Concepts in Clinical Nursing* (2nd ed.), K. C. Kintzel, ed., Philadelphia: J. B. Lippincott Company, 1977, pp. 606–617.

Newton, David W., Nichols, Arlene and Newton, Marion: You Can Minimize the Hazards of Corticosteroids. *Nursing '77*, June 1977, pp. 26–33.

Reichgott, Michael J., and Melmon, Kenneth L.: The Role of Corticosteroids in Shock. In *Steroid Therapy*, Daniel Azarnoff, ed., Philadelphia, W. B. Saunders Company, 1975 pp. 118–133.

● **DEXPANTHENOL** (Ilopan)

ACTIONS/ INDICATIONS	DOSAGE	PREPARATION AND STORAGE	DRUG INCOMPATIBILITIES	MODES OF IV ADMINISTRATION			CONTRAINDICATIONS; WARNINGS; PRECAUTIONS; ADVERSE REACTIONS
				INJECTION	INTERMITTENT INFUSION	CONTINUOUS INFUSION	
Coenzyme A precursor. Converts to a compound essential to normal intestinal motility. For prophylactic use immediately after	ADULTS: 1–2 ml (250–500 mg) by slow infusion until symptoms subside. CHILDREN: 11 mg/kg. Administer as in adults.	Store at room temperature. Supplied in 2-ml and 10-ml vials (250 mg/ml), and disposable syringes of 2 ml (250 mg/ml).	Do not mix with any other medication in infusion fluid.	NO	NO	YES Slow infusion is the only acceptable mode of administration. Use D5W or RL. Add dose to 250–1000 ml	CONTRAINDICATIONS None known WARNINGS 1. There have been reports of allergic reactions when this drug is used concomitantly with antibiotics, narcotics, and barbiturates. 2. Do not administer full-strength into the vein.

major abdominal surgery to minimize the possibility of paralytic ileus.

Used to treat distention secondary to gas retention.

PRECAUTIONS
1. If the patient has received neostigmine or similar stimulation drugs, wait at least 12 hours before administering this drug.
2. These same patients should not receive this drug until 1 hour has passed after withdrawal of succinylcholine.
3. Do not use if ileus has a mechanical etiology.
4. Effectiveness is reduced in the presence of hypokalemia.

ADVERSE REACTIONS
Increased frequency of bowel movements

of fluid

Titrate with patient response.

NURSING IMPLICATIONS
1. Take anaphylaxis precautions: see page 118.
2. Monitor for drug effectiveness (i.e., active bowel sounds, expulsion of flatus or stool). If drug fails to relieve symptoms, or if ileus occurs while drug is being administered, discontinue the infusion and notify the physician at once.
3. Apply other means of preventing postoperative ileus; e.g, early ambulation.
4. Monitor stool count carefully in infants. Notify physician if diarrhea occurs.

● DEXTRAN-40 (Rheomacrodex, L.M.D. — Low Molecular Weight Dextran)

ACTIONS/INDICATIONS	DOSAGE	PREPARATION AND STORAGE	DRUG INCOMPATIBILITIES	MODES OF IV ADMINISTRATION			CONTRAINDICATIONS; WARNINGS; PRECAUTIONS; ADVERSE REACTIONS
				INJECTION	INTERMITTENT INFUSION	CONTINUOUS INFUSION	
A polymer of glucose that can simulate the colloidal properties of albumin, that is, draw fluid from the cellular and intercellular spaces into the blood to expand blood volume and thus increase blood pressure. Used as a *temporary* blood substitute in hemorrhagic and traumatic shock or shock due to burns until whole	Must be individualized based on amount of fluid lost, and resultant hemoconcentration. This preparation of dextran can expand plasma volume to almost twice the volume infused. This expansion decreases in 3–4 hrs. ADULTS AND CHILDREN: Do not exceed 20 ml/kg of a 10% solution in the first 24 hrs.	Supplied in 500-ml bottles, a 10% solution in NS or D5W. Solution may crystallize over time or when stored at a temperature greater than 25°C (77°F). If flakes are seen in solution, heat to 100°C (210°F) until dissolution occurs. Cool to body or room temperature before use. Store at a constant temperature, not over 25°C.	Do not mix with any other medication. Do not add medications to the solution bottle.	NO	YES First 500 ml can be infused rapidly; subsequent doses more slowly (20 ml/min)	YES Titrated with blood pressure or according to clinical need and dosage guidelines.	CONTRAINDICATIONS 1. Known hypersensitivity 2. Bleeding disorders due to qualitative or quantitative defects in clotting factors 3. Renal disease with oliguria or anuria 4. Oliguria secondary to hemorrhagic shock that does not improve after the first dose 5. Severe congestive heart failure WARNINGS 1. Anaphylaxis and other allergic reactions can occur but are less frequent than with the use of dextran-70; usually seen within first 15–20 minutes of infusion. 2. Administer nonosmotically active fluids to prevent dehydration and to maintain adequate urine output. 3. The renal excretion of dextran increases urine viscosity and specific gravity (minor elevation). 4. To assess the state of the patient's hydration, use serum or urine osmolari-

DEXTRAN-40 (Rheomacrodex, L.M.D. — Low Molecular Weight Dextran) (Continued)

ACTIONS/ INDICATIONS	DOSAGE	PREPARATION AND STORAGE	DRUG INCOMPAT- IBILITIES	MODES OF IV ADMINISTRATION			CONTRAINDICATIONS; WARNINGS: PRECAUTIONS; ADVERSE REACTIONS
				INJECTION	INTERMITTENT INFUSION	CONTINUOUS INFUSION	
blood and plasma can be given. May be used for priming of extra-corporeal circulation.[1] Also used in certain clinical situations to enhance microcirculation and to decrease platelet aggregation.	hrs. Subsequent doses on following days should not exceed 10 ml/kg. Do not extend infusions beyond 5 days. *Usual dose*—500 ml. *For extracorporeal priming* —10–20 ml/ kg. Do not exceed 20 ml/ kg.	Use only if seal is intact, solution is clear and vacuum is detectable.					ty. Administer additional fluids accordingly. 5. Mannitol may be used to maintain an adequate urine flow. 6. Renal failure occurring during use of dextran-40 has been reported. 7. Abnormal renal and hepatic function values can sometimes be seen following the use of dextran. The cause of this is unknown. 8. Administer with caution in the presence of hemorrhage. Increased blood pressure and microperfusion may increase bleeding. 9. Safety for use in pregnancy has not been established. PRECAUTIONS 1. Dosages of this drug at 15 ml/kg of body weight will cause a prolonged bleeding time, a decreased blood factor VIII, decreased fibrinogen, factor V and factor IX to a greater extent than with hemodilution alone. 2. Dextran may also facilitate lysis of fibrin by plasmin. 3. Watch for early signs of abnormal bleeding. 4. Infusion of this solution can cause circulatory overload. This is especially likely in patients with decreased renal clearance of the dextran. Use with caution in these patients and in patients who are susceptible to or have pre-existing congestive heart failure. 5. Falsely high blood glucose results may be seen when the laboratory uses a technique involving high concentrations of acids (sulfuric or acetic). 6. Dextran may interfere with blood-typing procedures. Obtain blood samples for typing before infusion. If this is not possible, inform the laboratory that the patient has been given dextran. 7. Prevent depression of the hematocrit below 30, by administering whole blood or packed RBC's. ADVERSE REACTIONS 1. Allergic reactions ranging from urtica-

ria to anaphylaxis; antihistamines may relieve mild allergic reactions
2. Nausea, vomiting, fever, joint pain
3. Renal failure (rare)

a. Fall in blood pressure
b. Rise in pulse rate
c. Rise in central venous pressure or pulmonary artery (wedge) pressure
d. Rises in respiratory rate and effort
e. Onset rales in the lungs
f. Fall in PaO_2;
Slow infusion and notify the physician immediately
4. Monitor for bleeding disorders:
a. Oozing at incision lines
b. Oozing at venipuncture sites
c. Bleeding from any orifice or drainage system
d. Fall in blood pressure, rise in pulse, diaphoresis, and other signs and symptoms of shock

REFERENCE
1. Buchanan, E. Clyde: Blood and Blood Substitutes for Treating Hemorrhagic Shock. *American Journal of Hospital Pharmacy*, 34:634, June 1977.

NURSING IMPLICATIONS
1. Monitor for anaphylaxis and discontinue infusion at the earliest signs, see page 118 for anaphylaxis precautions and treatment. Notify physician.
2. Monitor for effectiveness of infusion when used in the treatment of shock:
a. Blood pressure (direct arterial or indirect), frequency depending on the clinical situation
b. Heart and respiratory rate (should decrease as blood pressure rises)
c. If available, pulmonary artery pressure (preferable) or CVP to assess the expansion of blood volume, and the heart's ability to pump
d. Urine output (at least hourly). Output should increase with the blood pressure (to at least 30 ml/hour). If it has not after the first 500 ml of dextran has infused, notify the physician and do not infuse dextran without further orders
e. Specific gravity of urine; if specific gravity does not decrease with increased urine output, or if a high value (greater than 1.030) is accompanied by oliguria, discontinue infusion and notify physician. Keep the patient hydrated with nonosmotically active fluids (D5W, RL, NS)
3. Monitor for onset of cardiac failure:

● DEXTRAN-70 (Macrodex)

ACTIONS/ INDICATIONS	DOSAGE	PREPARATION AND STORAGE	DRUG INCOMPAT- IBILITIES	MODES OF IV ADMINISTRATION			CONTRAINDICATIONS; WARNINGS; PRECAUTIONS; ADVERSE REACTIONS
				INJECTION	INTERMITTENT INFUSION	CONTINUOUS INFUSION	
Polymer of glucose that can simulate the colloidal properties of albumin, that is, draw fluid from the cellular and intercellular spaces into the blood to expand blood volume and thus increase blood pressure. Used as a *temporary* blood substitute in hemorrhagic shock, shock due to burns, or trauma, un-	Must be individualized, based on the amount of fluid lost and the resultant hemoconcentration. ADULTS: Do not exceed 20 ml/kg in the first 24 hrs, and 10 ml/kg thereafter. *Usual dose—* 500 ml. CHILDREN: Do not exceed 20 ml/kg in the first 24 hrs or 10 ml/kg	Supplied in 500-ml bottles, a 6% solution, in NS or D5W. This solution may crystallize if stored for long periods. If flakes are present, heat to 100°C (210°F) until dissolution occurs. Cool to body temperature before using. Store away from extremes of temperature. Use only if seal is intact, solution is clear,	Do not mix with any other medication. Do not add any medication to solution bottle.	NO	YES At a rate of 20–40 ml/ min, titrated with blood pressure or other clinically appropriate parameter.	YES At a rate of 20–40 ml/ min, titrated with blood pressure or other clinically appropriate parameter.	CONTRAINDICATIONS 1. Known hypersensitivity 2. Bleeding disorders due to qualitative or quantitative defects in clotting factors 3. Renal disease with oliguria or anuria 4. Oliguria secondary to hemorrhagic shock that does not improve after the first dose 5. Severe congestive heart failure WARNINGS 1. Anaphylaxis can occur, usually during the first 15–20 minutes of the infusion. 2. May interfere with platelet adhesiveness, resulting in a transient prolonged bleeding time, especially in doses greater than 1000 ml. 3. Prevent depression of the hematocrit below 30 secondary to hemodilution by administering whole blood or packed RBC's. 4. When large volumes are given, plas-

DEXTRAN-70 (Macrodex) (Continued)

ACTIONS/INDICATIONS	DOSAGE	PREPARATION AND STORAGE	DRUG INCOMPATIBILITIES	MODES OF IV ADMINISTRATION			CONTRAINDICATIONS; WARNINGS; PRECAUTIONS; ADVERSE REACTIONS
				INJECTION	INTERMITTENT INFUSION	CONTINUOUS INFUSION	
til whole blood or plasma can be given. This form of dextran increases plasma volume by slightly more than the volume infused, depending on fluid available to be drawn into the vascular space, and the rate of dextran clearance in the kidney.[1] This agent is also known to enhance microcirculation and to decrease platelet aggregation.	thereafter each 24 hrs.	and vacuum detectable.					ma protein levels will be decreased. 5. Safety for use in pregnancy has not been established. PRECAUTIONS 1. Dosages of this drug at 15 ml/kg of body weight will cause a prolonged bleeding time, a decreased blood factor VIII, decreased fibrinogen, factor V and factor IX to a greater extent than with hemodilution alone. 2. Dextran may also facilitate lysis of fibrin by plasmin. 3. Watch for early signs of abnormal bleeding. 4. Infusion of this solution can cause circulatory overload. This is especially likely in patients with decreased renal clearance of the dextran. Use with caution in these patients and in patients who are susceptible to or have pre-existing congestive heart failure. 5. Falsely high blood glucose results may be seen when the laboratory uses a technique involving high concentrations of acids (sulfuric or acetic). 6. Dextran may interfere with blood-typing procedures. Obtain blood samples for typing before infusion. If this is not possible, inform the laboratory that the patient has been given dextran. ADVERSE REACTIONS 1. Allergic reactions ranging from urticaria to anaphylaxis; antihistamines may relieve mild allergic reactions 2. Nausea, vomiting, fever, joint pain

NURSING IMPLICATIONS

1. Monitor for anaphylaxis and discontinue infusion at the earliest signs; see page 118 for anaphylaxis precautions and treatment. Notify physician.
2. Monitor for effectiveness of infusion when used in the treatment of shock:
   a. Blood pressure (direct arterial or indirect), frequency depending on the clinical situation
   b. Heart and respiratory rate (should decrease as blood pressure rises)
   c. If available, pulmonary artery pressure (preferable) or CVP to assess the expansion of blood volume, and the heart's ability to pump
   d. Urine output (at least hourly). Output should increase with the blood pressure (to at least 30 ml/hour). If it has not after the first 500 ml of

pansion:
   a. Fall in blood pressure
   b. Rise in pulse
   c. Rise in central venous pressure or pulmonary artery (wedge) pressure
   d. Rise in respiratory rate and effort
   e. Rales in the lungs
   f. Fall in PaO$_2$
   Slow infusion and notify the physician immediately.
4. Monitor for bleeding disorders:
   a. Oozing at incision lines
   b. Oozing at venipuncture sites

dextran has infused, notify the physician and do not infuse dextran without further orders
e. Specific gravity of urine; if specific gravity does not decrease with increased urine output, or if a high value (greater than 1.030) is accompanied by oliguria, discontinue infusion and notify physician. Keep the patient hydrated with nonosmotically active fluids (D5W, RL, NS)
3. Monitor for onset of cardiac failure that can be precipitated by volume ex-

c. Bleeding from any orifice or drainage system
d. Worsening signs and symptoms of shock.

REFERENCE
1. Buchanan, E. Clyde: Blood and Blood Substitutes for Treating Hemorrhagic Shock. *American Journal of Hospital Pharmacy,* 34:634, June 1977.

DIAZEPAM (Valium)

ACTIONS/ INDICATIONS	DOSAGE	PREPARATION AND STORAGE	DRUG INCOMPAT- IBLITIES	MODES OF IV ADMINISTRATION			CONTRAINDICATIONS; WARNINGS; PRECAUTIONS; ADVERSE REACTIONS
				INJECTION	INTERMITTENT INFUSION	CONTINUOUS INFUSION	
Short-acting CNS depressant, tranquilizer, anticonvulsant, skeletal muscle relaxant. Used in symptomatic relief of tension and anxiety states, psychoneurotic states. In acute alcohol withdrawal, it may be useful in relieving agitation, tremor, impending or overt delirium tremens. For endoscopic or operative procedures to decrease anxiety and recall. Adjunct to the treatment of status epilepticus and recurrent seizures. In tetanus, as a muscle relaxant.	Dosage must be individualized according to age and the condition being treated. ADULTS AND OLDER CHILDREN (OVER 12): 2–20 mg every 3–4 hrs. Use lower doses (2–5 mg) in the elderly or when other sedatives are used. Maximum of 30 mg in 8 hrs. INFANTS OVER 30 DAYS OF AGE AND CHILDREN UP TO 5 YEARS: *Tetanus*—1–2 mg, repeated every 3–4 hrs, as needed to control spasms. *Status epilepticus and recurrent seizures*—0.2	Do not mix with IV solutions; the drug precipitates. It is not currently known what effect the crystallized drug may have in the body. Protect vials from light in manufacturer's box.	Do not mix with any other medication.	YES Only acceptable mode of administration. Inject, undiluted, directly into the vein, cannula or into an IV tubing injection site that is *immediately* above the junction between the cannula and the tubing. This prevents the drug from mixing with fluid. After injection flush vein and tubing with NS to prevent thrombophlebitis. Inject *slowly,* no more rapidly than 5 mg/ min.	NO Drug will precipitate upon dilution in *any* solution.	NO Drug will precipitate upon dilution in *any* solution.	CONTRAINDICATIONS 1. Known hypersensitivity 2. Acute narrow-angle glaucoma; and open-angle glaucoma unless controlled by appropriate therapy 3. Parenterally in children under 30 days of age 4. In the presence of jaundice in children WARNINGS 1. Procedures must be applied to prevent venous thrombosis, tissue and vascular damage: a. Inject slowly: 1 minute for each 5 mg b. Use large veins c. Avoid intra-arterial administration d. Prevent extravasation e. Flush vein with NS following injection 2. Do not mix with intravenous solutions. 3. Extreme caution must be exercised when administering to patients with limited pulmonary reserve, to prevent apnea and cardiac arrest. 4. Concomitant use of barbiturates or other central nervous system depressants increases the risk of apnea. Respiratory support equipment must be readily available. 5. Do not administer to patients in shock, coma, or in acute alcoholic intoxication with depression of vital signs. 6. Use in pregnancy: There is an increased risk of congenital malformation associated with the use of this drug during the first trimester. Use

DIAZEPAM (Valium) (Continued)

ACTIONS/INDICATIONS	DOSAGE	PREPARATION AND STORAGE	DRUG INCOMPATIBILITIES	MODES OF IV ADMINISTRATION			CONTRAINDICATIONS; WARNINGS; PRECAUTIONS; ADVERSE REACTIONS
				INJECTION	INTERMITTENT INFUSION	CONTINUOUS INFUSION	
	—0.5 mg slowly, every 2–5 min. up to a maximum of 5 mg.						must be avoided.
							7. This drug enters cord blood. Obstetrical use is not recommended.
	CHILDREN 5 YEARS OR OLDER:						8. Use in children: Safety for use in infants less than 30 days of age has not been established. Use in older infants has been associated with prolonged central nervous system depression secondary to an inability to metabolize the drug.
	Tetanus—5–10 mg every 3–4 hrs. as needed to control spasms.						9. Apnea and hypotension can result from rapid injection.
	Status epilepticus and recurrent seizures—1 mg every 2–5 min. up to a maximum of 10 mg. slowly, every 2–4 hrs.						10. When diazepam is administered with a narcotic analgesic, the dosage of either drug must be reduced and administered with caution.
							11. Tonic status epilepticus has been precipitated in patients treated with IV diazepam for petit mal status or petit mal variant status.

PRECAUTIONS
1. Do not use for *maintenance* control of seizures.
2. Certain other drugs may potentiate the action of this drug, such as phenothiazines, narcotics, barbiturates, MAO inhibitors and antidepressants. Hypotension and severe muscle weakness may occur.
3. In highly anxious patients with accompanying depression, protective measures should be taken to prevent suicidal behavior.
4. Patients with impaired liver or renal function will require reduced dosage and monitoring for signs of toxicity for longer periods of time. This also applies to elderly and debilitated patients.
5. There may be an increase in the cough reflex and a greater likelihood of laryngospasm in per oral endoscopic procedures. Topical anesthetics should be used and countermeasures available.
6. Abrupt withdrawal after several days administration can precipitate convulsions and delirium.

ADVERSE REACTIONS

1. Thrombophlebitis at IV injection site
2. Central nervous system disturbances: drowsiness, fatigue, ataxia, depression, slurred speech, syncope, vertigo
3. Genitourinary: incontinence, urinary retention
4. Respiratory depression with large doses, can lead to apnea
5. Cardiovascular: bradycardia, hypotension, shock (most often with rapid injection)
6. Blurred vision, diplopia, and nystagmus
7. Skin rash and urticaria
8. Psychological: paradoxical reactions such as hyperexcited states, anxiety, confusion, insomnia. If any of these occur, the drug should be discontinued.
9. Hepatic: jaundice
10. Hematologic: neutropenia
11. In peroral endoscopic procedures, coughing, depressed respiration, dyspnea, hyperventilation, laryngospasm and pain in the throat or chest have been reported

NURSING IMPLICATIONS

1. Respiratory depression is the greatest hazard associated with intravenous administration of this drug. The respiratory status of all patients must be monitored frequently during the first few hours after injection:
   a. Count the respiratory rate every 2–5 minutes for the first 30 minutes and then every 15 minutes for the next hour and one-half.
   b. Observe for pallor or cyanosis of the mucous membranes and nail beds during this time.
   c. Be prepared to provide respiratory support. Have oxygen, suction equipment, an airway and manual breathing bag at the bedside ready for use. Endotracheal tubes and laryngoscope should also be readily available.
   d. Do not leave the patient unattended during the first hour after injection.
   e. Respiratory depression is more likely to occur in the following types of patients: those with pre-existing cardiac, pulmonary, renal, hepatic or neuromuscular disease (myasthenia gravis); patients with chest trauma or deformities; patients who have received other respiratory depressing drugs (see Precaution No. 2); and the elderly or very young.
2. If respiratory depression occurs, i.e., if the respiratory rate falls below 8/minute in an adult (see chart on page 545 for normal respiratory rates in children), take the following actions:
   a. If the patient can be aroused, verbally instruct him to breathe; repeat command to produce a respiratory rate of 10–12/minute.
   b. Stay with the patient until depressant effects have subsided.
   c. If the patient cannot be aroused, maintain an open airway and ventilate the patient with the manual breathing bag at a rate of 10–12/minute. The physician will determine whether the patient requires intubation. If cyanosis is present, begin administration of oxygen via the breathing bag.
3. Monitor blood pressure every 15–30 minutes during the first 2 hours following injection. If hypotension occurs, notify the physician and place the patient in a Trendelenburg position if it is not contraindicated. Vasopressors may be prescribed.
4. The patient should be kept at bed rest for the first 2 hours after injection. Ambulate with caution thereafter.
5. Monitor for urinary retention in susceptible patients (those with a history of prostatic hypertrophy or urethral stricture). Palpate bladder size every 4 hours and monitor urinary output.
6. Monitor psychiatric patients for exacerbation of depression or anxiety, take suicide precautions as indicated.
7. If this drug is used to control ventilation in the patient on a respirator:
   a. Because the patient will be respirator-dependent following a ventilation-controlling dose, check respirator connections frequently; they must be tight
   b. Set all available respirator alarm systems (apnea and pressure-sensitive) and keep them in continual operation
   c. Check arterial blood gases frequently for adequacy of ventilation
   d. Some hospital policies require constant attendance of a registered nurse for such patients

279

● **DIAZOXIDE** (Hyperstat IV)

ACTIONS/ INDICATIONS	DOSAGE	PREPARATION AND STORAGE	DRUG INCOMPAT- IBILITIES	MODES OF IV ADMINISTRATION				CONTRAINDICATIONS; WARNINGS; PRECAUTIONS; ADVERSE REACTIONS
				INJECTION	INTERMITTENT INFUSION	CONTINUOUS INFUSION		
Rapid-acting antihypertensive agent. Produces prompt reduction in blood pressure by relaxing the smooth muscles in the peripheral arterioles. Cardiac output increases; coronary and cerebral blood flow is maintained. Renal blood flow is increased. Pressure falls within one minute. Effect lasts less than 12 hours. Is indicated in the emergency reduction of blood pressure in malignant hypertension in hospitalized patients, when prompt reduction is needed.	ADULTS: Administer only in *peripheral* veins. With patient recumbent, inject 300 mg over 15 seconds time. If first dose fails to reduce pressure within 30 min, administer second dose (furosemide 40 mg is usually given with the second dose). Repeat as necessary at 4- to 24-hr intervals. CHILDREN, SMALL, OR VERY LARGE ADULTS: 5 mg/kg.[1] Follow directions above for administration.	Protect from light. Store away from heat or extreme cold. Do not use darkened solutions. Supplied in 20-ml ampuls (300 mg), 15 mg/ml.	Do not mix with any other medication.	YES Only effective when injected rapidly. Administer undiluted.	NO The drug must be injected rapidly. Slow rates and dilution are less effective in reducing blood pressure.	NO The drug must be injected rapidly. Slow rates and dilution are less effective in reducing blood pressure.		CONTRAINDICATIONS 1. Do not use in the treatment of compensatory hypertension associated with coarctation of the aorta or arteriovenous shunt. 2. Do not use in patients hypersensitive to diazoxide or other thiazide derivatives, unless possible benefits outweigh the risks. 3. Dissecting aortic aneurysm. WARNINGS 1. Safety for use in pregnancy has not been established. 2. Information is not available concerning the passage of diazoxide in breast milk. The drug does cross the placental barrier to appear in cord blood and can produce fetal or neonatal hyperbilirubinemia, thrombocytopenia, altered carbohydrate metabolism and other adverse effects. When given for eclampsia, this drug may stop labor; oxytocin may be used in this event. 3. Safety for use in children has not been established (see Dosage column). 4. Hypotension may (rarely) result from administration of this drug. If it occurs and requires therapy, it usually responds to sympathomimetic agents (norepinephrine). 5. Hyperglycemia occurs in the majority of patients but usually requires treatment only in patients with diabetes mellitus. It responds to insulin. 6. Cataracts have been reported after repeated daily doses. 7. This drug causes sodium retention. Repeated doses may cause edema and precipitate congestive heart failure. If adequate renal function exists, diuretics will remedy this. 8. Concurrently administered thiazide diuretics may potentiate the antihypertensive, hyperglycemic and hyperuricemic effects of diazoxide. 9. When diazoxide is administered with propranolol or to a patient recently treated with propranolol or guanethidine, its dose must be lower than

usual to prevent possible excessive hypotension.[2]

10. Effectiveness of diazoxide will be improved if extracellular fluid is shifted into the vascular compartment and eliminated with the use of a diuretic such as furosemide.

11. Patients concomitantly on coumarin or its derivatives may require a reduction in the anticoagulant dose.

12. Hypertensive crises due to pheochromocytoma or monoamine oxidase inhibitor therapy should not be treated by diazoxide; these conditions respond more specifically to an alpha-adrenergic receptor blocking drug such as phentolamine.[3]

PRECAUTIONS

1. Close monitoring of the patient's blood pressure must be carried out. Hypotension may occur and may require treatment (see Warning No. 4).

2. Use only peripheral veins for injection, avoid extravasation. If extravasation occurs, treat conservatively.

3. Rapid injection is required for effective antihypertensive action; slower injection will fail to reduce the blood pressure or will produce only a brief response.

4. Use with caution in patients with impaired cerebral or cardiac circulation. When abrupt reduction in blood pressure occurs, may cause ischemia.

5. Use with caution in patients with renal impairment or congestive heart failure because of the salt and water retention induced by this drug.

6. Patients with impaired renal function usually do not require a reduction in dosage.

7. Use with caution in patients with diabetes mellitus; there may be a transient rise in blood glucose. This is treatable with insulin. Nondiabetic patients will also show a rise in glucose, which is transient.

8. Hemo- and peritoneal dialysis will remove some diazoxide from the blood. These patients will require more than one injection.

ADVERSE REACTIONS
Frequently seen:
1. Sodium and water retention after repeated injections
2. Hyperglycemia

DIAZOXIDE (Hyperstat IV) (Continued)

ACTIONS/ INDICATIONS	DOSAGE	PREPARATION AND STORAGE	DRUG INCOMPATIBILITIES	MODES OF IV ADMINISTRATION			CONTRAINDICATIONS; WARNINGS; PRECAUTIONS; ADVERSE REACTIONS
				INJECTION	INTERMITTENT INFUSION	CONTINUOUS INFUSION	

CONTRAINDICATIONS; WARNINGS; PRECAUTIONS; ADVERSE REACTIONS

Infrequently seen:
1. Hypotension to shock levels
2. Transient myocardial ischemia which may lead to infarction, manifested by angina, atrial and ventricular arrhythmias, and ST segment changes
3. Cerebral ischemia, usually transient, but possibly leading to thrombosis, manifested by unconsciousness, seizures, paralysis, confusion or focal neurologic deficits
4. Increased BUN
5. Sensitivity reactions such as rashes, leukopenia, fever

Other reactions:
1. Extensive vasodilation
2. Postural hypotension
3. Bradycardia, tachycardia
4. Headache
5. Tightness in the chest and nonanginal chest discomfort
6. Many other somatic sensations

fall in blood pressure not related to medication administration
d. Left ventricular failure: shortness of breath, orthopnea, elevated central venous pressure, tachycardia, onset of third and/or fourth heart sounds, rales
e. Renal failure: oliguria, rising BUN.[4]
These complications can also occur if the blood pressure is overly reduced by medication.
12. After the hypertensive emergency has passed, the patient will require intensive hypertension education and follow-up to prevent subsequent crises and complications.

REFERENCES
1. Koch-Weser, Jan: Diazoxide. *New England Journal of Medicine,* 294(23): 1272, June 3, 1976.
2. Ibid.
3. Ibid.
4. Romankiewicz, J. A.: Pharmacology and Clinical Use of Drugs in Hypertensive Emergencies. *American Journal of Hospital Pharmacy,* 34(2):185, February 1977.

SUGGESTED READINGS
American Medical Association Committee on Hypertension: The Treatment of Malignant Hypertension and Hypertensive Emergencies, *JAMA,* 228:1673–1679, 1974.
Dhar, Sisir K., and Freeman, Philip: Clinical Management of Hypertensive Emergencies. *Heart and Lung,* 5(4):571–575, July–August 1976 (references).
Fleischmann, L. E.: Management of Hypertensive Crises in Children. *Pediatric*

NURSING IMPLICATIONS
1. Of primary importance is the frequent monitoring of the blood pressure. Generally, blood pressure starts to decrease within 1 minute. The lowest blood pressure will be reached within 2–5 minutes. The pressure will rise rapidly over the next 10–30 minutes, and then more slowly over the following 2–12 hours, reaching but rarely exceeding pretreatment levels.
2. During the first 10 minutes, record the blood pressure at least once every 1–2 minutes; then once every 5 minutes over the next hour; followed by once every hour for the next 2 hours; then once every 2 hours for the 2 hours and finally once every 4 hours for the next 12 hours. This cycle should only be interrupted by additional injections, at which time the cycle should begin again.
3. The patient should be kept recumbent during and for at least 1 hour after an injection. Check the lying and standing pressures before allowing a patient to become ambulatory. If there is a significant fall of pressure on standing, keep the patient at bed rest for an additional hour. Recheck lying and standing pressures again. Warn the patient against standing rapidly from bed or chair. (See No. 11).
4. Monitor for signs and symptoms of fluid and sodium retention in patients with a history of congestive heart failure or renal impairment:
   a. Increased weight (weigh daily)
   b. Rise in heart rate (take pulse every 4 hours)
   c. Dyspnea, orthopnea, rales, onset of third and/or fourth heart sound
   d. Rising jugular venous distension
   e. Peripheral pitting edema
   f. Decreased urinary output (record every 4–8 hours)
5. Nausea and vomiting occur frequently. Be prepared to prevent aspiration.
6. Do not leave the patient alone during the first hour, and then only when

Annals, 6(6):410–414, June 1977.

Jones, L. N.: Symposium on Teaching and Rehabilitation of the Cardiac Patient. Hypertension: Medical and Nursing Implications. *Nursing Clinics of North America,* 11:283–295, June 1976.

Keith, Thomas: Hypertension Crisis, Recognition and Management. *JAMA,* 237(15):1570–1577, April 11, 1977.

Koch-Weser, Jan: Diazoxide. *New England Journal of Medicine,* 294(23):1271–1274, June 3, 1976 (references).

———: Hypertensive Emergencies. *New England Journal of Medicine,* 290:211, 1974.

Long, M. L., et al.: Hypertension: What the Patient Needs to Know. *American Journal of Nursing,* 76:765–770, May 1976.

McDonald, W. J., et al.: Intravenous Diazoxide Therapy in Hypertensive Crisis. *American Journal of Cardiology,* 40(3):409–415, September 1977.

Romankiewicz, J. A.: Pharmacology and Clinical Use of Drugs in Hypertensive Emergencies. *American Journal of Hospital Pharmacy,* 34(2):185–193, February 1977 (references).

Tanner, Gloria: Heart Failure in the MI Patient. *American Journal of Nursing,* 77:230–234, February 1977 (discusses signs and symptoms of the onset of congestive heart failure).

vital signs have stabilized.

7. Be prepared to treat hypotension:
   a. Trendelenberg position
   b. A vasopressor should be on hand
   c. Fluids
8. Prevent extravasation (see page 96).
9. Monitor urine fractionals in diabetic patients during the first 24 hours. Insulin coverage may be ordered.
10. Monitor for the onset of cardiac problems. Instruct the patient to report chest pain of any type, or palpitations. Patients with a history of arrhythmias or previous myocardial infarction should be observed continuously via a bedside ECG monitor. Be prepared to treat arrhythmias:
    a. Drugs: lidocaine, atropine, oxygen
    b. An open intravenous line
    c. Defibrillator
11. Patients in hypertensive crisis should be kept at rest in bed. Monitor for the consequences of an acute and extreme elevation of blood pressure:
    a. Encephalopathy: confusion, stupor
    b. Cerebrovascular accident
    c. Myocardial ischemia and/or infarction: chest pain, arrhythmias, sudden

DIETHYLSTILBESTEROL DIPHOSPHATE (Stilphostrol)

ACTIONS/INDICATIONS	DOSAGE	PREPARATION AND STORAGE	DRUG INCOMPATIBILITIES	MODES OF IV ADMINISTRATION			CONTRAINDICATIONS; WARNINGS; PRECAUTIONS; ADVERSE REACTIONS
				INJECTION	INTERMITTENT INFUSION	CONTINUOUS INFUSION	
Synthetic estrogen. A potent, long-lasting nonsteroidal estrogen. Used for palliative treatment of prostatic and male breast cancer, estrogen-deficiency states, stimulation of secondary sex characteristics at puberty, postpartum suppression of lactation, amenorrhea, dysmenorrhea, hemostasis in uterine bleeding.	ADULTS ONLY: 500 mg on first day, followed by 1 gm daily for 5 days. *Maintenance*—250–500 mg, 1–2 times weekly.	Add only to D5W or NS for infusion.	Do not mix with any other medication.	NO	YES Usually 0.5 gm in 300 ml NS or D5W at a rate of 20–30 macrodrops/min during the first 10–15 min, and then at a rate so that the entire amount is given in 1 hour.	NO	CONTRAINDICATIONS 1. Markedly impaired liver function 2. Thrombophlebitis, thromboembolic disorders, cerebral thrombosis or embolism, or past history of any one of these disorders WARNINGS 1. Do not administer during pregnancy; it may cause vaginal cancer in female offspring. 2. Avoid use in presence of cancerous or precancerous lesions of the breast or genital tract in females unless the patient is at least 5 years postmenopausal. 3. Administer with caution to patients with a history of thrombophlebitis, thromboembolism, asthma, epilepsy, migraine, congestive heart failure, renal insufficiency, calcium or phosphorus metabolism problems. This drug may precipitate an acute exacerbation of these disorders. 4. Do not give to patients with blood dyscrasias, hepatic disease, or thyroid dysfunction.

DIETHYLSTILBESTEROL DIPHOSPHATE (Stilphostrol) (Continued)

ACTIONS/INDICATIONS	DOSAGE	PREPARATION AND STORAGE	DRUG INCOMPAT-IBILITIES	MODES OF IV ADMINISTRATION			CONTRAINDICATIONS; WARNINGS; PRECAUTIONS; ADVERSE REACTIONS
				INJECTION	INTERMITTENT INFUSION	CONTINUOUS INFUSION	

CONTRAINDICATIONS; WARNINGS; PRECAUTIONS; ADVERSE REACTIONS

5. Do not administer in patients who have not completed bone growth.
6. Discontinue therapy at the earliest sign of thrombophlebitis, cerebrovascular disorders, pulmonary embolism or retinal thrombosis.
7. Discontinue therapy at onset of proptosis (of the eye), double vision, migraine headache. If an examination reveals papilledema or retinal vascular lesions, do not restart therapy.
8. There may be a decrease in glucose tolerance; monitor diabetic patients carefully.
9. Certain liver and endocrine function tests may be affected by treatment with estrogen. If such tests are abnormal in a patient taking this drug, it is recommended that they be repeated after the drug has been withdrawn for 2 months.

ADVERSE REACTIONS
1. Gastrointestinal: anorexia, nausea, vomiting, diarrhea, cholestatic jaundice
2. Central nervous system: headache, malaise, depression, anxiety, dizziness
3. Breast engorgement (male and female)
4. Hypersensitivity reactions including anaphylaxis
5. Renal: salt and water retention, edema, rise in BUN
6. Skin: acne, purpura, hair loss, erythema nodosum, itching
7. Endometrial hyperplasia and bleeding have been reported in prolonged use of the drug
8. In males, gynecomastia, decreased libido, arrest of spermatogenesis, and testicular atrophy (usually only seen with prolonged use)
9. This drug may increase the incidence of thrombophlebitis, pulmonary embolism, cerebral thrombosis, coronary thrombosis, neuro-ocular lesions

NURSING IMPLICATIONS
1. Monitor for signs and symptoms of:
   a. Thrombophlebitis—pain, swelling, positive Homan's sign in the legs
   b. Cerebral thrombosis—change in mental status, weakness and numb-

   c. Increased respiratory rate, dyspnea, orthopnea
   d. Rales
   e. Increased heart rate
   f. Increased distention of the jugular veins

ness of the face or extremities, seizures

  c. Coronary thrombosis—chest pain, diaphoresis, fall in blood pressure
  d. Neuro-ocular lesions—changes in vision
  Report findings immediately to the physician; hold the next dose of the drug until further instructions from the physician.
2. There may be an increase in seizure activity; take seizure precautions when appropriate.
3. Monitor vulnerable patients for exacerbation of congestive heart failure secondary to fluid retention in susceptible patients:
  a. Increased weight
  b. Peripheral edema
4. Monitor patients with renal insufficiency for signs of worsening of the condition:
  a. Weigh daily
  b. Record intake and output every 8 hours. Compare findings with pretherapy values; report changes to the physician.
  c. Be aware of the patient's pretherapy BUN and changes during therapy
5. Notify the physician immediately at the onset of proptosis (downward displacement of the eyeball; double vision, migraine headache, head pain accompanied by visual changes, nausea, vomiting). The drug should be discontinued.

● DIGITOXIN (Digitaline, Crystodigin)

ACTIONS/ INDICATIONS	DOSAGE	PREPARATION AND STORAGE	DRUG INCOMPATIBILITIES	MODES OF IV ADMINISTRATION			CONTRAINDICATIONS; WARNINGS; PRECAUTIONS; ADVERSE REACTIONS
				INJECTION	INTERMITTENT INFUSION	CONTINUOUS INFUSION	
Cardiac glycoside; increases the force of myocardial contraction (positive inotropic effect), slows the discharge of the sinus node, slows conduction through the A-V node by its effect on the refractory period of these tissues via the autonomic nervous system.

After IV injection, therapeutic action starts in 25 minutes to 2 hours, peaks in 4–12 hours, and falls in 2–3 days. Effects are nil after 2–3 weeks.

Used in the treatment of all degrees of | ADULTS: *Digitalizing dose for rapid digitalization*— 0.6 mg initially, followed by 0.4 mg and then 0.2 mg at intervals of 4–6 hrs. A single digitalizing dose is not recommended. Average total digitalizing dose: 1.2–1.6 mg.

Maintenance —0.05–0.3 mg daily.

Dosage must be reduced in the presence of myocardial fibrosis, conduction defects, or renal failure.

INFANTS AND CHILDREN: *Digitalizing Doses* Newborns un- | Supplied in ampuls of 1 ml, 0.2 mg/ml. Do not add to IV fluids; this drug is unstable when diluted. | Do not mix with any other medication. | YES

Inject as close to the IV cannula as possible, either into the cannula hub or into the Y injection site closest to the vein. Inject SLOWLY. | NO

Do not mix with IV fluids. | NO

Do not mix with IV fluids. | CONTRAINDICATIONS
1. Ventricular tachycardia or fibrillation
2. Digitalis intoxication, known or suspected
3. Hypersensitivity to cardiac glycosides

WARNINGS
1. Many of the arrhythmias for which digitoxin is indicated can be caused by digitalis intoxication.
2. Patients receiving this drug who are in congestive heart failure may complain of nausea and vomiting. These symptoms must be differentiated from intoxication by further studies. Do not administer the drug until intoxication has been ruled out.
3. This drug is usually not given in the presence of idiopathic hypertrophic subaortic stenosis.
4. Administer with caution to patients adults and children with glomerulonephritis and congestive heart failure. Low total dosage, divided, with the concomitant use of reserpine or other antihypertensive, is recommended. Monitor ECG constantly, arrhythmias are likely to occur.
5. Patients with rheumatic carditis are usually very sensitive to this drug. Reduce dosage and monitor ECG. If this drug fails to produce improvement after trial doses, discontinue.
6. Premature, immature or infants with renal failure are very sensitive to digitalis titrate dosage carefully. |

DIGITOXIN (Digitaline, Crystodigin) (Continued)

ACTIONS/ INDICATIONS	DOSAGE	PREPARATION AND STORAGE	DRUG INCOMPAT- IBILITIES	MODES OF IV ADMINISTRATION			CONTRAINDICATIONS; WARNINGS; PRECAUTIONS; ADVERSE REACTIONS
				INJECTION	INTERMITTENT INFUSION	CONTINUOUS INFUSION	
congestive heart failure; to control, by slowing the conduction rate to the ventricles and by slowing discharge in the atria, atrial flutter and fibrillation and paroxysmal tachycardia; and used in cardiogenic shock, especially when there is accompanying pulmonary edema.	der 2 weeks, premature infants and those with reduced renal function or myocarditis— 0.022 mg/kg (0.30–0.35 mg/M²) *Under 1 year* —0.045 mg/ kg *1–2 years*— 0.040 mg/kg *Over 2 years*— 0.03 mg/kg This total dose should be divided into 3, 4 or more portions, and given with 6 or more hours between doses. The maintenance dose should be ¹⁄₁₀ of the digitalizing dose.						PRECAUTIONS 1. Administer with caution if the patient has recently received this or other digitalis preparations. 2. Administer with caution in the presence of hypercalcemia. 3. Administer with caution in the presence of premature ventricular contractions or any form of heart block. 4. Patients receiving any form of digitalis should not receive intravenous calcium. 5. Hypokalemia produced by diarrhea, thiazide diuretics, corticosteroids, hemodialysis, or any other cause sensitizes the heart to digitalis intoxication and may produce arrhythmias at normal doses. It also decreases the positive inotropic effect of the drug. 6. Patients with acute myocardial infarction, severe pulmonary disease, or advanced heart disease will be more sensitive to digitalis and more prone to arrhythmias. 7. Reduce dosage in myxedema and renal and hepatic failure. ADVERSE REACTIONS (Chiefly due to Overdosage) 1. Anorexia, nausea, vomiting, diarrhea 2. Mental depression, restlessness, headache, weakness, visual disturbances, confusion 3. Nearly any disturbance in cardiac rhythm can be produced by digitalis; the most common are premature contractions (atrial and ventricular), heart block, and sinus bradycardia 4. Gynecomastia (rare) TREATMENT OF DIGITALIS TOXICITY 1. Discontinue the drug at the first suspicion of toxicity and do not reinitiate until signs and symptoms of toxicity subside. 2. Initiate continuous ECG monitoring if not already present. 3. Maintain a normal serum potassium (3.5–5.5 mEq/liter), but do *not* administer intravenous potassium in the presence of advanced or complete

heart block secondary to digitalis tox-icity; the block may increase.[1]

4. Pharmacologic treatment of toxicity should be guided by the arrhythmia produced. Phenytoin (Dilantin) is usu-ally the drug of choice. Quinidine, li-docaine, procainamide, and proprano-lol can also be used depending on the clinical situation. (If propranolol is used, monitor atrioventricular conduc-tion closely; this drug may cause in-creasing A-V block.) Atropine can be used to treat bradyarrhythmias. (See entries for each drug for further de-tails on their use.)

5. If profound bradycardia and/or com-plete A-V block occur, transvenous temporary pacing may be necessary until toxicity resolves.

NURSING IMPLICATIONS

1. Patients receiving this medication intravenously should in most instances be observed for arrhythmias via continuous ECG monitoring. Observe for improvement if the drug is given to treat an arrhythmia, and observe for ar-rhythmias which may be produced by the drug. Some of the more common arrhythmias produced by toxic levels of digitoxin are: sinus bradycardia, premature ventricular and atrial contractions, atrioventricular block of all degrees, paroxysmal atrial tachycardia. Notify the physician of improve-ment in arrhythmia being treated, and document with an ECG tracing. If ar-rhythmias of toxicity appear, notify the physician, document with an ECG tracing, and hold the next dose of digitoxin until the physician decides what course of action is appropriate.

2. Be prepared to administer immediate care in the event of arrhythmias due to toxicity. (See treatment of Digitalis Toxicity above.) Atropine 0.5–1.0 mg can be given for a heart rate less than 50–60/minute. (In units where regis-tered nurses are expected to administer drugs in such an event, the unit physician should decide at what heart rate atropine should be administered and in what amount.) See page 194 for details on atropine.

   For premature ventricular contractions or ventricular tachycardia, lido-caine 50–100 mg can be given by intravenous injection. Again, unit policy should dictate when and how much drug is given. See page 365 for details on lidocaine.

3. Observe for noncardiac symptoms of digitalis toxicity: anorexia; nausea; vomiting and diarrhea; visual disturbances, e.g., rainbow vision or yellow vi-sion (rare); in children, poor feeding and irritability; headache (rare); confu-sion; severe fatigue.[2]

4. Monitor for signs of improvement if the patient is being treated for conges-tive heart failure:
   a. Reduction in weight (weigh the patient daily)
   b. Reduction in peripheral edema
   c. Increased urine output (measure every 8 hours)
   d. Decreased resting heart rate to normal limits (record every 4–8 hours)
   e. Decreased respiratory rate, disappearance of rales
   f. Increased exercise tolerance
   Note that worsening congestive failure despite digitalis administration may be a sign of digitalis toxicity.

5. Be aware of the patient's serum potassium. Hypokalemia can precipitate digitalis toxicity. Administer potassium supplements as ordered. These may produce nausea and vomiting (liquid preparations especially) usually soon after administration. The nurse's observations will be needed to differenti-ate between potassium-induced nausea and vomiting and that due to digi-talis toxicity. (Normal serum potassium: 3.5–5.5 mEq/liter)

6. Rarely, elderly patients experience hallucinations, anxiety, and delusions secondary to toxic levels of digitalis preparations. Monitor for onset of this complication, notify the physician, and initiate safety measures such as side rails, restraints as needed, close observation, reorientation, and reassur-ance.

7. Patients who will require this drug on a chronic basis must be instructed on safe self-administration of the digitalis. Points that must be presented are:
   a. The actions of the drug, what it can and cannot do for the patient
   b. Correct daily dosage
   c. Pulse-taking (if possible, not absolutely required), and actions to take with changes in rate and rhythm
   d. Signs and symptoms of toxicity and what to do if they appear
   e. Need for follow-up care
   f. Potassium intake
   g. Diet, activity, etc., necessary for general care of congestive heart failure
   The patient and/or family should be able to demonstrate and verbalize knowledge of these areas.

REFERENCES

1. Davis, Richard H., and Fisch, Charles: Potassium and Arrhythmias, *Geriat-rics*. November 1970, p. 110.
2. Lely, A. H., and van Enter, C. H. J.: Noncardiac Symptoms of Digitalis Intoxi-cation. *American Heart Journal*, 83(2):150, February 1972.

SUGGESTED READINGS

Amsterdam, Ezra A., et al.: Systemic Approach to the Management of Cardi-ac Arrhythmias. *Heart and Lung*, 2(5):747–753, September–October 1973 (references).

Arbeit, Sidney, et al.: Recognizing Digitalis Toxicity. *American Journal of Nursing*, 77(12):1936–1945, December 1977 (references).

Isacson, Lauren Marie, and Schultz, Klaus: Treating Pulmonary Edema. *Nurs-ing '78*, February 1978, pp. 42–46.

James, Frederick W., and Love, Ervena: Congestive Heart Failure in Infants and Children. *Heart and Lung*, 3(3):396–400, May–June 1974.

Lely, A. H., and van Enter, C. H. J.: Noncardiac Symptoms of Digitalis Intoxi-cation. *American Heart Journal*, 83(2):149–152, February 1972.

DIGITOXIN (Digitaline, Crystodigin) *(Continued)*

SUGGESTED READINGS (Continued)
Rosen, Michael R., Wit, Andrew, and Hoffman, Brian F.: Electrophysiology and Pharmacology of Cardiac Arrhythmias. IV Cardiac Antiarrhythmic and Toxic Effects of Digitalis. *American Heart Journal,* 89(3):391–399, March 1975 (references).

———— Treatment of Cardiac Arrhythmias. *Medical Letter on Drugs and Therapeutics,* 16(25):101–108, December 6, 1974.

Tanner, Gloria: Heart Failure in the MI Patient. *American Journal of Nursing* 77:230–234, February 1977.

DIGOXIN (Lanoxin Injection, Lanoxin Injection–Pediatric)

ACTIONS/ INDICATIONS	DOSAGE	PREPARATION AND STORAGE	DRUG INCOMPATIBILITIES	MODES OF IV ADMINISTRATION			CONTRAINDICATIONS; WARNINGS; PRECAUTIONS; ADVERSE REACTIONS
				INJECTION	INTERMITTENT INFUSION	CONTINUOUS INFUSION	
Cardiac glycoside, which increases the force of myocardial contraction, slows the discharge of the sinus node, slows conduction through the A-V node, by its effect on the refractory period of these tissues via the autonomic nervous system. Initial effect occurs within 5–10 minutes with maximal effect in 1–2 hours. Used in the treatment of all degrees of congestive heart failure; to control heart rate in atrial tachycardia, flutter, and fibrillation by slowing impulse formation and A-V conduction;	Recommended doses are practical, average figures; but dosage must be determined by the patient's sensitivity to the drug (See Warnings and Precautions), renal status, and body size. ADULTS AND CHILDREN OVER 10 YEARS OF AGE: Full digitalization may require 1.0 mg total dosage. Maintenance dosage is 0.125–0.5 mg daily. Therapeutic serum levels—0.5–2.5 ng*/ml. Dosage should be decreased in the presence of renal failure. *Nanograms	Do not add to IV fluid; drug is unstable when diluted. Supplied in 2-ml ampules, 0.25 mg/ml. Store at room temperature. (Pediatric Injection: 0.1 mg/ml ampuls)	Do not mix with any other medication in any manner.	YES Give slowly at a rate of 0.125–0.25 mg/min undiluted. Inject as close to the IV cannula as possible, either into the cannula hub or into the lowest Y injection site. In pulmonary edema, give dose over 10–15 min.	NO Do not mix with IV fluids.	NO Do not mix with IV fluids.	CONTRAINDICATIONS 1. Digitalis toxicity 2. Hypersensitivity to cardiac glycosides 3. In the presence of ventricular fibrillation WARNINGS 1. Titrate dosage carefully, monitoring heart rate, ECG, and serum levels to avoid intoxication. 2. Newborns vary in their tolerance to digitalis depending on their maturity. Premature and immature infants are very sensitive to this drug. Dosage must be individualized. 3. Many arrhythmias for which digitalis is prescribed can also be the result of digitalis intoxication. Rule out intoxication prior to administration. 4. Patients in congestive heart failure may complain of nausea and vomiting. Exclude the possibility of digitalis intoxication before continuing with drug administration. 5. Patients with renal insufficiency will require lower dosage due to drug accumulation in the body. Creatinine clearance can be used to help estimate the rate of digoxin excretion by the kidneys, and thus the dosage in the presence of renal failure. 6. Use in the treatment of obesity is unwarranted and dangerous. PRECAUTIONS 1. Atrial arrhythmias associated with hyperthyroidism and febrile states are resistant to digoxin. Avoid toxicity

and in cardiogenic shock when accompanied by pulmonary edema to improve myocardial contractility.

CHILDREN UNDER AGE 10: *Premature and newborn*

Total digitalizing dose—25–40 mcg/kg. ½ dose stat; ¼ dose in 4–6 hours; ½ dose in 4–6 hours.

Maintenance—1/10–1/5 of digitalizing dose divided into 2 doses daily.

Two weeks to 2 years

Total digitalizing dose—35–50 mcg/kg divided into 3–6 doses with 6 or more hrs between each dose.

Maintenance—1/5 of digitalizing dose divided into 2 doses daily.

Over 2 years–10 years

Total digitalizing dose—25–40 mcg/kg divided into 3–6 doses with 6 or more hrs between each dose.

Maintenance—1/5 of digitalizing dose.

with high doses; monitor ECG and serum levels carefully. (See Dosage column.)

2. The following clinical situations make the myocardium more prone to toxicity and require careful dosage management:
   a. Hypokalemia (even at usual digitalis dosage levels)
   b. Long-standing cardiac disease (extensive myocardial fibrosis)
   c. Acute myocardial infarction
   d. Severe pulmonary disease (chronic obstructive or fibrotic disease)
   e. Rheumatic carditis

3. The following clinical situations require reduction and careful titration of dosage in adults and children:
   a. Renal insufficiency
   b. Myxedema
   c. Following electrical conversion of arrhythmias
   d. Congestive heart failure accompanying acute glomerulonephritis (antihypertensives such as reserpine should be given at the same time)

4. Administer with caution in the following clinical situations:
   a. Advanced or complete heart block (cardiac pacing may be needed)
   b. Ventricular tachycardia
   c. If the patient has received digitalis within the last 2–3 weeks

5. Do not administer in the presence of idiopathic hypertrophic subaortic stenosis or constrictive pericarditis; a fall in cardiac output may result.

6. Avoid administering intravenous calcium to patients on digitalis drugs; fatal arrhythmias have resulted.

ADVERSE REACTIONS
1. Hypersensitivity: rash, urticaria, anaphylaxis (rare)
2. Gynecomastia
3. Toxic effects in children: bradycardia, premature ventricular contractions, vomiting, poor feeding
4. Toxic effects in adults:
   a. Gastrointestinal—anorexia, nausea, vomiting, diarrhea
   b. Central nervous system —headache, weakness, apathy, blurred vision, yellow vision, rainbow vision, confusion
   c. Arrhythmias—the most commonly seen are premature ventricular contractions and sinus bradycardia; however, almost any arrhyth-

● DIGOXIN (Lanoxin Injection, Lanoxin Injection–Pediatric) (Continued)

ACTIONS/ INDICATIONS	DOSAGE	PREPARATION AND STORAGE	DRUG INCOMPAT- IBILITIES	MODES OF IV ADMINISTRATION			CONTRAINDICATIONS; WARNINGS; PRECAUTIONS; ADVERSE REACTIONS
				INJECTION	INTERMITTENT INFUSION	CONTINUOUS INFUSION	
							mia may be produced by digitalis toxicity

TREATMENT OF DIGITALIS TOXICITY

1. Discontinue the drug at the first suspicion of toxicity and do not reinitiate until signs and symptoms of toxicity subside.

2. Initiate continuous ECG monitoring if not already present.

3. Maintain a normal serum potassium (3.5–5.5 mEq/liter), but do *not* administer intravenous potassium in the presence of advanced or complete heart block secondary to digitalis toxicity; the block may increase.[1]

4. Pharmacologic treatment of toxicity should be guided by the arrhythmia produced. Phenytoin (Dilantin) is usually the drug of choice. Quinidine, lidocaine, procainamide, and propranolol can also be used depending on the clinical situation. (If propranolol is used, monitor atrioventricular conduction closely. This drug may cause increasing A-V block.) Atropine can be used to treat bradyarrhythmias. See entries for each drug for further details on their use.

5. If profound bradycardia and/or complete A-V block occur, transvenous temporary pacing may be necessary until toxicity resolves.

NURSING IMPLICATIONS

1. Patients receiving this medication intravenously should, in most instances, be observed for arrhythmias via continuous ECG monitoring. Observe for improvement if the drug is given to treat an arrhythmia, and observe for arrhythmias which may be produced by the drug. Some of the more common arrhythmias produced by toxic levels of digoxin: sinus bradycardia, premature ventricular and atrial contractions, atrioventricular block of all degrees, paroxysmal atrial tachycardia. Notify the physician of improvement in arrhythmia being treated, and document with an ECG tracing. If arrhythmias of toxicity appear, notify the physician, document with an ECG tracing, and hold the next dose of digoxin until the physician decides what course of action is appropriate.

2. Be prepared to administer immediate care in the event of arrhythmias due to toxicity. See Treatment of Digitalis Toxicity above. Atropine 0.5–1.0 mg can be given for a heart rate less than 50–60/minute. (In units where registered nurses are expected to administer drugs in such an event, the unit physician should decide at what heart rate the atropine should be adminis-

secondary to toxic levels of digitalis preparations. Monitor for onset of this complication, notify the physician, and initiate safety measures, such as side rails, restraints (as necessary), close observation, reorientation, and reassurance.

7. Patients who will require this drug on a chronic basis must be instructed on safe self-administration of the digitalis. Points that must be presented are:
   a. The actions of the drug, what it can and cannot do for the patient
   b. Correct daily dosage
   c. Pulse-taking (if possible, not absolutely required), and actions to take with changes in rate and rhythm
   d. Signs and symptoms of toxicity and what to do if they appear
   e. Need for follow-up care
   f. Potassium intake
   g. Diet, activity, etc., necessary for general care of congestive heart failure
   The patient and/or family should be able to demonstrate and verbalize knowledge of these areas.

tered and in what amount.) See page 194 for details on atropine.

For premature ventricular contractions or ventricular tachycardia, lidocaine 50–100 mg can be given by intravenous injection. Again, unit policy should dictate when and how much drug is given. See page 365 for details on lidocaine.

3. Observe for noncardiac symptoms of digitalis toxicity: anorexia; nausea; vomiting and diarrhea; visual disturbances, e.g., rainbow vision or yellow vision (rare); in children, poor feeding and irritability; headache (rare); confusion; severe fatigue.[2]

4. Monitor for signs of improvement if the patient is being treated for congestive heart failure:
   a. Reduction in weight (weigh the patient daily)
   b. Reduction in peripheral edema
   c. Increased urine output (measure every 8 hours)
   d. Decreased resting heart rate to normal limits (record every 4 to 8 hours)
   e. Decreased respiratory rate; disappearance of rales
   f. Increased exercise tolerance
   Note that worsening congestive failure, despite digitalis administration, may be a sign of digitalis toxicity.

5. Be aware of the patient's serum potassium. Hypokalemia can precipitate digitalis toxicity. Administer potassium supplements as ordered. These may produce nausea and vomiting (liquid preparations especially), usually soon after administration. The nurse's observations will be needed to differentiate between potassium-induced nausea and vomiting and that due to digitalis toxicity. (Normal serum potassium: 3.5–5.5 mEq/liter.)

6. Rarely, elderly patients experience hallucinations, anxiety, and delusions

REFERENCES
1. Davis, Richard H., and Fisch, Charles: Potassium and Arrhythmias. *Geriatrics*, November 1970, p. 110.
2. Lely, A. H., and van Enter, C. H. J.: Noncardiac Symptoms of Digitalis Intoxication. *American Heart Journal*, 83(2):150, February 1972.

SUGGESTED READINGS
Amsterdam, Ezra A., et al.: Systemic Approach to the Management of Cardiac Arrhythmias. *Heart and Lung*, 2(5):747–753, September–October 1973 (references).
Arbeit, Sidney, et al.: Recognizing Digitalis Toxicity. *American Journal of Nursing*, 77(12):1936–1945, December 1977 (references).
Isacson, Lauren Marie, and Schultz, Klaus: Treating Pulmonary Edema. *Nursing '78*, February 1978, pp. 42–46.
James, Frederick W., and Love, Ervena: Congestive Heart Failure in Infants and Children. *Heart and Lung*, 3(3):396–400, May–June 1974.
Lely, A. H., and van Enter, C. H. J.: Noncardiac Symptoms of Digitalis Intoxication. *American Heart Journal*, 83(2):149–152, February 1972.
Rosen, Michael R., Wit, Andrew, and Hoffman, Brian F.: Electrophysiology and Pharmacology of Cardiac Arrhythmias. IV Cardiac Antiarrhythmic and Toxic Effects of Digitalis. *American Heart Journal*, 89(3):391–399, March 1975 (references).
———Treatment of Cardiac Arrhythmias. *Medical Letter on Drugs and Therapeutics*, 16(25):101–108, December 6, 1974.
Tanner, Gloria: Heart Failure in the MI Patient. *American Journal of Nursing*, 77:230–234, February 1977.

● DIHYDROERGOTAMINE MESYLATE (D.H.E.-45)

ACTIONS/ INDICATIONS	DOSAGE	PREPARATION AND STORAGE	DRUG INCOMPATIBILITIES	MODES OF IV ADMINISTRATION			CONTRAINDICATIONS; WARNINGS; PRECAUTIONS; ADVERSE REACTIONS
				INJECTION	INTERMITTENT INFUSION	CONTINUOUS INFUSION	
Alpha adrenergic blocking agent Directly stimulates smooth muscle of peripheral and cranial blood vessels to cause their constriction and produces depression of central vasomotor centers. Used to abort or prevent vascular head-	ADULTS ONLY: Usual dose is 1 mg (1 ml) with a maximum of 2 mg, first warning of a headache. Total weekly dosage should not exceed 6 mg (6 ml). Optimal dose for each patient should be sought.	Store away from heat and light. Discard if solution is discolored. Available in 1-ml ampuls with a concentration of 1 mg/ml.	Do not mix with any other medication.	YES Slowly, at a rate of 1 mg/2 min. Can be given undiluted.	NO	NO	CONTRAINDICATIONS Because of its vasoconstrictive effects, this drug is contraindicated in the presence of the following conditions: 1. Peripheral vascular disease 2. Coronary artery disease 3. Severe hypertension 4. Impaired hepatic or renal function 5. Sepsis Also contraindicated in the presence of known hypersensitivity. ADVERSE REACTIONS 1. Numbness and tingling of fingers and toes 2. Muscle pains in extremities 3. Muscular weakness in legs 4. Chest discomfort 5. Transient tachycardia or bradycardia 6. Nausea and vomiting

● DEHYDROCHOLATE, SODIUM (Decholin Sodium) (Continued)

ACTIONS/INDICATIONS	DOSAGE	PREPARATION AND STORAGE	DRUG INCOMPATIBILITIES	MODES OF IV ADMINISTRATION			CONTRAINDICATIONS; WARNINGS; PRECAUTIONS; ADVERSE REACTIONS
				INJECTION	INTERMITTENT INFUSION	CONTINUOUS INFUSION	
ache (migraine and its variants).							7. Itching and edema at injection site Discontinue the drug if any of the first four reactions occur; these symptoms indicate that undue vasoconstriction is occurring in the affected areas, i.e., peripheral blood vessels, including the coronary arteries.

NURSING IMPLICATIONS
1. Avoid extravasation; see page 96.
2. Monitor for tachycardia and bradycardia.
3. Instruct the patient on the origin of adverse reactions and give supportive care. Reactions are transient, usually lasting less than 4 hours.
4. If Adverse Reactions Numbers 1–4 above occur, notify the physician *immediately*. The drug should be discontinued.

● DIMENHYDRINATE (Dramamine)

ACTIONS/INDICATIONS	DOSAGE	PREPARATION AND STORAGE	DRUG INCOMPATIBILITIES	MODES OF IV ADMINISTRATION			CONTRAINDICATIONS; WARNINGS; PRECAUTIONS; ADVERSE REACTIONS
				INJECTION	INTERMITTENT INFUSION	CONTINUOUS INFUSION	
Mode of action unknown; has a depressant action on hyperstimulated inner ear function. Used to prevent and treat the nausea, vomiting, and vertigo of motion sickness. Duration of action is 4 hrs.	ADULTS: *Usual dose*—50–100 mg. May be repeated in 4 hrs. CHILDREN: Intravenous mode is not recommended.	Supplied ampuls of 1 ml containing a solution of 50 mg/ml; and multidose vials of 5 ml (50 mg/ml).	Do not mix with any other medication.	YES Each 50 mg. should be diluted in 10 ml of NS and injected over 2 min.	NO	NO	WARNINGS When used in conjunction with certain antibiotics that are capable of producing toxicity (streptomycin, gentamicin, kanamycin, neomycin), dimenhydrinate may mask the symptoms of ototoxicity. Irreversible auditory and vestibular damage may occur without warning. PRECAUTIONS, ADVERSE REACTIONS Drowsiness is a frequent side effect. The patient should be ambulated with assistance following an injection.

NURSING IMPLICATIONS
1. Ambulate the patient with caution if drowsiness and dizziness are a problem.
2. Monitor for effectiveness and report findings to the physician.

Take necessary precautions for patients who cannot follow directions.

DIPHENHYDRAMINE HYDROCHLORIDE (Benadryl)

ACTIONS/ INDICATIONS	DOSAGE	PREPARATION AND STORAGE	DRUG INCOMPAT- IBILITIES	MODES OF IV ADMINISTRATION			CONTRAINDICATIONS; WARNINGS; PRECAUTIONS; ADVERSE REACTIONS
				INJECTION	INTERMITTENT INFUSION	CONTINUOUS INFUSION	
Potent antihistaminic, anticholinergic (antispasmotic), antiemetic and sedative agent. Used for: • Prevention and treatment of allergic reactions to blood and plasma • Anaphylaxis along with other measures • Uncomplicated allergic reaction when oral route cannot be used • Motion sickness • Parkinsonism, including drug-induced extrapyramidal reactions • Insomnia	ADULTS: 10–50 mg (maximum daily dose is 400 mg; maximum single dose is 100 mg), for all indications. CHILDREN: 5 mg/kg/24 hrs or 150 mg/M²/24 hrs; divided into 4 doses. Maximum dose is 300 mg in 24 hours for all indications.	Supplied in multi-dose vials of 10 mg/ml; 50 mg/ml; 1-ml ampuls of 50 mg/ml and prefilled syringes of 50 mg/ml.	Do not mix with: Potassium iodide Amphotericin B Cephalothin Hydrocortisone	YES Slowly.	YES Use any fluid, 50–100 ml. Drip rate should be set according to hourly dose prescribed and patient response.	YES Use any fluid in any volume. Drip rate should be set according to hourly dose prescribed and patient response.	CONTRAINDICATIONS 1. Do not use in premature or newborn infants. 2. Do not use in patients with: a. Hypersensitivity to this drug b. An asthmatic attack, or other lower respiratory illness c. Narrow-angle glaucoma d. Prostatic hypertrophy e. Stenosing peptic ulcer f. Pyloroduodinal obstruction g. Bladder-neck obstruction 3. Do not administer to patients receiving MAO inhibitors. 4. Should not be used by nursing mothers. WARNINGS 1. Overdosage may produce convulsions and death, especially in infants and children. Correct dosage can produce excitation in young children. 2. Drowsiness is a frequent occurrence; take precautions when ambulating the patient. This occurs more often in the elderly. 3. Administer with caution during pregnancy; there exists potential harm to the fetus. 4. Anaphylaxis can occur. 5. This drug has additive effects when given with other CNS depressants. PRECAUTIONS 1. Avoid extravasation. 2. This drug has anticholinergic effects such as tachycardia, dry mouth, blurring of vision, and urinary retention. 3. Use with caution in patients with a history of asthma. (See Contraindication No. 2b.) ADVERSE REACTIONS 1. Drowsiness 2. Confusion 3. Nervousness 4. Nausea, vomiting, diarrhea 5. Visual disturbances 6. Difficulty in urination 7. Constipation

293

DIPHENHYDRAMINE HYDROCHLORIDE (Benadryl) (Continued)

ACTIONS/ INDICATIONS	DOSAGE	PREPARATION AND STORAGE	DRUG INCOMPATIBILITIES	MODES OF IV ADMINISTRATION			CONTRAINDICATIONS; WARNINGS; PRECAUTIONS; ADVERSE REACTIONS
				INJECTION	INTERMITTENT INFUSION	CONTINUOUS INFUSION	
							8. Chest tightness and wheezing 9. Dizziness, headache 10. Palpitations, insomnia 11. Dryness of mucous membranes, thickening of bronchial secretions 12. Tingling, weakness and a sensation of heaviness of the hands 13. Rash, urticaria, photosensitivity 14. Hemolytic anemia, thrombocytopenia, agranulocytosis 15. Anaphylaxis

3. Monitor all patients for urinary retention, i.e., urinary output and bladder size every 2–4 hours.
4. Notify the physician of the onset of any adverse reactions.
5. Administer supportive care to patients being treated for allergic reactions. See page 118 on anaphylaxis.
6. Be prepared to manage vomiting in a drowsy patient, to prevent aspiration.
7. Take precautions to prevent extravasation; See page 96.

NURSING IMPLICATIONS
1. Ambulate patients with care following injection to prevent injury; the patient may be dizzy as well as drowsy.
2. Be prepared to manage confusion. Keep side rails up for elderly patients or those who develop confusion or excitement, e.g. children. These patients may require one-to-one care until the adverse effects subside. Reassurance, reorientation and mild restraints should be used as necessary.

DIPHENIDOL (Vontrol)

ACTIONS/ INDICATIONS	DOSAGE	PREPARATION AND STORAGE	DRUG INCOMPATIBILITIES	MODES OF IV ADMINISTRATION			CONTRAINDICATIONS; WARNINGS; PRECAUTIONS; ADVERSE REACTIONS
				INJECTION	INTERMITTENT INFUSION	CONTINUOUS INFUSION	
Antivertigo agent. Has a specific action on the inner ear to control vertigo; inhibits the chemoreceptor trigger zone to control nausea and vomiting. Indicated in vertigo in Meniere's disease, middle- or inner-ear surgery; nausea and vomiting in surgery, neoplas-	ADULTS: For nausea, vomiting, and vertigo—Administer IV only to hospitalized patients for rapid control of acute symptoms; 20 mg followed by 20 mg in 1 hr if necessary. Then use IM or oral route. Not for IV use in children of any age.	Supplied in 2-ml ampuls in a concentration of 20 mg/ml.	Do not mix with any other medication in any manner.	YES Slowly, through the Y injection site; dilution is not necessary.	NO	NO	CONTRAINDICATIONS 1. Hypersensitivity 2. Renal failure, anuria (drug is excreted in the urine) WARNINGS 1. May cause hallucinations and confusion. Patients must be under constant observation. Discontinue the drug if mental changes occur. Benefits should be weighed against this risk. 2. Use in pregnancy, lactation, or in women of childbearing age requires that benefits be weighed against possible hazards to the mother and child. Not for use in treating the nausea and vomiting of pregnancy. PRECAUTIONS 1. The antiemetic action may mask signs

tic disease and inner-ear disturbances.

of drug overdose (digitalis), or may obscure the diagnosis of intestinal obstruction or brain tumor.
2. Monitor for the onset of any idiosyncratic blood dyscrasias.
3. Has a weak peripheral anticholinergic effect. Use with caution in patients with:
   a. Glaucoma (may increase intraocular pressure)
   b. Obstructive lesions of the gastrointestinal or genitourinary tracts (may increase obstruction)
4. May precipitate sinus tachycardia in patients with a history of this arrhythmia.
5. Hypotension has been reported.

ADVERSE REACTIONS
1. Auditory and visual hallucinations have been reported.
2. Drowsiness, overstimulation, depression, sleep disturbances, dry mouth, nausea, and blurred vision may occur.
3. Skin rash.
4. Transient hypotension.

NURSING IMPLICATIONS
1. Monitor patients closely for onset of mental disturbances. Take protective precautions. If they occur, support the patient as necessary; he will be frightened and agitated. Restrain as needed; use side rails at all times. Patient may need one-to-one care.
2. Monitor for signs of drug toxicity, intestinal obstruction, and increased intracranial pressure—other than nausea and vomiting (symptoms which this drug supresses).
   a. Patients concomitantly receiving digitalis drugs should be closely monitored for pulse rate and ECG changes as signs of digitalis toxicity.
   b. When intestinal obstruction is a possibility, monitor stool count, bowel sounds, abdominal girth.
   c. In patients with suspected increased intracranial pressure, monitor neu-

rologic signs such as pupil reaction to light, equality of hand grip, mental status.
3. In patients with glaucoma, observe for signs of increased intraocular pressure: dull headache, decreasing vision beginning at the periphery, severe eye pain, rainbow vision, dilated pupils.[1]
4. Monitor pulse rate and blood pressure closely following injection and for the next 4 hours.
5. Ambulate with caution; the patient may experience dizziness.

REFERENCE
1. Newell, Frank W., and Ernest J. Terry: *Ophthalmology—Principles and Concepts* (3rd ed.). St. Louis: C. V. Mosby Company, 1974, p. 329.

● DOPAMINE HYDROCHLORIDE (Intropin)

ACTIONS/ INDICATIONS	DOSAGE	PREPARATION AND STORAGE	DRUG INCOMPATIBILITIES	MODES OF IV ADMINISTRATION			CONTRAINDICATIONS; WARNINGS; PRECAUTIONS; ADVERSE REACTIONS
				INJECTION	INTERMITTENT INFUSION	CONTINUOUS INFUSION	
A sympathomimetic amine, precursor of norepinephrine. In-	ADULTS (starting doses): *Septic shock* —2–5 mcg/	Supplied in 5-ml ampuls, of a 40 mg/ml concentration.	Do not add any other medication to a solution bottle containing	NO	NO	YES Use any of the following fluids:	CONTRAINDICATIONS 1. Hypotension due to hypovolemia (may be used for a short time to maintain vital organ perfusion while fluids are being replaced, but volume replace-

DOPAMINE HYDROCHLORIDE (Intropin) (Continued)

ACTIONS/ INDICATIONS	DOSAGE	PREPARATION AND STORAGE	DRUG INCOMPATIBILITIES	MODES OF IV ADMINISTRATION			CONTRAINDICATIONS; WARNINGS; PRECAUTIONS; ADVERSE REACTIONS
				INJECTION	INTERMITTENT INFUSION	CONTINUOUS INFUSION	
creases cardiac output by direct (beta adrenergic receptor stimulation) inotropic effect on the heart muscle; and indirectly by stimulating the release of norepinephrine.[1] This drug also has a weak vasoconstrictor action (alpha adrenergic receptor stimulation) in peripheral blood vessels. There is no drastic increase in peripheral vascular resistance as a result of this action in intermediate doses.[2] There is also a nonadrenergic mediated dilation of renal and mesenteric vessels at low and intermediate doses.[3]

Onset of action is rapid, within 5 min. The duration is about 10 min. Specific actions are dose-dependent.

LOW DOSE (1–2 mcg/kg/min) Dilatation of renal and | kg/min.

Titrate to maintain an adequate systolic blood pressure (direct arterial), pulmonary artery wedge pressure, CVP and urinary output (see Nursing Implications).

Acute myocardial infarction —2–6 mcg/kg/min.

Titrate as described above.

Chronic congestive heart failure —1–2 mcg/kg/min.

Titrate to produce an adequate urine output (at least 30–50 ml/hr) and tissue perfusion.

Renal perfusion alone —0.5–2.0 mcg/kg/min.

Titrate to obtain desired urine output without undesirable changes in heart rate and blood pressure.

At any dosage | SEE TABLE BELOW FOR SOLUTION PREPARATION.

Solutions utilizing the fluids listed in the Continuous Infusion column are stable for 48 hours.[4]

Do not use solutions that are discolored.

As with all drugs that must be titrated, dopamine must not be mixed with other drugs in the same solution bottle; infuse it as a secondary IV line. | dopamine.

The following drugs CAN be piggy-backed into IV lines containing dopamine:[5]
Heparin
Lidocaine
Cephalothin
Oxacillin
Gentamicin
Potassium chloride
Calcium chloride
Calcium gluconate
Carbenicillin
Chloramphenicol
Kanamycin
Potassium penicillin
Tetracycline
Hydrocortisone
Methylprednisolone
Procainamide
Vitamins.

Do NOT mix in any manner with:
Amphotericin B[6]
Sodium bicarbonate | | | D5W
D5/NS
D5/0.45 saline
D5/RL
1/6 Molar Sodium Lactate
RL
20% Mannitol

Use no other fluids.

See Preparation column for solution preparation

USE AN INFUSION PUMP. | ment is mandatory)
2. Pheochromocytoma
3. Uncorrected tachyarrhythmias or ventricular fibrillation

WARNINGS
1. Use with caution and in reduced dosage in patients who are on or have received within the last 14 days MAO inhibitor drugs. The manufacturer suggests a dose 1/10 of the normal calculated dose.
2. Use in pregnancy requires that the possible benefits to the mother be weighed against possible risks to the fetus.
3. This drug is not recommended for use in children.
4. The shorter the time period between onset of signs and symptoms and the initiation of dopamine therapy, the better the prognosis.

PRECAUTIONS
1. In the presence of shock, the pulmonary artery wedge pressure should be in the 14–18 range prior to the administration of this drug.
2. Decrease the infusion rate if the diastolic blood pressure rises disproportionately (with a resultant lowering of the pulse pressure) to the systolic pressure. This indicates the presence of predominate vasoconstriction, and can be undesirable in certain clinical situations.
3. Avoid extravasation, which can lead to tissue necrosis and sloughing. Do not use small veins for infusion if at all possible. If extravasation occurs, immediately infiltrate the area with 10–15 ml of a solution of normal saline containing 5–10 mg of phentolamine (Regitine). Using a syringe with a 25 or 26 gauge needle, infiltrate liberally. The area will become red secondary to the vasodilatation produced by the phentolamine. Protect the area from subsequent trauma and monitor for signs of necrosis (see page 97).
4. In patients with a history of occlusive vascular disease (arteriosclerosis, arte- |

mesenteric vessels, no change in heart rate, blood pressure or cardiac output.

INTERMEDI-ATE DOSE (2–10 mcg/kg/min)

Increased cardiac output, increased systolic blood pressure, increased perfusion of the abdominal viscera, increased perfusion of the kidneys with secondary increase in glomerular filtration and sodium excretion, and minimal increase in myocardial oxygen requirements.

HIGH DOSE (greater than 20 mcg/kg/min)

Pronounced peripheral, renal and mesenteric vasoconstriction.

Indicated in the management of:
• Septic shock unresponsive to fluid challenge and steroids
• Acute myocardial infarction or immediate postoperative

level, once the desired response is obtained, maintain the infusion rate at the lowest level that produces optimal results.

CHILDREN: Not currently recommended for use in children.

PREPARATION OF DOPAMINE SOLUTIONS

Fluid Volume (ml)	Ampuls Of Dopamine (200 mg/ampul)	Resultant Concentration (mcg/ml)	mcg/Microdrop
500	2 (400 mg)	800	13
500	4 (800 mg)	1600	26
500	6 (1200 mg)	2400	40
500	8 (1600 mg)	3200	53

rial embolism, Raynaud's disease, cold injury, diabetic endarteritis. Buerger's disease, etc.) monitor closely for changes in circulation to the extremities. (See Nursing Implications.)
5. Use with extreme caution in patients receiving cyclopropane or halogenated hydrocarbon anesthetics. There may be increased myocardial irritability and resultant arrhythmias.

ADVERSE REACTIONS
1. Arrhythmias—premature ventricular contractions and ventricular tachycardia (both responsive to lidocaine)
2. Angina pectoris
3. Nausea and vomiting
4. Headache
5. Dyspnea
6. Hypotension (usually seen in high dosage)
7. Decreased urine output (usually seen in high dosage)

TREATMENT OF OVERDOSAGE (THE APPEARANCE OF ADVERSE REACTIONS)
1. Slow or stop the infusion and stay with the patient.
2. Monitor blood pressure every 1–2 minutes.
3. Usually additional measures are not necessary due to the short duration of action.
4. If the patient does not stabilize, a short-acting alpha adrenergic blocking agent (Phentolamine) can be administered as an intravenous infusion.
5. If the patient is able, instruct him, prior to the initiation of the infusion, to report chest pain of any kind. If it occurs, slow the infusion and monitor heart rate and blood pressure carefully. Observe for arrhythmias.
6. Be prepared to manage nausea and vomiting to prevent aspiration.
7. See Nursing Implications section for further details.

● DOPAMINE (Intropin) (Continued)

ACTIONS/ INDICATIONS	DOSAGE	PREPARATION AND STORAGE	DRUG INCOMPAT- IBILITIES	MODES OF IV ADMINISTRATION			CONTRAINDICATIONS; WARNINGS; PRECAUTIONS; ADVERSE REACTIONS
				INJECTION	INTERMITTENT INFUSION	CONTINUOUS INFUSION	
cardiac surgery with shock unresponsive to volume expanders
• Chronic congestive heart failure unresponsive to diuretics and digitalis, with or without vasodilator therapy
• Severe cirrhosis with renal insufficiency (this is a possible indication)							

NURSING IMPLICATIONS
1. Before therapy, weigh the patient for dosage determination.
2. Use an infusion pump at all times during the administration of this drug, to prevent over- or underdosage. If a pump is not available, microdrop intravenous infusion tubing must be used. (Always monitor ml's, or *volume* delivered, therefore mcg's delivered, *not* drops of fluid, to keep dosage accurate.)
   Whether using a pump or microdrop tubing, monitor the infusion rate frequently. With microdrop tubing the drip rate should be counted with each blood pressure determination. Prevent changes in drip rate secondary to patient movement, arm position, etc. with restraints and armboards. When the frequency of blood pressure determinations decreases with stabilization of the patient's condition, count the drip rate again at least every 15 to 30 minutes.
   Extreme caution must be exercised when using highly concentrated solutions of dopamine. Small changes in the infusion rate can change the dosage of the drug drastically.
3. Monitoring the patient's condition and drug effectiveness:
   a. It is recommended that the following parameters be continually evaluated and used to guide the dosage of dopamine during therapy:[7,8]
      1. Continuous direct arterial blood pressure via arterial cannulation (rather than by the less accurate and at times deceptive sphygmomanometry)
      2. Central venous pressure
      3. Pulmonary artery wedge pressure (especially in patients with or who are likely to develop left ventricular failure)
      4. Arterial blood gases and acid-base balance
      5. Urine output and specific gravity
      6. In some instances, cardiac output
      7. Heart rate and rhythm
      When using these parameters it is helpful to have pretreatment values

the downward titration until a desirable pressure is reached. Note the dosage of dopamine that produced the rise in pressure, notify the physician.

b. Hypotension:

High doses of this drug (greater than 20 mcg/kg/minute) can cause hypotension. If this occurs with such a dosage, reduce the infusion rate by 0.5 mg/kg/min (or 5 drops/min) increments until the arterial pressure begins to rise. If a rise is not seen, notify the physician. Note the dosage of dopamine that produced this effect. Low-dose therapy can also produce hypotension in some patients; see Nursing Implication No. 3d above.

Hypotension can also be the result of deterioration in the patient's condition, due to hypovolemia, sepsis, increasing cardiac decompensation, etc. Changing the dosage (increasing or decreasing, depending on the situation) may remedy this; if not, notify the physician.

c. Chest pain (angina), nausea, headache, dyspnea:

Instruct the patient to report the onset of any of these symptoms, if he is able. The patient who is unable to complain of the symptoms may become restless, or show an increase in heart or respiratory rate. In either case, stay with the patient. Reassure him that the situation can be controlled. Decrease the infusion rate by 0.5 mcg/kg increments every 5 minutes and monitor the arterial pressure. If these symptoms were due to the dopamine, they will usually subside within 10 minutes. If they do not subside with a decrease in dosage, notify the physician at once. Be prepared to manage vomiting to prevent aspiration.

d. Arrhythmias: Dopamine is capable of causing sinus and ventricular tachycardia and premature ventricular contractions. These arrhythmias can also be caused by the patient's underlying pathology that has neces-

for comparison.

b. Initial dosage and titration routine must be ordered by the physician. The dosage must be prescribed in mcg/kg/min terms, based on the response desired (see Actions/Indications column). Arterial blood pressure and other parameter goals of therapy must also be set by the physician. Ideal levels must be determined for each patient depending on the clinical situation. However, an adequate arterial systolic pressure is considered to be approximately 80 to 90 mm Hg,[9] the CVP 12 to 14 mm Hg, the pulmonary artery wedge pressure 14 to 18 mm Hg[10] (see Precaution No. 1), and a urine output of at least 30 ml per hour.

c. Begin titration with the prescribed initial dosage. The onset of action will be within 5 minutes, the duration up to 10 minutes. Increase the dose of dopamine by 0.5 mg/kg/min (or 5 drops/min) increments every 5 minutes until the arterial pressure and other parameter goals are reached. It is recommended to use the lowest dosage of dopamine that can maintain the desired response (see Dosage column).

d. Obtain arterial pressures every 2 to 5 minutes during the initial titration phase, whenever the patient becomes unstable, or during the weaning phase of administration. Keep blood pressure monitor alarms set at appropriate levels. During the maintenance phase of administration of this drug, when the patient's parameters are stable and at adequate levels, the frequency of blood pressure readings can be reduced to every 15 to 30 minutes. The patient may require dopamine therapy for several days; careful titration and monitoring will be required throughout this therapy.

As the patient's condition improves to the point where the dosage of dopamine can be decreased, the arterial pressure may fall as the low-dose range is reached (see Actions/Indications column). It may be advisable to stop the infusion at this point. The pressure may then rise back to a more desirable level. Continue to monitor pressures frequently for the next several hours to evaluate the patient's response. Be prepared to restart the infusion.

e. Monitor heart rate with each blood pressure determination. The ECG should be monitored throughout therapy for the onset of arrhythmias.

f. The central venous pressure and pulmonary artery wedge pressure should be obtained as frequently as the patient's condition dictates, usually hourly during the initial phase of therapy.

g. Measure urine output via a Foley catheter every hour during the initial titration phase, when the patient is unstable, if the patient is being treated for acute tubular necrosis, has pre-existing renal disease, and during the weaning phase of drug titration. As the cardiac output and arterial blood pressure increase, the urine output will also increase. In low-dose therapy, this drug causes dilatation of the renal arteries, increasing glomerular filtration and thus increase the urine output (see Actions/Indications column).

Monitor urine specific gravity at least every 4 hours and report changes to the physician. The value should stay within normal limits in most patients.

h. Monitor arterial blood gases every 2 to 4 hours via the arterial cannula, as the patient's condition dictates. Improvement in circulation with the rise in cardiac output and blood pressure should bring the pH and pCO_2 values within normal limits where they had previously indicated an acidotic state secondary to shock.

i. Monitor cardiac output as necessary under physician order.

4. Management of adverse reactions:

a. Excessive elevation in arterial pressure (greater that the target pressure prescribed by the physician):

Decrease the infusion rate by 0.5 mcg/kg/min increments every 5 minutes and monitor the arterial pressure every 1 to 2 minutes. Continue

sitated the use of dopamine. Fever, hypoxemia, pain, fear, physical exertion (struggling against a respirator, restlessness) can also cause them. If these other causes have been ruled out, reduce the infusion rate of dopamine by 0.5 mcg/kg/min (or 5 drops/min) increments, monitor the arterial pressure and notify the physician.

Ventricular irritability (premature ventricular contractions and ventricular tachycardia) can be controlled by lidocaine. Be prepared to administer a 100 mg bolus of lidocaine if either one of these arrhythmias occurs. Document the arrhythmia, the amount of lidocaine given, and notify the physician (follow hospital policy on the administration of lidocaine). If these arrhythmias continue to occur, a lidocaine infusion may be ordered (see page 365).

e. Peripheral vasoconstriction:

This can occur during high-dose therapy, see Actions/Indications column. A disproportionate rise in diastolic blood pressure will occur with a reduction in pulse pressure. The blood pressure via sphygmomanometry will be reduced. Other signs will be mottling of the skin, reduction in skin temperature, cyanosis of the nail beds, pallor, and diaphoresis (see Precaution No. 4).

If these signs appear, reduce the dosage of dopamine by 0.5 mg/kg/min (or 5 drops/min) increments every 5 minutes. Observe the arterial pressure frequently and watch for changes in the presenting signs. If an improvement is not seen, notify the physician (see Precaution No. 2).

f. Oliguria:

High-dose therapy (greater than 20 mcg/kg/minute) can produce renal artery constriction with a resultant fall in renal perfusion and urine output.[11] Deterioration in the patient's condition will also reduce the urine output. If output decreases below 30 ml/minute, notify the physician and continue careful monitoring. The physician may order a change in the dosage of dopamine, the administration of a diuretic, mannitol or fluids as needed.

5. Take all precautions to prevent extravasation; see page 96. Keep phentolamine readily available; see Precaution No. 3. If extravasation is even suspected (blanching of the skin around the intravenous cannula, swelling, etc.) notify the physician at once. Infiltration of the affected area with phentolamine must be carried out as soon as possible to help prevent tissue necrosis. After treatment, protect the area from further trauma and observe for sloughing of the tissue.

6. If this drug is administered during advanced life support, take all precautions to avoid mixing the dopamine with sodium bicarbonate. Flush the intravenous line with plain fluid before injecting the sodium bicarbonate and after, before restarting the dopamine infusion. If possible, use a separate intravenous line for the administration of the bicarbonate. These drugs are incompatible (see Drug Incompatibility column).

REFERENCES

1. Lee, W. C., and Yoo, C. S.: Mechanism of Cardiac Activities of Sympathomimetic Amines on Isolated Auricles of Rabbits. Archives International of Pharmacodynamics (French), 151:93, 1964.
2. Horwitz, David, Fox, Samuel, and Goldberg, Leon I.: Effects of Dopamine in Man. Circulation Research, 10:239, February 1962.
3. Meyer, M. B., McNay, John L., and Goldberg, Leon I.: Effects of Dopamine on Renal Function and Hemodynamics in the Dog. Journal of Pharmacology and Experimental Therapeutics, 156(1):187, 1967.
4. Gardella, L. A., et al.: Intropin (Dopamine Hydrochloride) Intravenous Admixture Compatibility. American Journal of Hospital Pharmacy, 36(6):577,

DOPAMINE (Intropin) (Continued)

REFERENCES (No. 4 continued)

5. Ibid, p. 578.
6. Gardella, L. A., et al.: Intropin (Dopamine Hydrochloride) Intravenous Admixture Compatibility. Part 3: Stability With Miscellaneous Additives. American Journal of Hospital Pharmacy, 35(5):582, May 1978.
7. Jahre, Jeffery A., et al.: Medical Approach to the Hypotensive Patient and the Patient in Shock. Heart and Lung, 4(4):578, July–August 1975.
8. Ayers, Stephen M., et al.: Care of the Critically Ill (2nd ed.). New York: Appleton-Century-Crofts, 1974, p. 259.
9. Tarazi, Robert C.: Sympathomimetic Agents in the Treatment of Shock. Annals of Internal Medicine, 81, September, 1974.
10. Ayers, p. 262.
11. Ibid.

SUGGESTED READINGS

Amsterdam, Ezra A., et al.: Evaluation and Management of Cardiogenic Shock, Part I: Approach to the Patient. Heart and Lung, 1(3):402–408, May–June 1972 (references).
———: Evaluation and Management of Cardiogenic Shock, Part II: Drug Therapy. Heart and Lung, 1(5):663–671, September–October 1972 (references).
Goldberg, Leon I., and Hsieh, Y.: Clinical Use of Dopamine. Rational Drug Therapy, 11:1–5, November 1977 (references).
Jahre, Jeffery, et al.: Medical Approach to the Hypotensive Patient and the Patient in Shock. Heart and Lung, 4(4):577–587 (references).
Tarazi, Robert C.: Sympathomimetic Agents in the Treatment of Shock. Annals of Internal Medicine, 81:364–371, September 1974.
Woods, Susan L.: Monitoring Pulmonary Artery Pressure. American Journal of Nursing, 76(11):1765–1771, November 1976 (references).
Dopamine for the Treatment of Shock. The Medical Letter, 17:13–14, 1975 (references).
Intravenous Infusion of Vasopressors—Programmed Instruction. American Journal of Nursing, 65(11):129–152, November 1965 (useful information on theories behind drug titration).

DOXAPRAM HYDROCHLORIDE (Dopram Injectable)

ACTIONS/INDICATIONS	DOSAGE	PREPARATION AND STORAGE	DRUG INCOMPATIBILITIES	MODES OF IV ADMINISTRATION			CONTRAINDICATIONS; WARNINGS; PRECAUTIONS; ADVERSE REACTIONS
				INJECTION	INTERMITTENT INFUSION	CONTINUOUS INFUSION	
Respiratory stimulant, through direct effects on central respiratory centers. Onset of action 20–40 seconds; peak 1–2 minutes; duration 5–12 minutes. Used as adjunct to therapy for: • Postanesthesia respiratory apnea or depression other than that due to muscle relaxant drugs • Stimulating deep breathing postop-	POSTANESTHESIA: Injection—0.5–1.0 mg/kg, repeat if necessary at 5-min intervals. Infusion—initiate at a 1 mg/ml solution at 5 mg/min until desired response is seen. Maintain infusion rate of 1–3 mg/min. Recommended total dosage is 4 mg/kg, not to exceed 3 gm. DRUG-INDUCED CNS DEPRESSION Injection—Give a priming	Do not add to any infusion fluid other than those listed. Suggested method of preparation of infusion: Add 250 mg of doxapram (12.5 ml) to 250 ml infusion fluid. Concentration produced is 1 mg/ml. To make a 2 mg/ml solution, add 400 mg of drug to 180 ml of fluid.	Do not mix with any other medication. Admixture with alkaline solutions such as thiopental or sodium bicarbonate will result in precipitation.	YES Slowly, no further dilution necessary.	YES Use one of the following infusion fluids: NS D5W D10W D5/NS D10/NS Follow recommended infusion rates; rapid infusion can cause hemolysis. Use an infusion pump.	YES Use one of the following infusion fluids: NS D5W D10W D5/NS D10/NS Follow recommended infusion rates; rapid infusion can cause hemolysis. Use an infusion pump.	CONTRAINDICATIONS 1. Convulsive states 2. Respiratory failure due to muscle weakness, flail chest, pneumothorax, airway obstruction or asthma, dyspnea (extreme). 3. Severe hypertension 4. Acute CVA 5. Hypersensitivity 6. Children under 12 years 7. Evidence of a head injury 8. Suspected or confirmed pulmonary embolus 9. Coronary artery disease 10. Frank uncompensated congestive heart failure 11. Pulmonary fibrosis WARNINGS 1. This drug is not antagonistic to muscle relaxants nor a specific antagonist to narcotics. 2. Respiratory support must be carried out in conjunction with this drug; see Nursing Implication No. 2. 3. Administer oxygen concomitantly if narcosis is present.

eratively
- Hastening return of pharyngeal reflexes secondary to drug overdose
- Drug-overdose respiratory depression
- Chronic pulmonary disease associated with acute hypercapnia (as a temporary measure), in hospitalized patients.

dose of 2.0 mg/kg; repeat in 5 min. Repeat same dose every 1–2 hrs until patient awakens. Watch for relapse into unconsciousness, or development of respiratory depression.

If a relapse occurs, resume 1- to 2-hr doses until arousal is sustained or maximum dosage (3 gm) is reached. If maximum dosage is reached, maintain respiration mechanically.

Do not repeat doses to patients who do not respond to the first dose; evaluate CNS for the cause of sustained depression.

Infusion— Give a priming dose of 1 mg/kg.

If patient awakens, watch for relapse. If there is no response, continue mechanical ventilation and repeat priming dose in 1–2 hrs.

If some respiratory response is

4. Administer with great caution to patients with cerebral edema, bronchial asthma, severe tachycardia or other arrhythmias, severe cardiac disease, hyperthyroidism, pheochromocytoma.
5. Safe use in pregnancy has not been established.
6. Discontinue if hypotension or dyspnea develops.

PRECAUTIONS
1. This drug will increase the work of breathing which can increase oxygen consumption and carbon dioxide production. Provide necessary supportive therapy.
2. Excessive dosage produces hyperventilation which leads to respiratory alkalosis, hypocapnia with tetany, and eventually apnea.
3. This drug may mask the residual effects of muscle relaxants.
4. The possibility of airway obstruction and hypoxia must be eliminated prior to the administration of this drug.
5. Administer with caution if patient has received sympathomimetics or MAO inhibitors. The combination may produce hypertension.
6. Use with care in patients with peptic ulcer disease or those undergoing gastric surgery.
7. Avoid extravasation or repeated use of single injection site.
8. Delay administration for 10 minutes after discontinuing halothane or cyclopropane anesthetics.
9. Monitor arterial blood gases carefully.
10. When used in acute respiratory insufficiency secondary to chronic obstructive pulmonary disease, use only for a short time (2 hours) as an aid to prevent elevation of arterial pCO_2 when oxygen is being given. Do not use with mechanical ventilation. Do not exceed suggested infusion rate to increase pCO_2 reduction; this drug increases the work of breathing and will cause fatigue.

ADVERSE REACTIONS
1. CNS: hyperactivity, sweating, clonus, muscle spasm, pyrexia, confusion, pupillary dilatation, headache
2. Respiratory: cough, dyspnea, laryngospasm, bronchospasm, rebound hypoventilation

● DOXAPRAM HYDROCHLORIDE (Dopram Injectable) (Continued)

ACTIONS/ INDICATIONS	DOSAGE	PREPARATION AND STORAGE	DRUG INCOMPATIBILITIES	MODES OF IV ADMINISTRATION			CONTRAINDICATIONS; WARNINGS; PRECAUTIONS; ADVERSE REACTIONS
				INJECTION	INTERMITTENT INFUSION	CONTINUOUS INFUSION	
	seen, begin infusion of the 1 mg/ml solution, at a rate of 1–3 mg/min (1–2 mg/min if depression is mild, 2–3 mg/min in moderate CNS depression. Discontinue if patient awakens, or at the end of 2 hrs. Then, continue supportive therapy for 1/2–2 hrs and repeat above infusion. Do not exceed a total daily dose of 3 gm.

CHRONIC OBSTRUCTIVE PULMONARY DISEASE ASSOCIATED WITH HYPERCAPNIA: Obtain baseline arterial blood gases. Using a 2 mg/ml solution, begin an infusion at a rate of 1–2 mg/min. If necessary, increase dose to a maximum of 3 mg/min.

Monitor blood gases every 1/2 hr during infusion to detect the onset of | | | | | | 3. Cardiovascular: increased blood pressure, sinus tachycardia, bradycardia, PVC's, lowered T-waves, tightness in chest, chest pain
4. GI: Nausea, vomiting, diarrhea
5. GU: Spontaneous voiding, urinary retention
6. Rash
7. Hematologic: decreased hematocrit, increased WBC count, elevated BUN

SYMPTOMS AND TREATMENT OF OVERDOSAGE
Signs: hypertension, tachycardia, skeletal muscle hyperactivity, increased deep tendon reflexes.
Duration of effects is short; monitor and support until signs disappear. Do not administer follow-up dose until at least 15 minutes after signs return to normal. Short-acting barbiturates may relieve these effects. Be prepared to assist ventilation mechanically. |

carbon dioxide retention and acidosis. Titrate oxygen administration and drug with arterial blood gases. If patient's respiratory condition deteriorates despite above regimen, discontinue drug infusion.

In these patients, additional infusions beyond the single maximum 2-hr administration period are not recommended. This drug is not recommended for use in children under 12 yrs of age.

NURSING IMPLICATIONS

1. Monitor blood pressure before the injection and at least every 2–3 minutes for one-half hour following. Overdosage causes marked elevation in blood pressure; see Symptoms and Treatment of Overdosage above. Report elevations to the physician.
2. The respiratory stimulant action produced by this drug is an increase in tidal volume and respiratory rate. Monitor the respiratory rate with each blood pressure determination. Also examine for the presence or absence of cyanosis. Maintain a patent airway and oxygen administration according to arterial blood gases. It is suggested that blood gases be obtained every 30 minutes to determine changes in pCO_2, pO_2, pH, and $pHCO_3$. Report abnormalities to the physician. Usually a marked rise in pCO_2 or fall in pO_2 is treated with mechanical ventilation. Doxapram should be discontinued at this time.
3. Patients with a history of cardiac disease and/or arrhythmias should be observed on a continuous ECG monitor. Be prepared to treat tachy- and bradyarrhythmias.
4. Maintain seizure precautions.
5. Be prepared to manage vomiting to prevent aspiration.
6. Monitor for the neurologic signs of overdosage, i.e., skeletal muscle hyperactivity and increased deep tendon reflexes. Notify the physician of the onset.
7. Take precautions to prevent injury, e.g., side rails, close observation, restraints as needed.
8. Monitor for urinary retention for the first 8–10 hours after the drug has been given. Palpate bladder size and record urine output every 2–4 hours. This is especially likely to occur in elderly males and any patient with a history of obstructive uropathy.
9. Extravasation can cause local tissue irritation. Take measures to prevent this; see page 96. If it occurs, conservative treatment with warm compresses may be indicated.
10. Adhere strictly to suggested infusion rate. An infusion pump is advisable to control the flow rate.
11. Patients with chronic pulmonary disease being treated with this drug are usually apprehensive. Provide close observation and reassurance. Be prepared at all times to assist breathing mechanically. Keep airways, suction, and a manual breathing bag at the bedside.

DOXORUBICIN HYDROCHLORIDE (Adriamycin, Hydroxydaunomycin Hydrochloride)

ACTIONS/ INDICATIONS	DOSAGE	PREPARATION AND STORAGE	DRUG INCOMPATIBILITIES	MODES OF IV ADMINISTRATION			CONTRAINDICATIONS; WARNINGS; PRECAUTIONS; ADVERSE REACTIONS
				INJECTION	INTERMITTENT INFUSION	CONTINUOUS INFUSION	
Cytotoxic antibiotic, cell-cycle specific. Use in the management of: • Acute leukemias (lymphocytic and myelogenous) • Lymphomas (Hodgkin's and non-Hodgkin's) • Sarcomas (Ewing's, osteogenic and soft tissue) • Breast cancer • Bladder and bronchogenic carcinomas (especially oat cell) • Wilms' tumor • Neuroblastoma	ADULTS: 60–75 mg/M^2 at 21-day intervals. (Alternate schedule: 30 mg/M^2 for 3 successive days repeated every 4 weeks). Total dose limit: 550 mg/M^2. CHILDREN: 30–35 mg/ M^2, same frequency as listed above for adults. Total dose limit: 400 mg/M^2. In the presence of liver impairment, see Warning No. 5. When this drug is used concomitantly with cyclophosphamide or in patients with a history of radiotherapy to the heart, the total dose limit should be 450 mg/M^2 (adults).	To reconstitute from powder, use sterile water for injection, D5W or NS. To the 10-mg vial add 5 ml of diluent; to the 50-mg vial, add 25 ml. SHAKE UNTIL DISSOLUTION IS SEEN. Resulting solution provides concentration of 2 mg/ml. Discard after 24 hours if stored unrefrigerated or after 48 hours if refrigerated. Take precautions to avoid skin contact with this drug during preparation; skin reactions have occurred.	Do not mix with heparin. If using a heparin lock device, flush system with saline both before and after injecting. Do not mix with any other medication in any manner.	YES Inject the reconstituted solution, into the tubing of a running IV of NS or D5W, over at least 5 minutes time. Rapid injection will cause facial flushing.	YES Add reconstituted solution dose to 50– 150 ml D5W or NS; infuse over 15–30 minutes.	NO	CONTRAINDICATIONS 1. Bone marrow depression secondary to other drugs or radiation 2. Pre-existing heart disease 3. History of previous cumulative doses of this drug or daunorubicin that have reached or exceeded total dose limits WARNINGS 1. This drug can cause severe acute left ventricular failure that does not respond to usual therapies unless caught in its early stages. This usually occurs in patients who have received doses exceeding total dose limits (550 mg/M^2). This limit seems to be lower (400 mg/M^2) in patients who have received radiotherapy or other cardiotoxic drugs. 2. The ECG sign of cardiac toxicity is reduced voltage of the QRS complex. Irreversible cardiac damage may occur if administration of the drug is continued after this sign appears. Cardiac toxicity can occur up to 6 months post-treatment, and is not favorably affected by any current therapy. 3. Transient, nonsignificant ECG changes may occur. These changes include supraventricular tachyarrhythmias, premature ventricular contractions and ST-T wave changes. These are seen in 10–30% of patients receiving therapy and occur during the first few days of administration. 4. Bone marrow suppression is seen in all patients achieving objective tumor remission. Leukopenia (WBC as low as 1000/cu mm) and thrombocytopenia occur maximally during the second week of administration and return to normal by the third week. Significant suppression (WBC less than 1000/cu mm) should prompt a dosage reduction or discontinuation of the drug. 5. Dosage should be reduced in the presence of liver impairment:

Serum Bilirubin	or	BSP Retention	Dosage
1. 2–3.0 mg%		9–15%	½ normal dose
>3.0 mg%		>15%	¼ normal dose

6. Dosage reduction is required in patients with bone marrow impairment secondary to tumor infiltration.
7. This drug may potentiate the toxicity of other anticancer therapies.

PRECAUTIONS

1. Manufacturer recommends hospitalization of the patient during the first phase of therapy.
2. This drug may alter fertility of male and female patients.
3. Mutations and fetal death have been produced by this drug in experimental animals.
4. Hyperuricemia may be produced by this agent secondary to lysis of tumor cells. Monitor serum uric acid levels. Pharmacologic agents may be necessary to control this effect.
5. Urine will be discolored red for 1–2 days after administration.
6. This is not an antimicrobial agent.
7. During injection, local erythematous streaking along the vein tract as well as facial flushing may indicate too rapid an administration; injection rate should be reduced.
8. Stinging or burning sensation during administration signifies a small degree of extravasation and even if blood return is good from needle aspiration, injection or infusion should be immediately terminated. Local tissue necrosis will result from extravasation.
9. Handle powder and solution with care. Contact with skin or mucosal tissues can result in vesication of those tissues if thorough cleansing with soap and water is not carried out.

ADVERSE REACTIONS

1. Dose-limiting toxicities: bone marrow suppression (leukopenia), myocardial failure.
2. Skin: hair loss in 80% of all patients (reversible, occurs 3–4 weeks after first dose); increased pigmentation of palms, soles of feet and proximal nailbeds in black patients (rare); increase in skin changes produced by

● **DOXORUBICIN HYDROCHLORIDE** (Adriamycin, Hydroxydaunomycin Hydrochloride) *(Continued)*

ACTIONS/ INDICATIONS	DOSAGE	PREPARATION AND STORAGE	DRUG INCOMPAT- IBILITIES	MODES OF IV ADMINISTRATION			CONTRAINDICATIONS; WARNINGS: PRECAUTIONS: ADVERSE REACTIONS
				INJECTION	INTERMITTENT INFUSION	CONTINUOUS INFUSION	

CONTRAINDICATIONS; WARNINGS: PRECAUTIONS: ADVERSE REACTIONS (continued):

radiation if the two therapies are administered concomitantly.

3. Gastrointestinal: nausea, vomiting and diarrhea in 50% of all patients; stomatitis and esophagitis with severe ulcerations (80% of all patients), begins with a burning sensation with erythema leading to ulceration within 2–3 days.

4. Vascular: sclerosis of small veins used for injection; facial flushing with too rapid an injection.

5. Hypersensitivity (there may be cross-allergenicity with lincomycin).

NURSING IMPLICATIONS

1. The patient receiving this medication will be experiencing the emotional and physical effects of the malignancy. Knowledge of the patient's feelings about his disease and its implications will assist in helping him tolerate the chemotherapy. The incidence of uncomfortable side effects and adverse reactions is high. It is within the nurse's ro e to assist the patient in coping with the discomforts of the disease and its treatment, and to help him work through depression and anger toward acceptance of the disease at his own pace. Despite the unpleasantness this drug may bring, it can be a source of hope for the patient.

2. Monitor for signs and symptoms of acute left ventricular failure: increased respiratory rate, dyspnea, tachycardia, orthopnea, appearance of third and fourth heart sounds, bilateral, basilar rales, elevation of jugular venous pulse, and frank pulmonary edema. Notify physician with the appearance of any one of these signs and symptoms. Place patient at rest in a semi-Foweler's position. Monitor vital signs and above signs and symptoms for deterioration in patient's condition. The doxorubicin will be discontinued with the onset of this complication.

3. Warn the patient that the urine will be red 1–2 days after each dose.

4. Avoid extravasation; see page 96. If a stinging or burning sensation is felt during administration, stop the injection, relocate the needle and complete the dosage. Sclerosis may occur in small veins used for injection.

5. *Management of gastrointestinal effects:*

   a. Administer antiemetics at appropriate times to prevent nausea and vomiting, before injection and/or before meals.

   b. Small frequent meals, timed with periods when the patient feels his best, are advisable. Bland foods are usually better tolerated. Carbohydrate and protein content should be high.

   c. If the patient is anorexic, encourage high nutrient liquids and water to maintain hydration.

   d. Keep accurate measurements of emesis volume and total intake and output to guide the physician in ordering parenteral fluids when necessary.

   e. Monitor onset of diarrhea; notify the physician. Administer antiperistaltics as ordered. Maintain hydration and monitor for signs of hypokalemia (if diarrhea is severe), e.g., muscle cramps and weakness.

6. *Management of hematologic effects:*

   a. This is a dose-limiting toxic effect. The drug is usually discontinued or

8. *Management of stomatitis:*

   a. Administer preventive oral care every 4 hours and/or after meals.

   b. For preventive care, use a very soft toothbrush (child's) and toothpaste; avoid trauma to tissues.

   c. Examine oral membranes at least once daily (instruct patient and/or family) to detect the onset of inflammation or ulceration.

   d. If stomatitis occurs, notify the physician and begin therapeutic oral care.[1] *Mild Inflammation:* Remove dentures, use a soft toothbrush and a hydrogen peroxide solution (1 part peroxide and 4 parts saline). Do not use toothpaste. Rinse with the peroxide solution and then water. Replace dentures. This procedure should be carried out every 4 hours and/or after meals.
   Severe Inflammation: Remove dentures; use soft gauze pads rather than a toothbrush. Use the peroxide solution as described above. Rinse with water using an asepto syringe and gentle suction until returns are clear. Do not replace dentures. It may be necessary to give this care every 2–4 hours.

   e. Order a bland, mechanical diet for patients with mild inflammation. If stomatitis is severe, the patient may be placed on NPO status by the physician.

   f. For patients who can tolerate oral intake, administer Xylocaine Viscous or acetaminophen elixir as a mouthwash prior to meals to decrease pain (do not use aspirin rinses) as ordered by the physician.

   g. Patients with severe stomatitis may require parenteral analgesia.

REFERENCE

1. Bruya, Margaret Auld, and Madeira, Nancy Powell: Stomatitis After Chemotherapy. *American Journal of Nursing,* 75(8):1351, August 1975.

SUGGESTED READINGS

Bolin, Rose Homan, and Auld, Margaret E.: Hodgkin's Disease. *American Journal of Nursing,* 74:1982–1966, November 1974.

Bruya, Margaret Auld, and Madeira, Nancy Powell: Stomatitis After Chemotherapy. *American Journal of Nursing,* 75(8):1349–1352, August 1975.

Foley, Genevieve V., and McCarthy, Ann Marie: The Child with Leukemia In a Special Hematology Clinic. *American Journal of Nursing,* 76:1115–1119, July 1976.

reduced as the white cell count falls toward 2000/cu mm, and should be restarted as the white count rises. The lowest white cell count is usually seen on the 14th day after the administration and returns to normal by the 21st day.

b. Be aware of the patient's white blood cell count prior to each dose.

c. If the WBC falls below 2000/cu mm, take measures to protect the patient from infection, such as protective (reverse) isolation, avoidance of traumatic procedures, maintaining bodily (especially perineal) cleanliness, carrying out strict urinary catheter care when appropriate, etc. Monitor for infection by recording temperatures every 4 hours; examine for rashes, swellings, drainage and pain. Explain these procedures to the patient.

d. Instruct the patient and/or family on the importance of follow-up blood studies if the drug is being administered on an outpatient basis.

7. *Management of hair loss:*

a. Use a scalp tourniquet during the injection, if ordered, to help prevent hair loss.

b. Counsel the patient on the possibility of hair loss to enable him to prepare for this disfigurement.

c. Reassure him of regrowth of hair following discontinuation of the drug.

d. Provide privacy, and time for the patient to discuss his feelings.

Foley, Genevieve, and McCarthy, Ann Marie: The Disease (Hodgkin's) and Its Treatment. *American Journal of Nursing,* 76:1109–1114, July 1976 (references).

Giadquinta, Barbara: Helping Families Face the Crisis of Cancer. *American Journal of Nursing,* 77:1583–1588, October 1977.

Gullo, Shirley: Chemotherapy—What to Do About Special Side Effects. *RN,* 40:30–32, April 1977.

Hannan, Jeanne Ferguson: Talking is Treatment, Too. *American Journal of Nursing,* 74:1991–1992, November 1974.

LeBlanc, Dona Harris: People with Hodgkin's Disease: The Nursing Challenge. *Nursing Clinics of North America,* 13(2):281–300, June 1978.

Marrow, Mary: Nursing Management of the Adolescent: The Effect of Cancer Chemotherapy on Psychosocial Development. *Nursing Clinics of North America,* 13(2):319–335, June 1978.

Martinson, Ida: The Child With Leukemia: Parents Help Each Other. *American Journal of Nursing,* 76:1120–1122, July 1976.

Showfety, Mary Patricia: The Ordeal of Hodgkin's Disease. *American Journal of Nursing,* 74:1987–1991, November 1974.

Vietti, Teresa J., and Valeriote, Frederick: Conceptual Basis for the Use of Chemotherapeutic Agents and Their Pharmacology. *Pediatric Clinics of North America,* 23:67–92, February 1976.

DOXYCYCLINE HYCLATE (Vibramycin)

ACTIONS/ INDICATIONS	DOSAGE	PREPARATION AND STORAGE	DRUG INCOMPATIBILITIES	MODES OF IV ADMINISTRATION			CONTRAINDICATIONS; WARNINGS; PRECAUTIONS; ADVERSE REACTIONS
				INJECTION	INTERMITTENT INFUSION	CONTINUOUS INFUSION	
Broad-spectrum tetracycline antibiotic. Indicated in the treatment of infections secondary to: • Rickettsiae • *Mycoplasma pneumoniae* • Agents of psittacosis, ornithosis, lymphogranuloma venereum, relapsing fever • *Haemophilus ducreyi* • *Pasteurella pestis* • *Pasteurella tularensis* • *Bartonella bacilliformis*	ADULTS: 100–200 mg/24 hrs, depending on the causative organism. *Primary and secondary syphilis*—300 mg daily for at least 10 days. CHILDREN: *100 lbs or less*—2 mg/lb on the first day, then 1–2 mg/lb every 24 hrs (see Contraindications). *Over 100 lbs* —use adult dose.	Reconstitute with sterile water for injection in the following amounts: 100-mg vial: 10 ml 200-mg vial: 20 ml The resulting solution will contain 10 mg/ml. Use the following fluids for infusion: NS D5W Invert sugar 10% Ringers injection Normosol-M in D5W Normosol-R in D5W	Do not mix with any other medication	NO	YES Add the dose to at least 100 ml of infusion fluid (see Preparation column) or make a solution of 0.5 mg/ml. Infuse over 1–4 hours. Protect the solution from direct sunlight. Do not exceed recommended rate of infusion to avoid adverse reactions.	YES Total 24-hr dose can be added to 1000 ml of fluid. (see Preparation column) Protect the solution from direct sunlight. Use an infusion pump to maintain uniform flow.	CONTRAINDICATIONS Hypersensitivity to any tetracycline WARNINGS 1. May cause permanent discoloration of a child's teeth when administered during the last half of pregnancy or during infancy through the first 8 years of life. Enamel hypoplasia has also been seen. 2. This drug is secreted in breast milk. 3. Exposure to ultraviolet light may produce an exaggerated sunburn reaction. PRECAUTIONS 1. Overgrowth infections due to nonsusceptible organisms may occur. 2. This drug may depress plasma prothrombin activity, thus making it necessary to decrease the dosage of a concomitantly prescribed anticoagulant. 3. Monitor hematopoietic and hepatic function during therapy. (This drug does not accumulate in patients with renal dysfunction, nor does it cause

DOXYCYCLINE HYCLATE (Vibramycin) (Continued)

ACTIONS/ INDICATIONS	DOSAGE	PREPARATION AND STORAGE	DRUG INCOMPATIBILITIES	MODES OF IV ADMINISTRATION			CONTRAINDICATIONS; WARNINGS; PRECAUTIONS; ADVERSE REACTIONS
				INJECTION	INTERMITTENT INFUSION	CONTINUOUS INFUSION	
• *Bacteroides* • *Vibrio comma* • *Vibrio fetus* • *Brucella* • *H. influenzae* • gonococci • Some gram-negative and gram-positive organisms. Sensitivity testing is advisable.		Plasma-Lyte 56 Plasma-Lyte 148. RL* D5/RL* Infuse within 12 hours of solution preparation. Reconstituted vials should be discarded after 72 hours. *If RL or D5/RL are used for infusion, infuse within 6 hours of preparation.					further renal impairment.[1,2] 4. Avoid administering this drug with penicillin. The actions of penicillin can be reduced by this drug. ADVERSE REACTIONS 1. Gastrointestinal: anorexia, nausea, vomiting, diarrhea, dysphagia, enterocolitis (these are rarely seen) 2. Skin: *Candida albicans* infection in the mouth (thrush) or perineum (monilia), causing a red, maculopapular, itching rash; exaggerated sunburn when skin is exposed to ultraviolet light 3. Hypersensitivity reactions of all forms ranging from rashes to anaphylaxis 4. Hematologic: Hemolytic anemia, thrombycytopenia (rare) 5. Thrombophlebitis at the injection site 6. *In infants*: bulging fontanels, papilledema (pseudotumor cerebri); usually disappears on discontinuation of the drug.

NURSING IMPLICATIONS

1. Take anaphylaxis precautions; see page 118.
2. If gastrointestinal disturbances occur, notify the physician. If disturbances such as nausea, vomiting and diarrhea are pronounced, the drug will probably be discontinued. Antiemetics, antacids, and constipating agents can be ordered to control symptoms. Monitor intake and output to assist the physician in planning for parenteral fluid replacement. Maintain hydration orally when possible.
3. If the patient will be taking the oral form of this drug as an outpatient, instruct him on the possibility of photosensitivity and the advisability of avoiding exposure to the sun (sun-block lotions may be of help if exposure cannot be avoided).
4. Women of childbearing age and potential, and mothers of children who may receive this drug, should be informed of Warning No. 1 and 2 by the physician. Assist in the interpretation of these warnings to the patient.
5. Even though blood dyscrasias are infrequently caused by this agent, be aware of the patient's complete blood cell count during therapy. If the platelet count begins to fall, the drug will probably be discontinued. Bleeding secondary to a low platelet count usually begins only after the count falls below 100,000/cu mm.
6. Monitor for signs and symptoms of overgrowth infections:

  a. Fever (take rectal temperature at least every 4–6 hours in all patients)
  b. Increasing malaise
  c. Newly appearing localized signs and symptoms: redness, soreness, pain, swelling, drainage (increased volume or change in character of pre-existing drainage)
  d. Monilial rash in perineal area (reddened areas with itching)
  e. Cough (change in pre-existing cough or sputum production)
  f. Diarrhea
7. Report the onset of any rash to the physician. Keep the patient's environment comfortably cool and the skin clean. Diphenhydramine (Benadryl) may be ordered to relieve itching.
8. Report the onset of jaundice to the physician.
9. Report the onset of bulging fontanels, and other signs of increasing intracranial pressure, to the physician.

REFERENCES

1. Barza, Michael, and Schiefe, Richard T.: Antimicrobial Spectrum, Pharmacology and Therapeutic Use of Antibiotics, Part I: Tetracyclines. *American Journal of Hospital Pharmacy,* 34:51, January 1977.
2. Appel, Gerald B., and Neu, Harold C.: The Nephrotoxicity of Antimicrobial Agents. *New England Journal of Medicine,* 296(13):722, March 31, 1977.

● DROPERIDOL (Inapsine; also contained in Innovar)

ACTIONS/ INDICATIONS	DOSAGE	PREPARATION AND STORAGE	DRUG INCOMPAT- IBILITIES	MODES OF IV ADMINISTRATION			CONTRAINDICATIONS; WARNINGS; PRECAUTIONS; ADVERSE REACTIONS
				INJECTION	INTERMITTENT INFUSION	CONTINUOUS INFUSION	
Tranquilizer, sedative antiemetic. Also causes peripheral vasoconstriction. Onset of action is 3–10 minutes after injection. Full effect is seen in 30 minutes, duration is 4–12 hours.

Indicated as:
• Premedication for induction to anesthesia
• In neuroleptanalgesia in which droperidol is given with a narcotic analgesic to aid in producing tranquility, decreasing anxiety and pain | ADULTS: *Premedication prior to surgery*—2.5–10 mg, 30–60 min prior to surgery.

Adjunct to general anesthesia: Induction—220–275 mcg/kg (2.5 mg/20–25 lbs) Titrate to obtain desired result. *Maintenance*—1.25–2.5 mg as needed. *Sedation*—2.5–10 mg

Adjunct to local anesthesia—2.5–5.0 mg 30–60 min prior to surgery.

CHILDREN (2–12 years of age): *Induction of anesthesia*—88–165 mcg/kg *Premedication*—45–55 mcg/kg (1.0–1.5 mg/20–25 lbs) | Supplied in 2-ml and 5-ml ampuls, 2.5 mg/ml. | Do not mix with any other medication in any manner. | YES

May be injected without further dilution, over 2–3 minutes. | NO | NO | CONTRAINDICATIONS
Hypersensitivity to droperidol or Innovar (fentanyl-droperidol combination drug).

WARNINGS
1. If administering Innovar, see page 325 for complete details on fentanyl.
2. Means of managing hypotension, e.g., fluids and vasopressor agents, must be readily available.
3. When this drug is used in conjunction with other central nervous system depressant drugs, respiratory support equipment and a narcotic antagonist agent (naloxone) must be readily available in the event of respiratory depression.
4. Dosage of narcotic drugs should be reduced when administered concomitantly with droperidol.
5. Safety for use of this drug in children under 2 years of age has not been established.
6. Safety for use in pregnancy has not been established.

PRECAUTIONS
1. Dosage of droperidol must be reduced when administering to the elderly, debilitated, poor-risk or patients also receiving one or more of the following drugs: barbiturates, tranquilizers, general anesthetics.
2. This drug can cause hypotension in all patients but is more likely to in those receiving spinal or peridural anesthesia. If this occurs, treat with vasopressors and fluids and elevation of the legs (if possible).
3. Administer with caution to patients with renal or hepatic impairment. The duration of action of this drug will be prolonged in these two conditions.
4. This drug may decrease pulmonary arterial pressure.

ADVERSE REACTIONS
1. Mild to moderate hypotension
2. Tachycardia
3. Postoperative drowsiness
4. Dizziness |

DROPERIDOL (Inapsine; also contained in Innovar) (Continued)

ACTIONS/ INDICATIONS	DOSAGE	PREPARATION AND STORAGE	DRUG INCOMPAT- IBILITIES	MODES OF IV ADMINISTRATION			CONTRAINDICATIONS; WARNINGS; PRECAUTIONS; ADVERSE REACTIONS
				INJECTION	INTERMITTENT INFUSION	CONTINUOUS INFUSION	
							5. Restlessness 6. Hallucinations TREATMENT OF OVERDOSAGE (EXTENSION OF EXPECTED PHARMACOLOGIC ACTIONS) 1. Support respirations with oxygen and mechanical assistance as necessary. Maintain an open airway. 2. Maintain body warmth. 3. Maintain adequate hydration. 4. Monitor blood pressure frequently. Use vasopressors as necessary. Duration of action is 4–12 hours.

NURSING IMPLICATIONS
1. Obtain a preinjection blood pressure. Monitor blood pressure every 5–10 minutes after administration—hypotension may occur. See Treatment of Overdosage above. Vasopressor agents (dopamine, metaraminol, etc.) should be readily available.
2. Monitor heart rate with blood pressure. Tachycardia may occur. If the patient has a history of cardiac problems, observe for cardiac decompensation if tachycardia is excessive or prolonged: increasing respiratory rate, restlessness, rales, jugular venous distention. Notify the physician if any one of these appear. Continue to monitor carefully.
3. Initiate safety precautions to prevent patient injury, e.g., side rails, frequent observation, restraints as needed. Ambulate the patient with caution, after recovery from major drug effects.
4. Be prepared to manage hallucinations with safety precautions, patient reassurance and orientation.
5. Be prepared to support respiration.

EDROPHONIUM CHLORIDE (Tensilon)

ACTIONS/ INDICATIONS	DOSAGE	PREPARATION AND STORAGE	DRUG INCOMPAT- IBILITIES	MODES OF IV ADMINISTRATION			CONTRAINDICATIONS; WARNINGS; PRECAUTIONS; ADVERSE REACTIONS
				INJECTION	INTERMITTENT INFUSION	CONTINUOUS INFUSION	
Cholinesterase inhibitor, short- and rapid-acting. Increases the activity of the parasympathetic nervous system. Onset of action is 30–60 seconds after injection; duration is 10 min. Used in the differential diagnosis of my-	Tensilon Test for Myasthenia Gravis: ADULTS: Inject 2 mg over a 15- to 30-second period. Leave the needle in place. If no reaction occurs after 45 seconds, inject 8 mg. If a cholinergic reaction occurs, the	Supplied in multiple-dose vials of 10 ml and ampuls of 1 ml (10 mg/ml)	Do not mix with any other medication in any manner.	YES Can be injected undiluted.	NO Pharmacologically inappropriate.	NO Pharmacologically inappropriate.	CONTRAINDICATIONS 1. Hypersensitivity to any anticholinesterase drug 2. Mechanical urinary or intestinal obstruction WARNINGS 1. Keep atropine 2.0 mg at the bedside during the use of this drug to counteract severe cholinergic reactions. 2. Use with caution in patients with asthma or cardiac arrhythmias (except those being treated by this agent). Transient bradycardia can occur (treat with atropine). Cardiac and respiratory arrest have occurred. 3. Safety for use in pregnancy and lacta-

tion has not been established.

PRECAUTIONS
Some patients may develop anticholinesterase insensitivity for brief or prolonged periods, and may need respiratory assistance. These patients should either not receive such drugs, or should receive reduced dosages. See Nursing Implications.

ADVERSE REACTIONS
The reactions that can be seen with this drug are common to all cholinesterase inhibitors. Those that occur are of rapid onset and short duration because of the drug's activity time:

1. Cardiovascular: bradycardia, fall in cardiac output (decreased blood pressure), cardiac arrest (usually only after high doses, or in hypersensitive patients)
2. Respiratory: (in order of progression): increased tracheobronchial secretions, laryngospasm, bronchiolar constriction, respiratory muscle paralysis, central respiratory paralysis, apnea
3. Central nervous system: difficulty speaking and swallowing, seizures
4. Eye: increasing output of tears, constricted pupils, blurred vision, diplopia (double vision), intense redness of conjunctiva
5. Gastrointestinal: increased salivation, nausea, vomiting, diarrhea, abdominal cramps
6. Urinary frequency and incontinency
7. Diaphoresis, skeletal muscle weakness

OVERDOSAGE
1. Signs and symptoms: Nausea, vomiting, diarrhea, sweating, increased bronchial and oral secretions, bradycardia. Secretions can produce airway obstruction.
2. Maintain an open airway and adequate oxygenation.
3. Administer atropine 0.4–0.5 mg IV. Repeat every 3–10 minutes until signs and symptoms are controlled.
4. Pralidoxime chloride may also be given, 50–100 mg/min with a maximum dose of 1000 mg. Titrate dose until signs and symptoms are controlled.
5. Be prepared to manage seizures.

asthenia gravis, and also used to differentiate a myasthenic crisis from a cholinergic crisis.

Can be used when a curare antagonist is needed to reverse the neuromuscular block produced by curare, tubocurarine, gallamine triethiodide or d-tubocurarine. It is *not* effective against decamethonium or succinylcholine.

Paroxysmal atrial tachycardia unresponsive to carotid massage can sometimes be terminated with this agent.

test is terminated. (See chart in Nursing Implications section.)

If the patient's reaction appears as listed under "Adequate" in the chart, the test is also stopped. In this case, the test can be repeated in 30 minutes.

CHILDREN:
Up to 75 lbs, give 1 mg. For children over 75 lbs, give 2 mg. If there is no response in 45 seconds, titrate doses of 0.1 mg every 30–45 seconds. Maximum dose for children under 75 lbs is 5 mg; for children over 75 lbs it is 10 mg.

INFANTS:
Start with 0.1 mg and if there is no response, increase up to a maximum of 0.5 mg.

Tensilon Test During Crisis
In crisis with severe respiratory distress, use no more than 2 mg. Respirations must be adequately supported before the drug is given.

EDROPHONIUM CHLORIDE (Tensilon) (Continued)

ACTIONS/ INDICATIONS	DOSAGE	PREPARATION AND STORAGE	DRUG INCOMPAT- IBILITIES	MODES OF IV ADMINISTRATION			CONTRAINDICATIONS; WARNINGS; PRECAUTIONS; ADVERSE REACTIONS
				INJECTION	INTERMITTENT INFUSION	CONTINUOUS INFUSION	
	This test is performed to differentiate increased severity of the myasthenia gravis from overtreatment with a cholinesterase inhibitor. The 2-mg dose of drug is given once respiratory support is adequate. If the patient has had an overdose of medication, symptoms of increased oropharyngeal secretions and further weakness of respiratory muscles will appear. If the crisis is due to increased severity of the disease, the symptoms will improve. See Nursing Implications.

As a curare antagonist (adults) — 10 mg injected over 30–45 seconds; repeat as necessary. Maximum dose is 40 mg.

In paroxysmal atrial tachycardia — 10 mg; | | | | | | |

repeat up to 40 mg to convert to normal sinus rhythm.[1]

NURSING IMPLICATIONS
1. During the Tensilon test
   a. Keep atropine 1.0 mg at the bedside, ready to administer, to combat above listed adverse effects of this drug, especially bradycardia.
   b. Be prepared to support respirations (the patient's condition and/or the drug can cause respiratory distress). Begin respiratory support, if the adult patient, with encouragement, cannot breathe at a rate greater than 8–10/minute (see page 545 for normal respiratory rates in children; support the respiratory effort if the child's rate falls below normal).
   c. Be prepared to manage vomiting to prevent aspiration. Tracheal suction equipment must be at the bedside, ready for use.
   d. Patients with a history of cardiac arrhythmias should be monitored electrocardiographically during administration of this drug. Watch for slowing heart rate.
   e. Patients diagnosed as having myasthenia will need complete instruction on self-care, e.g., signs and symptoms of crisis, medications, etc. They should wear a medical identification appliance.

Expected Responses and Diagnostic Findings for the Tensilon Test for Myasthenia Gravis

SIGNS AND SYMPTOMS	MYASTHENIC RESPONSE (Seen in untreated myasthenic patients; response can establish the diagnosis of myasthenia gravis, or inadequately treated myasthenia gravis.)	ADEQUATE RESPONSE (In adequately treated myasthenics, and in normal persons.)	CHOLINERGIC RESPONSE (In myasthenics who are over-treated with a cholinesterase inhibitor.)
Muscular strength (Ptosis; diplopia, difficulty speaking, difficulty swallowing, respiratory strength, limb strength)	Increased*	No change	Decreased†
Muscle twitching (Facial muscles, limb muscles, eye movement)	Absent	Present or absent	Present or absent
Adverse effects (Nausea, vomiting, abdominal cramps, increasing tears, diaphoresis)	Absent	Minimal	Severe

* Improvement in signs and symptoms
† Exacerbation of signs and symptoms
(Courtesy of Roche Products, Inc.)

REFERENCE
1. Harrison's Principles of Internal Medicine (7th ed.), New York: McGraw-Hill Book Company, 1974, p. 1134.

SUGGESTED READINGS
Guyton, Arthur C.: Textbook of Medical Physiology (5th ed.), Philadelphia: W. B. Saunders Company, 1976, Chapter 12, Neuromuscular Transmission; Function of Smooth Muscle, pp. 148–157; Chapter 15, The Autonomic Nervous System; The Adrenal Medulla, pp. 768–781.
Jones, LeAnna: Myasthenia and Me. RN, June 1976, pp. 51–55.
Brunner, Lillian Sholtis, and Suddarth, Doris Smith: The Lippincott Manual of Nursing Practice (2nd ed.), Philadelphia: J. B. Lippincott Company, 1978, pp. 934–937.

EPHEDRINE SULFATE

ACTIONS/ INDICATIONS	DOSAGE	PREPARATION AND STORAGE	DRUG INCOMPATIBILITIES	MODES OF IV ADMINISTRATION				CONTRAINDICATIONS; WARNINGS; PRECAUTIONS; ADVERSE REACTIONS
				INJECTION	INTERMITTENT INFUSION	CONTINUOUS INFUSION		
Adrenergic drug. Elevates blood pressure, relaxes bronchospasm, stimulates CNS.	ADULTS: 10–50 mg. Repeat 25 mg every 3–4 hours.	Supplied in ampuls, 50 mg/ml. Read label carefully; use only the preparation designed for IV use. Store at room temperature.	Do not inject into an IV line containing hydrocortisone.	YES Slowly over 1 min through Y-site or 3-way stopcock.	NO Do not add to IV solution.	NO Do not add to IV solution.		CONTRAINDICATIONS 1. Hypersensitivity 2. Glaucoma (the drug can increase intraocular pressure) 3. Patients receiving cyclopropane or halothane anesthetics (arrhythmias may result)
Used in the treatment of allergic disorders; as a vasopressor; in complete heart block to increase the ventricular rate; and to elevate blood pressure during spinal anesthesia.	CHILDREN: 3 mg/kg daily in 3–4 divided doses.							PRECAUTIONS 1. Administer with caution to patients with congestive heart failure, angina pectoris, diabetes, hyperthyroidism, prostatic hypertrophy, or hypertension. This drug may cause exacerbation of these conditions. 2. Administer with caution to patients on digitalis; arrhythmias may occur. 3. Administer with caution to patients on MAO inhibitors (Eutonyl, pargyline). 4. Prolonged use or overdosage will produce a syndrome resembling an anxiety state. 5. Do not use to increase blood pressure in acute hemorrhage or cardiogenic shock.

ADVERSE REACTIONS
Most adverse reactions are extreme forms of therapeutic actions and are due to overdosage.
1. Headache
2. Restlessness
3. Insomnia
4. Anxiety
5. Weakness
6. Dizziness
7. Confusion
8. Hallucinations
9. Chest pain
10. Nausea and vomiting
11. Repeated injection may cause urinary retention

Numbers 1 through 10 can usually be managed with rest.

NURSING IMPLICATIONS
1. Monitor blood pressure and heart rate before and after injection. After injection, take readings every 5 minutes until stabilization occurs.
2. Monitor patients with the following pre-existing conditions for worsening of the conditions:
   a. Congestive heart failure (daily weights, heart rate, central venous pressure, urine output)
   b. Angina pectoris (patient should report any chest pain)
   c. Diabetes (monitor urine glucose)
   d. Hyperthyroidism (tremulousness, increased heart rate)
   e. Prostatic hypertrophy (urinary retention)
   f. Hypertension (further elevation of blood pressure)
3. Monitor ECG continuously when administering to patients on digitalis.
4. Read label carefully; there are several preparations. Intravenous preparation contains no procaine or other compounds.

EPINEPHRINE HYDROCHLORIDE (Adrenalin)

ACTIONS/ INDICATIONS	DOSAGE	PREPARATION AND STORAGE	DRUG INCOMPATIBILITIES	MODES OF IV ADMINISTRATION			CONTRAINDICATIONS; WARNINGS; PRECAUTIONS; ADVERSE REACTIONS
				INJECTION	INTERMITTENT INFUSION	CONTINUOUS INFUSION	

The principle product of the adrenal medulla. A potent sympathomimetic drug that imitates all of the actions of the sympathetic nervous system by stimulating the adrenergic receptor cells both alpha and beta. Effects produced include:
• Increased cardiac output and heart rate
• Increased systolic blood pressure
• Relaxation of bronchial spasm
• Mobilization of liver glycogen stores.
 	
Indicated in:
• Hypersensitivity reactions, including anaphylaxis
• Bronchial spasm, i.e., acute asthmatic attacks
• Cardiac asystole to assist in the restoration of a cardiac rhythm
	ADULTS:
	Bradyarrhythmias, bronchospasm and allergic disorders (anaphylaxis)—0.5–1.0 ml of a 1:1000 solution; repeat as necessary, via injection.
	
	Cardiac arrest —5 ml of a 1:10,000 solution* as an intracardiac injection, use concomitantly with basic and advanced life support measures (CPR).
	
	CHILDREN:
	Bradyarrhythmias, bronchospasm and allergic disorders (anaphylaxis)— 0.01 ml/kg or 0.3 ml/M² up to 0.5 ml of a 1:1000 solution,† repeat every 4 hours as needed.
	
	Cardiac arrest —0.3–2.0 ml diluted to a 1:10,000 solution† (or 0.1 ml/kg)
	
	NEONATES:
	For all indications— 0.1– 0.5 ml/kg of a 1:10,000 so-
		Supplied in ampuls of 1 ml, 1:1000 solution. To make a 1:10,000 solution, add 9 ml NS to 1 ml of the 1:1000 solution.
		
		Also supplied in 5-ml prefilled syringes of a 1:10,000 solution.
		
		Protect vials from light. Do not use a solution that is discolored or contains a precipitate.
		NOTE: There are several preparations of this drug, some with additives such as oil. USE ONLY EPINEPHRINE LABELED FOR INTRAVENOUS USE.
			Do not add to sodium bicarbonate or Ionosol solutions.
			
			Do not mix with: Novobiocin Warfarin Calcium-containing preparations
				YES
				
				Most commonly used mode. Inject dose over 1 minute.
					YES
					
					Use D5W or NS in any amount.
					
					Use microdrop tubing or an infusion pump to control rate. Adjust rate with patient response.
						YES
						
						Use D5W or NS in any amount.
						
						Use microdrop tubing or an infusion pump to control rate. Adjust rate with patient response.
							CONTRAINDICATIONS
							1. Shock (other than anaphylaxis)
							2. During anesthesia with cyclopropane or halogenated hydrocarbons (arrhythmias can result).
							3. Coronary insufficiency, acute myocardial infarction. (This drug increases myocardial oxygen demands.)
							
							WARNINGS
							1. This drug can further increase the intraocular pressure in persons with narrow-angle glaucoma by causing pupillary dilation.
							2. Use only in life-threatening situations during labor; this drug can cause serious arrhythmias in the infant.
							3. Use with caution in patients with the following conditions:
							  a. Congestive heart failure
							  b. Arrhythmias of ventricular or atrial irritability
							  c. Angina pectoris
							  d. Hyperthyroidism
							  e. Emphysema
							  Epinephrine may cause an exacerbation of the problem.
							4. Inadvertent rapid injection or infusion may produce a sharp rise in blood pressure which may precipitate cerebrovascular hemorrhage.
							5. When this drug must be administered in the presence of congestive heart failure, the peripheral vasoconstriction and cardiac stimulation may precipitate pulmonary edema. Nitrates or alpha adrenergic blocking agents may counteract these effects.
							6. Arrhythmias may occur in patients concomitantly receiving digitalis, mercurial diuretics, or thiazide diuretics.
							
							ADVERSE REACTIONS
							1. Central nervous system: anxiety, fear, tremulousness, headache
							2. Cardiovascular: palpitations, premature atrial and ventricular contractions, supraventricular tachycardia, ventricular tachycardia, and ventricular fibrillation; pulmonary edema in susceptible patients

315

EPINEPHRINE HYDROCHLORIDE (Adrenalin) (Continued)

ACTIONS/ INDICATIONS	DOSAGE	PREPARATION AND STORAGE	DRUG INCOMPAT- IBILITIES	MODES OF IV ADMINISTRATION			CONTRAINDICATIONS; WARNINGS; PRECAUTIONS; ADVERSE REACTIONS
				INJECTION	INTERMITTENT INFUSION	CONTINUOUS INFUSION	
• Bradycardia, to increase heart rate	lution.† (In allergic disorders, brady- arrhythmias or broncho- spasm, repeat above dose every 2–4 hrs as needed.) * When this drug is given via intra- cardiac injection, the 1:10,000 so- lution must al- ways be used. The 1:1000 solu- tion can be giv- en by IV injec- tion. †A 1:10,000 solution should be used for chil- dren regardless of indication or mode of admin- istration.						

NURSING IMPLICATIONS
1. Bedside supportive care as indicated for the condition being treated; moni- tor blood pressure and heart rate before and every 2–5 minutes after injec- tion until stabilization, then every 15–30 minutes as needed.
2. Continuous ECG monitoring is advisable in all patients. Be prepared to man- age arrhythmias; keep lidocaine 100 mg at the bedside.
3. Do not leave the patient unattended during the infusion.
4. Signs of overdosage: cold, diaphoretic skin, cyanosis of the nailbeds, change in mental status, tachypnea. Stop the infusion, continue to monitor vital signs, and notify the physician.
5. This is an essential drug to keep on hand in any patient care area where medications or treatments are being dispensed, to treat anaphylaxis.

SUGGESTED READING
Guyton, Arthur C.: Textbook of Medical Physiology. Philadelphia: W. B. Saunders Company, 1976, Chapter 57, The Autonomic Nervous System; The Adrenal Medulla, pp. 768–781; Chapter 7, Immunity and Allergy, pp. 77–87.

ERGONOVINE MALEATE (Ergotrate Maleate)

ACTIONS/ INDICATIONS	DOSAGE	PREPARATION AND STORAGE	DRUG INCOMPAT- IBILITIES	MODES OF IV ADMINISTRATION			CONTRAINDICATIONS; WARNINGS; PRECAUTIONS; ADVERSE REACTIONS
				INJECTION	INTERMITTENT INFUSION	CONTINUOUS INFUSION	
Oxytocic drug; produces firm contraction of the uterus.	IV route used for emergency treatment of uterine hemor-	Supplied in am- puls of 0.2 mg/ ml.	Do not mix in IV tubing with: Amobarbital Ampicillin	YES Give thru Y in- jection site	NO Do not add to IV solutions.	NO Do not add to IV solutions.	CONTRAINDICATIONS 1. For the induction of labor 2. In threatened spontaneous abortion 3. Hypersensitivity

Produces an initial tetanic contraction, followed by a succession of minor relaxations and contractions. The extent of relaxation increases over 1–1½ hrs but rigorous contractions continue for 3 or more hrs.

The strong initial contraction can control uterine hemorrhage. Use to prevent or treat *postpartum* or postabortal hemorrhage.

rhage. 0.2 mg may be repeated in 2–4 hrs.

Cephalothin
Chloramphenicol
Chlortetracycline
Epinephrine
Heparin
Methicillin
Nitrofurantoin
Novobiocin
Pentobarbital
Protein hydrolysate
Sulfadiazine
Sulfisoxazole diolamine
Thiopental
Warfarin

or 3-way stopcock.

PRECAUTIONS
1. Not usually recommended for routine use prior to the delivery of the placenta.
2. Avoid prolonged use.
3. Hypocalcemia may reduce uterine response, but can be remedied by the IV administration of a calcium salt.

ADVERSE REACTIONS
1. Nausea and vomiting are rare.
2. Allergic reactions include anaphylaxis.
3. Hypertension (responds to 15 mg of chlorpromazine intravenously).
4. Overdosage produces abortion, convulsions, excitement, shock, tachycardia, thirst.

NURSING IMPLICATIONS
1. Overdosage is treated with discontinuation of the drug, vasodilators, sedatives, and calcium gluconate to relieve resulting muscular pain.
2. Monitor blood pressure every 3–5 minutes after injection for 1–2 hours to detect possible secondary hypertension. Notify physician if blood pressure rises. Chlorpromazine is prescribed in some instances to lower blood pressure, see Adverse Reaction No. 3.
3. Be prepared to manage vomiting, to prevent aspiration.
4. Postpartum patients receiving this drug should be kept on bedrest during therapy.
5. Maintain usual peripartum and postpartum care:
   a. Monitoring location of fundus
   b. Lochia checks
   c. Presence of cramping

● ERYTHROMYCIN LACTOBIONATE AND GLUCEPTATE (Erythrocin Lactobionate, Ilotycin Gluceptate)

ACTIONS/ INDICATIONS	DOSAGE	PREPARATION AND STORAGE	DRUG INCOMPAT- IBILITIES	MODES OF IV ADMINISTRATION			CONTRAINDICATIONS; WARNINGS; PRECAUTIONS; ADVERSE REACTIONS
				INJECTION	INTERMITTENT INFUSION	CONTINUOUS INFUSION	
Antibiotic. Used to treat infections due to the following organisms: • Group A beta hemolytic streptococcus*	ADULTS AND OLDER CHILDREN: 15–20 mg/ kg/24 hrs. Up to 4/gm/day may be given in divided doses, every 6	Reconstitute from powder using *only* sterile water for injection (*Do not* use water for injection, bacteriostatic). Add 10 ml to the	Do not mix with any other medication in the IV bottle. Do not mix in auxiliary lines containing: Metaraminol	NO	YES Add ¼ daily dose to D5W or NS for infusion, 100–250 ml. Use prepared solutions within 4	YES Usually 1 gm is added to 1000 ml of fluid. Dilute and infuse according	CONTRAINDICATIONS Hypersensitivity WARNINGS Safety for use in pregnancy has not been established. PRECAUTIONS 1. Reduced dosage may be advisable in

● ERYTHROMYCIN LACTOBIONATE AND GLUCEPTATE (Erythrocin Lactobionate, Ilotycin Gluceptate) (Continued)

ACTIONS/ INDICATIONS	DOSAGE	PREPARATION AND STORAGE	DRUG INCOMPATIBILITIES	MODES OF IV ADMINISTRATION			CONTRAINDICATIONS; WARNINGS; PRECAUTIONS; ADVERSE REACTIONS
				INJECTION	INTERMITTENT INFUSION	CONTINUOUS INFUSION	
• Alpha hemolytic streptococcus,* Staphylococcus aureus • Streptococcus pneumoniae • Mycoplasma pneumoniae • Hemophilus influenzae • Corynibacterium diphtheriae • Listeria monocytogenes • Neisseria gonorrhoeae* • The organism of Legionnaire's disease • Penicillin is usually considered the drug of choice in the treatment of infections due to these organisms, but erythromycin is an acceptable substitute in the presence of positive sensitivity tests, for patients who are sensitive to penicillin.	hrs, or by continuous infusion. NEONATES: 30–50 mg/kg/24 hrs. ADULTS WITH ACUTE PELVIC INFLAMMATORY DISEASE CAUSED BY N. GONORRHOEAE: 500 mg every 6 hrs for 3 days followed by 250 mg erythromycin stearate or base (oral preparation) every 6 hrs for 7 days. LEGIONNAIRE'S DISEASE: Optimal doses have not been established. Current recommendation—1–4 gm/day in divided doses.	500-mg vial and 20 ml to the 1000-mg vial, concentration will be 50 mg/ml. Store the reconstituted solution in the refrigerator. Discard after 2 weeks.	Cephalothin Cephaloridine Cefazolin Aminophylline Tetracyclines Streptomycin		hrs, infuse over 20–60 min. A more rapid infusion may cause irritation of the vein.	to the dosage and fluid volume, and the following information: When adding erythromycin gluceptate to a volume of solution which must be infused over a time greater than 4 hrs, the solution should be buffered to a pH of 7 using a sodium bicarbonate 4% solution (Abbott Lab's. Neut) or a phosphate-carbonate solution (Buff). Add 1 ampul of Buff or 5 ml of Neut to 500 or 1000 ml D5W or NS. When adding erythromycin lactobionate to the following fluids: D5W D5 in lactated Ringer's D5/NS Normosol-M in D5W Normosol-R in D5W, buffering compounds must first be added to the solution. Add 5 ml of 4% sodium bicarbonate (Abbott Lab's., Neut) to	patients with hepatic impairment. 2. Monitor hepatic function during therapy. ADVERSE REACTIONS 1. Allergic reactions ranging in severity from rashes to anaphylaxis. 2. Overgrowth infections secondary to nonsusceptible organisms.

each 500–1000 ml of solution used. When using NS, lactated Ringer's or Normosol-R without D5W, buffering is not required. Infuse all solutions within 8 hours.

b. Increasing malaise
c. Newly appearing localized signs and symptoms: redness, soreness, pain, swelling, drainage (increased volume or change in character of pre-existing drainage)
d. Monilial rash in perineal area (reddened areas with itching)
e. Cough (change in pre-existing cough or sputum production)
f. Diarrhea

NURSING IMPLICATIONS
1. Monitor effectiveness of drug therapy:
   a. Temperature every 4 hours (rectal if possible)
   b. Sputum production, quality and quantity
   c. The appearance of the wound
2. Take anaphylaxis precautions: see page 118.
3. Monitor for signs and symptoms of overgrowth infections:
   a. Fever (take rectal temperature at least every 4–6 hours in all patients)

ESTROGENS, CONJUGATED (Premarin Intravenous)

ACTIONS/ INDICATIONS	DOSAGE	PREPARATION AND STORAGE	DRUG INCOMPAT-IBILITIES	MODES OF IV ADMINISTRATION			CONTRAINDICATIONS; WARNINGS; PRECAUTIONS; ADVERSE REACTIONS
				INJECTION	INTERMITTENT INFUSION	CONTINUOUS INFUSION	
Female sex hormone, a mixture of estrogens. Used to control abnormal uterine bleeding due to hormonal imbalance in the absence of pathology. Also used to control spontaneous capillary bleeding and oozing during surgery and to decrease postoperative bleeding by increasing serum prothrombin levels, and decreasing antithrombin activity.	ADULTS: Usually one 25-mg injection, can be repeated in 6–12 hrs. CHILDREN: (To reduce blood loss during surgery.) 5–10 mg repeated as necessary.	To reconstitute powder, withdraw air from estrogen vial; using the diluent provided by the manufacturer (use no other), inject slowly against the vial wall, then agitate gently to dissolve. Store all forms in refrigerator and protect from light. Reconstituted form should be discarded after 60 days. Do not use if discoloration or precipitation occurs.	Do not inject into an IV line containing protein hydrolysate, vitamins, or Ringer's Lactate.	YES. May be injected into the tubing of a running IV, slowly to avoid inducing estrogen flush, 5 mg/min.	NO	NO	CONTRAINDICATIONS Do not use in women with any one of the following conditions: 1. Known or suspected cancer of the breast, except in patients being treated for metastatic disease 2. Known or suspected estrogen-dependent neoplasia 3. Known or suspected pregnancy (see Warnings) 4. Undiagnosed abnormal genital bleeding 5. Active thrombophlebitis, or thromboembolic disease 6. Past history of thrombophlebitis, thrombosis, or thromboembolic disorders associated with previous estrogen use (except when used in the treatment of breast malignancy) WARNINGS The following effects usually apply to long-term estrogen therapy. The risk of their occurring in short-term intravenous use is unknown; however, they should be kept in mind when this drug is administered. 1. Long-term continuous administration

● ESTROGENS, CONJUGATED (Premarin Intravenous) *(Continued)*

| ACTIONS/ INDICATIONS | DOSAGE | PREPARATION AND STORAGE | DRUG INCOMPAT- IBILITIES | MODES OF IV ADMINISTRATION | | | CONTRAINDICATIONS; WARNINGS: PRECAUTIONS; ADVERSE REACTIONS |
				INJECTION	INTERMITTENT INFUSION	CONTINUOUS INFUSION	
							of estrogen may increase the likelihood of carcinomas of the breast, cervix, vagina and liver, and may increase the risk of endometrial carcinoma. Cyclic administration of low doses may carry less risk than continuous therapy. Close clinical surveillance is required. Administer with caution in women with a strong family history of breast cancer or who have breast nodules, fibrocystic disease, or abnormal mammograms.

2. Use of this drug in pregnancy (early) may seriously damage the offspring. Females exposed in utero have an increased risk of developing a vaginal or cervical cancer. Vaginal adenosis and epithelial changes of the vagina and cervix may also occur, and may be precursors to malignancy. There may also be fetal abnormalities (limb and heart) due to this drug.

3. There may be an increased risk of gallbladder disease in women receiving postmenopausal estrogens.

4. There is an increased risk of thromboembolic disease in patients receiving estrogen therapy. If feasible, estrogens should be discontinued at least 4 weeks before surgery (of the type associated with an increased risk of thromboembolism) or during periods of prolonged immobilization. See Contraindication No. 6. Use with caution in the presence of cerebral vascular accidents or coronary artery disease. Male patients may have an increased risk of nonfatal myocardial infarction, pulmonary embolism and thrombophlebitis while on this drug in large doses (5 mg/day).

5. Benign hepatic adenomas have occurred (rarely) in patients on estrogen therapy. Signs and symptoms of this lesion may be abdominal pain (upper right quadrant), tenderness over the liver and a palpable mass. Rupture of this lesion will produce hypovolemic shock and intraperitoneal hemorrhage.

6. There may be an elevation in blood pressure, especially when high doses

are used.
7. There may be a decrease in glucose tolerance in diabetic and nondiabetic patients. Monitor serum glucose.
8. The administration of estrogens may lead to a severe hypercalcemia in patients with breast cancer and bone metastases. If this occurs, the drug should be stopped and appropriate measures taken to reduce serum calcium level.

PRECAUTIONS
1. Thorough family and patient medical history, and a physical examination must be carried out prior to use of this drug.
2. There may be an increase in fluid retention.
3. Patients with a past history of mental depression should be carefully observed for exacerbation of that illness.
4. Pre-existing uterine leiomyomata may increase in size during estrogen use.
5. Administer with caution to patients with impaired liver function; reduced dosage is advisable.
6. Use with caution in patients with incomplete bone growth; this drug effects epiphyseal closure with long-term therapy.
7. Alterations in organ function studies may occur with this drug:
   a. Increased sulfobromophthalein retention
   b. Increased prothrombin and factors VII, VIII, IX, and X; decreased antithrombin 3; increased norepinephrine-induced platelet aggregability. Increased: PBI, T_4 by column method, or T_4 by radioimmunoassay. Free T_3 resin uptake is decreased. Free T_4 is unaltered
   c. Impaired glucose tolerance
   d. Decreased pregnanediol excretion
   e. Reduced response to metyrapone test
   f. Reduced serum folate concentration
   g. Increased serum triglyceride and phospholipid concentration
8. This drug may be excreted in breast milk.

ADVERSE REACTIONS
1. Genitourinary: vaginal bleeding, spotting, change in menstrual flow, dysmenorrhea, premenstruallike syndrome, amenorrhea during and after treatment, increase in size of uterine

ESTROGENS, CONJUGATED (Premarin Intravenous) (Continued)

ACTIONS/ INDICATIONS	DOSAGE	PREPARATION AND STORAGE	DRUG INCOMPAT- IBILITIES	MODES OF IV ADMINISTRATION			CONTRAINDICATIONS; WARNINGS; PRECAUTIONS; ADVERSE REACTIONS
				INJECTION	INTERMITTENT INFUSION	CONTINUOUS INFUSION	

CONTRAINDICATIONS; WARNINGS; PRECAUTIONS; ADVERSE REACTIONS

fibromyomata, vaginal candidiasis, change in cervical erosion and degree of secretion, cystitislike syndrome
2. Breasts: tenderness, enlargement, secretion
3. Gastrointestinal: nausea, vomiting, abdominal cramps, bloating. Cholestatic jaundice may occur only in long-term therapy
4. Skin: cholasma or melasma, which may persist after the drug is discontinued, erythema multiforme, erythema nodosum, hemorrhagic eruption, loss of scalp hair, hirsutism
5. Eyes: steepening of corneal curvature, intolerance to contact lenses, usually with long-term therapy
6. Central nervous system: headache, migraine, dizziness, mental depression, chorea
7. Miscellaneous: increased weight, decreased glucose tolerance, aggravation of porphyria, peripheral edema, changes in libido (these effects may be seen in short-term therapy)

NURSING IMPLICATIONS
1. Be aware of all contraindications to the use of this agent; assist in taking a detailed history from patient and/or family.
2. Weigh the patient daily during therapy, notify physician of weight gain over 5 pounds in the course of a week. Patients with congestive heart failure or renal impairment may retain additional fluid. Monitor patients with congestive heart failure for signs and symptoms of further cardiac decompensation:
a. Sudden weight gain over 1-2 days
b. Dyspnea, increased resting respiratory rate, orthopnea, rales
c. Resting tachycardia
d. Elevation of jugular venous distention
e. Peripheral edema
f. Liver enlargement
g. Onset of third and fourth heart sounds
3. Monitor blood pressure every 2-4 hours or as patient's condition dictates. Elevations may occur.
4. Be aware of serum and urine glucose values. Diabetic patients may require larger doses of insulin due to decreased glucose tolerance.
5. When administering this drug to patients with breast cancer and bone metastasis, monitor for signs and symptoms of hypercalcemia:
a. Weakness
b. Anorexia, nausea and vomiting
c. Polyuria
6. If the patient has a history of mental depression, monitor for signs and symptoms of exacerbation. Explain cause to the patient, and provide support.

ETHACRYNATE, SODIUM (Edecrin)

ACTIONS/ INDICATIONS	DOSAGE	PREPARATION AND STORAGE	DRUG INCOMPAT- IBILITIES	MODES OF IV ADMINISTRATION			CONTRAINDICATIONS; WARNINGS; PRECAUTIONS; ADVERSE REACTIONS
				INJECTION	INTERMITTENT INFUSION	CONTINUOUS INFUSION	CONTRAINDICATIONS
Potent diuretic	ADULTS AND	Reconstitute by	Do not mix in	YES	YES	NO	

acts on the ascending limb of the loop of Henle, the proximal and distal tubules, to produce excretion of water, chloride, hydrogen, sodium, and potassium ions. Onset of action is within 5 min after injection.

Used for the treatment of:
- Edema in congestive heart failure, cirrhosis, renal disease
- Ascites of malignancy, idiopathic edema, lymphedema
- Short-term management of hospitalized older children with heart disease or nephrotic syndrome (not used in infants)
- Pulmonary edema: magnitude of diuresis depends on degree of fluid accumulation

OLDER CHILDREN (average weight): 50 mg (0.5–1.0 mg/kg); do not exceed single doses of 100 mg. May be repeated. Use small doses when giving over prolonged period.

Not recommended for use in infants.

adding 50 ml of D5W or NS. Do not use if solution is hazy or opalescent.

Discard after 24 hours.

IV line or syringe with any other medication.

May be given through Y-site. Inject *slowly* over at least 5 min. Use new injection site for each dose or flush well with IV fluid after injection.

Add reconstituted form to 50 ml NS. Run over 20–30 min. Do not use if solution is hazy.

1. Anuria
2. Discontinue if electrolyte imbalance, azotemia, and/or oliguria occur during treatment of renal disease
3. Discontinue if diarrhea occurs and do not readminister
4. Use in infants is not recommended
5. Pregnancy of any stage
6. Nursing mothers

WARNINGS
1. Produces profound diuresis with water and electrolyte depletion.
2. When used in cirrhotic patients, hospitalization is advised; hepatic coma may be precipitated.
3. Acute hypotension may occur.
4. Loss of serum potassium may precipitate arrhythmias in patients concomitantly receiving digitalis. Replace potassium according to serum concentration.
5. Lithium should not be given concomitantly, to prevent lithium toxicity.

PRECAUTIONS
1. Liberalization of sodium intake may be necessary during therapy.
2. Metabolic alkalosis may occur in patients with cirrhosis.
3. Safety and efficacy in hypertension has not been established.
4. Orthostatic hypotension may occur in patients on other antihypertensive agents.
5. Transient increase in BUN may occur. This reverses after discontinuation of the drug.
6. Monitor hearing when administering to critically ill patients or those receiving other ototoxic drugs (gentamycin, kanamycin, streptomycin, neomycin, cephaloridine).
7. Reduction in anticoagulant dosage may be required.

ADVERSE REACTIONS
1. Gastrointestinal: anorexia, nausea, vomiting, dysphagia, diarrhea
2. Renal: reversible hyperuricemia and acute gout
3. Carbohydrate metabolism—hyperglycemia in patients with cirrhosis; can potentiate oral hypoglycemic agents
4. Hematologic: agranulocytosis or severe neutropenia
5. Hepatic: jaundice, altered liver function

ACTIONS/ INDICATIONS	DOSAGE	PREPARATION AND STORAGE	DRUG INCOMPAT- IBILITIES	MODES OF IV ADMINISTRATION			CONTRAINDICATIONS; WARNINGS: PRECAUTIONS: ADVERSE REACTIONS
				INJECTION	INTERMITTENT INFUSION	CONTINUOUS INFUSION	
							6. Ear: vertigo, deafness, and tinnitus have occurred usually in renal patients; usually reversible within 24 hours; rarely is damage permanent (see Precaution No. 6.)

NURSING IMPLICATIONS
1. Monitor for onset of diarrhea, notify physician. Drug is usually discontinued if this occurs.
2. Monitor for signs of:
   a. Sodium depletion — mental confusion, weakness, abdominal cramps, stupor, hypotension.
   b. Potassium depletion — muscle cramps, weakness
   c. Dehydration — weight loss greater than 2 lbs/day, dry mucous membranes, decreased skin turgor (tenting), weakness, lethargy, decreasing venous pressure, decreased urine output.
   d. Hepatic encephalopathy — confusion, muscle tremors.
3. Patients also receiving digitalis should be observed via continuous ECG monitoring for onset of digitalis toxicity arrhythmias (sinus bradycardia and premature ventricular contractions most frequently seen). (See page 288 on digoxin for more detailed information on digitalis toxicity.)
4. Monitor blood pressure before and immediately after injection and every 5 minutes for the next hour. Fluids and vasopressors may be ordered to treat hypotension.
5. Ambulate with caution if patient is on any other antihypertensive agent; there may be postural hypotension.
6. Monitor for loss of hearing, tinnitus, and vertigo. Notify physician.

SUGGESTED READINGS
Kemp, Ginny, and Kemp, Doug: Diuretics. *American Journal of Nursing*, June 1978, pp. 1007–1010.
Plumb, Vance J., and James, Thomas N.: Clinical Hazards of Powerful Diuretics, Furosemide and Ethacrynic Acid. *Modern Concepts of Cardiovascular Disease*, July 1978, pp. 91–94.

● FAT EMULSION, 10% (Intralipid 10%)

ACTIONS/ INDICATIONS	DOSAGE	PREPARATION AND STORAGE	DRUG INCOMPAT- IBILITIES	MODES OF IV ADMINISTRATION			CONTRAINDICATIONS; WARNINGS: PRECAUTIONS: ADVERSE REACTIONS
				INJECTION	INTERMITTENT INFUSION	CONTINUOUS INFUSION	
Fatty acids in emulsion form used as a source of calories and to provide essential fatty acids. To prevent fatty acid deficiency for patients requiring parenteral nutrition, and to reverse a known deficiency state characterized by scaly skin	ADULTS: 100 mg/min (1 ml/min) for the first 15–30 min then increase to 2–3 ml/min if no reaction. Give only 500 ml (50 gm) first 24 hrs; if no reaction, increase following day. Do not exceed 2.5 gm/kg/day. Should not make up more than 50–60%	Store in refrigerator. Discard unused portion. *Use the administration set provided by the manufacturer.* Do not use if there is any separation of the solution. Keep the bottle and tubing higher than all other IV bottles and tubing in a piggyback system. This will	Do not add any other medication to the infusion; must be infused alone.	NO	YES Infuse separately from any other IV, if possible. *Do not mix* with IV fluids. Can be infused in same vein as parenteral nutrition fluids by Y-site. Rate of each infusion should be controlled by separate pumps. *Do not* use filters.	YES Infuse separately from any other IV, if possible. *Do not mix* with IV fluids. Can be infused in same vein as parenteral nutrition fluids by Y-site. Rate of each infusion should be controlled by separate pumps. *Do not* use filters.	CONTRAINDICATIONS Fat metabolism disturbances (hyperlipidemia, lipoid nephrosis, acute pancreatitis if accompanied by hyperlipidemia). WARNINGS Administer with caution to patients with severe liver damage, pulmonary disease, anemia or blood coagulation disorders, or when there is a pre-existing danger of fat embolism. PRECAUTIONS 1. Monitor the patient's ability to remove infused fat from circulation. The lipemia must clear between daily infusions. 2. Liver function must be monitored. If impairment develops, the emulsion

prevent the lighter-than-water fat solution from floating up into other IV lines and bottles.

If possible, use a separate IV site for this infusion alone.

10% solution- 100 mg/ml

should not be continued; transient increases in LDH and SGOT following infusion usually return to normal within 4–8 hrs.[1]
3. Daily platelet counts should be done on neonates.

ADVERSE REACTIONS
1. Thrombophlebitis at infusion site
2. Rarely: dyspnea, cyanosis, allergic reactions, vomiting, headache, flushing, hyperlipidemia, hypercoagulability
3. Delayed reactions: hepatomegaly, splenomegaly, thrombocytopenia, leukopenia, transient elevation of liver function tests
4. Overload of fat syndrome: focal seizure, fever, leukocytosis, splenomegaly, shock

NURSING IMPLICATIONS
1. Extreme caution must be exercised to prevent contamination of infusion, tubing, and IV site.
2. Monitor infusion site for signs of thrombophlebitis. Adhere to suggested infusion rates to decrease vein irritation, despite the fact that this solution is isotonic.

3. Stop infusion if any adverse reaction occurs; see above list. Notify the physician if any one of these complications arises.

REFERENCE
1. Jeffrey, L. P., et al.: Intravenous Fat Emulsion: An Innovative Concept. *Hospital Formulary,* 12(1):772–773 (references).

● FENTANYL (Sublimaze; also contained in Innovar)

ACTIONS/ INDICATIONS	DOSAGE	PREPARATION AND STORAGE	DRUG INCOMPAT- IBILITIES	MODES OF IV ADMINISTRATION			CONTRAINDICATIONS; WARNINGS; PRECAUTIONS; ADVERSE REACTIONS
				INJECTION	INTERMITTENT INFUSION	CONTINUOUS INFUSION	
Narcotic, analgesic. Actions similar to morphine and meperidine. Indications: • Preanesthetic • To maintain anesthesia • Postoperative pain A dose of 0.1 mg is approximately equivalent in analgesic activity to 10 mg of	Dosage must be individualized by age, weight, pathology, and other drugs, and anesthesia to be used. ADULTS: *Premedication* —0.05–0.1 mg *Adjunct to general anesthesia* —0.05– 0.1 mg repeated at 2- to 3-min intervals *Maintenance*	Store at room temperature. Keep in packaging to protect from light. This is a Schedule II under the Controlled Substances Act of 1970. Maintain hospital or institutional regulations guiding its use.	Do not mix with any other medication.	YES Slowly, over 2–3 min.	NO	NO	CONTRAINDICATIONS Hypersensitivity WARNINGS 1. Resuscitative equipment must be readily available, including a narcotic antagonist to manage apnea. 2. Patients receiving this drug must not be left alone. 3. Be prepared to treat hypotension. 4. Respiratory depression occurs and lasts longer than the analgesic effects. Large doses can cause apnea. 5. When other narcotics are used, administer 1/4 to 1/3 of the usual dose. 6. Muscle rigidity may occur with rapid injection. 7. Drug dependence can occur. 8. Severe and unpredictable potentiation by MAO inhibitors has been

● **FENTANYL** (Sublimaze; also contained in Innovar) (*Continued*)

ACTIONS/ INDICATIONS	DOSAGE	PREPARATION AND STORAGE	DRUG INCOMPAT- IBILITIES	MODES OF IV ADMINISTRATION			CONTRAINDICATIONS; WARNINGS: PRECAUTIONS; ADVERSE REACTIONS
				INJECTION	INTERMITTENT INFUSION	CONTINUOUS INFUSION	
morphine and 75 mg of meperidine.

Onset of action is almost immediate after IV injection. Maximal analgesic and respiratory depressant effects are seen after 5–15 min. The usual duration of the analgesic effect is 30–60 min. | *of anesthesia* —0.025–0.05 mg as needed *Regional anesthesia*—0.05– 0.1 mg *Postop*— 0.05 –0.1 mg every 2 hrs | | | | | | reported; they should not be administered for 14 days prior to use of fentanyl.
9. Use with caution in patients who are susceptible to respiratory depression, e.g., increased intracranial pressure, brain tumor. This drug may also obscure clinical signs of these conditions.
10. Safety for use in children less than 2 years of age has not been established.
11. Safety for use in pregnancy and during delivery has not been established.

PRECAUTIONS
1. The initial dose must be reduced in the elderly, debilitated and other poor-risk patients. Reaction to initial dose should determine subsequent doses.
2. Respiratory depression can occur and is additive to the depression caused by local and systemic anesthesia.
3. Hypotension can occur; treat with head-down position if possible, and fluids. Pressor agents can also be used (except epinephrine).
4. Use with caution in patients with pulmonary disease.
5. If respiratory depression occurs with postoperative administration, use a narcotic antagonist (nalorphine, naloxone) and assisted ventilation.
6. Pulmonary arterial pressure can be reduced if the droperidol-fentanyl form of this drug is used.
7. Other central nervous system depressant drugs will need to be given in reduced dosage when used with fentanyl.
8. Administer with caution in the presence of liver or kidney impairment.
9. Bradycardia may occur. Atropine may be used to reverse this. Use with caution in patients with preexisting bradyarrhythmias.

ADVERSE REACTIONS
1. Most common: respiratory depres- |

sion, apnea, bradycardia, muscle rigidity. If these are untreated, cardiac arrest can result.
2. Dizziness, hypotension, blurred vision, nausea, vomiting, laryngospasm.
3. With the droperidol-fentanyl combination: chills, restlessness postop.; can be controlled with antiparkinson agents, if severe.

MANAGEMENT OF OVERDOSAGE
1. Manifestations of overdosage:
   a. Respiratory depression—hypoventilation and apnea
   b. Muscle rigidity
   c. Bradycardia, circulatory depression (hypotension)
2. Treatment:
   a. Assisted ventilation, oxygen, maintenance of patent airway.
   b. If muscle rigidity is present, an intravenous neuromuscular blocking agent may be needed to allow assisted ventilation.
   c. A narcotic antagonist such as nalorphine, levallorphan, or naloxone should be used for respiratory depression after the above emergency supportive measures have been initiated. Follow individual narcotic antagonist instructions: nalorphine (Nalline), page 415; levallorphan (Lorfan), page 360; naloxone (Narcan), page 417. The duration of respiratory depression may exceed the duration of effectiveness of the antagonist.

Monitor for onset of laryngospasm (dyspnea, wheezing, stridor). If the respiratory rate falls (adults: less than 8–10/minute; children: see chart of normal values on page 545), attempt to verbally stimulate the patient to increase the respiratory rate. Frequency of stimulation should be such as to bring the rate to a normal level. If the patient cannot be aroused, begin assisted ventilation with a manual breathing bag (Ambu, Puritan, Hope). Maintain a patent airway with an oral-pharyngeal airway; administer oxygen if cyanosis develops. Notify physician. Have a narcotic antagonist agent at the bedside. Continue respiratory support until swallow, gag and cough reflexes return, and until the patient's spontaneous respiratory rate is 12–14/minute. Monitor blood gases and remain with the patient for the next several hours. Note that the duration of action of a narcotic antagonist may be less than that of the respiratory depression produced by the fentanyl; additional doses of the antagonist may be needed.
4. Be prepared to manage vomiting to prevent aspiration.
5. If this drug is given to patients who are ambulatory, assist as needed in the event of dizziness, to prevent injury.

NURSING IMPLICATIONS
1. Patients receiving this drug intravenously should be under constant observation to detect the possible onset of respiratory or circulatory depression. Resuscitative equipment and drugs should be readily available.
2. Monitor heart rate and blood pressure before and every 5–10 minutes after an injection, for 30 minutes. Then monitor these parameters every 15 minutes times 3. The duration of action is 30–60 minutes in patients with normal liver and kidney function and over 60 minutes in the presence of hepatic and renal impairment. Patients with pre-existing arrhythmias should be observed via continuous ECG monitoring during therapy with this drug. Bradycardia (adults: heart rate less than 60/minute; for children see chart of normal rates on page 545) can be treated with atropine 0.5–1.0 mg. Significant hypotension will probably be treated with vasopressors and/or a narcotic antagonist.
3. For patients not already receiving respiratory assistance, monitor respiratory rate at least every 3–5 minutes following an injection. At the same time, observe for the presence of cyanosis of the oral membranes and nail beds.

327

FLOXURIDINE (FUDR)

ACTIONS/ INDICATIONS	DOSAGE	PREPARATION AND STORAGE	DRUG INCOMPAT- IBILITIES	MODES OF IV ADMINISTRATION			CONTRAINDICATIONS; WARNINGS; PRECAUTIONS; ADVERSE REACTIONS
				INJECTION	INTERMITTENT INFUSION	CONTINUOUS INFUSION	
Antineoplastic antimetabolite. Used in the palliative management of carcinoma. For regional intra-arterial infusion only.	0.1–0.6 mg/ kg/day. Higher doses are recommended for liver perfusion: 0.4–0.6 mg/kg/day. Administer until adverse reactions appear, and resume when they disappear. Continue for as long as positive effects are seen.	Reconstitute the 500-mg vial with 5 ml sterile water for injection. This yields a solution containing 100 mg/ml. Store in refrigerator. Discard after 2 weeks.	Do not mix with any other medication.	NO	NO	YES For continuous *intra-arterial* infusion only. Daily dose is diluted in D5W or NS 1000 ml (smaller volumes can be used in fluid-restricted patients). Use an infusion pump to overcome arterial pressure and insure uniform rate of infusion.	CONTRAINDICATIONS 1. Poor nutritional status 2. Depressed bone marrow function 3. Serious infection WARNINGS 1. Patients should be hospitalized during first course of treatment. 2. Use with extreme caution in poor risk patients with: 　a. Impaired liver or renal function 　b. History of high-dose pelvic irradiation 　c. Previous therapy with alkylating agents 3. This drug is not intended as an adjuvant to surgery. 4. Safety for use in pregnancy has not been established with respect to adverse effects in fetal development. Teratogenicity and mutagenicity have been demonstrated in animals. 5. Any other agent which adds stress, interferes with nutrition or depresses bone marrow will increase the toxicity of floxuridine. 6. *Signs of toxicity:* Stomatitis, esophagopharyngitis, leukopenia (WBC less than 3500/cu mm), vomiting (intractable), diarrhea, gastrointestinal ulceration and bleeding, thrombocytopenia (platelets less than 100,000/cu mm), hemorrhage from any site. Therapy must be promptly discontinued until signs disappear. PRECAUTIONS 1. The highly toxic nature of this drug must be explained to the patient prior to therapy. A therapeutic response is unlikely to occur without some evidence of toxicity. 2. White blood cell count and platelet count should be monitored daily during initial stages of therapy. Severe hematologic toxicity, gastrointestinal hemorrhage and death can occur even in carefully selected and monitored patients. The drug must be discontinued when toxic signs occur.

ADVERSE REACTIONS

1. Gastrointestinal: nausea, vomiting (intractable in toxicity), diarrhea, enteritis, stomatitis
2. Blood: marrow depression producing leukopenia and thrombocytopenia
3. Hepatic: elevation of liver function tests (SGOT, bilirubin)
4. Skin: hair loss, rashes, pruritus, skin ulceration
5. Neurologic: ataxia, blurred vision, seizures, depression
6. Urologic: dysuria
7. Fever and malaise
8. Hypoadrenalism
9. Vascular damage (chemical)

NURSING IMPLICATIONS

1. A pump will be required to infuse the medication against arterial pressure and to insure correct infusion rate.
2. Administer care to arterial catheter daily using sterile technique. (See care of subclavian IV catheter, page 50.) Monitor for signs of vascular infection or vessel irritation (drainage, swelling, redness, pain, fever), bleeding, aneurysm formation (pulsatile mass in incisional area); infuse at correct rates to decrease likelihood of vessel damage.
3. Take extra precaution to prevent dislodgement of the catheter. Be prepared to manage arterial bleeding if dislodgement occurs. If patient is able, instruct him on emergency care. Keep equipment at bedside (sterile 4 × 4 gauze pads, phlebotomy tray, tourniquet).
4. Extravasation must be avoided (see page 96). If it occurs, notify the physician immediately and discontinue perfusion. Apply warm compresses and prevent further trauma to the affected area, and administer care as ordered by the physician.
5. *Management of gastrointestinal effects:*
   a. Administer antiemetics at times to produce the greatest symptomatic relief such as prior to the infusion and/or prior to meals, whichever is more effective.
   b. Small frequent meals, timed with periods when the patient feels his best, are advisable. Bland foods are more easily tolerated. Carbohydrate and protein content should be high.
   c. If the patient is anorexic, encourage high nutrient liquids and water to maintain hydration.
   d. Keep accurate measurements of emesis volume and total intake and output to guide the physician in ordering parenteral fluids when necessary.
6. *Management of hematologic effects:*
   a. Be aware of the patient's white blood cell and platelet count prior to each injection.
   b. If the WBC falls below 2000/cu mm, take measures to protect the patient from infection, such as protective (reverse) isolation, avoidance of traumatic procedures, maintenance of bodily (especially perineal) cleanliness, carrying out strict urinary catheter care when appropriate, etc. Monitor for infection by recording temperatures every 4 hours, examining for rashes, swellings, drainage and pain. Explain these measures to the patient.
   c. If the platelet count falls below 100,000/cu mm, monitor for thrombocytopenic bleeding: petechiae, purpura, hematuria, melena, blood in stools, gum bleeding, vaginal bleeding, epistaxis, hematemesis, etc.

Avoid trauma. Transfusions may be ordered.
7. *Management of hair loss:*
   a. Counsel the patient on the possibility of hair loss to enable him to prepare for this disfigurement.
   b. Reassure him of regrowth of hair following discontinuation of the drug.
   c. Provide privacy, and time for the patient to discuss his feelings.
8. If rashes occur, administer cool compresses as ordered. Turn the patient frequently, if on bed rest, to prevent skin breakdown. Notify the physician if skin ulceration occurs. Prevent injury to affected areas. If the patient experiences pruritus, keep the environmental temperature around 70-72 degrees. Diphenhydramine (Benadryl) may be ordered to decrease the itching.
9. *Management of neurologic effects:*
   a. Ataxia: Protect the patient from injury; ambulation should be assisted.
   b. Blurred vision: Take safety precautions; reassure the patient of the temporary nature of the visual changes.
   c. Seizures: Initiate seizure precautions; notify physician of occurrence.
   d. Mental depression: Reassure the patient that this is a drug-induced symptom that is transient; provide time for the patient to express concerns; educate family of the problem, elicit their help.
10. Maintain adequate fluid (especially water) intake to help prevent dysuria secondary to the drug and its metabolite in the bladder. Encourage the patient to void every 2 hours.
11. *Management of stomatitis:*
    a. Administer preventive oral care every 4 hours and/or after meals.
    b. For preventive care use a very soft toothbrush (child's) and toothpaste; avoid trauma to tissues.
    c. Examine oral membranes at least daily (instruct patient and/or family) to detect the onset of inflammation or ulceration.
    d. If stomatitis occurs, notify the physician and begin therapeutic oral care:[1]
       (1) *Mild Inflammation:* Remove dentures; use a soft toothbrush and a hydrogen peroxide solution (1 part peroxide and 4 parts saline). Do *not* use toothpaste. Rinse with the peroxide solution and then water. Replace dentures. This procedure should be carried out every 4 hours and/or after meals.
       (2) *Severe Inflammation:* Remove dentures; use soft gauze pads rather than a toothbrush. Use the peroxide solution as described above. Rinse with water using an asepto syringe and gentle suction until returns are clear. Do not replace dentures. It may be necessary to give this care every 2-4 hours.

● FLOXURIDINE (FUDR) (Continued)

NURSING IMPLICATIONS (No. 11 continued)
  e. Order a mechanical soft, bland diet for patients with mild inflammation. If the stomatitis is severe, the patient may be placed on a liquid diet or NPO status by the physician.
  f. For patients who can tolerate oral intake, administer Xylocaine Viscous or acetaminophen elixir as a mouthwash prior to meals to decrease pain (do not use aspirin rinses), as ordered by the physician.
  g. Patients with severe stomatitis may require parenteral analgesia.

REFERENCE

1. Bruya, Margaret Auld, and Madeira, Nancy Powell: Stomatitis After Chemotherapy. *American Journal of Nursing,* 75:1351, August 1975.

SUGGESTED READINGS
  Bruya, Margaret Auld, and Madeira, Nancy Powell: Stomatitis After Chemotherapy. *American Journal of Nursing,* 75(8):1349–1352, August 1975.
  Giadquinta, Barbara: Helping Families Face the Crisis of Cancer. *American Journal of Nursing,* 77:1583–1588, October 1977.
  Gullo, Shirley: Chemotherapy—What To Do About Special Side Effects. *RN,* 40:30–32, April 1977.

● FLUOROURACIL (5-FU, 5-Fluorouracil)

ACTIONS/ INDICATIONS	DOSAGE	PREPARATION AND STORAGE	DRUG INCOMPATIBILITIES	MODES OF IV ADMINISTRATION			CONTRAINDICATIONS; WARNINGS; PRECAUTIONS; ADVERSE REACTIONS
				INJECTION	INTERMITTENT INFUSION	CONTINUOUS INFUSION	

Antineoplastic, antimetabolite, cell-cycle specific. For palliative management of carcinoma of colon, rectum, breast, stomach and pancreas when considered incurable by surgery or other means.	ADULTS AND CHILDREN: Dosage must be based on weight (use ideal weight if there has been weight gain due to edema).
	
	12–15 mg/kg/day once a day, for 4 successive days. *Daily dose must not exceed 800 mg.* If no toxicity is observed, 6 mg/kg is given on 6th, 8th, 10th, and 12th days. Discontinue after 12th day dose.
	
	Patients in poor nutritional state (see Contraindications) should receive 6 mg/kg/day for 3 successive days. If no toxicity is seen, 3 mg/kg may be
		Available in 10-ml ampuls containing 500 mg of drug (50 mg/ml).
		
		Slight discoloration does not affect the use of the drug. Protect from light. If a precipitate occurs due to exposure to low temperatures, resolubilize by heating to 140°F (60°C) and shake.
		
		Cool to body temperature before administering.
			Do not mix with any other medication in any manner.	YES
				
				No dilution is required
					YES
					
					Use D5W or NS 100–200 ml.
					
					Infuse over 30–60 min.
						NO	CONTRAINDICATIONS
							1. Poor nutritional state
							2. Depressed bone marrow function
							3. Presence of serious infection
							
							WARNINGS
							1. Patient must be hospitalized during initial treatment.
							2. Use with extreme caution in patients with a history of high-dose pelvic irradiation, previous use of alkylating agents, those who have bone marrow involvement by metastatic tumors, or who have impaired hepatic or renal function.
							3. Safety for use in pregnancy has not been established.
							4. There may be mutagenic effects on germinal cells of males and females.
							5. Any form of therapy that adds stress, interferes with nutrition, or depresses bone marrow, will increase the toxicity of fluorouracil.
							6. Therapy should be discontinued if any one of the following signs of toxicity appear:
							  a. Stomatitis, esophagopharyngitis
							  b. Leukopenia, WBC <3500/cu mm
							  c. Vomiting (intractable)
							  d. Diarrhea
							  e. GI ulceration or bleeding
							  f. Platelet count <100,000/cu mm
							  g. Hemorrhage from any site
							
							PRECAUTIONS
							1. WBC with differential should be taken prior to each dose.

2. Death has resulted from fluorouracil due to GI hemorrhage or bone marrow depression.
3. Avoid extravasation.

ADVERSE REACTIONS
1. Gastrointestinal: anorexia, nausea, vomiting, diarrhea, stomatitis, esophagopharyngitis (usually seen on fourth day of a loading dose therapy and subsides 2–3 days after discontinuation (50% of all patients)
2. Blood: bone marrow depression producing leukopenia and thrombocytopenia (leukopenia nadir—maximum depression—at 9–21 days, and thrombocytopenia nadir at 7–17 days)
3. Skin: hair loss (reversible), loss of finger- and toenails, rashes (usually seen on trunk, maculopapular), photosensitivity, Addisonian hyperpigmentation
4. Photophobia
5. Neurologic: reversible cerebellar ataxia (1% incidence, may last several weeks after discontinuation)

b. Be prepared to administer antiemetics around the fourth day of loading dose therapy. These drugs can be given prophylactically prior to the onset of symptoms.
c. Small frequent meals, timed with periods when the patient feels his best, are advisable. Bland foods are usually tolerated better than others. Carbohydrate and protein content should be high.
d. If the patient is anorexic, encourage high nutrient liquids and water to maintain nutrition and hydration.
e. Keep accurate measurements of emesis volume and total intake and output to guide the physician in ordering parenteral fluids when necessary.
f. Monitor for the onset of diarrhea. Notify the physician and administer antiperistaltic drugs as ordered. Observe for signs and symptoms of hy-

given on 5th, 7th, and 9th days. Daily dose should not exceed 400 mg.

If no toxicity, continue on following schedules:
1. Repeat dosage of first course every 30 days after the last day of the previous course.
2. When toxic signs have subsided, administer a maintenance dose of 10–15 mg/kg/week as a single dose. Do not exceed 1 gm/week.

Upper limit for daily dose in poor-risk patients is 400 mg.

Dosage reduction in the presence of renal impairment must be based on individual patient response.[1]

NURSING IMPLICATIONS
1. The patient receiving this medication will be experiencing the emotional and physical effects of the malignancy. Knowledge of the patient's feelings about his disease and its implications will assist in helping him tolerate the chemotherapy. The incidence of uncomfortable side effects and adverse reactions is high. It is within the nurse's role to assist the patient in coping with the discomforts of the disease and its treatment, and to help him work through depression and anger toward acceptance of the disease at his own pace. Despite the unpleasantness this drug may bring, it can be a source of hope for the patient.
2. *Management of gastrointestinal effects:*
   a. See Adverse Reactions No. 1.

331

FLUOROURACIL (5-FU, 5-Fluorouracil) (Continued)

NURSING IMPLICATIONS (No. 2 continued)

g. Monitor for signs and symptoms of esophagopharyngitis: sore throat, dysphagia, burning pain in the chest. Notify the physician. Administer antacids as ordered. A bland, mechanical soft diet is advisable.

3. *Management of stomatitis:*

a. Administer preventive oral care every 4 hours and/or after meals.

b. For preventive oral care use a very soft toothbrush (child's) and toothpaste; avoid trauma to the tissues.

c. Examine oral membranes at least once daily (instruct patient and/or family) to detect the onset of inflammation or ulceration.

d. If stomatitis occurs, notify the physician and begin therapeutic oral care:[2]

   Mild Inflammation: Remove dentures: use a soft toothbrush and a hydrogen peroxide solution (1 part peroxide and 4 parts saline). Do not use toothpaste. Rinse with the peroxide solution and then water. Replace dentures. This procedure should be carried out every 4 hours and/or after meals.

   Severe Inflammation: Remove dentures; use soft gauze pads rather than a toothbrush. Use the peroxide solution as described above. Rinse with water using an asepto syringe and gently suction until returns are clear. Do not replace dentures. It may be necessary to give this care every 2–4 hours.

4. *Management of hematologic effects:*

a. The greatest degree of bone marrow depression occurs usually on day 7–14; the time of recovery varies.

b. Be aware of the patient's white blood cell and platelet count prior to each injection.

c. If the WBC falls to 2000/cu mm, take measures to protect the patient from infection such as protective (reverse) isolation, avoidance of traumatic procedures, maintaining bodily (especially perineal) cleanliness, carrying out strict urinary catheter care when appropriate, etc. Monitor for infection by recording temperature every 4 hours, and examining for rashes, swellings, drainage and pain. Explain these measures to the patients.

d. If the platelet count falls below 100,000/cu mm, monitor for thrombocytopenic bleeding: petechiae, purpura, hematuria, melena, blood in stools, gum bleeding, vaginal bleeding, epistaxis, hematemesis, etc. Avoid trauma. Transfusion may be ordered.

e. Instruct the patient and family on the importance of follow-up blood studies if the drug is being administered on an outpatient basis.

5. *Management of hair loss:*

a. Use a scalp tourniquet during injection, if ordered, to help prevent hair loss.

b. Counsel the patient on the possibility of hair loss to enable him to prepare for this disfigurement.

c. Reassure him of regrowth of hair following discontinuation of the drug.

d. Provide privacy, and time for the patient to discuss his feelings.

6. *Management of skin problems:*

a. If rashes occur, administer cool compresses as ordered. Turn the patient on bed rest frequently to prevent skin breakdown.

b. Reassure the patient that finger- and toenails will grow back after discontinuation of the drug. Protect fingers and toes from trauma.

c. Warn the patient to avoid exposure to the sun to prevent sunburn. If exposure is unavoidable, suggest the use of a sunblock lotion.

d. Inform the patient of the transient nature of skin pigmentation changes.

7. If the patient develops ataxia, initiate measures to protect him from injury during dangerous activities such as climbing stairs.

REFERENCES

1. Shinn, Arthur F., et al.: Dosage Modification of Cancer Chemotherapeutic Agents in Renal Failure. *Drug Intelligence and Clinical Pharmacy,* 11:141, March 1977.

2. Bruya, Margaret Auld, and Madeira, Nancy Powell: Stomatitis After Chemotherapy. *American Journal of Nursing,* 75(8):1351, August 1975.

SUGGESTED READINGS

Bruya, Margaret Auld, and Madeira, Nancy Powell: Stomatitis After Chemotherapy. *American Journal of Nursing,* 75(8):1349–1352, August 1975.

Giadquinta, Barbara: Helping Families Face the Crisis of Cancer. *American Journal of Nursing,* 77:1583–1588, October 1977.

Gullo, Shirley: Chemotherapy—What To Do About Special Side Effects. *RN,* 40:30–32, April 1977.

Laatsch, Nancy: Nursing the Woman Receiving Adjuvant Chemotherapy for Breast Cancer. *Nursing Clinics of North America,* 13(2):337–349, June 1978.

FOLIC ACID (Folate Sodium, Folvite, Pteroylglutamic Acid)

ACTIONS/ INDICATIONS	DOSAGE	PREPARATION AND STORAGE	DRUG INCOMPAT- IBILITIES	MODES OF IV ADMINISTRATION			CONTRAINDICATIONS; WARNINGS; PRECAUTIONS; ADVERSE REACTIONS
				INJECTION	INTERMITTENT INFUSION	CONTINUOUS INFUSION	
Vitamin, required for the formation of DNA and RNA, thereby promotes growth, stimulates production of red	ADULTS: 0.25–1.0 mg daily. Resistant cases may require larger doses. Daily maintenance dosage after	Store in original packaging to protect from light.	Do not mix with any solution or medication containing a calcium salt or heavy metal salt.	YES Over 1 minute. Use a 100 mcg/ml solution (add 5 mg folic acid to 49 ml of sterile	YES In any IV fluid in any amount.	YES In any IV fluid in any amount.	WARNINGS Administration of folic acid alone is not correct therapy for pernicious anemia and other megaloblastic anemias in which vitamin B_{12} is deficient. PRECAUTIONS Folic acid may obscure pernicious ane-

blood cells. Used to treat megaloblastic anemias, macrocytic anemias secondary to malabsorption states (sprue trauma, worm infestation). Combined with iron, it alleviates secondary or iron deficiency anemia.

RBC count is normal: 0.4 mg

Pregnancy or lactation— 0.8 mg.

CHILDREN: IV administration not recommended.

mia in that blood counts may be normal with continued advancement of neurological degeneration.

ADVERSE REACTIONS
Hypersensitivity reactions.

water for injection to make this solution).

NURSING IMPLICATIONS
Take anaphylaxis precautions; see page 118.

● FUROSEMIDE (Lasix)

ACTIONS/ INDICATIONS	DOSAGE	PREPARATION AND STORAGE	DRUG INCOMPAT- IBILITIES	MODES OF IV ADMINISTRATION			CONTRAINDICATIONS; WARNINGS; PRECAUTIONS; ADVERSE REACTIONS
				INJECTION	INTERMITTENT INFUSION	CONTINUOUS INFUSION	
Potent diuretic. Effect begins within 5 min of injection, peaks in 30 min, lasts 2 hrs.

Used in the treatment of edema in congestive heart failure, cirrhosis, and renal disease. Emergency treatment of pulmonary edema. | ADULTS: *Initial*—20-40 mg. A second dose can be given 2 hrs later. If no response, increase dose by 20-mg increments, no sooner than 2 hrs after last dose.

Pulmonary edema—40 mg followed by another 40 mg in 1-1½ hours.*

CHILDREN: 1 mg/kg. If no response, increase by 1 mg/kg in 2 hrs. Doses | Store at room temperature. Do not use if solution is yellow.

Use filtering needle (or syringe filter) when removing from ampuls. | Do not mix with any other medication. | YES

Slowly over 1-2 min. Most effective mode to produce diuresis. | YES

Use NS, RL, or D5W *only.* Administer at 1 mg/min. | YES

Use NS, RL, or D5W *only.* Infuse within 24 hrs.

Use this mode for large doses to avoid hearing loss, 2000 -3000 mg over 8-10 hrs; do not exceed a rate of 4 mg/ min. | CONTRAINDICATIONS
1. May cause fetal abnormalities; do not use in pregnancy or in women who may be pregnant without weighing benefits against risk
2. Anuria
3. If BUN or oliguria increases during therapy, discontinue drug
4. Hepatic coma or electrolyte imbalance
5. Hypersensitivity

WARNINGS
1. Excessive diuresis may result in dehydration, reduction of blood volume, or circulatory collapse. The possibility of vascular thrombosis exists, especially in elderly patients.
2. Excessive loss of potassium may precipitate digitalis toxicity.
3. Sudden alterations of fluid and electrolyte balance may precipitate hepatic coma.
4. Observe for blood dyscrasias, liver damage, and idiosyncratic reactions.
5. There may be cross-allergenicity with sulfonamides. |

● **FUROSEMIDE** (Lasix) (*Continued*)

ACTIONS/ INDICATIONS	DOSAGE	PREPARATION AND STORAGE	DRUG INCOMPAT- IBILITIES	MODES OF IV ADMINISTRATION			CONTRAINDICATIONS; WARNINGS; PRECAUTIONS; ADVERSE REACTIONS
				INJECTION	INTERMITTENT INFUSION	CONTINUOUS INFUSION	
	greater than 6 mg/kg are not recommended. *Very high doses are sometimes used in renal failure, up to 3000 mg.						**CONTRAINDICATIONS; WARNINGS; PRECAUTIONS; ADVERSE REACTIONS** PRECAUTIONS 1. There will be loss of sodium, water and potassium. 2. Patients concomitantly receiving antihypertensive agents may need reduced dosage of those agents while on furosemide. 3. Asymptomatic hyperuricemia may occur. 4. Reversible elevations of BUN have been reported, usually secondary to dehydration. This should be avoided in renal patients. 5. Tinnitus and reversible hearing impairment have been reported. Some cases of irreversible hearing loss have been seen. Ototoxicity has usually been evident following rapid injection of doses exceeding the recommended level, in patients with renal failure. Slow infusion of this drug is recommended when renal impairment is present. (Do not exceed 4 mg/min.) 6. Alterations in glucose tolerance can occur in diabetics and latent diabetics; hyperglycemia has been reported. 7. Salicylate toxicity may occur in patients on high doses of salicylates in conjunction with furosemide. 8. Furosemide may increase the nephrotoxicity of cephaloridine. 9. This drug may decrease arterial responsiveness to pressor amine drugs. 10. There may be an enhanced response to curare and its derivatives. Patients who will be undergoing surgery should have furosemide discontinued 2 days before. ADVERSE REACTIONS 1. Dermatitis: urticaria, pruritus, exfoliative dermatitis 2. Nausea, vomiting, diarrhea 3. Postural hypotension 4. Blurred vision 5. Hematologic changes 6. Hearing loss (see Precautions No. 5) 7. Children: abdominal pain following injection

8. Diuresis may be accompanied by weakness, fatigue, dizziness, muscle cramps, thirst, diaphoresis, urinary urgency

a. Excessive weight loss
b. Decreased skin turgor (tenting)
c. Weakness, lethargy
d. Decreased urine output
e. Increased specific gravity
5. Monitor blood pressure every 30 minutes after injection and then every 2 hours or as indicated by the patient's condition. Hypovolemia and fall in cardiac output with subsequent hypotension is likely to occur with excessive diuresis. Fluids will be used to re-establish blood volume. Utilize central circulatory monitoring devices if available, such as pulmonary artery pressure and central venous pressure.

SUGGESTED READINGS
Kemp, Ginny, and Kemp, Doug: Diuretics. *American Journal of Nursing,* 78:1007–1010, June 1978 (references).
Plumb, Vance J.: Clinical Hazards of Powerful Diuretics, Furosemide and Ethacrynic Acid. *Modern Concepts of Cardiovascular Disease,* 47(7), July 1978.

NURSING IMPLICATIONS
1. Weigh the patient prior to therapy and daily thereafter.
2. Monitor urine output every 8 hours or more frequently as indicated. Observe for oliguria (adults: less than 30 ml/hour for 2 or more consecutive hours; children: see page 546). Observe for bladder distention in susceptible patients. Use a urinary collection device in infants and small children.
3. Monitor for electrolyte imbalance, i.e., hyponatremia, hypokalemia. Signs and symptoms:

Hyponatremia
Headache
Nausea, diarrhea
Abdominal cramps
Confusion and stupor
Hypotension (late)

Hypokalemia
Weakness
Muscle cramps
Lethargy
Irritability
Abdominal distention
Cardiac arrhythmias (late)
Poor feeding in infants.

Administer potassium supplements as ordered.
4. Monitor for dehydration:

● GENTAMICIN SULFATE (Garamycin 40 mg/ml and Garamycin Pediatric 10 mg/ml)

ACTIONS/ INDICATIONS	DOSAGE	PREPARATION AND STORAGE	DRUG INCOMPATIBILITIES	MODES OF IV ADMINISTRATION				CONTRAINDICATIONS; WARNINGS; PRECAUTIONS; ADVERSE REACTIONS
				INJECTION	INTERMITTENT INFUSION	CONTINUOUS INFUSION		
Aminoglycoside antibiotic to treat serious infections due to susceptible strains of the following organisms: • *Pseudomonas aeruginosa* • *Proteus* • *E. coli* • *Klebsiella-Enterobacter-Serratia* Effective in septicemia, infections of the CNS, urinary tract, respiratory tract, GI	IN THE PRESENCE OF NORMAL RENAL FUNCTION ADULTS: 3 mg/kg/day in equally divided doses every 8 hrs. In life-threatening infections, up to 5 mg/kg/day (reduce as soon as clinically indicated). See page 337 for dosage in the presence of renal failure.	Mix in D5W or NS only. Supplied in the following forms: 2-ml vials (80 mg) 1.5-ml vials (60 mg) 2-ml prefilled syringes (80 mg) Concentration is 40 mg/ml. Pediatric form: 2-ml vials (20 mg) Concentration is 10 mg/ml.	Do not mix with: Carbenicillin Cephalosporins Heparin Oxacillin Choramphenicol Nafcillin Vitamin B complex	NO Nephrotoxicity, ototoxicity increased with rapid injection.	YES Use 100–200 ml NS or D5W. Do not exceed a concentration of 1 mg/ml. *Infuse over 1–2 hours.*	NO Therapeutically inappropriate.		CONTRAINDICATIONS Hypersensitivity WARNINGS 1. This drug is nephrotoxic; use with caution in patients with pre-existing renal impairment. Monitor renal function in all patients. Discontinue if BUN or creatinine rises. 2. This drug produces both vestibular and auditory damage. That occurs most frequently in patients with renal disease or those receiving higher than recommended doses. Monitor eighth cranial nerve function. Discontinue at first signs. 3. Peritoneal or hemodialysis will remove drug from the blood. 4. Monitor serum concentration when possible. (Keep peak <12 mcg/ml, valleys <2 mcg/ml.) 5. Concurrent use of streptomycin, neomycin, kanamycin, cephaloridine, vio-

GENTAMICIN SULFATE (Garamycin 40 mg/ml and Garamycin Pediatric 10 mg/ml) (Continued)

ACTIONS/ INDICATIONS	DOSAGE	PREPARATION AND STORAGE	DRUG INCOMPAT- IBILITIES	MODES OF IV ADMINISTRATION			CONTRAINDICATIONS; WARNINGS; PRECAUTIONS; ADVERSE REACTIONS
				INJECTION	INTERMITTENT INFUSION	CONTINUOUS INFUSION	
tract, skin, and soft tissues	CHILDREN: 3–6 mg/kg/ day given in equally divided doses every 8 hours. INFANTS AND NEONATES: < 1 week of age—5 mg/ kg/24 hrs, in equally divided doses every 12 hrs. 1–6 weeks of age—7.5 mg/ kg/24 hrs, in equally divided doses every 8 hrs. > 6 weeks— 5.0–7.5 mg/ kg/24 hrs,in equally divided doses every 6 hrs. PREMATURE: Not recom- mended un- less infection is life-threaten- ing; then fol- low dosage listed for in- fants and neo- nates above. In the presence of renal failure in adults:[1] 1. Select Loading Dose in mg/kg [LEAN WEIGHT] to provide peak serum level desired. Approxi- mate peak levels from commonly used loading doses are indicated below:						mycin, polymyxin B, or polymyxin E should be avoided. 6. Avoid use of potent diuretics. 7. Safety for use in pregnancy has not been established. PRECAUTIONS 1. May potentiate the effects of succinyl- choline and tubocurarine. 2. Overgrowth of nonsusceptible organ- isms can occur. ADVERSE REACTIONS 1. Nephrotoxicity, usually due to larger than recommended doses 2. Neurotoxicity: damage to vestibular and auditory branches of the eighth cranial nerve. Numbness, skin tin- gling, muscle twitching and seizures have been reported 3. Hypersensitivity: fever, rash, itching urticaria 4. Anemia and other blood dyscrasias 5. Nausea, vomiting, anorexia, transient hepatomegaly 6. Hypo- and hypertension 7. Neuromuscular blockade, may poten- tiate other agents with neuromuscu- lar-blocking properties.

LOADING DOSE	EXPECTED PEAK SERUM LEVEL BASED UPON ONE-HALF HOUR IV INFUSION
2.0 mg/kg	6–8 μg/ml
1.75 mg/kg*	5–7 μg/ml
1.5 mg/kg	4–6 μg/ml
1.25 mg/kg	3–5 μg/ml
1.0 mg/kg	2–4 μg/ml

*(Recommended for most moderate to severe systemic infections.)

2. Select Maintenance Dose (as percentage of chosen loading dose) to continue peak serum levels indicated above according to patient's creatinine clearance and desired dosing interval.

PERCENTAGE OF LOADING DOSE REQUIRED FOR DOSAGE INTERVAL SELECTED:

Cr. Clear.	8 hrs.	12 hrs.	24 hrs.
90	90%	—	—
80	88	—	—
70	84	—	—
60	79	91%	—
50	74	87	—
40	66	80	—
30	57	72	92%
25	51	66	88
20	45	59	83
15	37	50	75
10	29	40	64
7	24	33	55
5	20	28	48
2	14	20	35
0	9	13	25

Hull and Sarubbi do not recommend adjustments of gentamicin dosage in patients with mild to moderate renal impairment who are receiving carbenicillin concomitantly.[2]

NURSING IMPLICATIONS
1. Take anaphylaxis precautions; see page 118.
2. Monitor renal function:
   a. BUN and creatinine—be aware of these values, daily.
   b. Urinary output—monitor for oliguria every 8 hours or as condition indicates.
   c. Urine specific gravity—fall in value may indicate impending failure. Weight—weigh patients before initiating and daily throughout therapy. Notify physician of changes in renal status.
3. Monitor for eighth cranial nerve damage:
   a. *Auditory damage*—High-frequency hearing, loss as determined by audiometric testing, general hearing loss.
   b. *Vestibular damage*—dizziness, vertigo, tinnitus (ringing in the ears), roaring in the ears.

4. Monitor for signs and symptoms of nonsusceptible organism overgrowth infection:
   a. Fever (take rectal temperature at least 4–6 hours)
   b. Increasing malaise
   c. Signs and symptoms of localized infection: redness, soreness, pain, swelling, drainage (change in volume or character of pre-existing drainage)
   d. Cough (change in volume or character or pre-existing sputum)
   e. Diarrhea
   f. Oral lesions (thrush) or perineal itching and rash (monilia) secondary to *Candida albicans*

REFERENCES
1. Hull, J. Heyward, and Sarubbi, Felix A.: Gentamicin Serum Concentrations:

REFERENCES (Continued)
1. Pharmacokinetic Predictions. Annals of Internal Medicine, 85:188, August 1976. (Used by permission.)
2. Ibid.

SUGGESTED READING
Vanderveen, Timothy W.: Aminoglycoside Antibiotics. American Journal of IV Therapy, July 1977, pp. 5–13.

● **GLUCAGON HYDROCHLORIDE**

ACTIONS/ INDICATIONS	DOSAGE	PREPARATION AND STORAGE	DRUG INCOMPATIBILITIES	MODES OF IV ADMINISTRATION			CONTRAINDICATIONS; WARNINGS; PRECAUTIONS; ADVERSE REACTIONS
				INJECTION	INTERMITTENT INFUSION	CONTINUOUS INFUSION	
Produced in the pancreas; causes an increase in blood glucose. Used to treat hypoglycemic states. Liver glycogen must be present for drug to be effective. Juvenile-type diabetes may also need carbohydrate injection in addition. Used by some groups to reverse the adverse effects of propranolol and enhance the effect of digitalis when used for congestive heart failure. (Glucagon has a mild positive inotropic effect; that is, it can increase the force of myocardial contractility and increase cardiac output.)	*In hypoglycemia—* ADULTS: 0.5–1.0 unit. If patient does not respond, repeat twice and *administer glucose, 50% by intravenous injection.* CHILDREN: 0.025–1.0 mg/kg/dose. Repeat in 20 min. Maximum total dose is 1 mg. Administer 50% dextrose in water concomitantly. NEONATES: (The symptomatic newborn of a diabetic mother) 0.30 mg/kg/dose, repeated once in 20 min. Give 50% dextrose in addition.	Use diluent provided by manufacturer and no other. Use entire diluent vial. Solution produced is 1 mg/ml. Refrigerate and discard after 90 days.	Do not mix with any other medication in any manner.	YES. May administer through Y-injection site over 1 min.	NO. Pharmacologically inappropriate.	NO. Pharmacologically inappropriate.	CONTRAINDICATIONS Hypersensitivity PRECAUTIONS Liver glycogen stores must be available. If not, supplements of glucose must be given to treat the hypoglycemia. ADVERSE REACTIONS Nausea and vomiting on awakening from hypoglycemic state

NURSING IMPLICATIONS
Hypoglycemia:
1. Stay with the patient with hypoglycemia. Monitor time of awakening. Repeat dose in 20 minutes if there is no response.
2. Maintain an open intravenous line.
3. Have 50% dextrose at the bedside.
4. Prevent aspiration by turning patient on his side. Keep tracheal suction equipment at bedside. Use airways (manual breathing bags, etc.) and assist breathing as needed.
5. Observe seizure precautions.
6. If patient does not awaken after 20 minutes and full doses of glucagon and glucose, unconscious state may be due to something other than hypoglycemia.
7. Determine what precipitated the hypoglycemia.
8. Instruct patient and family on:
   a. causes and prevention of hypoglycemia
   b. signs and immediate treatment
   c. Use of glucagon at home (if prescribed by physician)
   d. Complete diabetic self-care

HEPARIN, SODIUM (Lipo-Heparin, Panheparin, Sodium Heparin from Beef Lung, Sodium Heparin from Porcine Intestinal Mucosa)

ACTIONS/ INDICATIONS	DOSAGE	PREPARATION AND STORAGE	DRUG INCOMPATIBILITIES	MODES OF IV ADMINISTRATION			CONTRAINDICATIONS; WARNINGS; PRECAUTIONS; ADVERSE REACTIONS
				INJECTION	INTERMITTENT INFUSION	CONTINUOUS INFUSION	
Anticoagulant, a mucopolysaccharide formed by the mast cells and present in the human body in minute amounts.	Titrate dosage with clotting time and/or partial thromboplastin time (PTT). Maintain PTT at 1.5–2 times a control value.	Supplied in beef lung and porcine intestinal mucosa derivations in the following concentrations: 1000 units/ml 5000 units/ml 10,000 units/ml 20,000 units/ml	Do not mix with: Gentamicin Procainamide Prochlorperazine Diphenhydramine Promazine Narcotics Barbituates Erythromycin Cephalothin	YES Give undiluted.	YES Use 50–100 ml of any IV fluid (usually D5W or NS).	YES *Preferred mode of administration.* Add 24-hr dose to 1000 ml of any fluid (usually D5W or NS).	CONTRAINDICATIONS 1. Hypersensitivity 2. Peptic ulcer disease (active) 3. Inability to perform suitable blood coagulation tests 4. Uncontrollable bleeding 5. Cerebral hemorrhage 6. Advanced liver disease 7. Threatened abortion 8. Splenomegaly
Heparin is thought to exert its anticoagulant effect by potentiating the action of a circulating heparin co-factor (antithrombin III) in neutralizing the activator forms of clotting factors VII, IX, X, XI and XII as well as thrombin. May also block the action of bioactive amines released from platelets at the surface of the thromboembolus. These	ADULTS: Initially, 10,000 units. Follow with 5,000–10,000 units every 4–6 hrs by injection or intermittent infusion; or 20,000 to 40,000 units/ 24 hrs via continuous infusion, 1000 units/hr. In total body perfusion, 150 units/kg, guided by appropriate coagulation studies throughout the procedure.		If an intermittent scalp-vein needle infusion set is used, flush the system with NS before these drugs are given.			Use an infusion pump.	WARNINGS 1. Use with caution in disease states in which there is an increased chance of hemorrhage, such as subacute bacterial endocarditis, arterial sclerosis, increased capillary permeability; during and immediately following major surgery, especially of brain, spinal cord and eye; hemophilia; thrombocytopenia; tube drainage of any organ. 2. Appropriate coagulation studies (usually partial thromboplastin time) should be done after initial dose and after any change in dosage. 3. Salicylates may induce bleeding because of their effect on platelet aggregation (the main hemostatic defense of heparinized patients), and the ulcerative action they have on gastric mucosa. 4. Use with caution any drug which prolongs prothrombin time or delays coagulation in any way. 5. Because this agent is derived from an-

HEPARIN, SODIUM (Lipo-Heparin, Panheparin, Sodium Heparin from Beef Lung, Sodium Heparin from Porcine Intestinal Mucosa) (*Continued*)

ACTIONS/INDICATIONS	DOSAGE	PREPARATION AND STORAGE	DRUG INCOMPATIBILITIES	MODES OF IV ADMINISTRATION			CONTRAINDICATIONS; WARNINGS; PRECAUTIONS; ADVERSE REACTIONS
				INJECTION	INTERMITTENT INFUSION	CONTINUOUS INFUSION	
amines are responsible in part for local constriction of bronchi and blood vessels in a pulmonary embolus. • Used for prophylaxis and treatment of: 1. Venous thrombosis 2. Pulmonary embolism 3. Atrial fibrillation with embolus • Prevention of cerebral thrombosis • Diagnosis and treatment of disseminated intravascular coagulation defects • Prevention of intravascular clotting after arterial or cardiac surgery • Anticoagulation in: hemodialysis, peritoneal dialysis, transfusion, and extracorporeal circulation.	CHILDREN: Initially, 50 units/kg; maintenance, 100 units/kg every 4 hrs. See Management of Overdosage for protamine neutralization of heparin.						imal tissue, it should be used with caution in patients with a history of allergy. Before a therapeutic dose is given to such a patient, a trial dose of 1000 units should be given. 6. Use with caution during pregnancy, especially during the last trimester (heparin does not cross the placental barrier), and in the immediate postpartum period when bleeding could take place. There is no adequate information on whether this drug may cause fetal abnormalities. 7. Larger than normal doses of heparin may be necessary in febrile states. 8. The use of digitalis, tetracyclines, nicotine, and antihistamines may partially counteract the anticoagulant action of heparin. 9. An increased resistance to heparin is frequently encountered in cases of thrombosis, thrombophlebitis, infections with thrombosing tendency, myocardial infarction, cancer, and in the postoperative patient. Increased dosage and careful monitoring of coagulation studies may be needed. PRECAUTIONS 1. Use with caution in the presence of mild hepatic or renal disease, hypertension, and during menstruation. 2. Caution should be used when administering ACD-converted blood (blood collected in heparin sodium and later converted to ACD blood), since heparin anticoagulant activity persists without decline for up to 22 days following the conversion when stored under refrigeration. The coagulation mechanism of the recipient may be altered by such blood, especially if large amounts are given. 3. Patients receiving this drug should be hospitalized. ADVERSE REACTIONS 1. Hemorrhage (see section on overdosage)

2. Hypersensitivity: chills, fever, urticaria, asthma, anaphylaxis
3. Acute reversible thrombocytopenia (abnormally low platelet count), reverses with discontinuation of the drug
4. Osteoporosis following long-term high-dose administration
5. Aldosterone suppression, causing an increase in sodium and water in the urine, and an increased retention of potassium
6. Transient hair loss (may be delayed after therapy), rare
7. Rebound hyperlipidemia following discontinuation of the drug
8. Priapism (acute, sustained erection of the penis), rare

MANAGEMENT OF OVERDOSAGE
1. Overdosage is indicated by excessively prolonged clotting or partial thromboplastin times or the onset of acute bleeding.
2. Protamine sulfate (1% solution) by slow infusion will neutralize the heparin. See page 476 for detailed description of use.
3. Blood or plasma transfusions may be necessary. These dilute heparin and add to the hemostatic properties of the blood but do not neutralize heparin.

bleeding occurs, hold the next dose of heparin and notify the physician. Monitor vital signs.
4. Monitor for signs and symptoms of allergic reaction.
5. Avoid IM injections and trauma-producing procedures such as catheterizations.
6. Keep protamine on hand; see Management of Overdosage and page 476 for its use.

SUGGESTED READINGS
Caprini, J. A., Zoelline, J. L. and Weisman, M.: Heparin Therapy, Part 1. *Cardiovascular Nursing*, 13:13–16, May–June 1977 (references).
Geske, Cheryl S.: Anticoagulant Therapy in Acute Myocardial Infarction. *Heart and Lung*, 1:639–648, September–October 1972 (references).
Stein, Myron, Stevens, Paul, and Saffer, Alfred: Recognition and Management of Pulmonary Embolism. *Heart and Lung*, 1:650–654, September–October 1972.

NURSING IMPLICATIONS
1. Monitor coagulation studies (partial thromboplastin time) with the physician. Be certain that the values are within therapeutic range before administering subsequent doses.
2. Use correct heparin lock technique (see page 149) for heparin injections. Use an infusion pump for continuous infusions.
3. Monitor for signs of bleeding:
   a. Hematuria (may be the earliest sign)
   b. Melena, red blood in the stools, positive guaiac (examine all stools)
   c. Hematemesis
   d. Nose bleeding
   e. Gum bleeding
   f. Prolonged bleeding after venipunctures or IM injections
   g. Ecchymosis
   h. Swelling of any muscle group associated with pain and tenderness
   i. Vaginal bleeding (advise patients to report the onset of menstruation). If

HISTAMINE PHOSPHATE (Histamine Test for Pheochromocytoma)

ACTIONS/ INDICATIONS	DOSAGE	PREPARATION AND STORAGE	DRUG INCOMPAT-IBILITIES	MODES OF IV ADMINISTRATION				CONTRAINDICATIONS; WARNINGS; PRECAUTIONS; ADVERSE REACTIONS
				INJECTION	INTERMITTENT INFUSION	CONTINUOUS INFUSION		
A diagnostic agent. Used for presumptive diagnosis of pheochromocytoma. Used for the patient with paroxysmal signs of excessive catecholamine secretion but with negative urine tests.	Test procedure: 1. Withhold antihypertensives, sympathomimetics, sedatives, and narcotics for 24 hrs before the test. 2. Do *not* withhold food. 3. Resting blood pressure must be less than 150/110. 4. Epinephrine should be available in case of hypotensive response. 5. Phentolamine should be available to depress BP if it rises. 6. While resting in bed, patient should receive a slow infusion of D5W or NS. 7. A 2-hr urine test is performed for catecholamines.	Supplied in 1-ml ampuls, equivalent to 0.275 mg/ml of histamine phosphate or 0.1 mg/ml of histamine base; from ampul No. 338. NOTE: Histamine Phosphate Injection for *Gastric* Histamine Test is to be injected subcutaneously.	Do not mix with any other medications.	YES Rapid injection through Y-injection site.	NO	NO		CONTRAINDICATIONS 1. In the elderly 2. Hypertension (blood pressure exceeding 150/100) WARNINGS Attacks of severe asthma or other serious allergic conditions may be precipitated. Use with caution in patients with a history of asthma or allergy. PRECAUTIONS 1. May cause flushing, dizziness, headache, nervousness, local or generalized allergic manifestations, marked hypertension or hypotension, tachycardia and abdominal cramps. 2. Increases secretion of gastric acid and may cause symptoms of peptic ulcer. 3. Frequent monitoring of blood pressure and heart rate should be carried out during administration of this drug. If there is a pronounced fall in blood pressure, epinephrine should be given promptly. 4. A large dose may cause severe occipital headache, blurred vision, anginal (chest) pain, a rapid drop in blood pressure, and cyanosis of the face. Overdosage may cause vasomotor collapse, shock, and death. ADVERSE REACTIONS (Besides those listed under Precautions) 1. Bronchial constriction, dyspnea 2. Visual disturbances 3. Faintness, syncope 4. Urticaria 5. Nervousness 6. Palpitations 7. Diarrhea and vomiting 8. Metallic taste 9. Seizures

8. At the end of the 2 hrs, the first dose is given of 0.01 mg histamine base (or 0.0275 mg of histamine phosphate).

9. A second 2-hr urine collection is started.

10. A second dose of 0.05 mg histamine base (0.1375 mg of histamine phosphate) is given if there is no response within 5 min.

11. Record BP and pulse every 30 seconds for 15 min.

12. Positive test:
    a. Increase in BP of at least 20/10 mm Hg greater than that obtained in a cold pressor test.
    b. Increase in BP of at least 60/40 mm Hg above the base-

343

HISTAMINE PHOSPHATE (Histamine Test for Pheochromocytoma) (*Continued*)

ACTIONS/ INDICATIONS	DOSAGE	PREPARATION AND STORAGE	DRUG INCOMPAT- IBILITIES	MODES OF IV ADMINISTRATION			CONTRAINDICATIONS; WARNINGS; PRECAUTIONS; ADVERSE REACTIONS
				INJECTION	INTERMITTENT INFUSION	CONTINUOUS INFUSION	
	line and greater than that of the cold pressor test. c. Elevation of urinary catecholamines above pretest.						

NURSING IMPLICATIONS
1. Monitor BP during test as indicated. Have epinephrine on hand for hypotension and phentolamine for hypertension.
2. Be prepared to treat allergic reaction; see page 118.

3. Follow test procedure as described under Dosage.
4. Assist in interpreting test results to the patient. Surgery is often indicated for patients with pheochromocytoma.

HYDRALAZINE HYDROCHLORIDE (Apresoline Hydrochloride)

ACTIONS/ INDICATIONS	DOSAGE	PREPARATION AND STORAGE	DRUG INCOMPAT- IBILITIES	MODES OF IV ADMINISTRATION			CONTRAINDICATIONS; WARNINGS; PRECAUTIONS; ADVERSE REACTIONS
				INJECTION	INTERMITTENT INFUSION	CONTINUOUS INFUSION	
Antihypertensive. Produces vascular smooth muscle relaxation to decrease peripheral vascular resistance.

Increases cardiac output and renal blood flow. Used to treat severe essential hypertension, but is not predictably ef- | ADULTS: 20–40 mg, repeat as necessary. Patients with renal impairment will require lower doses. Blood pressure will fall within a few minutes after injection; maximal decrease within 10–80 min. *Maximum daily dose* — 300 –400 mg. | Available in 1-ml ampuls, 20 mg/ml. Discard unused portions. | Do not inject into IV tubing containing: Aminophylline Ampicillin Chlorothiazide Edetate calcium disodium Ethacrynate Hydrocortisone Mephentermine Methohexital | YES

May be given undiluted through Y injection site. Inject at a rate of 10 mg/min. | NO

Do not mix with fluids. | NO

Do not mix with fluids. | CONTRAINDICATIONS
1. Hypersensitivity
2. Coronary artery disease
3. Rheumatic mitral valve disease

WARNINGS
1. High, prolonged doses may produce a syndrome resembling systemic lupus erythematosus. Drug should be discontinued in this event. Symptoms will regress with some residual.
2. Complete blood count, LE prep., and antinuclear antibody titers should be done before and periodically during therapy. Positive results require consideration for discontinuing the drug.
3. Use MAO inhibitors with caution in patients receiving this drug.
4. Use in pregnancy only when essential |

fective in hypertensive emergencies.

CHILDREN: 1.7–3.5 mg/kg/day divided into 4–6 equal doses.

Intravenous route should be used only when the oral route is inappropriate.

for the welfare of the patient.
5. Profound hypotension may occur when this drug is administered with diazoxide.

PRECAUTIONS
1. Produces reflex myocardial stimulation which increases myocardial oxygen consumption and can precipitate angina and ECG changes of ischemia. Do not use in patients with coronary artery disease.
2. May cause postural hypotension.
3. Use with caution in patients with acute cerebral vascular accident; reduced blood pressure may cause relative cerebral ischemia.
4. Use with caution in the presence of advanced renal disease; reduced dosage will be required.
5. Monitor hemoglobin, RBC count, WBC count during *prolonged* therapy.
6. Will induce sodium and water retention.
7. This drug does not reduce renal blood flow[1]

ADVERSE REACTIONS
1. Reactions are reversible with discontinuation of the drug or reduction of dosage.
2. Common side effects:
   a. Headache
   b. Flushing of the face
   c. Peripheral neuritis (numbness, tingling; may be relieved with pyridoxine)
   d. Dizziness
   e. Tremors
   f. Muscle cramps
   g. Psychotic reactions
   h. Rashes
   i. Constipation
   j. Blood dycrasias
   k. Fever and chills
   l. Hypotension

OVERDOSAGE
1. Signs: hypotension, tachycardia, headache, myocardial ischemia, chest pain, arrhythmias, shock.
2. Treatment: Support blood pressure with volume expanders; avoid use of pressor agents. If vasopressor is used, select one least likely to produce cardiac arrhythmias. Digitalize as needed. Monitor renal function.

NURSING IMPLICATIONS
1. Expect the blood pressure to begin to decrease from 10–80 minutes after each injection. Monitor the blood pressure (indirect measurements will suffice) every 5 to 10 minutes after the injection for 1 hour, then once an hour for 2 hours, and then every 4 hours until the next injection. Repeat cycle for each dose unless the patient has complications.

HYDRALAZINE HYDROCHLORIDE (Apresoline Hydrochloride) (Continued)

NURSING IMPLICATIONS (Continued)

2. If the patient has had a recent myocardial infarction or cerebrovascular accident, monitor the blood pressure more frequently than stated above. Report any fall in blood pressure below the goal set by the physician, to the physician. Be prepared to treat hypotension (see Overdosage above).

3. If the patient is able to cooperate, instruct him to report chest pain of any type. Anginal pain could indicate the onset of myocardial ischemia; notify the physician at once, and continue to monitor vital signs, including ECG, frequently.

4. Monitor for the consequences of severely elevated blood pressure if the patient is experiencing a hypertensive crisis:
   a. Encephalopathy—confusion, stupor, nausea, vomiting, visual disturbances, reflex asymmetries
   b. Cerebrovascular accident—paralysis or weakness
   c. Myocardial ischemia and/or infarction—chest pain, ECG changes (see Nursing Implication No. 3, previous page)
   d. Left ventricular failure—shortness of breath, orthopnea, elevated central venous pressure (or pulmonary artery pressure), tachycardia, rales, onset of a third and/or fourth heart sound.
   e. Renal failure—oliguria, rising BUN and creatinine[2]
   Overdosage of this drug can cause an extreme reduction in blood pressure which can also cause these complications.

5. If the patient is receiving this drug for a noncrisis situation, he may ambulate after the injection when the blood pressure has stabilized. Before the patient ambulates alone, determine if postural hypotension is occurring on rising. If it is, report the lying and standing pressures to the physician. Take the necessary safety precautions to prevent patient injury. Instruct the patient to rise from a lying position slowly and to stand only after having been in the sitting position for 3–5 minutes, and to then rise slowly.

6. Monitor for the onset of a lupus-type syndrome seen with this drug: joint pains and swelling, malaise.

7. If the patient is to receive this drug in its oral form on a chronic basis, he must be instructed on hypertensive self-care prior to discharge from the hospital.

REFERENCES
1. AMA Committee on Hypertension: The Treatment of Malignant Hypertension and Hypertensive Emergencies. *JAMA*, 228(13):1675, June 24, 1974.
2. Romankiewicz, J. A.: Pharmacology and Clinical Use of Drugs in Hypertensive Emergencies. *American Journal of Hospital Pharmacy*, 34(2):185–193, February 1977.

SUGGESTED READINGS
American Medical Association Committee on Hypertension: The Treatment of Malignant Hypertension and Hypertensive Emergencies. *JAMA*, 228:1673–1679, June 24, 1974.

Fleischmann, L. E.: Management of Hypertensive Crisis in Children. *Pediatric Annals*, 6(6):410–414, June 1977.

Jones, L. N.: Symposium on Teaching and Rehabilitation of the Cardiac Patient. Hypertension: Medical and Nursing Implications. *Nursing Clinics of North America*, 11:283–295, June 1976.

Keith, Thomas: Hypertensive Crisis. Recognition and Management. *JAMA*, 237(15):1570–1577, April 11, 1977.

Koch-Weser, Jan: Hypertensive Emergencies. *New England Journal of Medicine*, 290:211–214, January 24, 1974.

Long, M. L., et al.: Hypertension: What the Patient Needs to Know. *American Journal of Nursing*, 76:765–770, May 1976.

Romankiewicz, J. A.: Pharmacology and Clinical Use of Drugs in Hypertensive Emergencies. *American Journal of Hospital Pharmacy*, 34(2):185–193, February 1977 (references).

HYDROCORTISONE SODIUM SUCCINATE (Solu-Cortef) and HYDROCORTISONE SODIUM PHOSPHATE (Hydrocortone)

ACTIONS/INDICATIONS	DOSAGE	PREPARATION AND STORAGE	DRUG INCOMPATIBILITIES	MODES OF IV ADMINISTRATION			CONTRAINDICATIONS; WARNINGS; PRECAUTIONS: ADVERSE REACTIONS
				INJECTION	INTERMITTENT INFUSION	CONTINUOUS INFUSION	
Adrenocorticosteroid, with potent anti-inflammatory, metabolic and other numerous effects. Used in: • Endocrine disorders • Collagen diseases • Allergic states • Respiratory diseases	ADULTS: *Severe shock*—35–50 mg/kg every 30–60 min. for a maximum of 4 doses. *Other clinical situations:*—100–500 mg initially repeated as necessary to obtain an appropriate clinical re-	Supplied in 100-, 250-, 500-, and 1000-mg vials. 100-mg size can be reconstituted with 2 ml water for injection, bacteriostatic. For other vials use diluent provided by the manufacturer. Protect reconstituted form from light; dis-	Do not mix with: Methicillin Nafcillin Narcotics Kanamycin Tetracycline Cephalosporins Aminophylline Hydralazine Insulin is compatible for up to 8 hours in solution.	YES Undiluted 100 mg/min. Through Y injection site of a running IV.	YES Dilute to 2 mg/ml. Infuse over 15–20 min. Use D5W or NS.	YES Use D5W, NS or D5/NS. Use no less than 1 ml of IV fluid to dilute 1 mg of drug.	CONTRAINDICATIONS 1. Systemic fungal infections 2. In the absence of a life-threatening situation, avoid in: a. peptic ulcer disease b. viral diseases (especially ocular) c. infectious diseases without antibiotic treatment (especially TB) d. myasthenia gravis e. psychosis 3. Hypersensitivity WARNINGS 1. Additional stress during therapy (surgery, trauma, infection, etc.) may require larger doses.

Shock Overwhelming infections Adrenal insufficiency	sponse. CHILDREN: Governed by severity of condition and response to initial doses. Use no less than 25 mg/kg daily. *Gram-neg. shock*—initially, 50 mg/kg; then: 50–75 mg/kg day (maximum single dose 500 mg). *Status asthmaticus*— 10 mg/kg/day NEONATES: 2.5 mg/kg/dose	card after 3 days. Note that hydrocortisone sodium succinate and sodium phosphate are the only two hydrocortisone preparations that can be given intravenously. Read labels carefully.

2. There may be a decreased ability to localize infection.
3. There may be masking of signs of infection.
4. Prolonged use is known to produce cataracts, glaucoma, optic nerve damage, and enhance ocular infections.
5. Use in pregnancy and lactation requires that potential benefits be weighed against hazard to the fetus. Infants born to mothers on corticosteroids should be observed for signs of hypoadrenalism.
6. Large doses elevate BP, cause salt and water retention, and increase excretion of potassium. Dietary salt restriction and potassium supplements may be needed. There is also increased calcium excretion.
7. Do not vaccinate against smallpox or other diseases while patient is on therapy.
8. Use in TB must be limited to fulminating or disseminated types, patients with history of TB may have a reactivation of the disease.
9. Anaphylaxis has occurred secondary to this drug.

PRECAUTIONS
1. Drug-induced adrenocortical insufficiency can be avoided by tapering of doses to discontinue (this is usually important only in prolonged therapy).
2. There is an enhanced effect of corticosteroids in patients with hypothyroidism and cirrhosis. (Lower dosage is advisable.)
3. Psychosis can result from therapy. Pre-existing psychiatric problems may be exacerbated.
4. Use with caution in:
   a. Nonspecific ulcerative colitis, especially if there is a danger of abscess or perforation
   b. Diverticulitis
   c. Fresh intestinal anastomoses
   d. Peptic ulcer disease
   e. Renal insufficiency
   f. Hypertension
   g. Osteoporosis

ADVERSE REACTIONS SEEN IN SHORT-TERM INTRAVENOUS THERAPY
1. Fluid and electrolyte imbalance: sodium and water retention with possible secondary hypertension, hypokalemia, hypocalcemia
2. Gastrointestinal: peptic ulcer with possible perforation, pancreatitis, ulcerative eosophagitis

HYDROCORTISONE SODIUM SUCCINATE (Solu-Cortef) and HYDROCORTISONE SODIUM PHOSPHATE (Hydrocortone) (Continued)

ACTIONS/ INDICATIONS	DOSAGE	PREPARATION AND STORAGE	DRUG INCOMPAT- IBILITIES	MODES OF IV ADMINISTRATION			CONTRAINDICATIONS: WARNINGS: PRECAUTIONS: ADVERSE REACTIONS
				INJECTION	INTERMITTENT INFUSION	CONTINUOUS INFUSION	
							3. Dermatologic: impaired wound healing 4. Neurologic: increased intracranial pressure, seizures (increasing frequency in patients with pre-existing seizure disorder), vertigo, headaches, mental confusion, euphoria, exacerbation of psychosis. 5. Endocrine: decreased glucose tolerance, increase hypoglycemic agent and insulin requirements in diabetics 6. Eye: increased intraocular pressure. 7. Metabolic: negative nitrogen balance secondary to rapid muscle catabolism.

NURSING IMPLICATIONS

1. Take precautions to prevent infections in wounds by using strict aseptic technique in dressing changes, etc. Avoid traumatic procedures such as catheterizations. The skin may become more fragile because of the steroid therapy. Patients on bed rest and those with general body weakening secondary to an acute illness should be turned hourly (except during sleep, then every 2–3 hours) to prevent skin breakdown. Initiate the use of supportive measures such as flotation pads, water mattress, etc. Administer scrupulous skin care to prevent infection.

2. Monitor blood pressure every 2–4 hours, or as the patient's condition dictates. Monitor blood pressure before, during and immediately after intravenous injection; hypotension can occur.

3. Weigh the patient daily to detect for water and sodium retention. Dietary restrictions in sodium may be prescribed by the physician. Examine daily for peripheral edema. Monitor for exacerbation of congestive heart failure in susceptible patients (increasing dyspnea, increasing resting heart rate, fatigue, rales, etc.)

4. There may be delayed healing of wounds; take precautions to prevent dehiscence. Sutures may be left in longer than usual for this reason.

5. Monitor urine glucose in patients on high-dose therapy and with diabetes. Diabetic individuals may require a larger dosage of insulin or oral agent.

6. Administer antacid therapy as ordered to assist in preventing peptic ulcer. Monitor for signs of the development of an ulcer and/or acute intestinal bleeding: melena, positive stool guaiac, hematemesis, epigastric pain and/ or distention, anemia or falling hematocrit.

7. Monitor for signs and symptoms of hypokalemia: weakness, irritability, abdominal distention, poor feeding in infants, muscle cramps.[1] Dietary or pharmacologic potassium supplements may be ordered, guided by serum potassium levels.

8. Monitor for signs and symptoms of hypocalcemia: irritability, change in mental status, seizures, nausea, vomiting, diarrhea, muscle cramps, late effects—cardiac arrhythmias, laryngeal spasm and apnea.[2] Dietary or pharmacologic supplements may be ordered guided by serum calcium levels.

9. Patients with a history of seizure activity may have an increasing number of seizures while on steroid therapy. Apply appropriate safety precautions.

10. Monitor for behavioral changes, which may range from simple euphoria to depression and psychosis. Apply appropriate safety precautions. A change in dosage may relieve such symptoms.

11. Tuberculin testing should be carried out prior to initiation of steroid therapy, if possible. The patient's reactivity to the tuberculin is altered by the drug, giving a false result.

12. Ambulate the patient with caution if vertigo occurs, and initiate the use of side rails and other safety measures to prevent patient injury. Report the onset to the physician.

13. Be alert to the signs of increasing intraocular pressure: eye pain, rainbow vision, blurred vision, nausea and vomiting.[3] Notify the physician immediately.

REFERENCES

1. Beeson, Paul, and McDermott, Walsh (editors): *Cecil-Loeb Textbook of Medicine,* (14th ed.). Philadelphia: W. B. Saunders Company, 1975, p. 1587.
2. Ibid., p. 1815.
3. Newell, Frank W., and Ernest, J. Terry: *Ophthalmology—Principles and Concepts* (3rd ed.), St. Louis: C. V. Mosby Company, 1974, p. 329.

SUGGESTED READINGS

Glasser, Ronald J.: How the Body Works Against Itself: Autoimmune Diseases. *Nursing '77,* September 1977, pp. 34–38.
Melick, M. E.: Nursing Intervention for Patients Receiving Corticosteroid Therapy. In *Advanced Concepts in Clinical Nursing* (2nd ed.), K. C. Kintzel, ed., Philadelphia: J. B. Lippincott Company, 1977, pp. 606–617.
Newton, David W., Nichols, Arlene, and Newton, Marion: You Can Minimize the Hazards of Corticosteroids. *Nursing '77,* June 1977, pp. 26–33.
Reichgott, Michael J., and Melmon, Kenneth L.: The Role of Corticosteroids in Shock. In *Steroid Therapy* Daniel Azarnoff, ed., Philadelphia: W. B. Saunders Company, 1975, pp. 118–133.

HYDROMORPHONE HYDROCHLORIDE (Dihydromorphinone HCl, Dilaudid)

ACTIONS/ INDICATIONS	DOSAGE	PREPARATION AND STORAGE	DRUG INCOMPAT- IBILITIES	MODES OF IV ADMINISTRATION			CONTRAINDICATIONS; WARNINGS; PRECAUTIONS; ADVERSE REACTIONS
				INJECTION	INTERMITTENT INFUSION	CONTINUOUS INFUSION	
Morphine derivative; narcotic analgesic. Used for relief of moderate to severe pain in the following situations: • Postoperatively • Acute myocardial infarction • Any form of cancer	ADULTS: 2 mg usual; 3–4 mg in very severe pain every 4–6 hrs or as the duration of pain relief dictates. CHILDREN: Dosage not available for use in children. Adolescents can receive adult dosage.	Do not mix with IV fluids. This is a Schedule II drug under the Controlled Substances Act of 1970. Maintain hospital or institutional regulations guiding its use.	Do not inject into an IV line containing sodium bicarbonate or thiopental sodium.	YES Dilute dosage in 10 ml Sterile Water for Injection or NS, inject slowly over 3–5 min.	NO Do not mix with IV fluids.	NO Do not mix with IV fluids.	CONTRAINDICATIONS 1. Intracranial lesion producing increased intracranial pressure 2. Hypersensitivity to opiate derivatives 3. Respiratory depression WARNINGS 1. May be habit-forming. 2. Rapid injection can cause hypotension and respiratory depression. 3. Use in pregnancy requires that potential benefits outweigh risks to the fetus. 4. Administer with caution in the presence of bronchial asthma. PRECAUTIONS There is a possibility of respiratory depression. ADVERSE REACTIONS 1. Nausea, vomiting 2. Dizziness 3. Somnolence (seldom produces drowsiness) 4. Constipation (if given chronically) 5. Pain at injection site, especially if there is extravasation 6. Urinary retention 7. Postural hypotension 8. Bronchospasm (especially in patients with prior history of asthma) OVERDOSAGE 1. Symptoms: respiratory depression (decreased rate, tidal volume, Cheyne-Stokes respiratory pattern, cyanosis), extreme somnolence progressing to stupor or coma, skeletal muscle flaccidity, cold and clammy skin, bradycardia, hypotension; apnea may follow. 2. Treatment: re-establishment of an adequate airway and ventilation, followed by the administration of a narcotic antagonist (naloxone hydrochloride, nalorphine hydrochloride, levallorphan tartrate). The duration of action and thus respiratory depression of hydromorphone may exceed that of the antagonist. Repeat doses

HYDROMORPHONE HYDROCHLORIDE (Dihydromorphinone HCl, Dilaudid) (Continued)

ACTIONS/ INDICATIONS	DOSAGE	PREPARATION AND STORAGE	DRUG INCOMPAT- IBILITIES	MODES OF IV ADMINISTRATION			CONTRAINDICATIONS; WARNINGS; PRECAUTIONS: ADVERSE REACTIONS
				INJECTION	INTERMITTENT INFUSION	CONTINUOUS INFUSION	
							of the antagonist may be required. Oxygen, fluids, vasopressors and other supportive measures should be employed as indicated.

NURSING IMPLICATIONS

1. Schedule doses to prevent pain from reaching its maximum intensity. Never withhold an analgesic unless ordered by the physician.
2. Evaluate patient's response to the drug. Notify physician if dosage, frequency, or agent is apparently ineffective.
3. Administer one-half hour prior to treatments, ambulation, or other painful procedures such as coughing or chest physical therapy. Administer at bedtime to promote restful sleep.
4. Administer emotional support positioning and other care measures to enhance analgesic affect of the drug.
5. Monitor for respiratory depression:
   a. Count respiratory rate every 2–3 minutes during and for the first 15 minutes after intravenous injection and every 15–30 minutes for the next 2 hours. Repeat cycle with additional doses.
   b. If respiratory rate falls below 8–10/minute, attempt to arouse the pa-
   tient. If successful, coach him to breathe at a rate of 10–12/minute. Notify the physician; have naloxone or other antagonist at the bedside. Do not leave the patient alone.
   c. If the patient cannot be aroused to increase respiratory rate, begin ventilation with manual breathing bag at a rate of 10–12/minute. Monitor pulse. Administer oxygen if cyanosis develops. Notify the physician. Do not leave the patient alone until a spontaneous respiratory rate of 10–12/minute is reached, and other vital signs have stabilized.

SUGGESTED READINGS

McCaffery, Margo, and Hart, Linda L.: Undertreatment of Acute Pain with Narcotics. *American Journal of Nursing,* 76(10):1586–1591, October 1976 (references).

Wiley, Francis M., and Rhein, Marilee: Challenges of Pain Management: One Terminally Ill Adolescent. *Pediatric Nursing,* 3:26–27, July–August 1977.

HYOSCYAMINE (LEVO) SULFATE (Levsin)

ACTIONS/ INDICATIONS	DOSAGE	PREPARATION AND STORAGE	DRUG INCOMPAT- IBILITIES	MODES OF IV ADMINISTRATION			CONTRAINDICATIONS; WARNINGS; PRECAUTIONS: ADVERSE REACTIONS
				INJECTION	INTERMITTENT INFUSION	CONTINUOUS INFUSION	
Antispasmotic, anticholiner- gic. Used in the medical man- agement of peptic ulcer, to control gastric hypersecre- tion, intesti- nal hyper- motility and cramps. Also used in mild dysenteries and diverticuli- tis, biliary and renal colic. For	ADULTS: 0.5 mg. Do not exceed recommended dosage. CHILDREN: Not recom- mended.	Caution: There are two paren- teral forms of this drug. The preparation *without* pheno- barbital is the only form to be given IV.	Do not mix with any other medication in any manner.	YES Slowly, over at least 1–2 min. Inject into the tubing of a running IV.	NO Not recom- mended.	NO Not recom- mended.	CONTRAINDICATIONS 1. Glaucoma 2. Prostatic hypertrophy 3. Cardiac tachyarrhythmias 4. Diabetes mellitus PRECAUTIONS Discontinue with signs of hyper- sensitivity. ADVERSE REACTIONS Usually are secondary to overdosage: dry mouth, blurred vision, difficulty in urination, tachycardia, hypersensitivity.

preanesthesia to decrease respiratory secretions. To treat the symptoms of Parkinson's disease. May also be used in anticholinesterase poisoning.

NURSING IMPLICATIONS
1. Monitor patients with a history of tachyarrhythmias for recurrence. Keep lidocaine 100 mg at the bedside.
2. Monitor elderly male patients with or without prostatic hypertrophy for urinary retention by measuring 8-hourly output and palpating for bladder distention every 4 hours.

● INSULIN, REGULAR (Iletin)

ACTIONS/ INDICATIONS	DOSAGE	PREPARATION AND STORAGE	DRUG INCOMPAT- IBILITIES	MODES OF IV ADMINISTRATION			CONTRAINDICATIONS; WARNINGS; PRECAUTIONS; ADVERSE REACTIONS
				INJECTION	INTERMITTENT INFUSION	CONTINUOUS INFUSION	
Hypoglycemic hormone. Promotes the movement of glucose from blood to cell for oxidation; lowers blood glucose level; regulates the formation of glucose from noncarbohydrate sources.	ADULTS: Dosage must be determined and titrated with blood glucose and acetone levels.	Use U-80 or U-100 concentrations of regular insulin. Use appropriate syringes. DO NOT USE U-500 REGULAR INSULIN INTRAVENOUSLY.	Do not mix in infusion solution with other medications because of titration dosage. Do not mix in an intravenous line with:	YES Through Y injection.	YES	YES	PRECAUTIONS Do not allow blood glucose to fall below 100 mg/100 ml.
	Severe diabetic acidosis— 100–200 units initially, followed by additional doses of 20–50 units every 30 min, guided by hourly blood glucose (should not fall below 100 mg/100 ml).	Store in refrigerator. Discard if solution is cloudy or has a color change. These changes indicate loss of potency.	Aminophylline Phenytoin (Dilantin) Heparin Barbituates Chlorothiazide Nitrofurantoin Novobiocin Penicillin Sulfadiazine		When blood glucose is excessively high, NS is usually used as infusion fluid.	When blood glucose is excessively high, NS is usually used as infusion fluid.	ADVERSE REACTIONS 1. Hypoglycemia 2. Allergic reactions to either pork or beef
Used to treat hyperglycemia and diabetic ketoacidosis. Also used to induce hypoglycemic shock in psychotherapy and in polarizing solutions for treatment of acute myocardial infarction. When administered	Low-dose infusions can also be used at a rate of 5–10 units/hr, following an initial bolus of 100 units. During	There can be adsorption of insulin to the surfaces of glass and plastic solution containers. It has been suggested to add small amounts of nor-			D5W can be used when blood glucose is near normal.	D5W can be used when blood glucose is near normal.	
					Infusion rate is titrated with blood glucose values. Add a sufficient amount of insulin to make calculation of drip rate simple; e.g. 25 units in 500 ml (1 unit/20 ml).	Infusion rate is titrated with blood glucose values. Add a sufficient amount of insulin to make calculation of drip rate simple; e.g. 25 units in 500 ml (1 unit/20 ml).	

351

INSULIN, REGULAR (Iletin) (Continued)

ACTIONS/ INDICATIONS	DOSAGE	PREPARATION AND STORAGE	DRUG INCOMPAT- IBILITIES	MODES OF IV ADMINISTRATION			CONTRAINDICATIONS; WARNINGS; PRECAUTIONS; ADVERSE REACTIONS
				INJECTION	INTERMITTENT INFUSION	CONTINUOUS INFUSION	
with dextrose, potassium will move from the blood into the cell.	ing infusion, titrate drip rate with hourly blood and urine glucose levels.	mal serum human albumin to the infusion to prevent this. Regardless of this adsorption, infusion rates must be guided by serum glucose levels.					

NURSING IMPLICATIONS
1. Monitor blood and urine glucose and ketone levels, and serum carbon dioxide during administration of insulin. Do not allow blood glucose to fall below 100 mg/100 ml.
2. Monitor for signs and symptoms of hypoglycemia: diaphoresis; pallor in fair-skinned individuals and ashened color in dark-skinned persons; change in mental status, e.g., confusion, agitation, or lethargy; headache; hunger or nausea; tachycardia; tremors; seizure.
3. Administer supportive care to the comatose patient in ketoacidosis, i.e., prevention of aspiration, respiratory care, prevention of skin breakdown, fluid and electrolyte balance, monitoring of vital signs.
4. Use an infusion pump for intermittent and continuous infusions for precise control of rate. It is advisable for patients receiving such infusion to be cared for in an intensive care unit.

SUGGESTED READINGS
Heber, David, Molitch, Mark E., and Sperling, Mark A.: Low-Dose Continuous Insulin Therapy for Diabetic Ketoacidosis. *Archives of Internal Medicine,* 137:1377–1380, October 1977.
——————: Low-Dose Insulin Therapy in Diabetic Ketoacidosis. *Archives of Internal Medicine,* 137:1361–1362, October 1977.

IRON DEXTRAN (Imferon)

ACTIONS/ INDICATIONS	DOSAGE	PREPARATION AND STORAGE	DRUG INCOMPAT- IBILITIES	MODES OF IV ADMINISTRATION			CONTRAINDICATIONS; WARNINGS; PRECAUTIONS; ADVERSE REACTIONS
				INJECTION	INTERMITTENT INFUSION	CONTINUOUS INFUSION	
A ferric complex; a source of elemental iron, which is used by the body in the formation of hemoglobin for oxygen transport

Used to treat iron deficiency anemia when oral iron therapy is ineffective or impos- | To calculate dosage, use the formula below: | Available in 2- and 5-ml ampuls. NOTE: the multidose bottle is for IM use *only* (contains phenol). Use only NS as infusion fluid. | Do not mix with any other medication in any manner. | YES

Undiluted, slowly, 1 mg/ min may be injected into the venous side of a hemodialysis shunt or fistula needle.

Give a test dose of 25 mg (calculate into ml of solution) over 5 minutes' time. If | YES

Add total dose to 200–250 ml of NS. Give a test dose of 25 mg (calculate into ml of solution) over 5 minutes' time. If no reaction occurs, the remainder of the solution can be infused over 1–2 hrs. (500-ml solu- | NO | CONTRAINDICATIONS
1. Known hypersensitivity
2. Any anemia other than iron deficiency
3. Asthma and atopic (allergic) history

WARNINGS
1. Use with caution in the presence of hepatic disease.
2. Safety for use in pregnancy has not been established.

PRECAUTIONS
1. Unwarranted therapy with parenteral iron can cause excess storage of iron with the possibility of exogenous hemosiderosis. |

2. Patients with rheumatoid arthritis may have an exacerbation of joint pain.

ADVERSE REACTIONS
1. Anaphylaxis
2. Severe febrile reactions
3. Arthralgia and myalgia
4. Phlebitis at intravenous injection site
5. Peripheral vascular flushing with rapid intravenous injection
6. Hypotension during and immediately following injection
7. Headache, nausea, shivering, rash
8. Dyspnea
9. Facial edema
10. Staining of the skin at the injection site

tion is infused over 6–8 hrs.) Flush vein with saline after infusion.

no reaction occurs, the remainder of the solution can be injected at 1 mg/min.

$$0.3 \times \text{body weight (in pounds)} \times \left(100 - \frac{\text{patient's hemoglobin in gm/100 ml} \times 100}{14.8}\right) = \text{mg of iron dextran}$$

Dosage in ml is derived by dividing the above number by 50.

sible.

Intravenous use must be limited to cases where there is
• Insufficient muscle mass for IM injection
• Impaired IM absorption (e.g., edema)
• Hemophilia
• Chronic substantial blood loss (e.g., familial telangiectasia)
• Hemodialysis

ADULTS:
An 0.5-ml (25 mg) test dose should be administered on the first day to observe for toxic reactions. Then increase to calculated dose.

CHILDREN:
Initial test dose 0.5 ml (25 mg). Increase in 2–3 days to calculated dose.

Children less than 30 pounds should be given a dose 80% of the calculated dose.

Dosage in adults and

353

IRON DEXTRAN (Imferon) (Continued)

ACTIONS/INDICATIONS	DOSAGE	PREPARATION AND STORAGE	DRUG INCOMPATIBILITIES	MODES OF IV ADMINISTRATION			CONTRAINDICATIONS; WARNINGS; PRECAUTIONS; ADVERSE REACTIONS
				INJECTION	INTERMITTENT INFUSION	CONTINUOUS INFUSION	
	children must be guided by periodic hematologic studies. Iron storage may lag behind the appearance of normal blood morphology (cell formation) usually 3 weeks following first administration.						2. Be aware of the patient's hemoglobin prior to injection (see Precaution No. 1). 3. Warn arthritic patients of possible exacerbation of their condition.

NURSING IMPLICATIONS
1. Take anaphylaxis precautions; see page 118.

ISOPROTERENOL HYDROCHLORIDE (Isuprel, Iprenol)

ACTIONS/INDICATIONS	DOSAGE	PREPARATION AND STORAGE	DRUG INCOMPATIBILITIES	MODES OF IV ADMINISTRATION			CONTRAINDICATIONS; WARNINGS; PRECAUTIONS; ADVERSE REACTIONS
				INJECTION	INTERMITTENT INFUSION	CONTINUOUS INFUSION	
Sympathomimetic (produces the effects of epinephrine); a beta adrenergic stimulator. Produces the following effects: • Increased contractility of the heart • Improved myocardial conductivity • Increased heart rate • Increased systolic blood pres-	ADULTS: *Cardiac standstill or complete heart block*—bolus injection of 20–60 mcg (1–3 ml of the 1:50,000 solution), followed by 10–200 mcg as needed to elicit a response. OR Administer as an infusion; initial rate of 5 mcg/min adjusted to patient response.	Available in 1 ml and 5 ml vials of a 1:5000 solution (0.2 mg/ml) (200 mcg/ml). The following solutions are most commonly used: *1:50,000* (20 mcg/ml). Prepare by adding 1 ml of the 1:5000 solution to 9 ml diluent. *1:500,000* (2.0 mcg/ml). Prepare by adding	Do not mix with: Barbiturates Sodium bicarbonate Any calcium preparation Aminophylline	YES Use a 1:50,000 solution as described under Preparation and Storage. Inject over 1 min. This mode is recommended only for cardiac standstill or bronchospasm in *adults*.	YES Using a 1:500,000 solution, begin the infusion with the dosages recommended. Titrate with arterial pressure, heart rate, pulmonary artery pressure and urine flow. Use a volumetric infusion pump if available.	YES Using a 1:500,000 solution, begin the infusion with the dosages recommended. Titrate with arterial pressure, heart rate, pulmonary artery pressure and urine flow. Use a volumetric infusion pump if available.	CONTRAINDICATIONS 1. Pre-existing tachyarrhythmias (except those ventricular arrhythmias treated by increasing cardiac output by using this drug) 2. Tachyarrhythmias secondary to digitalis intoxication 3. Subaortic hypertrophic stenosis PRECAUTIONS 1. Do not administer at the same time as epinephrine; it may cause arrythmias. 2. This drug increases myocardial oxygen consumption; adjust dosage carefully in the presence of coronary insufficiency. These patients may have anginal pain at high cardiac rates. 3. Potential benefits to the mother must be weighed against risks to the

fetus if used during pregnancy.

ADVERSE REACTIONS
1. Flushing of the face
2. Sweating
3. Mild tremors
4. Nervousness
5. Headache
6. Palpitations—usually transient and do not require discontinuation of the drug
7. Pulmonary edema has been reported in patients extremely sensitive to sympathomimetic drugs
8. Precipitation of transient complete heart block
9. Postresuscitation tachycardia
10. Myocardial irritability producing premature ventricular contractions and ventricular tachycardia

sure and decreased diastolic pressure • Relaxation of bronchial and intestinal smooth muscle		OR As an intracardiac injection, 20 mcg (0.1 ml of the 1:50,000 solution). Repeat as necessary.
Used as an adjunct to the treatment of shock, cardiac standstill, carotid sinus hypersensitivity.		1 ml of the 1:5000 solution to 99 ml diluent to obtain 100 ml of infusion, or add 5 ml of drug to 495 ml diluent to obtain 500 ml for infusion.
Used in the temporary management of complete heart block and sinus bradycardia.	*Bronchospasm*—in anesthesia, or when an attack is unresponsive to inhalation drug administration, 10–20 mcg (0.5–1.0 ml at the 1:50,000 solution) as a direct IV injection.	A more concentrated solution can be used for patients requiring large dosage and a minimum of fluid: 2 mg of drug (10 ml of the 1:5000 solution) in 500 ml of diluent.
Also used in the management of bronchospasm during anesthesia.	*Shock, carotid sinus hypersensitivity, sinus bradycardia*—range, 0.5–30.0 mcg/min via an infusion (use the 1:500,000 solution). Volume rate = 0.25–15 ml/min. Dosage must be regulated by patient response.	Use D5W or NS for infusion.
	CHILDREN: *Bradyarrhythmias*—0.5–4.0 mcg/min (use the 1:500,000 solution). Titrate with heart rate.	
	Cardiac standstill—1–4 mcg/min (use the 1:500,000 solution). Titrate with patient response.	

● ISOPROTERENOL HYDROCHLORIDE (Isuprel, Iprenol) (Continued)

ACTIONS/INDICATIONS	DOSAGE	PREPARATION AND STORAGE	DRUG INCOMPAT-IBILITIES	MODES OF IV ADMINISTRATION			CONTRAINDICATIONS: WARNINGS; PRECAUTIONS: ADVERSE REACTIONS
				INJECTION	INTERMITTENT INFUSION	CONTINUOUS INFUSION	
	A bolus injection may also be used, 10–30 mcg (0.5–1.5 ml of a 1:50,000 solution), followed by an infusion of 200 mcg in 300 ml of fluid, titrated with patient response.\n\n*Status asthmaticus (investigational)*—0.8–1.7 mcg/kg/min by infusion. Monitor ECG and titrate with patient response.						

NURSING IMPLICATIONS

1. Adequate parameters must be available for monitoring to guide titration of this drug. At a minimum heart rate, ECG, central venous pressure, indirect blood pressure (by sphygmomanometer) and urine output must be utilized. If possible, it is advisable to use direct arterial blood pressure and central venous pressure readings. Because of this drug's vasoconstrictive actions, the indirectly obtained blood pressure may be significantly different from the more accurate intra-arterial blood pressure. The values of these parameters to strive for when titrating the drug must be determined by the physician.

2. Heart rate and blood pressure (direct or indirect) must be recorded prior to and every 2–3 minutes during the initial phase of titration. When the blood pressure stabilizes for at least 1 hour near or at the desired, preset value, frequency of monitoring can be reduced to every 15–30 minutes, or as indicated by the patient's general condition.

3. Central venous pressure or pulmonary artery pressure should be recorded prior to and every 30 minutes during titration. A continuous oscilloscopic display of arterial and pulmonary arterial pressures is ideal in this situation.

4. Urine output should be recorded hourly during the initial phase of therapy with this drug. Urine flow reflects indirectly the perfusion of the kidneys. A fall in urine output may indicate the need for a change in drug therapy, either an increase in isoproterenol drip rate, or its discontinuation and the initiation of another agent. Notify the physician if urine output falls below 30 ml/hour for 2 consecutive hours in an adult patient (see chart on page 546 for normal urine output in children).

5. Use a volumetric infusion pump if available. If a pump is not available, use

6. microdrop tubing and perform frequent drip counts.

7. Patients requiring therapy with this drug frequently require respiratory support. Monitor respiratory rate, effort and blood gases with other parameters. Be prepared to initiate manual ventilation.

8. Monitor ECG continuously during infusion; premature ventricular contractions are common during administration. If these occur, decrease infusion rate. If isoproterenol dosage cannot be decreased, a lidocaine infusion may be started at 1–4 mg/minute (dosage during the use of isoproterenol may be greater than normal because of drug-induced improved hepatic perfusion). Other causes for myocardial irritability such as hypoxia must be ruled out. If the heart rate exceeds 110 beats/min (adults), decrease infusion rate while monitoring other parameters.

9. Instruct the patient, if he is able to cooperate, to report chest pain.

10. Avoid extravasation.

SUGGESTED READINGS

Amsterdam, Ezra A., et al.: Evaluation and Management of Cardiogenic Shock. Part I. Approach to the Patient. *Heart and Lung*. 1(3):402–408, May–June 1972 (references).

———: Evaluation and Management of Cardiogenic Shock. Part II. Drug Therapy. *Heart and Lung*. 1(5):663–671, September–October 1972 (references).

Tarazi, Robert C.: Sympathomimetic Agents in the Treatment of Shock. *Annals of Internal Medicine*, 81:364–371, September 1974 (references).

Woods, Susan L.: Monitoring Pulmonary Artery Pressures. *American Journal of Nursing*, 76:1765–1771, November 1976 (references).

KANAMYCIN SULFATE (Kantrex and Kantrex Pediatric)

ACTIONS/INDICATIONS	DOSAGE	PREPARATION AND STORAGE	DRUG INCOMPATIBILITIES	MODES OF IV ADMINISTRATION			CONTRAINDICATIONS; WARNINGS; PRECAUTIONS; ADVERSE REACTIONS
				INJECTION	INTERMITTENT INFUSION	CONTINUOUS INFUSION	
Antibiotic used for short-term treatment of serious infections caused by susceptible strains of: • N. gonorrhoeae • H. influenzae • E. coli • Enterobacter aerogenes • Shigella • Salmonella • K. pneumoniae • Serratia marcescens • Proteus Sensitivity testing must be carried out.	ADULTS: *Maximum daily dose*—1.5 gm (or 15 mg/kg/day) Total dose should be divided into 2–3 equal doses, or administered via a continuous infusion. CHILDREN AND NEONATES 15 mg/kg/day in 2–3 equal doses. RENAL DYSFUNCTION Dosage can remain as stated above with an increase in the interval between doses calculated by: Serum creatinine (mg/100 ml) × 9 = interval in hrs.	Use D5W, NS or D5/NS for infusion. Supplied in 2-ml vials of 500 mg (250 mg/ml) and 1 gm in 3-ml vials (333 mg/ml) for use in adults; and 2-ml vials of 75 mg (37.5 mg/ml) for use in children.	Do not mix with any other antibiotic or barbiturates in any manner.	NO Dilute before administration.	YES For administration of divided doses. Dilute each 500 mg of drug in at least 200 ml D5W, NS, D5/NS. Administer at a rate of 2–3 ml/min.	YES Add a 12-hr dose to 1000 ml D5W, NS or D5/NS, and infuse over 12 hrs.	CONTRAINDICATIONS 1. Hypersensitivity 2. Previous therapy with ototoxic drugs that produced or may have produced damage 3. Not used for long-term therapy, as for the treatment of tuberculosis WARNINGS 1. Known to cause damage to the auditory portion of the eighth cranial nerve. High-frequency deafness occurs first. Tinnitus or vertigo indicate vestibular injury and impending irreversible deafness. 2. Renal impairment increases the likelihood of ototoxicity. Daily dosage and intervals between doses should be decreased in renal failure. 3. If renal function deteriorates during therapy, the drug should be discontinued. 4. Older patients receiving more than 15 gm total dose should be observed more closely for eighth cranial nerve damage. 5. Concurrent use of other ototoxic agents increases the likelihood of eighth nerve damage (streptomycin, polymyxin B and E, neomycin, gentamicin and viomycin) and permanent hearing loss. 6. Concomitant use with rapid-acting diuretics (furosemide, etc.) may also cause irreversible deafness. 7. Safety for use in pregnancy has not been established. PRECAUTIONS 1. Obtain a pretreatment audiogram when possible. Follow-up studies are also indicated. 2. Keep patient well hydrated to prevent chemical irritation to the renal tubules. Renal function should be determined before and during therapy. If signs of irritation appear (casts, white or red cells, and albumin), hydration should be increased and dosage reduced. Therapy must be stopped if BUN rises or urinary output decreases.

357

KANAMYCIN SULFATE (Kantrex and Kantrex Pediatric) (Continued)

ACTIONS/ INDICATIONS	DOSAGE	PREPARATION AND STORAGE	DRUG INCOMPAT- IBILITIES	MODES OF IV ADMINISTRATION			CONTRAINDICATIONS; WARNINGS; PRECAUTIONS; ADVERSE REACTIONS
				INJECTION	INTERMITTENT INFUSION	CONTINUOUS INFUSION	

NURSING IMPLICATIONS
1. Monitor for signs of ototoxicity:
   a. Vestibular damage—dizziness, vertigo, tinnitus, roaring in the ears
   b. Auditory damage—high-frequency hearing loss as determined by audio-metric testing, general hearing loss
2. Monitor renal function:
   a. Urine output at least every 8 hours. Notify the physician of an output less than 240 ml in 8 hours (see chart on page 546 for normal output volume in children).
   b. BUN, daily. Be aware of the BUN prior to daily dose.
   c. Send urine for analysis to detect casts, red cells, or albumin, at least every other day.
3. Maintain hydration based on patient's size, weight, presence or absence of extraordinary fluid losses or fluid intolerances.
4. Take anaphylaxis precautions; see page 118.
5. Monitor for signs and symptoms of nonsusceptible organism overgrowth infection:
   a. Fever (take rectal temperature at least every 4–6 hours)
   b. Increasing malaise
   c. Signs and symptoms of a newly developing localized infection: redness, soreness, pain, swelling, drainage (change in character or volume of pre-existing drainage)
   d. Cough (change in sputum character or volume)
   e. Diarrhea
   f. Oral lesions (thrush) or perineal rash (monilia) due to *Candida albicans*

SUGGESTED READING
Vanderveen, Timothy W.: Aminoglycoside Antibiotics *American Journal of IV Therapy,* July 1977, pp. 5–13.

ADVERSE REACTIONS
1. Nephrotoxicity
2. Ototoxicity
3. Hypersensitivity: rash, drug fever

KETAMINE HYDROCHLORIDE (Ketalar, Ketaject)

ACTIONS/ INDICATIONS	DOSAGE	PREPARATION AND STORAGE	DRUG INCOMPAT- IBILITIES	MODES OF IV ADMINISTRATION			CONTRAINDICATIONS; WARNINGS; PRECAUTIONS; ADVERSE REACTIONS
				INJECTION	INTERMITTENT INFUSION	CONTINUOUS INFUSION	
Nonbarbiturate. Produces profound analgesia, with *normal* pharyngeal-laryngeal reflexes, *normal* or enhanced skeletal muscle tone, cardiac and respiratory stimulation. Patent airway is maintained by unaffected reflexes. Used as: • Sole anesthetic agent for short procedures	ADULTS: Dosage must be individualized by patient response. *For induction* —1.0–4.5 mg/kg (0.5–2.0 mg/lb) produces anesthesia in 30 seconds, lasts 5–10 min. For maintenance, additional increments can be administered without cumulative effect. The larger the total dose, the long-	Supplied in the following forms (Ketaject and Ketalar): 20-ml vial (10 mg/ml) 50-ml vial (10 mg/ml) 10-ml vial (50 mg/ml) 5-ml vial (100 mg/ml) NOTE: The 100 mg/ml concentration must be diluted 1:1 with NS or D5W.	Do not mix with any other medication.	YES May be given undiluted, except the 100 mg/ml form, which should be mixed with an equal amount of sterile water for injection, NS or D5W. Inject slowly, over at *least* 1 min. Rapid administration can cause apnea.	YES Dilute in D5W or NS.	NO	CONTRAINDICATIONS 1. When an elevation in blood pressure could be hazardous 2. Hypersensitivity WARNINGS 1. Respiratory depression has been reported; equipment must be readily available to support respiration. 2. Cardiac function must be monitored during use of the drug, especially in hypertensives and patients with history of cardiac problems. 3. Barbiturates and narcotics prolong recovery. 4. Safety for use in pregnancy and obstetrics has not been established. PRECAUTIONS 1. This agent should not be used alone for procedures involving the pharynx, larynx, or bronchial tree. Muscle relaxants and respiratory support must be

- Induction of anesthesia
- Supplement to other anesthetic agents

er the recovery period.

CHILDREN: 9–13 mg/kg (4–6 mg/lb), usually given *intramuscularly*, produces anesthesia in 3–4 min, lasting 12–25 min.

PREOPERATIVE PREPARATION

1. Patient should be N.P.O. at least 6–12 hrs prior to administration.
2. Atropine, scopolamine, or other drying agents should be given prior to induction.
3. Patient should be in a supported position during administration of this drug.

given.

2. The incidence of emergence reactions (confusional states) can be reduced by avoiding verbal and touching stimulation during recovery. This does not preclude vital sign monitoring.
3. Rapid IV injection can result in apnea and elevated BP.
4. Surgery involving visceral pain pathways should be supplemented with additional appropriate agents.
5. Use with caution in patients with chronic alcoholism and in acute alcohol intoxication.
6. Use with caution in patients with elevated cerebrospinal fluid pressure; this drug may elevate it further.

ADVERSE REACTIONS

1. Cardiovascular: hyper- and hypotension, tachycardia and bradycardia arrhythmias
2. Respiratory: respirations are frequently stimulated, but depression laryngospasm and apnea can also occur
3. Eye: slight, increased intraocular pressure, diplopia, and nystagmus
4. Psychological: emergence confusion, anxiety, hallucinations, lasting from 2–24 hours, in about 12% of all cases; no residual effects have been seen
5. Neurological: tonic and clonic muscle movements resembling seizures
6. Gastrointestinal: anorexia, nausea and vomiting (rare).
7. Rash and anaphylaxis are also possible.

NURSING IMPLICATIONS

1. Position the patient prior to administration of this drug, to prevent injury, i.e., use straps, padding, etc. as indicated.
2. Patient should be N.P.O. prior to receiving ketamine as with any anesthetic.
3. Be prepared to manage respiratory insufficiency. Have equipment at the bedside to support ventilation.
4. Blood pressure, pulse and respirations must be monitored every 2–3 minutes during use of this drug.
5. *Postoperative care:* Keep verbal and tactile stimuli to a minimum during recovery phase to decrease likelihood and severity of an emergence reaction. If such a reaction occurs, be prepared to administer a short-acting barbiturate sedative to control excitement, confusion and irrational behavior. Take necessary precautions to prevent patient injury (e.g., restraints, padding, etc.). These reactions are less likely to occur in persons less than 15 years, or greater than 65 years of age.
   a. Maintain a patent airway with the endotracheal tube, followed by an oral-pharyngeal airway as necessary, if other anesthetic agents have been used with ketamine (ketamine alone usually does not alter oral-pharyngeal reflexes or cause airway obstruction secondary to the depression of these reflexes).
   b. Monitor the respiratory rate continuously until an adequate spontaneous rate has been reached and has stabilized.
   c. Monitor heart rate and blood pressure at a schedule dictated by recovery room or institutional policy, usually every 15 minutes for the duration of the stay of an uncomplicated patient.
   d. Be prepared to treat hypotension, pressor agents and/or fluids are usually prescribed.
   e. Take precautions to prevent aspiration, by patient positioning.
   f. Administer supportive care as indicated for drugs used concomitantly with this anesthetic agent such as neuromuscular blocking agents (succinylcholine, tubocurarine, etc.), and analgesics.
   g. An anesthesiologist usually decides when a patient can be discharged from the recovery area; follow institutional policy.
6. When this drug is used for outpatient procedures, the patient must remain at rest under close surveillance until recovery from anesthesia is complete. Return home must be supervised by a responsible adult. The patient should not drive a car for at least the next 8 hours.

LEVALLORPHAN TARTRATE (Lorfan)

ACTIONS/ INDICATIONS	DOSAGE	PREPARATION AND STORAGE	DRUG INCOMPATIBILITIES	MODES OF IV ADMINISTRATION			CONTRAINDICATIONS; WARNINGS; PRECAUTIONS; ADVERSE REACTIONS
				INJECTION	INTERMITTENT INFUSION	CONTINUOUS INFUSION	
Narcotic antagonist when used in the presence of a strong narcotic effect. In the absence of this effect, it can cause respiratory depression. Used to manage significant respiratory depression secondary to narcotic administration.	ADULTS: 1 mg initially, followed by 0.5 mg at 10- to 15-min intervals. Total dose must not exceed 3 mg. May be used during delivery. NEONATES: To decrease respiratory depression secondary to narcotic effects in the mother; inject 0.05–0.1 mg (0.02 mg/kg) into the umbilical cord vein, subcutaneously, or IM. PREMATURE INFANTS: 0.05 mg via the umbilical vein.	Supplied ready for injection. Discard unused portion of vial. Available in 1-ml ampuls, 10-ml vials (1 mg/ml).	Do not mix with any other medication.	YES Slowly, undiluted, over 2–3 min.	NO	NO	CONTRAINDICATIONS 1. Mild respiratory depression 2. Narcotic addiction—it may produce withdrawal symptoms WARNINGS This drug is ineffective against respiratory depression due to barbiturates, anesthetics, or other non-narcotic agents or due to pathologic causes, and may actually increase the depression. PRECAUTIONS 1. If used in the absence of narcotic effect, respiratory depression may result. 2. Respiratory support measures (airway, endotracheal tube, manual ventilation, oxygen) must also be employed when treating narcotic respiratory depression. 3. Repeated doses exceeding 3 mg will treat the narcotic depression, but may result in respiratory depression equal to or greater than that produced by the narcotic. ADVERSE REACTIONS 1. Therapeutic dose: depression, restlessness, lethargy, dizziness, drowsiness, gastric upset, sweating, pallor, nausea, sense of heaviness in the limbs 2. Higher doses: hallucinations, strange dreams, confusion

NURSING IMPLICATIONS

1. Respiratory depression can return if the duration of depressive effects of the narcotic lasts longer than the effects of nalorphine.
2. Place the following equipment at the bedside or nearby: oral-pharyngeal airways, endotracheal tubes and laryngoscope, suction, oxygen, manual breathing bag (Ambu, Hope, Puritan), arterial blood gas sampling equipment.
3. The patient should be under constant observation.
4. Monitor respiratory status; respiratory depression is the primary indication for the use of this drug and is diagnosed by the presence of hypercarbia (elevated pCO$_2$) and hypoxemia (reduced pO$_2$). Signs and symptoms of hypoxia include tachycardia, pallor, hypotension, confusion, restlessness.
5. Assist respirations until nalorphine is effective as indicated by an adequate spontaneous respiratory rate and return of gag, cough, and swallow reflexes.

cotic addict. Use side rails at all times; restraints may be necessary.
11. Signs of acute withdrawal in the neonate:[1]
   a. Excessive irritability, crying, etc.
   b. Increased appetite, yet poor feeding ability
   c. Reduced sleeping periods
   d. Tremulousness
   e. Rarely seizures
   f. Diarrhea and vomiting
   g. Tachypnea
   h. Fever
   i. Sneezing
   Report the onset of any one of these signs to the physician.
12. Support ventilation until the respiratory rate is adequate and the gag, cough and swallow reflexes have returned permanently. Withdrawal of any form of support should be supervised by a physician.

REFERENCE
1. Kandall, Stephen R.: Managing Neonatal Withdrawal. *Drug Therapy*, May 1976, p. 48.

SUGGESTED READINGS
Kandall, Stephen R.: Managing Neonatal Withdrawal. *Drug Therapy*, May 1976, pp. 47–58.
McCaffery, Margo, and Hart, Linda: Undertreatment of Acute Pain With Narcotics. *American Journal of Nursing*, 76(10):1586–1591, October 1976.
Rogers, Robert M., and Juers, John A.: Physiologic Considerations in the Treatment of Acute Respiratory Failure. *Basics of Respiratory Disease*, 3(4), March 1975.

6. Examine frequently for signs of vomiting. Take precautions to prevent aspiration (position patient on one side, keep suction equipment ready to use, gastric intubation if abdominal distention is present).
7. Patients should be intubated if there is vomiting, if ventilation via airway and mask is ineffective (no improvement in arterial blood pO_2 or pCO_2) or if such support will be required for a prolonged period of time.
8. Monitor blood pressure and heart rate (apical or via ECG monitor) every 3–5 minutes until the patient has recovered and/or vital signs have reached desirable levels and stabilized (as determined by the physician).
9. Patients with pre-existing ventricular irritability, secondary to pathology or drugs, should be placed on continuous ECG monitoring. Be prepared to treat ventricular tachycardia or fibrillation.
10. Be prepared to manage acute narcotic withdrawal symptoms in the nar-

LEVARTERENOL BITARTRATE (Levophed)

ACTIONS/ INDICATIONS	DOSAGE	PREPARATION AND STORAGE	DRUG INCOMPATIBILITIES	MODES OF IV ADMINISTRATION			CONTRAINDICATIONS; WARNINGS; PRECAUTIONS; ADVERSE REACTIONS
				INJECTION	INTERMITTENT INFUSION	CONTINUOUS INFUSION	
Alpha and beta adrenergic stimulant, norepinephrine which produces the following effects: • Increased myocardial contractility (increases cardiac output) • Dilatation of coronary arteries • Increased systemic blood pressure • Increased venous return to the heart Used to restore normal blood pressure in these hypotensive states: • Postpheochromocytomectomy • Postsympathectomy	ADULTS AND CHILDREN: (All indications) *Initial drip rate*—2–3 ml/ min (8–12 mcg/min). *Maintenance drip rate*— 0.5–1.0 ml/ min (2–4 mcg/min). Up to 68 mg/day have been given in in severe cases. Titrate to maintain arterial blood pressure, CVP, or pulmonary artery pressure at desired level. DO NOT ABRUPTLY STOP INFUSION; TAPER DOSAGE DOWN OVER SEVERAL HOURS.	Standard infusion solution: 4 ml (4 mg) of drug in 1000 ml D5W or D5/ NS. Concentration will be: 4 mcg/ml For patients requiring fluid restriction, add 4 ml (4 mg) to 500 ml solution. Concentration will be: 8 mcg/ml USE *ONLY* D5W OR D5/ NS FOR INFUSION FLUID.	Do not mix in any manner with: Aminophylline Sodium bicarbonate Sodium iodide Any cephalosporin Chlorothiazide Chlorpheniramine Novobiocin Barbiturates Phenytoin (Dilantin)	NO	YES Using the 4 or 8 mcg/ml solution, begin the infusion at the lowest suggested dosage rate. Increase dosage as necessary to elicit a patient response. Use a volumetric infusion pump.	YES Using the 4 or 8 mcg/ml solution, begin the infusion at the lowest suggested dosage rate. Increase dosage as necessary to elicit a patient response. Use a volumetric infusion pump.	CONTRAINDICATIONS 1. Untreated hypovolemia 2. Mesenteric or peripheral vascular thrombosis, unless given as a lifesaving measure 3. During cyclopropane and halothane anesthesia, may precipitate ventricular tachycardia and/or fibrillation WARNINGS Use with extreme caution in the presence of MAO inhibitors or antidepressants of the triptyline or imipramine types; concomitant use with levarterenol may precipitate hypertension. PRECAUTIONS 1. Blood depletion and hypovolemia must be corrected prior to or during administration of levarterenol. 2. Avoid producing hypertension with excessive administration of this drug. In previously hypertensive patients, it is recommended that the blood pressure be increased no higher than 40 mm Hg below the pre-existing systolic pressure. 3. Use a large vein for infusion. Avoid use of a cutdown site and use of lower extremity veins. 4. Prevent extravasation; this drug will cause tissue necrosis and sloughing if it comes in contact with tissue because of its intense vasoconstrictive action.

● **LEVARTERENOL BITARTRATE** (Levophed) (*Continued*)

ACTIONS/ INDICATIONS	DOSAGE	PREPARATION AND STORAGE	DRUG INCOMPAT- IBILITIES	MODES OF IV ADMINISTRATION			CONTRAINDICATIONS; WARNINGS; PRECAUTIONS; ADVERSE REACTIONS
				INJECTION	INTERMITTENT INFUSION	CONTINUOUS INFUSION	
• Acute myo- cardial in- farction • Sepsis • Anaphylaxis • Idiosyncratic reactions to drugs (or overdosage, e.g., antihy- pertensive agents) • Cardiac ar- rest							ADVERSE REACTIONS 1. Sinus bradycardia. 2. Overdosage can produce severe hy- pertension, reflex bradycardia, in- creased peripheral vascular resistance and resultant decreased cardiac out- put. 3. Prolonged administration of any vasopressor may produce plasma vol- ume depletion. This should be contin- uously corrected during therapy; if not on discontinuation of levarterenol, hypotension may recur, or poor tissue perfusion may result. 4. The intense vasoconstriction pro- duced by large doses of this drug has been known to be associated with ischemia of fingers and toes, leading to gangrene of these areas.

NURSING IMPLICATIONS

1. Adequate parameters must be available for monitoring to guide titration of this drug. At a minimum, heart rate, ECG, central venous pressure, indirect blood pressure (by sphygmomanometer) and urine output must be used. If possible, it is advisable to use direct arterial blood pressure and pulmonary artery pressure readings instead of indirect blood pressure and central ve- nous pressure readings. Because of this drug's vasoconstrictive actions, the indirectly obtained blood pressure may be significantly different from the intra-arterial blood pressure. The values of these parameters to strive for when titrating the drug must be determined by the physician.

2. Heart rate and blood pressure (direct or indirect) must be recorded prior to and every 2–3 minutes during the initial phases of titration. When the blood pressure stabilizes for at least 1 hour near or at the desired, preset value, frequency of monitoring can be reduced to every 15–30 minutes, or as indicated by the patient's general condition.

3. Central venous pressure or pulmonary artery pressure should be recorded prior to and every 30 minutes during titration. A continuous oscilloscopic display of arterial and pulmonary arterial pressures is ideal in this situation.

4. The patient should be observed for arrhythmias via continuous ECG moni- toring. Myocardial irritability as evidenced by premature ventricular contrac- tions and sinus bradycardia can occur. Be prepared to treat both. See No. 8 below.

5. Urine output should be recorded hourly during the initial phase of therapy with this drug for shock. Urine flow reflects indirectly the perfusion of the kidneys. A fall in urine output may indicate the need for a change in drug therapy, either an increase in levarterenol drip rate, or its discontinuation and the initiation of another agent. Notify the physician if urine output falls below 30 ml/hour for 2 consecutive hours in an adult patient (see chart on page 546 for normal urine output in children).

6. Use a volumetric infusion pump if available. If the device has an infiltration alarm system, use it.

site. Some physicians recommend the addition of the vasodilator phentol- amine (Regitine) 5–10 mg to each 1000 ml of levarterenol solution to de- crease tissue damage in the event of extravasation.[1] If extravasation does occur, the affected area must be infiltrated with a solution of phentolamine 5–10 mg in saline 5–10 ml, using a 25 gauge needle. This procedure should be carried out immediately upon discovery of the infiltration. In- volved areas of tissue will be severely blanched and cold. After the phentol- amine treatment, protect the area from additional trauma.

8. Observe for signs and symptoms of overdosage (too rapid an infusion rate): headache, tachycardia, premature ventricular contractions, diaphoresis, pal- lor (if not already present), chest pain. If any one of these appears, slow the infusion and notify the physician.

9. Patients requiring therapy with this drug frequently require respiratory sup- port. Monitor respiratory rate, effort and blood gases with other parame- ters. Be prepared to initiate manual ventilation.

REFERENCE
1. Tarazi, Robert C.: Sympathomimetic Agents in the Treatment of Shock. *An- nals of Internal Medicine,* 81:369, September 1974.

SUGGESTED READINGS
Amsterdam, Ezra A. et al.: Evaluation and Management of Cardiogenic Shock. Part I. Approach to Patient. *Heart and Lung,* 1(3):402–408, May–June 1972 (references).
——: Evaluation and Management of Cardiogenic Shock. Part II. Drug Ther- apy. *Heart and Lung,* 1(5):663–671, September–October 1972 (references).
Tarazi, Robert C.: Sympathomimetic Agents in the Treatment of Shock. *An- nals of Internal Medicine,* 81:364–371, September 1974 (references).
Woods, Susan L.: Monitoring Pulmonary Artery Pressures. *American Journal of Nursing,* 76:1765–1771, November 1976 (references).
Intravenous Infusion of Vasopressors—Programmed Instruction. *American*

7. Prevent extravasation, see page 96 for guidelines. Check the infusion site frequently for blood return and free flow of fluid. Observe for blanching of the skin along the course of the vein; if this occurs, change the infusion

Journal of Nursing, 65(11):129–152, November 1965. (Useful information on the theories behind titration.)

● LEVORPHANOL TARTRATE (Levo-Dromoran)

ACTIONS/ INDICATIONS	DOSAGE	PREPARATION AND STORAGE	DRUG INCOMPAT- IBILITIES	MODES OF IV ADMINISTRATION			CONTRAINDICATIONS; WARNINGS; PRECAUTIONS; ADVERSE REACTIONS
				INJECTION	INTERMITTENT INFUSION	CONTINUOUS INFUSION	
Potent narcotic, synthetic analgesic similar to morphine. For relief of moderate to severe pain in • Biliary colic • Renal colic • Myocardial infarction • Trauma • Cancer • Postoperative period Has sedative properties. Duration of action is 6–8 hrs in most patients.	ADULTS: 2–3 mg. No dosage recommendations for children.	Available in ampuls of 1 ml and in multidose bottles of 10 ml (2 mg/ ml). This is a Schedule II drug under the Controlled Substances Act of 1970. Maintain hospital or institutional regulation guiding its use.	Do not inject into an IV line containing: Aminophylline Ammonium chloride Chlorothiazide Heparin Methicillin Novobiocin Phenytoin Sodium bicarbonate Sodium iodide Barbiturates	YES *Slowly* into the Y-injection site of a running IV.	NO	NO	CONTRAINDICATIONS 1. Acute alcoholic intoxication or withdrawal 2. Bronchial asthma 3. Increased intracranial pressure 4. Respiratory depression, hypoxia WARNINGS 1. Potentially habit-forming 2. Should be used in pregnancy only when expected benefits to the mother outweigh risks to the fetus PRECAUTIONS Levallorphan tartrate (Lorfan) can be used as an antagonist to this drug in case of overdose and/or respiratory depression. The two drugs may be given in combination to prevent respiratory depression without decreasing analgesia. See below. ADVERSE REACTIONS 1. Nausea, vomiting, dizziness, especially in the ambulatory patient 2. Allergy: rash, urticaria 3. Hypotension, respiratory depression, cardiac arrhythmias 4. Urinary retention USE OF LEVALLORPHAN TARTRATE (LORFAN) AS ANTAGONIST 1 mg IV initially, followed by 0.5 mg every 3 min until desired effect is seen. This drug usually acts within 1 minute and its action lasts for 2–5 hours.

NURSING IMPLICATIONS
1. Monitor for respiratory depression. Do not administer to patients who are minimally alert or having respiratory problems; see Precautions.
2. Respiratory support equipment must be readily available: airways, endotracheal tubes/laryngoscope, oxygen, manual breathing bag (Hope, Ambu, Puritan), suction.
3. Onset of drug action is usually within 1–2 minutes and lasts for 6 hours.

Monitor the patient continuously for respiratory depression for the first hour after infection and every 15–20 minutes for the next 2 hours. If the respiratory rate falls below 8–10/minute, attempt to arouse the patient and to increase the respiratory rate to 12–14/minute. Stay with the patient until the effects of the drug have diminished either over time or through the use of a narcotic antagonist (levallorphan tartrate).

If the patient is apneic or unarousable, begin artificial ventilation using an

LEVORPHANOL TARTRATE (Levo-Dromoran) (Continued)

NURSING IMPLICATIONS (No. 3 continued)
airway and manual breathing bag (if this equipment is not immediately available, proceed with mouth-to-mouth breathing). Maintain a ventilation rate of 12–14/minute until a narcotic antagonist can be administered, and until spontaneous respirations of an adequate rate return.

If the patient develops respiratory depression to a normal dose of this drug, any subsequent doses should be reduced in amount.

4. Monitor for urinary retention, palpate bladder size, and measure urine output every 4 hours while the patient is receiving this drug.

5. Monitor for irregular pulse, bradycardia or tachycardia.
6. Patients receiving IV levorphanol should be kept at rest for at least one-half hour after injection, and then be ambulated with caution (assistance), especially the elderly or debilitated.

SUGGESTED READING
McCaffery, Margo, and Hart, Linda: Undertreatment of Acute Pain With Narcotics. *American Journal of Nursing,* 76:1586–1591, October 1976 (references).

LEVOTHYROXINE SODIUM (Synthroid)

ACTIONS/ INDICATIONS	DOSAGE	PREPARATION AND STORAGE	DRUG INCOMPAT- IBILITIES	MODES OF IV ADMINISTRATION			CONTRAINDICATIONS; WARNINGS; PRECAUTIONS; ADVERSE REACTIONS
				INJECTION	INTERMITTENT INFUSION	CONTINUOUS INFUSION	
A form of thyroxine, the principle hormone secreted by the thyroid gland. Used for replacement therapy for decreased to absent thyroid function. Intravenous administration is used for myxedematous coma and for thyroid hormone replacement when oral administration is not possible and a rapid onset of action is needed.	ADULTS AND CHILDREN: 0.2–0.5 mg Full effects will be evident 24 hrs later. A repeat injection of 0.1–0.2 mg can be given on the second day if significant improvement has not been seen. *Myxedematous coma*—0.2–0.5 mg. PBI levels should be monitored and used to guide subsequent dosage.	Supplied in vials containing 0.5 mg of drug in powder form. To reconstitute add 5 ml NS (do not use any diluents containing a bacteriostatic agent). Shake vial to insure thorough mixing. Solution will contain 0.1 mg/ml. Use immediately and discard unused portion.	No data. Do not mix with any other medication in any manner.	YES Use a solution containing 0.1 mg/ml over 1 min.	NO	NO	CONTRAINDICATIONS (RELATIVE) 1. Thyrotoxicosis 2. Acute myocardial infarction 3. Adrenal insufficiency WARNINGS 1. Use with caution in patients with cardiovascular disease, especially hypertension. Use a low initial dosage. Decrease dosage if chest pain or other sign of cardiac problems occur. 2. Careful observation is required if catecholamines (epinephrine) are administered to patients with cardiac problems on this drug. (This also applies during surgery.) Monitor for arrhythmias. 3. May potentiate anticoagulant effects of warfarin or coumarin. 4. Adrenal insufficiency must be corrected with corticosteroids prior to the administration of thyroid hormones. 5. Use for treatment of obesity is inappropriate and hazardous. PRECAUTIONS 1. Dosage must be delivered in small initial doses and gradual increments. 2. In patients with diabetes, insulin and oral hypoglycemia agent requirements may increase. The opposite is true if thyroid dosage is decreased. ADVERSE REACTIONS Excessive dosage may cause the symptoms of hyperthyroidism, e.g., weight

loss, palpitations, chest pain, leg cramps, nervousness, sweating, tachycardia and other arrhythmias, headache, insomnia, heat intolerance, fever. Dosage should be decreased.

NURSING IMPLICATIONS
1. Full effects of this drug will not be seen until the day after administration.
2. Patients with cardiac problems must be observed by continuous ECG monitoring during and following intravenous injection. Anticipate tachyarrhythmias (atrial fibrillation, paroxysmal atrial tachycardia and premature ventricular contractions).
3. When administering catecholamines or sympathomimetics to patients on this drug and with cardiac problems monitor ECG continuously and be prepared to treat ventricular irritability (premature ventricular contractions, ventricular tachycardia). Keep lidocaine 100 mg at the bedside.
4. If the patient is concomitantly on coumarin or warfarin anticoagulants,

monitor closely for bleeding. Be aware that the anticoagulant dosage should be decreased.
5. Monitor diabetics for hyperglycemia, e.g., with urine fractionals. Be aware of the fasting blood sugar. Insulin or oral hypoglycemic dosage may have to be increased.
6. Monitor for signs of hyperthyroidism (see Adverse Reactions). Instruct the patient to report symptoms, if he is capable.
7. Patients on IV therapy will eventually be placed on the oral form of thyroid.
8. Administer supportive care as indicated for the comatose patient, e.g. skin care, safety precautions.

● LIDOCAINE (Xylocaine Hydrochloride Intravenous for Cardiac Arrhythmias)

ACTIONS/INDICATIONS	DOSAGE	PREPARATION AND STORAGE	DRUG INCOMPATIBILITIES	MODES OF IV ADMINISTRATION			CONTRAINDICATIONS; WARNINGS; PRECAUTIONS; ADVERSE REACTIONS
				INJECTION	INTERMITTENT INFUSION	CONTINUOUS INFUSION	
				YES	YES	YES	
Antiarrhythmic. Increases the electrical stimulation threshold of the ventricular myocardium during diastole, with no change in contractility. Indicated in the acute management of: • Ventricular arrhythmias during surgery and during acute myocardial infarctions (PVC's and ventricular tachycardia) • Management of the above listed arrhythmias secondary to the use of	ADULTS: *Initial*—50–100 mg bolus. If no change in the arrhythmia in 5 min, repeat dose. Use *only* the 5-ml, 100-mg ampuls or prefilled syringes for direct IV injection. Do not administer more than 200–300 mg in 1 hr. (See precautions No. 1.) *Maintenance*—following an initial bolus, begin a continuous infusion if necessary. Dosage range is 1–4 mg/	This drug is supplied in several parenteral forms. Use *only* solutions labeled for cardiac arrhythmias, 40 mg/ml multidose vials for preparation of infusions; and 5-ml, 100-mg ampuls and prefilled syringes for direct IV injection. To prepare solutions for infusions: a 4 mg/ml concentration is the most convenient for infusion rate calculation. *Lidocaine* — *Vol. of Fluid* 2 gm — 500 ml 1 gm — 250 ml 600 mg — 150 ml	Do not mix with sodium bicarbonate in any manner.	At a rate of 25–50 mg/min; more rapid administration has caused seizure. May be given undiluted. Allow adequate time for the drug to reach the site of action before repeating dose (5 min.) Bolus injection insures rapid rise in blood level of the drug and should precede infusions.	Use any IV fluid (D5W preferred). Titrate with ECG response (i.e., suppression of premature ventricular contractions). USE AN INFUSION PUMP OR AT LEAST MICRODROP TUBING TO CONTROL FLOW RATE.	Use any IV fluid (D5W preferred). Titrate with ECG response (i.e., suppression of premature ventricular contractions). USE AN INFUSION PUMP OR AT LEAST MICRODROP TUBING TO CONTROL FLOW RATE.	CONTRAINDICATIONS 1. Known hypersensitivity to any local anesthetic 2. High grade sinoatrial or atrioventricular block, Wolff-Parkinson-White Syndrome WARNINGS 1. Constant ECG monitoring must be used when administering this drug for titration of drip rate. 2. Signs of prolongation of conduction, i.e., increasing P-R interval or widening of the QRS complex, should prompt discontinuation of the drug. This drug can increase the severity of A-V block. 3. Discontinue if arrhythmias appear or seem to be increased by the drug. 4. Emergency resuscitative equipment must be readily available, i.e. defibrillator. 5. Knowledge of dosage for children is limited. 6. This drug may increase the ventricular rate in the presence of atrial fibrillation. 7. Safety for use in pregnancy has not been established.

LIDOCAINE (Xylocaine Hydrochloride Intravenous for Cardiac Arrhythmias) (Continued)

ACTIONS/ INDICATIONS	DOSAGE	PREPARATION AND STORAGE	DRUG INCOMPAT- IBILITIES	MODES OF IV ADMINISTRATION			CONTRAINDICATIONS; WARNINGS; PRECAUTIONS; ADVERSE REACTIONS
				INJECTION	INTERMITTENT INFUSION	CONTINUOUS INFUSION	
other drugs (vasopressors, dopamine, etc.)	min. (20–50 mcg/kg/min in the average 70-kg person). Up to 7 mg/ min has been used for short periods; do not exceed this dosage, or 200–300 mg in 1 hr. Titrate with ECG monitoring. CHILDREN: *Initial* (using a 2% solution)— 0.5–1.0 mg/ kg/dose; repeat in 5–10 min as needed. *Maintenance* —20–50 mcg/kg/min. Do not exceed 100 mg in 1 hr. INFANTS: *Injection*— 0.5 mg/kg/dose, repeated every 5–10 min as needed.[1]	Yield: 4 mg/ml Rates: 4 mg/min = 1 ml/min = 60 microdrops/min = 60 ml/hr 3 mg/min = ¾ ml/min = 45 microdrops/min = 45 ml/hr 2 mg/min = ½ ml/min = 30 microdrops/min = 30 ml/hr 1 mg/min = ¼ ml/min = 15 microdrops/min = 15 ml/hr	Use D5W as infusion fluid.				PRECAUTIONS 1. Use with caution in patients with severe liver or renal impairment (drug is metabolized and excreted via these two systems). Accumulation may occur leading to toxicity. 2. Use with caution in the presence of hypovolemic shock. 3. Administration for PVC's in the presence of sinus bradycardia, without prior acceleration of the sinus rate (by isoproterenol or pacing), may increase the PVC's and lead to ventricular tachycardia. 4. Treat other factors which can produce premature ventricular contractions, e.g., hypoxia, pain, hypotension, digitalis toxicity, other drugs. 5. Older patients may develop adverse effects and toxicity more frequently than other age groups.[2] ADVERSE REACTIONS 1. NONCARDIAC SIGNS OF TOXICITY: a. Numbness of the lips, tongue, pharynx and face b. Dysarthria (difficulty in speaking) c. Tremors d. Parethesias e. Blurred or double vision f. Dizziness, mental changes, confusion, anxiety, restlessness g. Advanced toxicity — seizures, respiratory depression. h. Tinnitus i. Allergic reactions 2. CARDIAC SIGNS OF TOXICITY: a. Prolongation of P-R interval or widening of the QRS complex b. Bradycardia (sinus arrest may occur in the presence of sick sinus syndrome) c. *Increasing* frequency of premature ventricular contractions d. Hypotension, cardiovascular collapse Patients with severe hepatic disease or severe congestive heart failure, and the elderly, have a higher incidence of toxicity, especially of the central nervous system. These patients will ex-

2. Lie, K. I., et al.: Lidocaine in the Prevention of Primary Ventricular Fibrillation. *New England Journal of Medicine*, December 1974, p. 1235.

SUGGESTED READINGS

Andreoli, Kathleen G., et al.: *Comprehensive Cardiac Care* (3rd ed.), St. Louis: C. V. Mosby Company, 1975, pp. 169–177 on premature ventricular contractions and ventricular tachycardia; and pp. 312–313 on administration.

Collinsworth, Ken A., Kalman, Sumner M., Harrison, Donald C.: The Clinical Pharmacology of Lidocaine as an Antiarrhythmic Drug. *Circulation*, 50:1217–1230, December 1974 (references). This article is for advanced readers.

Intravenous Infusion of Vasopressors—Programmed Instruction. *American Journal of Nursing*, 65(11):129–152, November 1965. (Useful information on the theories behind titration that can be applied to all drugs.)

Levitt, Barrie, Borer, Jeffrey S. and Saropa, Arleen: The Clinical Pharmacology of Antiarrhythmic Drugs, Part I: Lidocaine and Procainamide. *Cardiovascular Nursing*, 10(5), September–October 1974.

Mattea, Judith and Mattea, Edward: Lidocaine and Procainamide Toxicity During Treatment of Arrhythmias. *American Journal of Nursing*, 76(9):1429–1431, September 1976.

hibit these signs and symptoms for a longer period of time after an infusion has been discontinued.

3. MANAGEMENT:
   a. Stop the infusion immediately with the onset of any one sign or symptom. Signs and symptoms will usually subside within 15–20 minutes.
   b. Continue to monitor for the arrhythmia being treated.
   c. Have the following drugs readily available to treat adverse reactions:
      (1) Hypotension—vasopressors such as metaraminol (Aramine), levarterenol (Levophed), dopamine (avoid the use of any agent that will increase ventricular irritability)
      (2) Bradycardia—atropine 0.5–1.0 mg. (average adult dose)
      (3) Seizures—diazepam 2.5–5.0 mg. (average adult dose)
   d. Monitor respiratory status: maintain an open airway and oxygenation.

NURSING IMPLICATIONS

1. Use a volumetric infusion pump to control flow rate and therefore dosage. If a pump is not available, use microdrop intravenous tubing and monitor the drip rate frequently. Record the total 8-hour dose in milligrams, and the milligram per minute dose required to control the arrhythmia on an hourly basis.
2. Examine the patient frequently for cardiac and noncardiac signs and symptoms of toxicity. See Adverse Reaction No. 3 above on the management of toxicity. Be prepared to manage seizures; keep the side rails up at all times. Instruct the patient to report any symptoms when they occur, if he is able. Notify the physician of the onset of toxicity.
3. Monitor blood pressure every 10–15 minutes until the infusion rate has stabilized with the control of the arrhythmia, then every hour. If hypotension occurs, slow the infusion and begin more frequent monitoring of the blood pressure. Notify the physician.
4. When titrating to control the arrhythmia, always use the least amount of drug necessary for control.

REFERENCES

1. *JAMA*, 227(7, Suppl.):859, February 18, 1974.

LINCOMYCIN (Lincocin)

ACTIONS/ INDICATIONS	DOSAGE	PREPARATION AND STORAGE	DRUG INCOMPAT- IBILITIES	MODES OF IV ADMINISTRATION				CONTRAINDICATIONS; WARNINGS; PRECAUTIONS; ADVERSE REACTIONS
				INJECTION	INTERMITTENT INFUSION	CONTINUOUS INFUSION		
Antibiotic, effective against most common gram-positive organisms. Used to treat serious infections due to susceptible strains of Streptococci, Pneumococci, Staphylococci, and anerobes, including Clostridium. Use should be reserved for penicillin-allergic patients, or for other patients for whom a penicillin is inappropriate.	ADULTS: (Depending on severity of the infection) 600–1000 mg every 8–12 hrs. This may be increased for severe infections. Up to 8 gms/day have been given. DOSAGE MODIFICATION IN THE PRESENCE OF RENAL IMPAIRMENT: *Mild renal failure*—no change in dose. *Uremia*—increase dose interval to every 12 hrs. *Hemo- and peritoneal dialysis*—same as in uremia. CHILDREN: (>1 mon. of age) 10–20 mg/kg/day depending on severity of infection; given in evenly divided doses every 8–12 hrs.	Available in prefilled 600-mg syringes and in 600-mg and 3-gm vials.	Do not mix with phenytoin, any other anitbiotics, or protein hydrolysate.	NO Must be diluted. Undiluted administration has precipitated cardiac arrest when given by direct injection.	YES Use: D5W, D10W, D5/NS, Ringer's solution, sodium, lactate ⅙ molar, Travert 10%- electrolyte No. 1, dextran in saline 6%, for infusion. Follow dilution table for volumes of infusion fluid and infusion time limits.	YES Use: D5W, D10W, D5/NS, Ringer's solution, sodium, lactate ⅙ molar, Travert 10% electrolyte No. 1, dextran in saline 6%, for infusion. Follow dilution table for volumes of infusion fluid and infusion time limits.		CONTRAINDICATIONS 1. Hypersensitivity to lincomycin or clindamycin 2. Minor bacterial infections 3. The newborn 4. Significant liver impairment WARNINGS 1. Intravenous administration can cause severe colitis which may end fatally and is characterized by severe, persistent diarrhea and abdominal pain. Drug must be discontinued if this occurs. Colitis may not occur for several weeks after last dose. Mild cases may respond to discontinuation of the drug. Moderate to severe cases would be managed with fluid, electrolyte and protein supplementation as indicated. Systemic corticosteroids and steroid enemas may help. 2. Safety for use in pregnancy has not been established. 3. This drug is secreted in breast milk. PRECAUTIONS 1. Use with caution in patients with a history of gastrointestinal disease, asthma, and significant allergies. 2. Overgrowth of nonsusceptible organisms, especially yeasts, can occur. 3. Monitor liver function during therapy. 4. This drug has neuromuscular blocking properties that may enhance the action of other blocking agents, use with caution in patients receiving such agents. ADVERSE REACTIONS 1. Gastrointestinal: stomatitis, nausea, vomiting, diarrhea, enterocolitis 2. Blood dyscrasias: neutropenia, leukopenia, agranulocytosis, and thrombocytopenic purpura, usually reversible 3. Hypersensitivity reactions of all forms 4. Syncope, hypotension, and cardiopulmonary arrest following rapid injection of large doses 5. Tinnitus and vertigo 6. Overgrowth infections

DOSE	VOL. DIL.	TIME
600 mg	100 ml	1 hr
1 gm	100 ml	1 hr
2 gm	200 ml	2 hrs
3 gm	300 ml	3 hrs
4 gm	400 ml	4 hrs

NURSING IMPLICATIONS

d. Cough (change in volume or character of sputum)
e. Diarrhea
f. Oral lesions (thrush) or perineal rash and itching (monilia) due to *Candida albicans*.

1. Monitor the patient for onset of colitis: increased frequency of stools, abdominal pain, diarrhea. At onset, do not administer the next dose. Notify physician. The drug should be discontinued. Patients who have received this drug should also be instructed to report the onset of any of the above symptoms if they occur during the first month after discontinuation of the drug.

4. Patients receiving this drug concomitantly with a neuromuscular blocking agent (*e.g.* tubocurarine, gallamine, succinylcholine, etc.) will require respiratory monitoring and support for a longer than normal period during recovery from the neuromuscular blocking agent. Lincomycin prolongs the paralytic effects of these drugs.

2. Take anaphylaxis precautions; see page 118.
3. Monitor for signs and symptoms of a nonsusceptible organism overgrowth infection:

a. Fever (take rectal temperature at least every 4–6 hours)
b. Increasing malaise
c. Signs and symptoms of a localized infection—redness, soreness, pain, swelling, drainage (change in volume or character of pre-existing drainage)

REFERENCE

1. Appel, Gerald B., and Neu, Harold C.: The Nephrotoxicity of Antimicrobial Agents. *New England Journal of Medicine*, 296:666, March 24, 1977.

● MAGNESIUM SULFATE

ACTIONS/ INDICATIONS	DOSAGE	PREPARATION AND STORAGE	DRUG INCOMPATIBILITIES	MODES OF IV ADMINISTRATION				CONTRAINDICATIONS; WARNINGS; PRECAUTIONS; ADVERSE REACTIONS
				INJECTION	INTERMITTENT INFUSION	CONTINUOUS INFUSION		
Central nervous system depressant. Also depresses smooth cardiac and skeletal muscle. Is an antagonist of calcium to the CNS. Used to treat: • Seizures in toxemia of pregnancy • Hypomagnesemia • Uterine tetany secondary to large doses of oxytocin • Cerebral edema (as an osmotic agent) • Barium poisoning • Hypertension or encephalopathy in children with	ADULTS: *Anticonvulsant* —1 gm repeated as needed. *Magnesium deficiency*—1 –2 gm. Repeat until relief of symptoms is seen or the serum level of magnesium has returned to normal. *Cerebral edema*—2.5 gm. Repeat as needed. *Eclampsia*— 10–14 gm total dose. Usually given by infusion, titrated with frequency of seizures: use a solution of 4–5 gm in 250	Supplied in the following concentrations and containers: 100 mg/ml (10% solution), 10 ml and 20 ml ampuls 250 mg/ml (25% solution), 10 ml ampuls 500 mg/ml (50% solution), 2 ml, 10 ml and 20 ml ampuls, and in 30 ml multidose vials (Also in disposable syringes of 10% and 50% concentrations.) Use a 5% solution for infusion, made by adding 5 gm of drug to 100 ml	Do not mix with: Aminophylline Sodium bicarbonate Any calcium preparation Novobiocin Vitamin B complex Clindamycin Tobramycin Polymyxin Chlorpromazine	YES Do not exceed a rate of 1.5 ml/min of a 10% solution (150 mg/min)	YES At a rate not to exceed 3 ml of a 5% solution/ min (150 mg/ min) until effects are obtained. Do not exceed 150 mg/min of a 10% solution.	YES At a rate not to exceed 3 ml of a 5% solution/ min (150 mg/ min) until effects are obtained. Do not exceed 150 mg/min of a 10% solution.		CONTRAINDICATIONS 1. Any degree of heart block 2. Myocardial damage (acute myocardial infarction, myocardopathy, etc.) PRECAUTIONS 1. Administer with caution in the presence of renal disease; no more than 2 gm should be given within a 48-hour period. Monitor serum levels. 2. High plasma magnesium levels will produce flushing, sweating, hypotension, shock, depressed cardiac and CNS function, weakness. 3. Overdosage will cause respiratory depression and eventually paralysis and apnea. 4. Decreases serum calcium. 5. Decrease dosage of barbiturates, narcotics, or other CNS depressants while administering magnesium to prevent overdepression. 6. Administer with extreme caution if the patient has received digitalis. Treating magnesium toxicity with calcium in the digitalized patient is hazardous. Serious alterations in A-V conduction including complete heart block can occur. 7. Calcium gluconate or calcium gluceptate should be readily available for IV administration as an antidote in

369

MAGNESIUM SULFATE (Continued)

ACTIONS/ INDICATIONS	DOSAGE	PREPARATION AND STORAGE	DRUG INCOMPAT- IBILITIES	MODES OF IV ADMINISTRATION			CONTRAINDICATIONS; WARNINGS; PRECAUTIONS; ADVERSE REACTIONS
				INJECTION	INTERMITTENT INFUSION	CONTINUOUS INFUSION	
acute nephri- tis Raises serum magnesium levels immedi- ately and the effects last 30 min.	ml D5/NS (2% solution), re- peating as necessary. Do not exceed a 24-hr dose of 30–40 gm. (May also be given IM.)

Uterine tetany— 1–2 gm by infusion titrated with uterine tone. (Use infusion described un- der eclampsia above.)

Barium poison- ing— 1–2 gm by infusion ti- trated with presence or absence of muscle spasms.

When giving this drug for the above indi- cations in re- peated doses or infusions, the patient's knee jerk re- flex should be tested before each addition- al dose, or pe- riodically dur- ing an infu- sion. If the reflex is ab- sent, the ad- ministration of the drug should be stopped until the reflex re- turns. | D5/NS. The concentration of the infusion should not ex- ceed 20%. | | | | | the event that high serum magnesium levels develop. (See Nursing Implica- tion No. 5.) |

Administration of the drug beyond the point where the knee jerk disappears may lead to apnea.

Total parenteral nutrition—1 gm (8.1 mEq)/day, depending on serum magnesium level.

CHILDREN:
Total parenteral nutrition—0.5 gm (4 mEq)/day, depending on serum magnesium level.

Magnesium deficiency—25 mg/kg every 6 hrs for 3-4 doses, depending on serum magnesium level.

Dosage for other indications not available.

NURSING IMPLICATIONS
1. Normal serum magnesium is 1.5-2.0 mEq/liter.
2. Low serum magnesium will produce: CNS irritability (seizures, spasicity), personality changes, tremor, cardiac tachyarrhythmias.
3. Do not leave the patient alone during infusion.
4. Monitor for effectiveness of the magnesium infusion:
   a. Anticonvulsant effect
   b. Relaxation of spastic muscles and tremors
   c. Resolution of arrhythmias
   Infusion is usually stopped when these signs appear.
5. Monitor for symptoms of high serum magnesium (usually begin at serum levels of 4 mEq/liter):
   a. Loss of knee-jerk reflex (check every 5 minutes or prior to each dose)
   b. Decreased respiratory rate (count every 5 minutes); respiratory paralysis may occur.
   c. Flushing of the skin (especially the face)
   d. Diaphoresis
   e. Flaccidity
   f. Hypotension (monitor blood pressure every 5-10 minutes during infusion)
   If one or more of these signs appear, slow or stop the infusion and notify physician.
6. Be prepared to manage respiratory failure. Keep the following equipment readily available: airways, suction, oxygen, endotracheal tubes and laryngoscope, manual breathing bag and mask.
7. Calcium gluconate or calcium gluceptate infusion can be a specific antidote to combat high magnesium levels and resultant respiratory failure. Keep a prepared infusion at the bedside. (See pages 211-215 on calcium infusions.) When using calcium infusions, place the patient on continuous ECG monitoring. Be prepared to manage arrhythmias, especially if the patient is on a digitalis preparation.

SUGGESTED READINGS
Butts, Priscilla: Magnesium Sulfate in the treatment of Toxemia. *American Journal of Nursing*, 77:1294-1928, August 1977 (reference).
Elbaum, Nancy: Detecting and Correcting Magnesium Imbalance. *Nursing '77*, August 1977, pp. 34-35.

● MANNITOL

ACTIONS/ INDICATIONS	DOSAGE	PREPARATION AND STORAGE	DRUG INCOMPATIBILITIES	MODES OF IV ADMINISTRATION			CONTRAINDICATIONS; WARNINGS; PRECAUTIONS; ADVERSE REACTIONS
				INJECTION	INTERMITTENT INFUSION	CONTINUOUS INFUSION	
Osmotic diuretic; a sugar-alcohol that increases the osmolarity of the blood to draw fluid from the intracellular and extracellular spaces. Prevents the reabsorption of water in the renal tubules. The result is obligatory diuresis. Uses: • Evaluation of glomerular filtration rate • To prevent or treat oliguria secondary to renal insufficiency • To reduce intracranial or intraocular pressure, therapeutically or prior to surgery • To promote the urinary excretion of toxic substances • To reduce intracranial pressure and to treat cerebral edema by reducing brain mass	ADULTS: *To prevent or treat oliguria* *Test dose—* 200 mg/kg (or 12.5 gm) given over 3–5 min. If there is an increase in urine output after 5 min, the full dose by infusion can be given. *Infusion—*50–200 gm, in 24 hrs. Rate is adjusted to maintain a urine flow of 30–50 ml/hr. Use 5, 10 or 15% solution. *Treatment of increased intracranial or intraocular pressure—*1.5–2.0 gm/kg over 30–60 min. Use a 15 or 20% solution. *To promote excretion of toxic substances—*up to 200 gm over 30–60 min, repeated until blood levels of the substance show clearance. Use a 5 or 10% solution.	Supplied in the following concentrations: *Percent solution* 5% 10% 15% 20% 25% *Grams/ 100 ml* 5 10 15 20 25 *mg/ml* 50 100 150 200 250 If crystals are present in the vial, place it in warm water (50°C) until the crystals are dissolved. Cool to body temperature or room temperature before administration. *Always* use an in-line IV filter, regardless of the mode of administration.	Do not mix in any manner with: Potassium chloride Blood Cephalosporins	YES Slowly, over 3–5 min. Use an in-line filter. See table under Preparation column to convert mg to ml.	YES Time of infusion is usually 30–60 min. Use an in-line filter. Titrate with desired result. 5, 10, 15 or 20% solutions are usually used. See table under Preparation column to convert mg to ml.	YES Titrate with desired result. Use an in-line filter. 5, 10, 15 or 20% solutions are usually used. See table under Preparation column to convert mg to ml.	CONTRAINDICATIONS 1. Well established anuria due to renal disease 2. Renal failure that fails to respond to a test dose within 3–5 min 3. Severe dehydration 4. Active intracranial bleeding except during craniotomy 5. Congestive heart failure and pulmonary edema (and pulmonary edema secondary to abnormal capillary permeability); or the appearance of failure during administration WARNINGS 1. Administer with caution to patients with compromised renal reserve. 2. Infusion should be stopped if oliguria or azotemia develops. 3. Large doses may produce circulatory overload and cardiac decompensation. 4. Water intoxication may occur if large doses are given to patients unable to excrete the drug rapidly enough. 5. There may be serious electrolyte and fluid imbalances secondary to this drug. Monitor serum sodium and potassium levels. 6. Reduction of intracranial pressure may increase intracranial bleeding if active bleeding exists. 7. Safe use in pregnancy has not been proven. 8. Dosage requirements for patients under 12 years of age have not been established. PRECAUTIONS 1. Monitor renal function (BUN and creatinine levels) and hydration (central venous pressure, blood pressure, urine specific gravity and skin turgor). 2. Reduction of urine output (less than 100 ml/hr) should prompt discontinuation of the drug unless oliguria is secondary to a nonrenal condition. Correct nonrenal causes. 3. Do not administer at the same time as whole blood is being infused. If unavoidable, add at least 20 mEq NaCl

To evaluate glomerular filtration—100 ml of a 20% solution added to 180 ml NS, infused over 30 min (normal urinary output response is 125 ml/min in males and 116 ml/min in females).

CHILDREN: (all indications):
Test dose—200 mg/kg or 6 gm/M² over 3–5 min.

Infusion—2 gm/kg or 60 gm/M² titrated with urine output (see chart of normal urine outputs on page 546). See Warnings no. 8.

NURSING IMPLICATIONS
1. Monitor renal function, i.e., responsiveness to the drug:
   a. Hourly or half-hourly urinary output. Drug infusion rate is usually titrated against urine output. Infusion is usually stopped if after a routine dose the output falls below 100 ml/hour. (The kidneys must be able to excrete the fluids drawn into the vascular compartment by the drug.)
   b. Specific gravity—use collection device in children if appropriate.
   c. Hydration via CVP, skin turgor.
   d. Be aware of the patient's BUN and creatinine levels, elevation of either value not due to other causes should prompt discontinuation of the mannitol.
   e. Monitor ability to urinate, check for bladder distention *hourly*. Use a pediatric collection device in children under 2 years or as indicated.
2. Monitor cardiac status:
   a. Blood pressure and pulse every hour.
   b. Observe for increased respiratory rate, orthopnea, dyspnea, rales.
   c. If there is known cardiac disease, CVP, arterial pressure or pulmonary artery (wedge) pressure should be monitored to indicate the onset of compromise in left ventricular function. Deviations should prompt discontinuation of the infusion and notification of the physician.
   d. Be prepared to treat cardiac decompensation—oxygen, rotating tourniquets, thiazide diuretics, digitalis.
3. Be aware of the patient's serum sodium and potassium. Monitor for signs of hyponatremia and hypokalemia:
   a. Hyponatremia—headache, nausea, abdominal cramps, disorientation, diarrhea, hypotension (late).
   b. Hypokalemia—weakness, lethargy, muscle cramps, irritability, abdominal distention, cardiac arrhythmias (late).
4. In the presence of head injury when mannitol is administered to reduce intracranial pressure, monitor change in neurologic signs that could indicate intracranial bleeding:
   a. Pupil reaction to light
   b. Hand grip
   c. Orientation
   d. Movement of extremities
   These signs may also be monitored to evaluate reduction in intracranial pressure secondary to the administration of mannitol.
5. Take extravasation precautions: see page 96.

to the mannitol.
4. Avoid extravasation.
5. Monitor cardiac status, i.e., heart rate, blood pressure, signs of congestive heart failure.
6. Can increase the chances of eighth cranial nerve damage when given with kanamycin.

ADVERSE REACTIONS
1. Rapid infusion leads to circulatory overload, pulmonary edema, water intoxication
2. Sodium and chloride loss in the urine may be excessive
3. Renal adverse reactions—osmotic nephrosis
4. Convulsions, dizziness
5. Headache, chest pain, arm pain
6. Nausea, vomiting, thirst
7. Hypo- and hypertension
8. Allergic reactions of all forms

MECHLORETHAMINE HYDROCHLORIDE (Mustargen, Nitrogen Mustard)

ACTIONS/ INDICATIONS	DOSAGE	PREPARATION AND STORAGE	DRUG INCOMPAT- IBILITIES	MODES OF IV ADMINISTRATION			CONTRAINDICATIONS; WARNINGS; PRECAUTIONS; ADVERSE REACTIONS
				INJECTION	INTERMITTENT INFUSION	CONTINUOUS INFUSION	
A nitrogen mustard cyto-toxic agent which inhibits rapidly prolif-erating cells. Used for palli-ative treatment of Hodgkin's disease (sta-ges III and IV), lymphosar-coma, chronic myelocytic or lymphocytic leukemia, poly-cythemia vera, mycosis fun-goides, and bronchogenic carcinoma.	ADULTS AND CHILDREN: Dosage varies with the dis-ease and clini-cal status of the patient. Usually 0.4 mg/kg for each course in a single dose or divided do-ses of 0.1–0.2 mg/kg/day depending on the specific protocol for each patient. Weight used must be minus estimated ede-ma weight. Duration and frequency of treatments vary with the disease being treated.	To prepare from powder, inject 10 ml of sterile water for injection or NS into the vial (do not remove the needle), shake to dissolve completely, withdraw dose. The resultant solution will contain 1 mg/ ml of the drug. Discard unused portion. Do not use if the solution is discolored or if droplets of wa-ter are in the vial with the powder prior to reconstitution.	Do not mix with any other medication in any manner.	YES Into the Y in-jection site of a running IV to prevent vein ir-ritation. Inject over 3–5 min. Flush the vein with 10 ml NS after the injec-tion.	NO	NO	CONTRAINDICATIONS 1. Because of the toxicity of this drug and the unpleasant side effects, the use in patients with inoperable neo-plasms or in the terminal stage of the disease must be balanced against the limited gain. 2. Use in widely disseminated neo-plasms. 3. Use in the presence of bone marrow depression secondary to tumor infil-tration that does not improve with the use of the drug. 4. In the presence of infectious dis-eases. WARNINGS 1. Avoid extravasation; if it occurs, painful inflammation and necrosis of the tissue can occur. When discov-ered, the area should be promptly in-filtrated with a sterile sodium thio-sulfate (⅙molar) solution. Ice compresses should then be applied for the next 6–12 hours. 2. An accurate tissue diagnosis of the disease, knowledge of its natural course and a comprehensive clinical history must be obtained to guide therapy. 3. Determine the patient's hematologic status prior to administration; see Adverse Reaction No. 4. 4. Use only in the absence of acute or chronic suppurative inflammation. 5. The possible benefits of administra-tion of this drug in women of child-bearing potential must be weighed against the risks. If use can be post-poned until the third trimester, it should; fetal malformations can oc-cur. PRECAUTIONS 1. Avoid inhalation of the dust or va-pors of this drug, or contact with skin, mucous membranes or eyes. Should accidental eye contact occur, copious irrigation with normal saline or balanced salt ophthalmic irrigat-ing solution should be done immedi-

ately. Possible damage must be evaluated by a physician. Accidental contact with the skin should be treated with copious water irrigation for 15 minutes, followed by application of a 2% sodium thiosulfate solution.

2. Neither this drug or x-ray therapy should be given until the bone marrow has recovered from other chemotherapy or x-ray therapy. Irradiation of the sternum, ribs and vertebrae shortly after a course of nitrogen mustard may lead to hematologic complications (bone marrow suppression).

3. There is a possibility of the development of a second malignancy, especially when this drug is combined with other antineoplastic agents or radiation.

4. Hyperuricemia may develop. Medication for this may be required. Adequate hydration may minimize this problem.

5. Use with caution in chronic lymphatic leukemia, if at all; there is a high incidence of bone marrow *failure* in this situation.

ADVERSE REACTIONS

1. Toxic manifestations are very common in the use of this agent.

2. Thrombosis and thrombophlebitis can occur secondary to IV injection. This problem is even more likely if the venous pressure is elevated secondary to central vein occlusion.

3. The side effects that will limit the dosage and duration of therapy are nausea, vomiting and bone marrow depression.

4. Bone marrow depression (the lowest level of depression occurs 2–3 weeks after administration of the drug), producing leukopenia, thrombocytopenia (may advance to hemorrhagic stage, i.e., platelet count less than 50,000/cu mm). Marrow recovery occurs usually 2 weeks after the last dose of the drug. Excessive dosage (greater than 0.4 mg/Kg) can cause severe forms of leukopenia and thrombocytopenia which have ended fatally.

5. Gastrointestinal: severe nausea and vomiting 1–8 hours after injection; lasts for several hours; stomatitis.

● MECHLORETHAMINE HYDROCHLORIDE (Mustargen, Nitrogen Mustard) (Continued)

ACTIONS/ INDICATIONS	DOSAGE	PREPARATION AND STORAGE	DRUG INCOMPAT- IBILITIES	MODES OF IV ADMINISTRATION			CONTRAINDICATIONS; WARNINGS; PRECAUTIONS; ADVERSE REACTIONS
				INJECTION	INTERMITTENT INFUSION	CONTINUOUS INFUSION	

							6. Immunosuppressive actions:
							  a. Are more likely to occur if the patient is also on steroids.
							  b. The patient becomes more susceptible to any kind of infection.
							7. Herpes zoster may occur secondary to immunosuppression and other factors. If this occurs, discontinue the drug until the rash is healed.
							8. Rashes can occur; most frequently seen is a maculopapular type.
							9. Reproductive abnormalities: chromosomal changes, menstrual disturbances, impaired spermatogenesis.
							10. Hepatotoxicity can occur and will be evidenced by jaundice (rare).
							11. Hair loss is fairly common.
							12. Neurotoxicity:
							  a. Can cause eighth cranial nerve damage.
							  b. Auditory changes will be tinnitus (ringing in the ears) and diminished hearing.
							  c. Vestibular damage will be evidenced by vertigo.

NURSING IMPLICATIONS

1. The patient receiving this medication will be experiencing the emotional and physical effects of the malignancy or other condition being treated. Knowledge of the patient's feelings about his disease and its implications will assist in helping him tolerate the chemotherapy. The incidence of uncomfortable side effects and adverse reactions is high. It is within the nurse's role to assist the patient in coping with the discomforts of the disease and its treatment, and to help him work through depression and anger toward acceptance of the disease at his own pace. Despite the unpleasantness this drug may bring, it can be a source of hope for the patient.

2. Many patients experience fewer injection side effects (e.g., nausea and vomiting) when they are placed in a prone or reclining position during the administration of this drug.

3. Take all precautions to prevent extravasation. If extravasation occurs or is suspected, follow directions under Warning No. 1. Keep sodium thiosulfate on hand.

4. Management of nausea and vomiting:
   a. Usually occurs 1–3 hours after injection. Vomiting may subside after 8 hours, but nausea can persist for 24 hours.
   b. Administer this drug at night if possible to correlate with normal sleep patterns, accompanied by sedation and an antiemetic.
   c. To be effective, antiemetics should be administered 1 hour prior to the injection of the drug.
   d. Small frequent meals, timed with periods when the patient feels his

   best, are most easily tolerated.

b. For preventive care use a very soft toothbrush (child's) and toothpaste; avoid trauma to tissues.

c. Examine oral membranes at least daily (instruct patient and/or family) to detect the onset of inflammation or ulceration.

d. If stomatitis occurs, notify the physician and begin theraputic oral care:[1]
   (1) *Mild Inflammation:* Remove dentures, use a soft toothbrush and a hydrogen peroxide solution (1 part peroxide and 4 parts saline). Do *not* use toothpaste. Rinse with the peroxide solution and then water. Replace dentures. This procedure should be carried out every 4 hours and/or after meals.
   (2) *Severe Inflammation:* Remove dentures, use soft gauze pads rather than a toothbrush. Use the peroxide solution as described above. Rinse with water using an asepto syringe and gentle suction until returns are clear. Do not replace dentures. It may be necessary to give this care every 2–4 hours.

e. Order a bland, mechanical soft diet for patients with mild inflammation. If stomatitis is severe, the patient may be placed on NPO status by the physician.

f. For patients who can tolerate oral intake, administer Xylocaine Viscous or acetaminophen elixir as a mouthwash prior to meals to decrease pain (do not use aspirin rinses), as ordered by the physician.

g. Patients with severe stomatitis may require parenteral analgesia.

9. If rashes occur, administer cool compresses as ordered. Turn the patient frequently to prevent skin breakdown.

10. Monitor for jaundice; notify physician at onset.

best, are advisable. Bland foods usually are tolerated. Carbohydrate and protein content should be high.
e. If the patient is anorexic, encourage high nutrient liquids and water to maintain hydration (hydration helps to avoid complications of hyperuricemia).
f. Keep accurate measurements of emesis volume and total intake and output to guide the physician in ordering parenteral fluids when necessary.

5. Management of hematologic effects:
a. Be aware of the patient's white blood cell and platelet counts prior to each injection.
b. If the WBC falls to 2000/cu mm, take measures to protect the patient from infection, such as protective (reversed) isolation, avoidance of traumatic procedures, maintenance of bodily (especially perineal) cleanliness, carrying out strict urinary catheter care when appropriate, etc. Monitor for infection by recording temperatures every 4 hours, examining for rashes, swellings, drainage and pain. Explain these measures to the patient.
c. If the platelet count falls below 100,000/cu mm, monitor for thrombocytopenic bleeding: petechiae, purpura, hematuria, melena, blood in stools, gum bleeding, vaginal bleeding, epistaxis, hematemesis, etc. Avoid trauma. Transfusions may be ordered.
d. Instruct the patient and family on the importance of follow-up blood studies, and the reporting of the signs and symptoms listed in "b" and "c" above if the drug is being administered on an outpatient basis.
6. Thrombophlebitis can occur at the injection site. Notify the physician at onset; apply warm compresses as ordered, elevate the extremity. Protect the area from trauma.
7. Management of hair loss:
a. Use scalp tourniquet during injection if ordered.
b. Counsel the patient on the possibility of hair loss to enable him to prepare for this disfigurement.
c. Reassure him of regrowth of hair following discontinuation of the drug.
d. Provide privacy, and time for the patient to discuss his feelings.
8. Management of stomatitis:
a. Administer preventive oral care every 4 hours and/or after meals.

11. Monitor for hearing loss, tinnitus, and vertigo which indicate the onset of auditory and vestibular nerve damage. Notify the physician.
12. The positive expected outcomes from therapy are: regression of tumor size, decreased pain, increased appetite and exercise tolerance.

REFERENCE
1. Bruya, Margaret Auld, and Madeira, Nancy Powell: Stomatitis After Chemotherapy. American Journal of Nursing. 75(8):1351, August 1975.

SUGGESTED READINGS
Bolin, Rose Homan, and Auld, Margaret E.: Hodgkin's Disease, American Journal of Nursing. 74(11):1982–1986, November 1974.
Bruya, Margaret Auld, and Madeira, Nancy Powell: Stomatitis After Chemotherapy. American Journal of Nursing. 75(8):1349–1352, August 1975 (references).
Denley, Diana L.: Nursing the Patient Who is Immunosuppressed. American Journal of Nursing.76(10):1619–1625, October 1976 (references).
Foley, Genevieve, and McCarthy, Ann Marie: The Child with Leukemia—The Disease and Its Treatment. American Journal of Nursing. 76(7):1109–1114, July 1976 (references).
———:"The Child with Leukemia—In a Specialty Hematology Clinic. American Journal of Nursing, 76(7):1115–1119, July 1976.
Hannan, Jeanne Ferguson: Talking is Treatment, Too. American Journal of Nursing, 74(11):1991–1992, November 1974.
Le Blanc, Dona Harris: People with Hodgkin Disease: The Nursing Challenge. Nursing Clinics of North America, :3(2):281–300, June 1978.
Martinson, Ida: The Child with Leukemia: Parents Help Each Other. American Journal of Nursing, 76(7):1120–1122, July 1976.
Morrow, Mary: Nursing Management of the Adolescent: The Effect of Cancer Chemotherapy on Psychosocial Development. Nursing Clinics of North America, 13(2):319–335, June 1978.
Showfety, Mary Patricia: The Ordeal of Hodgkin's Disease. American Journal of Nursing, 74(11):1987–1991, November 1974.

● MENADIOL SODIUM DIPHOSPHATE (Synkayvite Injectable, Vitamin K₄, Kappadione)

ACTIONS/ INDICATIONS	DOSAGE	PREPARATION AND STORAGE	DRUG INCOMPATIBILITIES	MODES OF IV ADMINISTRATION				CONTRAINDICATIONS; WARNINGS; PRECAUTIONS; ADVERSE REACTIONS
				INJECTION	INTERMITTENT INFUSION	CONTINUOUS INFUSION		
Vitamin K analog. Vitamin K is necessary for the synthesis in the liver of prothrombin (FACTOR II), proconvertin (FACTOR VII),	ADULTS: 5–15 mg once or twice daily. CHILDREN: 5–10 mg once or twice daily.	Store at room temperature, 59–86°F or 15 –30°C.	Do not mix with any other medication.	YES May be given undiluted over 1 min (preferred route of administration).	YES Use any IV fluid, in any volume.	YES Use any IV fluid, in any volume.		CONTRAINDICATIONS Do not administer to the mother during the last weeks of pregnancy to prevent physiologic hypoprothrombinemia or hemorrhagic disease in the newborn.

WARNINGS
1. Phytonadione is best used to prevent or treat hemorrhagic disease in the |

MENADIOL SODIUM DIPHOSPHATE (Synkayvite Injectable, Vitamin K₄, Kappadione) (Continued)

ACTIONS/ INDICATIONS	DOSAGE	PREPARATION AND STORAGE	DRUG INCOMPATIBILITIES	MODES OF IV ADMINISTRATION			CONTRAINDICATIONS; WARNINGS; PRECAUTIONS; ADVERSE REACTIONS
				INJECTION	INTERMITTENT INFUSION	CONTINUOUS INFUSION	
thromboplastin (FACTOR IX), and Stuart factor (FACTOR X), the major components of blood coagulation. Effects begin 1–2 hrs after injection. Used to treat the hypoprothrombinemia that results from decreased absorption or use of vitamin K (obstructive jaundice, biliary fistula, sprue, ulcerative colitis, celiac disease, intestinal resection, cystic fibrosis of the pancreas, regional enteritis, and antibacterial therapy). Also in hypoprothrombinemia secondary to salicylates.	PERINATAL DOSE: 1–5 mg, one dose (phytonadione is the *preferred* agent in this age group).						newborn. 2. This drug will *not* counteract the actions of heparin. 3. Knowledge on effects in the fetus or germinal cells is limited. Therefore, safety for use in pregnancy has not been established. PRECAUTIONS 1. Temporary resistance to prothrombin-depressing anticoagulants may occur. This may necessitate larger doses of the anticoagulant or initiating the use of heparin. 2. Hypoprothrombinemia secondary to hepatocellular liver disease will not respond to vitamin K therapy. ADVERSE REACTIONS 1. Prolongation of prothrombin time after maximum doses (NOTE: This is a reverse reaction in comparison to the basic action of the drug to normalize prothrombin time). 2. In infants (especially the premature) excessive doses may cause increased bilirubinemia in the first few days of life. This may lead to kernicterus which can then lead to brain damage and death (this drug is not recommended for use in this age group). 3. Erythrocyte hemolysis can occur in patients with a genetic deficiency of glucose-6-phosphate dehydrogenase (G6PD) in their RBC's. 4. This drug may further depress liver function in patients with liver disease. 5. Allergic reactions (rash and urticaria) have been reported.

NURSING IMPLICATIONS
1. Care of the patient with hypoprothrombinemia:
   a. Monitor for signs of bleeding—gum bleeding, nosebleeds, hematuria, melena, red blood in the stools, ecchymosis, petechiae, vaginal bleeding, etc.
   b. Protect the patient from injury (e.g., use electric razor, wear slippers or shoes at all times, prevent falls).
2. Be aware of the patient's prothrombin time and partial thromboplastin time (PTT). Prothrombin time should be the same as the laboratory control which is usually 11–16 seconds, but will be prolonged over control time in hypoprothrombinemia. The PTT will also be prolonged.
3. Report the onset of a rash or urticaria to the physician; administer comfort measures as indicated.

SUGGESTED READING
Guyton, Arthur C.: *Textbook of Medical Physiology* (5th ed), Philadelphia: W. B. Saunders Company, 1976, Chapter 9, Hemostasis and Blood Coagulation, pp. 99–111.

MEPERIDINE HYDROCHLORIDE (Demerol Injection)

ACTIONS/INDICATIONS	DOSAGE	PREPARATION AND STORAGE	DRUG INCOMPATIBILITIES	MODES OF IV ADMINISTRATION				CONTRAINDICATIONS; WARNINGS; PRECAUTIONS; ADVERSE REACTIONS
				INJECTION	INTERMITTENT INFUSION	CONTINUOUS INFUSION		
Narcotic analgesic. Actions similar to morphine. For relief of moderate to severe pain, as a preoperative medication, for support of anesthesia, for obstetrical analgesia.	ADULTS: *For pain*— 10– 100 mg every 2–4 hrs. *Preoperative*— 10–50 mg. *Anesthesia support*— injection or infusion, titrate to patient need and effects obtained. SEE PREPARATION COLUMN FOR SOLUTION. CHILDREN: IV administration not recommended.	Must be diluted prior to injection. Solution for infusion is prepared by adding enough meperidine to a desired volume of fluid to produce a concentration of 1 mg/ml. Use D5W or NS. This is a Schedule II drug under the Controlled Substances Act of 1970. Maintain hospital or institutional regulations guiding its use.	Do not mix with any other drug in IV bottle; and do not inject into an IV line containing: Aminophylline Heparin Methicillin Morphine Phenytoin Sodium bicarbonate Sodium iodide Barbiturates	YES Very slowly, diluted in an equal amount of NS. See Warning No. 4.	YES Only by anesthesiologist. Titrate to obtain desired effect without producing adverse reactions. Use a 1 mg/ml solution.	YES Only by anesthesiologist. Titrate to obtain desired effect without producing adverse reactions. Use a 1 mg/ml solution.		CONTRAINDICATIONS 1. Hypersensitivity 2. Patients who are receiving or have received MAO inhibitors (Marplan, etc.) in the past 2 weeks WARNINGS 1. Physical and psychic dependence occurs. Tolerance may also occur after repeated doses. 2. Use with caution and in reduced dosage in patients who are concurrently on other narcotic analgesics, general anesthetics, phenothiazines, other tranquilizers, sedative-hypnotics, and any other CNS depressants, including alcohol. Respiratory depression, hypotension and coma may result. 3. In the presence of a head injury, intracranial lesion, or in any case of increased intracranial pressure, this drug may further increase cerebrospinal fluid pressure and can depress respirations. Use caution in these situations. 4. Rapid IV injection can lead to severe respiratory depression, apnea, shock, and cardiac arrest. A narcotic antagonist and respiratory support equipment must be at the bedside. The patient must be lying down during administration. 5. Use with *extreme* caution in patients with an acute asthmatic attack, chronic obstructive lung disease, cor pulmonale, decreased respiratory reserve (chest trauma, surgery, cancerous lesions, malformations), pre-existing respiratory depression, hypoxia or hypercapnia (increased blood pCO_2). Apnea can result. 6. Administer with extreme caution to patients with hypovolemia, acute blood loss, or who have received phenothiazines. Severe hypotension can result. 7. May produce orthostatic hypotension; keep patient at rest. 8. Do not use in pregnant patients prior to the labor period, unless benefits

MEPERIDINE HYDROCHLORIDE (Demerol Injection) (Continued)

ACTIONS/ INDICATIONS	DOSAGE	PREPARATION AND STORAGE	DRUG INCOMPAT- IBILITIES	MODES OF IV ADMINISTRATION			CONTRAINDICATIONS; WARNINGS; PRECAUTIONS; ADVERSE REACTIONS
				INJECTION	INTERMITTENT INFUSION	CONTINUOUS INFUSION	
							outweigh risks to the fetus. Can produce respiratory depression in the infant when given during labor. Resuscitation of the infant may be required.
							9. This drug is secreted in breast milk.
							10. See Nursing Implications for treatment of overdosage and adverse reactions.
							PRECAUTIONS
							1. Use with caution in patients with atrial flutter and other supraventricular arrhythmias; increased ventricular response may result.
							2. May aggravate pre-existing seizure disorders.
							3. May obscure symptoms used to diagnose patients with acute abdominal symptoms.
							4. Reduce dosage and use with caution in the elderly or debilitated, in patients with severe hepatic or renal impairment, hypothyroidism, Addison's disease, prostatic hypertrophy or urethral stricture. These patients are more likely to have adverse reactions.
							ADVERSE REACTIONS
							1. Respiratory depression and apnea
							2. Circulatory depression, i.e., fall in blood pressure, cardiac arrest
							3. Light-headedness, dizziness, sedation
							4. Nausea, vomiting
							5. Diaphoresis
							6. Transient hallucinations, disorientation, euphoria, weakness
							7. Constipation, biliary tract spasm
							8. Tachycardia, bradycardia, palpitations
							9. Urinary retention
							10. Hypersensitivity reactions ranging from rashes to anaphylaxis
							11. Visual disturbances
							12. Dry mouth

NURSING IMPLICATIONS

1. Monitor closely for respiratory depression and extreme somnolence during the first hour after an injection. If the respiratory rate falls below 8 per

4. When used in patients with atrial tachyarrhythmias, monitor ECG continuously for increased ventricular response and possible subsequent cardiac decompensation (fall in blood pressure, signs of pulmonary edema).

minute, attempt to stimulate the patient to increase his respiratory rate. Firmly instruct him to breathe, repeating instructions to make him breathe at least 10–12 times a minute.[1] If the patient does not respond to this, begin to support respirations manually using mouth-to-mouth breathing or a manual breathing bag and mask. Call for the physician to administer a narcotic antagonist such as naloxone (Narcan). Prepare 0.1–0.4 mg for an initial dose. (See page 417 for full information on naloxone.) Fluids and vasopressors may be required for the patient who becomes hypotensive.

2. If the patient receiving meperidine has a pre-existing respiratory problem which makes him more vulnerable to breathing difficulties or depression (e.g., hypoxia, pulmonary infection, chest trauma, chest surgery, any patient immediately postanesthesia, chest malformations, those who have received neuromuscular blocking agents, other respiratory depressing agent or who are in shock), keep the following equipment at the bedside:
   a. Oxygen if not already in use
   b. Oral-pharyngeal airways
   c. Suction equipment
   d. Endotracheal tubes and a laryngoscope (if not already in use)
   e. Manual self-inflating breathing bag.
   Follow resuscitation guidelines as listed in No. 1 above. Such patients should not be left alone during the first hour after injection. Meperidine causes the same amount of respiratory depression as does morphine (contrary to popular belief). Peak depression will occur within 1 hour of injection (usually 15 minutes after an IV injection). Normal respirations return within 2 hours.[2]

3. Monitor for further rise in intracranial pressure in patients with a pre-existing problem. Neurologic signs, blood pressure and heart rate should be evaluated at least every 30 minutes.

5. Take seizure precautions for patients with pre-existing seizure disorders.
6. Monitor for urinary retention in patients with prostatic hypertrophy or urethral stricture. Palpate bladder size every 4 hours. Measure urine output every 8 hours or as patient's condition warrants.
7. Be prepared to manage nausea and vomiting. Take aspiration precautions in patients with weakened gag reflex. Keep suction at the bedside.
8. Take safety precautions in the elderly in the event of disorientation to prevent patient injury; use side rails and soft restraints as necessary.
9. Take precautions to prevent constipation in patients on prolonged therapy with this drug (hydration, stool softeners, enemas as necessary).
10. Administer successive doses when pain is just beginning to return. Do not wait until it returns to full intensity. Dosage intervals must be determined by patient response rather than time intervals. Notify physician if pain is returning before the time interval he has prescribed is reached.

REFERENCES
1. McCaffery, Margo, and Hart, Linda L.: Undertreatment of Acute Pain with Narcotics. American Journal of Nursing, 76:1589, October 1976.
2. Ibid.

SUGGESTED READINGS
McCaffery, Margo, and Hart, Linda L.: Undertreatment of Acute Pain with Narcotics. American Journal of Nursing, 76:1586–1591, October 1976 (references).
Smith, Dorothy W., and Germain, Carol P. Hanley: Care of the Adult Patient (4th ed.), Philadelphia: J. B. Lippincott Company, 1975, pp. 134–146 (references).

MEPHENTERMINE SULFATE (Wyamine Sulfate Injection)

| ACTIONS/ INDICATIONS | DOSAGE | PREPARATION AND STORAGE | DRUG INCOMPATIBLITIES | MODES OF IV ADMINISTRATION | | | | CONTRAINDICATIONS; WARNINGS; PRECAUTIONS; ADVERSE REACTIONS |
				INJECTION	INTERMITTENT INFUSION	CONTINUOUS INFUSION		
Sympathomimetic; increases blood pressure, cardiac output. Produces cerebral stimulation. Used to control hypotension secondary to ganglionic blockade and that occuring with spinal anesthesia.	ADULTS: *Hypotension during surgery after spinal anesthesia, or in severe illness* —30–45 mg with repeated doses of 30 mg as necessary, in single injection or by continuous infusion of a 0.1% solution. *Hypotension secondary to spinal anesthe-*	To prepare an 0.1% solution: add 600 mg to 500 ml of D5W. Supplied in vials of 15 mg/ml, 30 mg/ml, and in prefilled syringes of a 30 mg/ml concentration.	Do not mix with epinephrine or hydralazine in any manner.	YES No need to dilute, but inject over at least 1–2 min.	YES Titrate flow rate with patient response. Use a 0.1% solution and an infusion pump.	YES Titrate flow rate with patient response. Use a 0.1% solution and an infusion pump.		CONTRAINDICATIONS 1. Hypotension induced by chlorpromazine and other phenothiazines 2. In the presence of MAO inhibitors 3. Untreated hemorrhagic shock (see Precaution No. 1) 4. Hypersensitivity 5. In the presence of reserpine, guanethidine or tricyclic antidepressants WARNINGS 1. Hypovolemia must be corrected. 2. Use with caution in patients with cardiac disease. 3. If used during labor and delivery, caution must be exercised if the patient has received an oxytocic drug. Severe hypertension may result. 4. Use during pregnancy or lactation

MEPHENTERMINE SULFATE (Wyamine Sulfate Injection) (Continued)

ACTIONS/ INDICATIONS	DOSAGE	PREPARATION AND STORAGE	DRUG INCOMPAT- IBILITIES	MODES OF IV ADMINISTRATION			CONTRAINDICATIONS; WARNINGS; PRECAUTIONS; ADVERSE REACTIONS
				INJECTION	INTERMITTENT INFUSION	CONTINUOUS INFUSION	
	sia in cesarean section—15 mg, repeated as necessary. *Shock in acute myocardial infarction*—60 mg by injection, followed by a continuous 0.1% infusion. CHILDREN: 0.4 mg/kg as a single dose, IV slowly. Repeat as necessary or use a slow infusion of a 0.1% solution.						must be after balancing benefits to the mother against risks to the fetus. PRECAUTIONS 1. Can be used to maintain blood pressure in hemorrhagic shock while volume and blood replacement are in progress. 2. Rapid infusion can cause severe hypertension and acute cardiac decompensation. 3. When vasopressor drugs are used for long periods, the resulting vasoconstriction may prevent adequate expansion of circulating volume and may cause perpetuation of the shock state. 4. Use with caution in patients with cardiac disease, thyroid disease, hypertension or diabetes. There may be excessive reaction to the drug. 5. May cause relapse of malaria. ADVERSE REACTIONS Reactions are usually minimal, and result from CNS stimulation: 1. Anxiety 2. Hypertension (usually caused by overdosage). There may also be cardiac arrythmias such as PVC's, ventricular tachycardia and fibrillation.

NURSING IMPLICATIONS
1. The following parameters must be available for the monitoring of the effectiveness of this drug: central venous pressure, or pulmonary artery pressure; intra-arterial or indirect blood pressure, urine output. Values to strive for in the titration of this drug must be set by the physician. Monitor parameters every 3–5 minutes until desired levels are reached, and then every 15–30 minutes after stabilization.

2. Use an infusion pump to maintain an accurate infusion rate and to prevent overdosage.
3. Patients with active cardiac arrhythmias, or a past history of them, should be observed on a continuous ECG monitor. Be prepared to treat ventricular irritability, e.g., premature ventricular contractions or ventricular tachycardia. Keep lidocaine 100 mg readily available.
4. Prevent extravasation; see page 96.

METARAMINOL BITARTRATE (Aramine)

ACTIONS/ INDICATIONS	DOSAGE	PREPARATION AND STORAGE	DRUG INCOMPAT- IBILITIES	MODES OF IV ADMINISTRATION			CONTRAINDICATIONS; WARNINGS; PRECAUTIONS; ADVERSE REACTIONS
				INJECTION	INTERMITTENT INFUSION	CONTINUOUS INFUSION	
Potent sympathomimetic	ADULTS: *Initial*—When	To prepare solution add 100	Do not add other drugs to	YES	YES	YES	CONTRAINDICATIONS 1. Do not use with halothane or cyclo-

agent; increases systolic and diastolic blood pressure by its positive inotropic effect on the heart and by its peripheral vasoconstrictor action. Effects begin 1–2 minutes after intravenous injection and last 20 minutes.

a rapid response is needed, 0.5–5.0 mg by injection

Indicated primarily for prevention and treatment of conditions where there are changes in vasomotor tone.

Acute hypotensive states associated with spinal anesthesia, adjunctive treatment of hypotension due to hemorrhage, reactions to drugs, surgical complications, and shock secondary to brain damage due to tumor or trauma.

May also be effective as an adjunct in the treatment of hypotension due to cardiogenic shock or septicemia.

mg of drug to 500 ml D5W or NS.* This produces a solution of 0.2 mg/ml. Modifications in this solution can be made for patients needing more or less fluid.

Maintenance —0.2–0.6 mg/min infusion using an 0.2 mg/ml solution at a rate of 1–3 ml/min. Titrate with blood pressure, CVP, pulmonary artery pressure and urine flow. Allow at least 10 min to pass between changes in infusion rate.

CHILDREN:
Initial— 10 mcg/kg (300 mcg/M²)

Maintenance —0.2–0.6 mg/min infusion using an 0.2 mg/ml solution at 1–3 ml/min. Titrate with blood pressure, CVP, pulmonary artery pressure and urine flow.

IV bottle. Do not mix in IV tubing with:
Penicillin
Erythromycin
Nafcillin
Methicillin
Amphotericin B
Dexamethasone
Fibrinogen
Hydrocortisone
Prednisolone
Thiopental
Warfarin

USE INFUSION PUMP, FLOW CONTROL DEVICE, OR AT LEAST MICRODROP IV TUBING.

*Ringer's injection, lactated Ringer's, Dextran 6% in saline, Normosol-R and Normosol-M in D5W can also be used as infusion fluids.

Titrate with blood pressure, CVP and/or pulmonary artery pressure, and urinary output.

See Preparation column for preparation of solution.

Titrate with blood pressure, CVP and/or pulmonary artery pressure, and urinary output.

See Preparation column for preparation of solution.

Inject over at least 1–2 min undiluted.

propane anesthetics unless the patient's condition demands its use. Concomitant use may cause cardiac arrhythmias.
2. Hypersensitivity.

PRECAUTIONS
1. This drug can cause significant vasoconstriction which may decrease blood flow to vital organs if regional vascular resistance increases above perfusion pressure. This can be evidenced by fall in urine output. If this occurs another agent may be added to the regimen or metaraminol discontinued and another agent such as dopamine or isoproterenol substituted.
2. Titrate carefully to prevent hypertension. Excessive rise in blood pressure can precipitate pulmonary edema, angina pectoris, arrhythmias and cardiac arrest.
3. Concomitant use in digitalized patients may cause arrhythmias such as premature arterial and ventricular contractions. Titrate carefully.
4. Administer with caution to patients with cirrhosis; these patients may require lower dosage. Electrolyte imbalances secondary to the liver dysfunction should be corrected to prevent arrhythmias.
5. Rapid infusion can cause myocardial irritability and resultant arrhythmias. Reduction in drip rate usually remedies the situation.
6. Hypoxia and acidosis must be corrected during use with this drug to prevent arrhythmias.
7. Allow at least 10 minutes to pass between changes in drip rate, because the maximum effect of an increase or decrease in drip rate is apparent only after 8–10 minutes.
8. Because of the prolonged action of this drug, a cumulative effect can be seen. With an excessive vasopressor response there may be a prolonged elevation in blood pressure even after the infusion has been stopped.
9. MAO inhibitors potentiate the actions of metaraminol.
10. Prolonged use may result in vasoconstriction that prevents adequate expansion of circulating plasma volume. This can perpetuate the shock syndrome and requires the use of volume expanders as guided by cen-

METARAMINOL BITARTRATE (Aramine) (Continued)

ACTIONS/ INDICATIONS	DOSAGE	PREPARATION AND STORAGE	DRUG INCOMPAT- IBILITIES	MODES OF IV ADMINISTRATION			CONTRAINDICATIONS; WARNINGS; PRECAUTIONS; ADVERSE REACTIONS
				INJECTION	INTERMITTENT INFUSION	CONTINUOUS INFUSION	

CONTRAINDICATIONS; WARNINGS; PRECAUTIONS; ADVERSE REACTIONS

tral venous pressure or pulmonary artery pressure.

11. Because the vasoconstriction produced, administer with caution to patients with congestive heart failure, coronary artery disease, hyperthyroidism, hypertension, diabetes mellitus or peripheral vascular disease.

12. Avoid extravasation since tissue necrosis or sloughing may occur. Avoid use of lower extremities, scalp veins or small hand veins for infusion. If infiltration occurs, discontinue infusion immediately and apply warm compresses to the affected area or subcutaneously inject phentolamine (Regitine) 5–10 mg in saline.
5–10 ml using a 25 gauge needle.

13. This drug may cause a relapse of malaria.

ADVERSE REACTIONS
1. Cardiac: may cause myocardial irritability and resultant tachyarrhythmias such as premature atrial and ventricular contractions, ventricular tachycardia or rarely ventricular fibrillation. This may occur more frequently in the presence of an acute myocardial infarction, coronary artery disease, hypoxia and acidosis (metabolic or respiratory).

2. Hypertension secondary to excessive dosage or idiosyncratic response.

3. Oliguria secondary to decreased renal perfusion.

NURSING IMPLICATIONS
1. Adequate parameters must be available for monitoring to guide titration of this drug. At a minimum, heart rate, central venous pressure, indirect blood pressure (by sphygmomanometer) and urine output must be checked. If possible, it is advisable to use direct arterial blood pressure and pulmonary artery pressure readings instead of indirect blood pressure and central venous pressure readings. Because of this drug's vasoconstrictive actions, the indirectly obtained blood pressure may be significantly different from the more accurate intra-arterial blood pressure. The values of these parameters to strive for when titrating the drug must be determined by the physician.

2. Heart rate and blood pressure (direct or indirect) must be recorded prior to and every 2–3 minutes during the initial phases of titration. When the blood pressure stabilizes for at least 1 hour near or at the desired, preset

6. Use an infusion pump if available. If the device has an infiltration system, use it.

7. Prevent extravasation; see page 96 for guidelines. Check infusion site frequently for blood return and free flow of fluid. Observe for blanching of the skin along the course of the vein; if this occurs, change the infusion site (see Precaution No. 12). Protect affected area from trauma.

8. Observe for signs and symptoms of overdosage (too rapid an infusion rate): headache, tachycardia, premature ventricular contractions, diaphoresis, pallor (if not already present), chest pain, hypertension.
If one or more of these appear, decrease the infusion rate and notify the physician.

9. Patients requiring therapy with this drug frequently require respiratory support. Monitor respiratory rate, effort and blood gases with other parame-

value, frequency of monitoring can be reduced to every 15–30 minutes, or as indicated by the patient's general condition.

3. Central venous pressure or pulmonary artery pressure should be recorded prior to and every 30 minutes during titration. A continuous oscilloscopic display of arterial and pulmonary arterial pressures is ideal in this situation.

4. The patient should be observed for arrhythmias via continuous ECG monitoring.

5. Urine output should be recorded hourly during the initial phase of therapy with this drug for shock. Urine flow reflects indirectly the perfusion of the kidneys. A fall in urine output may indicate the need for a change in drug therapy, either a reduction in metaraminol drip rate, or its discontinuation and the initiation of another agent. Notify the physician if urine output falls below 30 ml/hour for 2 consecutive hours in an adult patient (see chart on page 546 for normal urine output in children).

ters. Be prepared to initiate manual ventilation.

SUGGESTED READINGS

Amsterdam, Ezra A. et al.: Evaluation and Management of Cardiogenic Shock. Part I. Approach to the Patient. *Heart and Lung.* 1(3):402–408, May–June 1972 (references).

_____: Evaluation and Management of Cardiogenic Shock. Part II. Drug Therapy. *Heart and Lung,* 1(5):663–671, September–October 1972 (references).

Tarazi, Robert C.: Sympathomimetic Agents in the Treatment of Shock. *Annals of Internal Medicine,* 81:364–371, September 1974 (references).

Woods, Susan L.: Monitoring Pulmonary Artery Pressures. *American Journal of Nursing,* 76:1765–1771, November 1976 (references).

● METHANTHELINE BROMIDE (Banthine)

ACTIONS/ INDICATIONS	DOSAGE	PREPARATION AND STORAGE	DRUG INCOMPAT- IBILITIES	MODES OF IV ADMINISTRATION			CONTRAINDICATIONS; WARNINGS; PRECAUTIONS; ADVERSE REACTIONS
				INJECTION	INTERMITTENT INFUSION	CONTINUOUS INFUSION	
Synthetic anti-cholinergic agent with atropinelike actions that slow gastroin-testinal propul-sion and de-crease gastric acid secretion. Used in the parenteral form as a pre-anesthetic dry-ing agent.	ADULTS: 25–50 mg can be repeat-ed in 6 hours. CHILDREN: Intravenous administration not recom-mended.[1]	Supplied in vials of 50 mg; discard unused portions.	Do not mix with any other drug in any manner.	YES Dilute in 10 ml NS; administer each 50 mg or less over at least 1 min.	NO	NO	CONTRAINDICATIONS 1. Glaucoma 2. Any obstructive disease of the gastro-intestinal tract 3. Obstructive uropathy 4. Intestinal atony in the elderly or debil-itated 5. Megacolon 6. Hiatal hernia associated with reflex esophagitis 7. Unstable cardiac status in acute hemorrhage WARNINGS 1. Use with caution in cardiac disease; this drug can cause tachycardia. 2. There may be anhidrosis (cessation of sweating) for 6 hours after injection. 3. Overdosage causes loss of control of voluntary muscles, particularly respi-ratory muscles. PRECAUTIONS 1. Have patient void prior to injection to avoid urinary retention. 2. This drug is potentiated by synthetic narcotic analgesics, tricyclic antide-pressants (Elavil, etc.), antihistamines, MAO inhibitors, nitrates, and pheno-thiazines. Patients receiving these drugs will require a lower dosage of methantheline.

METHANTHELINE BROMIDE (Banthine) (Continued)

ACTIONS/ INDICATIONS	DOSAGE	PREPARATION AND STORAGE	DRUG INCOMPAT- IBILITIES	MODES OF IV ADMINISTRATION			CONTRAINDICATIONS; WARNINGS; PRECAUTIONS; ADVERSE REACTIONS
				INJECTION	INTERMITTENT INFUSION	CONTINUOUS INFUSION	
							ADVERSE REACTIONS 1. Dry mouth 2. Blurred vision 3. Respiratory paralysis 4. Tachycardia 5. Hypotension 6. Constipation 7. Urinary retention In the event of respiratory paralysis, provide ventilatory support as needed, and administer neostigmine methylsulfate. See page 418.

NURSING IMPLICATIONS

1. Monitor carefully for respiratory paralysis. Keep respiratory support equipment readily available: oxygen, airways, endotracheal tubes and laryngoscope, suction, manual breathing bag. Begin to assist ventilation if the respiratory rate falls below 8–10 per minute or if the patient is exhibiting increasing respiratory effort. Keep neostigmine readily available.
2. Ambulate with caution; there may be postural hypotension and dizziness.
3. Monitor for urinary retention, especially in the elderly male, with or without

a history of prostatic disease. Have patient void prior to injection. After the injection, palpate bladder size every 2–4 hours for the next 8 hours.
4. Monitor pulse rate and blood pressure after each injection. Notify the physician of the onset of tachycardia or hypotension.

REFERENCE
1. Shirkey, Harry C.: *Pediatric Drug Handbook*, Philadelphia: W. B. Saunders Company, 1977, p. 138.

METHAPYRILENE HYDROCHLORIDE (Histadyl)

ACTIONS/ INDICATIONS	DOSAGE	PREPARATION AND STORAGE	DRUG INCOMPAT- IBILITIES	MODES OF IV ADMINISTRATION			CONTRAINDICATIONS; WARNINGS; PRECAUTIONS; ADVERSE REACTIONS
				INJECTION	INTERMITTENT INFUSION	CONTINUOUS INFUSION	
Antihistamine used to treat: • Allergic reaction to blood or plasma • Anaphylaxis, as an adjunct to epinephrine • Other uncomplicated allergic conditions when oral therapy is impossible or contraindicated.	Adjust to the response of the patient. ADULTS: 10–20 mg may increase to 40 mg if necessary. Best given by infusion. CHILDREN: 0.3–0.6 mg/kg.	Supplied in 10-ml vials, 20 mg/ml.	Do not mix with any other medication in any manner.	YES Slowly over 1 min. May be given undiluted.	YES Add dose to 250 ml NS and infuse over 30 min.	YES If continued therapy is needed, use NS, add dose to 250–500 ml and titrate drip rate with patient response.	CONTRAINDICATIONS 1. Newborn and premature infants 2. Nursing mothers 3. Lower respiratory tract disease; do not use to treat symptoms, including asthma 4. Hypersensitivity to this or similar antihistamines 5. In patients on MAO inhibitors 6. Glaucoma 7. Stenosing peptic ulcer or any gastrointestinal obstruction 8. Prostatic hypertrophy 9. Bladder neck obstruction WARNINGS 1. Overdosage in children causes hallucinations, convulsions and death.

Excitation may also be produced even at normal dosage.
2. Safety for use in pregnancy has not been established.
3. This drug may add to the depressant effects of alcohol and any other central nervous system depressant.

PRECAUTIONS

Use with caution when there is a history of bronchial asthma, increased intraocular pressure, hyperthyroidism, cardiac or renal disease, hypertension, diabetes. This drug can cause exacerbation of these conditions or complications.

ADVERSE REACTIONS

1. Most frequent: sedation, dry mouth, thickening of bronchial secretions, dizziness, disturbed coordination.
2. Less frequent: fatigue, confusion, restlessness, excitation, nervousness, nausea, vomiting, diarrhea, constipation, urinary retention, rashes, tachycardia, diplopia, tightness in the chest.

MANAGEMENT OF OVERDOSAGE

Reactions range from CNS depression in adults to excitation in children. There may also be fixed, dilated pupils, flushing and hypotension. Do not use stimulants. Discontinue administration. Levarterenol can be used for hypotension, 1 ml in 250 ml NS administered as a drip, titrated with blood pressure.

5. In patients with pulmonary disease, monitor respirations and the management by the patient of bronchial secretions. These secretions will thicken; increased frequency of suctioning may be required. Use humidity to keep secretions fluid. Auscultate the lungs for effectiveness of suctioning and coughing at least every 2 hours during therapy. Turn hourly. Monitor temperature.
6. Monitor for urinary retention.
7. Be prepared to manage vomiting. Have suction available.
8. Monitor pulse and blood pressure every 30–60 minutes, as indicated.

NURSING IMPLICATIONS

1. Monitor for excitation in children; take safety precautions to prevent injury.
2. Monitor for oversedation in patients concomitantly on other CNS depressants.
3. Carefully observe patients with bronchial asthma, increased intraocular pressure, hyperthyroidism, cardiac disease, renal disease, hypertension, diabetes for exacerbation of these conditions or complications such as cardiac arrhythmias in cardiac patients.
4. Monitor effectiveness of the drug and be prepared to render additional support to patients with anaphylaxis; see page 118.

METHICILLIN SODIUM (Staphcillin, Celbenin)

ACTIONS/INDICATIONS	DOSAGE	PREPARATION AND STORAGE	DRUG INCOMPATIBILITIES	MODES OF IV ADMINISTRATION			CONTRAINDICATIONS; WARNINGS; PRECAUTIONS; ADVERSE REACTIONS
				INJECTION	INTERMITTENT INFUSION	CONTINUOUS INFUSION	
Antibiotic, penicillinase-resistant. Synthetic penicillin. Used to treat infections due to penicillinase-producing staphylococci. Susceptibility tests must be performed.	ADULTS: 1 gm. every 6 hrs. Higher doses are used in severe infections. OLDER CHILDREN: 100–400 mg/kg/24 hrs in divided doses every 4–6 hrs.	Reconstitute powder with sterile water for injection or sodium chloride injection: 1-gm vial—add 1.5 ml 4-gm vial—add 5.7 ml 6-gm vial—add 8.6 ml The concentration of each preparation is 500 mg/ml.	Do not mix with any other medication in any manner.	YES Further dilute reconstituted form with 25 ml NS, inject at a rate of 10 ml/min.	YES Further dilute the reconstituted form with the following amounts of sterile water or compatible IV fluid (see Preparation column):	YES Add a 6- or 12-hr dose to 500–1,000 ml of the fluids listed in Preparation column. Infuse over the appropriate amount of time.	CONTRAINDICATIONS Hypersensitivity to any penicillin. WARNINGS There may be cross-allergenicity with cephalosporins. PRECAUTIONS 1. Use with caution in patients with allergies. 2. Monitor renal, hepatic, and hematopoietic systems during therapy. This drug rarely precipitates renal impairment in infants and adults.[2] The incidence is only slightly higher in children.[3]
Also effective in treating infection due to susceptible *Strep. pneumoniae*, Group A beta-hemolytic streptococci and penicillin G-resistant and penicillin G-sensitive staphylococci.	NEONATES:[1] *0–14 days of age, 2,000 gm or less in weight*—50 mg/kg/24 hrs in equally divided doses every 12 hrs.	Shake vial vigorously. Discard unused solution after 24 hours if stored at room temperature, or 4 days if stored in refrigerator.			DOSE / VOL. OF ADDED DILUENT: 1 gm — 50 ml 4 gm — 65 ml 6 gm — 97 ml Infuse over 30–60 min.		3. There is a possibility of overgrowth of non-susceptible organisms. 4. Safety for use during pregnancy has not been established. 5. Lower dosage and close blood level monitoring is necessary in premature or immature infants and patients with renal failure.
	0–14 days of age, over 2,000 gm in weight—75 mg/kg/24 hrs in equally divided doses every 8 hrs.	Use the following fluids for infusion of methicillin: NS D5W D5/NS 10% D-fructose in water 10% D-fructose in NS M/6 Sodium r-lactate Lactated Ringer's					ADVERSE REACTIONS 1. Hypersensitivity: rash, urticaria, anaphylaxis, serum sickness 2. Oral lesions: glossitis and stomatitis (rare) 3. Blood dyscrasias: hemolytic anemia, thrombocytopenia, leukopenia, agranulocytosis (usually only seen in high-dose, prolonged therapy)
	15–30 days of age, 2,000 gm or less in weight—75 mg/kg/24 hrs in equally divided doses every 8 hrs.	Lactated potassic saline 5% Plasma hydrolysate in water 10% Invert sugar in water 10% Invert sugar plus 0.3%					4. Signs of renal impairment: hematuria, casts, azotemia, oliguria, pyuria. These disappear with discontinuation of the drug 5. Overgrowth infection secondary to organisms not susceptible to methicillin
	15–30 days of age, over 2,000 gm in weight—100 mg/kg/24 hrs in equally divided doses every 6 hrs.						

Therapy should be continued for at least 48 hrs after the patient has become afebrile and asymptomatic and cultures are negative.	potassium chloride in water Travert 10% electrolyte #1, #2, #3 Solutions of 2 mg/ml, 10 mg/ml and 20 mg/ml of this drug in the above fluids are stable for 8 hours. Drug concentration and rate and volume of the solution used should be adjusted so that the total dose is administered before the drug loses its stability.

NURSING IMPLICATIONS

1. Take anaphylaxis precautions; see page 118.
2. Monitor for signs and symptoms of overgrowth infections:
   a. Fever (take rectal temperature at least every 4–6 hours in all patients)
   b. Increasing malaise
   c. Newly appearing localized signs and symptoms; redness, soreness, pain, swelling, drainage (increased volume or change in character of pre-existing drainage)
   d. Monilial rash in perineal area (reddened areas with itching)
   e. Cough (change in pre-existing cough or sputum production)
   f. Diarrhea
3. Complete blood counts should be performed during therapy. Patients on prolonged high-dose therapy may experience decreasing white cell and platelet counts. If this occurs, usually the drug is discontinued. Infections secondary to low white-cell counts usually occur only after the count reaches 2,000/cu mm or less. If this occurs, place the patient in protective (reversed) isolation, avoid traumatic procedures, and monitor for signs and symptoms of infection. Bleeding secondary to a low platelet count usually begins only after the count falls below 100,000/cu mm. If the count reaches this level, monitor for unusual bleeding and avoid traumatic procedures.
4. Monitor for signs of renal impairment (occurrence is rare):
   a. Be aware of the patient's BUN and serum creatinine.
   b. Send urine for analysis at least weekly while the patient is on intensive intravenous therapy (see Adverse Reaction No. 4).
   c. Notify the physician of the onset of hematuria.
   d. Monitor for oliguria, urine output less than 240 ml per 8-hour period. (See chart on page 546 for normal urine output in children.)
5. If stomatitis occurs, notify the physician and begin therapeutic oral care:[4]
   a. *Mild Inflammation:* Remove dentures; use a soft toothbrush and a hydrogen peroxide solution (1 part peroxide and 4 parts saline). Do *not* use toothpaste. Rinse with the peroxide solution and then water. Replace dentures. This procedure should be carried out every 4 hours and/or after meals.
   b. *Severe Inflammation:* Remove dentures. Use soft gauze pads rather than a toothbrush. Use the peroxide solution as described above. Rinse with water using an asepto syringe and gentle suction until returns are clear. Do not replace dentures. It may be necessary to give this care every 2–4 hours.
   c. Order a bland, mechanical, soft diet for patients with mild inflammation. If stomatitis is severe, the patient may be placed on NPO status by the physician.
   d. For patients who can tolerate oral intake, administer Xylocaine Viscous or acetaminophen elixir as a mouthwash prior to meals to decrease pain (do not use aspirin rinses) as ordered by the physician.
   e. Patients with severe stomatitis may require parenteral analgesia.

REFERENCES
1. McCracken, George H.: *Antimicrobial Therapy for Newborns,* New York: Grune and Stratton, 1977, p. 23.
2. Appel, Gerald, and Neu, Harold C.: The Nephrotoxicity of Antimicrobial Agents. *New England Journal of Medicine,* 296(12):644, March 24, 1977.
3. McCracken, p. 23.
4. Bruya, Margaret Auld, and Maderia, Nancy Powell: Stomatitis After Chemotherapy. *American Journal of Nursing,* 75(8):1351, August 1975.

METHOCARBAMOL (Robaxin Injectable)

ACTIONS/ INDICATIONS	DOSAGE	PREPARATION AND STORAGE	DRUG INCOMPATIBILITIES	MODES OF IV ADMINISTRATION			CONTRAINDICATIONS; WARNINGS; PRECAUTIONS; ADVERSE REACTIONS
				INJECTION	INTERMITTENT INFUSION	CONTINUOUS INFUSION	
Skeletal muscle relaxant, centrally acting. Produces general central nervous system depression. Used in addition to rest, physical therapy and other measures to treat acute, painful musculoskeletal problems, such as severe muscle strain, tetanus, strychnine poisoning, black widow spider bite, lead poisoning, opiate withdrawal. Mechanism of action is unknown.	Dosage and frequency should be based on the severity of the condition and the patient's response. Total *adult* dose should not exceed 3 gm/day for more than 3 days (except in tetanus). TETANUS: (In addition to usual supportive care) *Adults—* 1–2 gm injected as a bolus, followed by 1–2 gm via infusion. This is repeated every 6 hrs until an nasogastric tube can be inserted; then oral form can be given via tube. *Children—* minimum initial dose: 15 mg/kg repeated every 6 hrs via infusion, for tetanus; otherwise not recommended for children. OTHER CONDITIONS: Dosage and frequency must be based on the severity	Supplied in 10-ml ampuls, 100 mg/ml. Discard unused portions of vials. Use *only* NS or D5W for infusion fluid.	Do not mix with any other medication in any manner.	YES At a maximum rate of 3 ml/min. Inject into tubing of a running IV	YES Use NS or D5W. 1 gm of drug in 250 ml fluid. Infuse over 1–2 hours.	NO	CONTRAINDICATIONS 1. Renal disease (drug contains polyethylene glycol 300) 2. Hypersensitivity WARNINGS Safety for use in pregnancy has not been established. PRECAUTIONS 1. Avoid extravasation. 2. Keep patient recumbent during injection, and 10–15 minutes after, to reduce likelihood of adverse reactions. 3. Observe seizure precautions in known epileptic patients. 4. Not for use in children under 12 years of age except in the treatment of tetanus. 5. Drug may be secreted in milk; nursing should be stopped during therapy. ADVERSE REACTIONS 1. Dizziness, syncope, hypotension 2. Gastrointestinal: nausea, vomiting and diarrhea 3. At sight of injection: pain, thrombophlebitis, sloughing (with extravasation) 4. Hypersensitivity: ranging from urticaria to anaphylaxis 5. Visual changes, headache 6. Many of the above can be avoided with slow injection and recumbency during injection

of the condition and the response seen from initial doses.

Usual dose— 1–3 gm every 6 hrs.

NURSING IMPLICATIONS
1. Avoid extravasation; see page 96.
2. Keep patient recumbent during the injection and for 10–15 minutes after, depending on his condition. Then ambulate with caution.
3. Monitor for adverse affects; be prepared to manage anaphylaxis (see page 118).
4. Be prepared to manage vomiting to prevent aspiration.

● METHOHEXITAL SODIUM (Brevital Sodium)

ACTIONS/ INDICATIONS	DOSAGE	PREPARATION AND STORAGE	DRUG INCOMPAT- IBILITIES	MODES OF IV ADMINISTRATION			CONTRAINDICATIONS; WARNINGS; PRECAUTIONS; ADVERSE REACTIONS
				INJECTION	INTERMITTENT INFUSION	CONTINUOUS INFUSION	
Barbiturate anesthetic, rapid, ultra-short-acting. Used for induction of anesthesia for short procedures or for inducing a hypnotic state.	Individualize according to patient response. *Continuous drip anesthesia*—0.2% solution at 1 gt/second titrated with patient response. *Induction and intermittent injection*—1.0% solution, 5–12 ml (50–120 mg), effects will last 5–7 min. Maintain with 2–4 ml (20–40 mg) every 4–7 min, according to patient response.	To prepare from powder: Follow dilution instructions *exactly.* Do *not* use diluents containing bacteriostats. Sterile water for injection is the preferred diluent. Use *only* D5W or NS for infusion. *Preparation* *1% solution (10 mg/ml):* Amp #660 (500 mg)—add 50 ml diluent Amp #760 (500 mg)—add 50 ml of accompanying diluent Amp #664 (2.5 gm)—add 250 ml diluent	Do not mix with atropine, metocurine iodide, succinylcholine, scopolamine, or barbiturates.	YES A 1% solution at a rate of 1 ml in 5 seconds. (See Preparation column.)	YES Using a 0.2% solution at a rate individualized according to patient response.	YES Using a 0.2% solution at a rate individualized according to patient response.	CONTRAINDICATIONS 1. When general anesthesia is contraindicated 2. Latent or manifest porphyria 3. Known hypersensitivity to barbiturates WARNINGS 1. May be habit-forming. 2. Continuous infusion or repeated injections may cause cumulative effects, resulting in prolonged somnolence and respiratory-circulatory depression. 3. Safety for use in pregnancy has not been established. PRECAUTIONS 1. Respiratory depression, apnea or hypotension can occur even at normal doses. 2. Administer with caution to debilitated patients or those with renal, respiratory, circulatory, hepatic or endocrine impairment. 3. Use with *extreme* caution in patients with status asthmaticus. 4. Extravasation will cause pain, swelling, ulceration, and necrosis. DO NOT INJECT INTRA-ARTERIALLY; will cause gangrene of the extremity. 5. This drug's depressant effects will be additive to other central nervous system depressants.

METHOHEXITAL SODIUM (Brevital Sodium) (Continued)

ACTIONS/ INDICATIONS	DOSAGE	PREPARATION AND STORAGE	DRUG INCOMPAT- IBILITIES	MODES OF IV ADMINISTRATION			CONTRAINDICATIONS; WARNINGS; PRECAUTIONS; ADVERSE REACTIONS
				INJECTION	INTERMITTENT INFUSION	CONTINUOUS INFUSION	
		Amp #662 (5 gm)—add 500 ml diluent					ADVERSE REACTIONS 1. Circulatory depression 2. Thrombophlebitis and pain at injec- tion site 3. Respiratory depression and apnea 4. Laryngospasm and bronchospasm 5. Hiccups 6. Skeletal muscle hyperactivity 7. Emergence delirium 8. Headache, nausea, vomiting 9. Hypersensitivity ranging from rash to anaphylaxis
		Amp #663 (2.5 gm)—add 15 ml diluent and add to 250 ml for in- fusion					
		Amp #659 (5 gm)—add 30 ml diluent and add to 500 ml for in- fusion.					
		Amps #663 and 659 (first solution after addition of 30 ml may be light yellow; should be clear after adding to 250 ml).					
		To make a 0.2% solution for drip: Use amps #660 or #760 and add to 250 ml D5W or NS after ini- tial 50 ml dilu- tion.					
		After dilution with first small volume diluent this drug can be stored at room tempera- ture for 6 weeks. Large volume solution for infusion must be discarded after 24 hours. Dis- card any solu-					

tion if discolored.

This is a Schedule IV drug under the Controlled Substances Act of 1970. Maintain hospital or institutional regulations guiding the use of this drug.

NURSING IMPLICATIONS

1. Equipment necessary for respiratory support must be readily available, e.g., manual breathing bag, airways, suction, oxygen. Monitor respiratory rate continuously during anesthesia. See Nos. 6 and 7 below.
2. This drug is usually administered only by or under the direct supervision of an anesthesiologist. Follow hospital regulation.
3. Strictly adhere to maximum injection and infusion rate suggestions and maximum limits. Use an infusion pump to assist with rate control, to insure maximum benefit from the drug and to prevent overdosage. Patients with liver impairment should receive smaller doses and should be monitored more closely and for a longer period of time than usual.
4. Patients with porphyria are sensitive to barbiturates in that they may experience an acute attack of the disease secondary to the administration of a barbiturate (see Contraindications). The onset of an acute attack is indicated by severe colicky abdominal pain radiating to the back. There is usually severe vomiting, fever and leukocytosis in addition.[1]
5. Avoid extravasation; see page 96. Extravascular or intra-arterial injection of this drug can cause tissue necrosis and gangrene of the affected extremity, respectively. Thrombophlebitis can also occur during the course of an infusion. Examine for redness and pain along the nerve tract, and discontinue the infusion if signs and symptoms appear and notify the physician.
6. Take anaphylaxis precautions; see page 118.
7. Monitor for symptoms of acute overdosage (listed in order of progression):
   a. Respiratory depression, i.e., decreased respiratory rate and depth
   b. Peripheral vascular collapse, i.e., fall in blood pressure, pallor, diaphoresis, tachycardia
   c. Pulmonary edema (rare)
   d. Decreased or absent reflexes, pupillary constriction
   e. Stupor beyond anesthetic level, that does not resolve in expected 5–10 minutes.
   f. Coma
   Stop the injection or infusion immediately upon noting one of these symptoms. Notify the physician. Discontinuation of the infusion is usually all that is necessary to prevent further problems. If not, see item No. 8 below.
8. Management of acute overdosage:
   a. Continue to stay with the patient, and monitor vital signs
   b. Maintain an open airway and adequate ventilation
   c. Keep the patient as alert as possible by verbal and physical stimuli. Encourage the patient to breathe at an adequate rate (12–14 breaths/minute for an adult). If necessary, initiate artificial ventilation with a manual breathing bag (Puritan, Hope, Ambu, etc.) at a rate of 12–14 breaths/minute.
   d. Circulatory support in the form of fluids and drugs may be ordered.
9. The sedation produced by this drug may be preceded by transient changes in mental status, such as feelings of euphoria, and confusion. If this occurs, attempt to calm the patient and take measures to prevent injury until the patient returns to his normal status.
10. Postanesthesia Care:
    a. Monitor respiratory rate continuously until an adequate rate has been reached and stabilized.
    b. Maintain a patent airway with an endotracheal tube, followed by oral-pharyngeal airway until swallow, cough and gag reflexes and an adequate respiratory rate have returned.
    c. Respiratory support equipment must be readily available: oxygen, airways, endotracheal tube and laryngoscope, suction, manual breathing bag.
    d. The patient must be under constant observation until vital signs have stabilized, the patient is alert and there is full return of swallow, cough and gag reflexes.
    e. Monitor heart rate and blood pressure at a schedule dictated by recovery room policy (usually every 15 minutes for an uncomplicated patient). Be prepared to treat hypotension (pressor agents and fluids are usually prescribed).
    f. Be prepared to manage emergence delirium. Prevent injury, use side rails continuously, and restrain if indicated.
    g. Take precautions to prevent aspiration.
    h. An anesthesiologist usually decides when the patient can be discharged from the recovery room.

REFERENCE
1. Beeson, Paul B., and McDermott, Walsh (editors): Cecil-Loeb Textbook of Medicine (14th ed.). Philadelphia: W. B. Saunders Company, 1977, p. 1873.

● METHOTREXATE SODIUM (A.M.E., Amethopterin)

ACTIONS/ INDICATIONS	DOSAGE	PREPARATION AND STORAGE	DRUG INCOMPAT- IBILITIES	MODES OF IV ADMINISTRATION			CONTRAINDICATIONS; WARNINGS; PRECAUTIONS; ADVERSE REACTIONS
				INJECTION	INTERMITTENT INFUSION	CONTINUOUS INFUSION	
Antimetabo- lite. Used for antineoplastic chemotherapy in the follow- ing malignan- cies:	IV route is recommended for the follow- ing conditions and at the fol- lowing doses:	Use *only* sterile water for injec- tion for prepa- ration from powder:	Do not mix with any other medication.	YES	YES	YES	CONTRAINDICATIONS 1. Pregnancy 2. In psoriatic patients with severe renal, hepatic or bone marrow disorders, or pregnancy.
• Choriocar- cinoma	*Acute leuke- mia in chil-*	5-mg vial, add 2 ml.		Inject into the Y injection site of a running IV. Further di- lute reconsti-	Use 50–100 ml D5W or NS, and infuse over 30–60	Use 1000 ml D5W or NS for high-dose ther- apy. Infuse as	WARNINGS 1. This drug has many toxic side effects. Patients who are receiving the drug intravenously must be hospitalized.
• Chorioaden- oma destru- ens	*dren*— 3.3/M² daily to induce remission. To	50-mg vial, add 20 ml.		tuted solution with 2 cc ster- ile water for in- jection for ev-	min.	directed by the physician.	2. Patients and/or significant others must be informed of the severe and potentially fatal toxic reactions.
• Hydatidiform mole	maintain re- mission, 2.5 mg/kg every	The resultant solution con-		ery 5 mg of drug. Inject at a rate of 10			3. Use in psoriasis must be limited to se- vere, disabling forms, refractory to other drug therapy. Deaths have been
• Acute lym- phocytic and meningeal leukemia	14 days (usual- ly given with prednisone)	tains 2.5 mg/ ml.		mg/min. Rapid injection can cause syncope. Flush vein with			reported with the use of this drug for psoriasis. 4. Monitor renal, hepatic and hematolog-
• Acute lym- phoblastic leukemia	*Psoriasis*— 10 –25 mg/week until response	Avoid contact of drug with skin. Flush with water for 10		15–20 ml ster- ile water for in- jection.			ic systems before and frequently dur- ing therapy. 5. Administer with extreme caution in
• Lymphosar- coma	is seen; then begin oral dos-	minutes if it oc- curs.		Do not use leg veins if at all			the presence of hepatic dysfunction. Concomitant use of other drugs that cause liver damage, including alcohol,
• Mycosis fun- goides	age.			possible.			must be avoided. 6. Fetal death has occurred in pregnant
• Breast can- cer	In all condi- tions dosage must be indi-						women receiving this agent. 7. High-dose regimens should not be initi- ated without providing for folinic acid
• Severe pso- riasis	vidualized.						(leukovorin) rescue. See Dosage col- umn. This is a manufacturer's sugges-
• Epidermoid cancer of the head and neck	*High-dose ther- apy*— 20–300 mg/kg every 2–3 weeks.						tion. High-dose regimens are investi- gational and hazardous.
• Some groups also use high- dose therapy for osteo- genic sarco- ma.	Leukovorin cal- cium (folinic acid, citrovo- rum factor) can then be administered 2–12 hrs lat-						PRECAUTIONS 1. Use with caution in the presence of infections and pre-existing bone mar- row depression. 2. Concomitant use with other marrow- depressing drugs should be avoided.
• Lung cancer, especially squamous cell and small cell types.	er. Dose is 6– 16 mg/M² giv- en IM or orally, repeated every 6 hrs for 72 hours. (Leuko- vorin is thought to pro- tect normal cells from damage from						3. Discontinue with first signs of oral er- ythema, ulceration, bleeding from any point, chills and fever, hematologic depression. 4. Tests to perform before, during and after therapy: complete hemogram, hematocrit, urinalysis, hepatic and re- nal function, chest x-ray. 5. Do not administer the following drugs concomitantly with methotrexate: sul- fonamides (antibacterial, hypoglyce- mic or diuretic); salicylates.

the methotrex-
ate. This pro-
cedure is cur-
rently consid-
ered to be ex-
perimental).[1,2]

6. Use with extreme caution in the presence of infection, peptic ulcer, ulcerative colitis, debility, extremes of age.
7. Calcium leukovorin should be available to treat overdosage. Usual dose is 3–6 mg IM administered within 4 hours of methotrexate dose. See Dosage Column.
8. The reader is encouraged to read suggested references on high-dose therapy at the end of this section.

ADVERSE REACTIONS
1. Blood: luekopenia, thrombocytopenia, anemia
2. Gastrointestinal: nausea, vomiting, diarrhea, enteritis, intestinal ulceration, stomatitis, liver damage
3. Skin: rashes, hair loss, depigmentation, itching
4. General: malaise, fatigue, chills, fever
5. Genitourinary: renal impairment, cystitis, impaired spermatogenesis and oogenesis, menstrual irregularities, abortion, fetal defects
6. Central nervous system: headaches, dizziness, seizures, neurologic deficits such as paresis
7. Pneumonitis
8. Osteoporotic effects

the most uncomfortable symptoms occur.
c. Small frequent meals, timed with periods when the patient feels his best, are advisable. Bland foods are usually tolerated most easily. Carbohydrate and protein content should be high.
d. If the patient is anorexic, encourage high nutrient liquids and water. Maintain hydration.
e. Keep an accurate measurement of emesis and stool volumes and total intake and output to guide the physician in ordering parenteral fluids when necessary.
f. Administer constipating agents as needed for diarrhea. Monitor for signs of hypokalemia (weakness, muscle cramps).
g. Monitor for the onset of obstructive ileus (abdominal pain, distention, obstipation).
h. Monitor stools for visible and occult blood.
i. Administer laxatives and stool softeners as ordered if constipation occurs.

9. Management of hematologic effects:
a. Be aware of the patient's white blood cell and platelet count prior to each injection.
b. If WBC falls to 2000/cu mm, take measures to protect the patient from infection, such as protective (reversed) isolation, avoidance of traumatic procedures, maintenance of bodily (especially perineal) cleanliness, carrying out strict urinary catheter care when appropriate, etc. Monitor for infection: temperatures every 4 hours, examination for rashes, swellings, drainage and pain. Explain measures to the patient.
c. If platelet count falls below 100,000/cu mm, monitor for thrombocytopenic bleeding: petechiae, purpura, hematuria, melena, blood in stools, gum bleeding, vaginal bleeding, epistaxis, hematemesis, etc. Avoid trauma. Transfusions may be ordered.
d. Instruct the patient and/or family on the importance of follow-up blood work and reporting of the signs and symptoms listed in "b" and "c" if

NURSING IMPLICATIONS
1. The patient receiving this medication will be experiencing the emotional and physical effects of the malignancy or the psoriasis. Knowledge of the patient's feelings about his disease and its implications will assist in helping him tolerate the chemotherapy. The incidence of uncomfortable side effects and adverse reactions is high. It is within the nurse's role to assist the patient in coping with the discomforts of the disease and its treatment, and to help him work through depression and anger toward acceptance of the disease at his own pace. Despite the unpleasantness this drug may bring, it can be a source of hope for the patient.
2. Notify the physician if jaundice develops.
3. Administer supportive care for generalized discomforts such as fatigue, malaise, fever and chills. These reactions will be depressing and frustrating for the patient.
4. Monitor urine output during intensive therapy. Oliguria can be an indication of renal impairment. Notify the physician if the urine output falls below 240 ml for an 8-hour period (see chart on page 546 for normal urine values for children). Be aware of the patient's BUN.
5. Keep the patient hydrated and encourage frequent fluid intake (at least every 2 hours) to prevent cystitis secondary to drug metabolites in the urine. Encourage voiding every 2–3 hours to remove the drug-containing urine from the bladder. Signs and symptoms of chemical cystitis include: frequency, urgency, dysuria, hematuria (micro- and macroscopic). Report these to the physician.
6. Instruct the patient to report neurologic changes such as dizziness, unilateral weakness, etc. Monitor for seizures, especially in high-dose therapy.
7. Report any signs or symptoms of pneumonitis to the physician: cough, shortness of breath, rales, changes on x-ray, chest pain.
8. Management of gastrointestinal disturbances:
a. Nausea and vomiting are usually mild and of short duration.
b. Administer an antiemetic, if needed, to correspond to the time when

● **METHOTREXATE SODIUM (A.M.E., Amethopterin) (Continued)**

NURSING IMPLICATIONS (No. 9 continued)

10. Management of neurologic side effects:
    a. Instruct the patient and/or family to report numbness, paresthesias, pain, headaches. Inform the physician at the onset.
    b. If the patient is on high-dose therapy, monitor for seizures.
    c. Monitor for signs and symptoms of mental depression that are related to drug administration. Inform the physician and administer supportive care. Knowing the etiology can relieve the patient of some anxiety.

11. Management of stomatitis:
    a. Onset of stomatitis may indicate the presence of more serious intestinal ulceration.
    b. Administer preventive oral care every 4 hours and/or after meals.
    c. For preventive care use a very soft toothbrush (child's) and toothpaste; avoid trauma to tissues.
    d. Examine oral membranes at least daily (instruct patient and/or family) to detect the onset of inflammation and erythema.
    e. If stomatitis occurs, notify the physician and begin therapeutic oral care:[3]
       (1) *Mild Inflammation:* Remove dentures, use soft toothbrush and a hydrogen peroxide solution (1 part peroxide and 4 parts saline). Do *not* use toothpaste. Rinse with peroxide solution and then water. Replace dentures. This procedure should be carried out every 4 hours and/or after meals.
       (2) *Severe Inflammation:* Remove dentures, use soft gauze pads rather than a toothbrush. Use peroxide solution described above. Rinse with water using an asepto syringe and gentle suction until returns are clear. Do not replace dentures. It may be necessary to carry out this procedure every 2–4 hours.
    f. Order a soft, bland diet for patients with inflammation. If stomatitis is severe, the patient may be placed on NPO status by the physician.
    g. For patients who can tolerate oral intake, administer Xylocaine Viscous or acetaminophen elixir as a mouthwash prior to meals to decrease pain (do not use aspirin rinses), as ordered by the physician.
    h. Patients with severe stomatitis may require parenteral analgesia.

12. If rashes occur, administer cool compresses and topical agents as ordered. Keep the patient's environment cool. Turn frequently to prevent skin breakdown.

13. Management of hair loss:
    a. Use scalp tourniquet, if ordered, to help prevent hair loss.
    b. Counsel the patient on the possibility of hair loss to enable him to prepare for this disfigurement.
    c. Reassure him of regrowth of hair following discontinuation of the drug.
    d. Provide privacy, and time for the patient to discuss his feelings.

REFERENCES

1. Silver, Richard T., Lauper, R. David and Jarowski, Charles I.: *A Synopsis of Cancer Chemotherapy.* The York Medical Group, Dun-Donnelley Publishing Corporation, 1977, p. 59.
2. Bender, John F., Grove, William R., and Fortner, Clarence L.: High-Dose Methotrexate with Folinic Acid Rescue. *American Journal of Hospital Pharmacy,* 34:962, September 1977.
3. Bruya, Margaret Auld and Madeira, Nancy Powell: Stomatitis After Chemotherapy. *American Journal of Nursing,* 75(8):1351, August 1975.

SUGGESTED READINGS

Asperheim, Mary K. and Eisenhaur, Laurel: *The Pharmacology Basis of Patient Care* (3rd ed.), Philadelphia: W. B. Saunders Company, 1977, p. 476.
Bender, John F., Grove, William R., and Fortner, Clarence L.: High-Dose Methotrexate with Folinic Acid Rescue. *American Journal of Hospital Pharmacy,* 34:961–965, September 1977.
Bruya, Margaret Auld and Madeira, Nancy Powell: Stomatitis After Chemotherapy. *American Journal of Nursing,* 75(8):1349–1352, August 1975.
Giadquinta, Barbara: Helping Families Face the Crisis of Cancer. *American Journal of Nursing,* 77:1583–1588, October 1977.
Gullo, Shirley: Chemotherapy—What To Do About Special Effects. *RN,* 40:30–32, April 1977.
Laatsch, Nancy: Nursing the Woman Receiving Adjuvant Chemotherapy for Breast Cancer. *Nursing Clinics of North America,* 13(2):337–349, June 1978.
Morrow, Mary: Nursing Management of the Adolescent: The Effect of Cancer Chemotherapy on Psychosocial Development. *Nursing Clinics of North America,* 13(2):319–335, June 1978.
Nirenberg, Anita: High-Dose Methotrexate for the Patient with Osteogenic Sarcoma. *American Journal of Nursing,* 76:1776–1780, November 1976.
Sovik, Corinne: The Nursing Care of Lung Cancer Patients, Emphasizing Chemotherapy. *Nursing Clinics of North America,* 13(2):301–317, June 1978.
Vietti, Teresa J., and Valeriote, Frederick: Conceptual Basis for the Use of Chemotherapeutic Agents and Their Pharmacology. *Pediatric Clinics of North America,* 23:67–92, February 1976.

● **METHOXAMINE HYDROCHLORIDE (Vasoxyl)**

ACTIONS/ INDICATIONS	DOSAGE	PREPARATION AND STORAGE	DRUG INCOMPATIBILITIES	MODES OF IV ADMINISTRATION				CONTRAINDICATIONS; WARNINGS; PRECAUTIONS; ADVERSE REACTIONS
				INJECTION	INTERMITTENT INFUSION	CONTINUOUS INFUSION		
Vasopressor which produces prompt and prolonged rise in blood pressure; does	ADULTS: *Anesthesia*— 3–5 mg for emergency IM route use. should be	Store in the refrigerator. Discard unused portions of vial.	Do not mix with any other medication in any manner.	YES Slowly at a rate of 5 mg/ min.	YES 40 mg of drug in 250 ml D5W.	YES 40 mg of drug in 250 ml D5W.		CONTRAINDICATIONS As a combination with local anesthetics to prolong their action at local sites. PRECAUTIONS 1. Do not use this drug to substitute for

not increase heart rate. Has no central nervous system action; has a direct vaso-constrictive action on the arterioles. Used to support blood pressure during anesthesia and in terminating paroxysms of supraventricular tachycardia.

used for routine situations. A second dose may be given in 15 min. if necessary.

Supraventricular tachycardia—10 mg.

CHILDREN: 0.8 mg/kg or 0.2 mg/M²

Supplied in 1-ml ampuls, 20 mg/ml.

Titrate flow rate with BP response.

Use microdrop infusion tubing and infusion pump.

Titrate flow rate with BP response.

Use microdrop infusion tubing and infusion pump.

replacement of blood, plasma, or fluids if loss has occurred and resulted in hypotension.
2. High dosage will cause undesirably high blood pressure and bradycardia.
3. Intravenous route should be reserved for emergencies.
4. Use with caution in the presence of hyperthyroidism, or severe hypertension (even though patients with hypertension sometimes have a greater fall in BP during spinal anesthesia), or during the use of ergot alkaloids.
5. The increase in peripheral vascular resistance produced by this drug may exacerbate congestive heart failure.
6. Potentiated by MAO inhibitors such as isocarboxazid; reduced dosage will be required.

ADVERSE REACTIONS
May produce sustained, excessive elevated blood pressure accompanied by headaches, urinary urgency, and projectile vomiting. Usually seen after high dosage.

NURSING IMPLICATIONS
1. Monitor blood pressure by indirect or direct (arterial pressure) measurements every 2 minutes during administration until stabilized, then every 5–10 minutes. Decrease drip rate or frequency of injections before blood pressure reaches near undesirable levels; this drug has a prolonged action. If hypertension develops, discontinue the drug, notify the physician. Antihypertensive agents such as hydralazine may be ordered.
2. Monitor heart rate. If rate falls below 60 per minute, atropine sulfate 0.5 mg may be prescribed. When treating supraventricular tachycardias, use continuous ECG monitoring.
3. If the patient has a history of congestive heart failure, monitor closely for signs of decompensation:
a. Tachycardia (may or may not occur)
b. Elevated CVP (engorgement of external jugular veins)
c. Increased respirations (may not be observable if patient is under anesthesia)
d. Decreased pO₂
e. Bilateral rales.
Notify the physician on the appearance of any of these signs. Be prepared to treat with potent diuretics (furosemide), rotating tourniquets, oxygen, morphine, etc., as prescribed by the physician.

METHYLDOPATE HYDROCHLORIDE (Aldomet Ester HCl Injection)

ACTIONS/ INDICATIONS	DOSAGE	PREPARATION AND STORAGE	DRUG INCOMPAT- IBILITIES	MODES OF IV ADMINISTRATION			CONTRAINDICATIONS; WARNINGS; PRECAUTIONS; ADVERSE REACTIONS
				INJECTION	INTERMITTENT INFUSION	CONTINUOUS INFUSION	
Antihypertensive. Reduces both supine and standing blood pressure. Used to manage hypertensive crisis	ADULTS: *Range*—100–1000 mg. *Usual adult dose*—250–500 mg at 6 hour intervals.	Supplied in 5-ml vials, 50 mg/ml. Add only to D5W for infusion.	Do not combine with any other drug in IV bottle; do not add to an IV line containing antibiotics.	NO Not recommended.	YES Add dose to 100 ml D5W. Infuse over 30–60 min.	NO Maximum effects cannot be achieved via this route.	CONTRAINDICATIONS 1. Active hepatic disease 2. If previous therapy with methyldopa has been associated with liver impairment 3. Hypersensitivity 4. Eclampsia

METHYLDOPATE HYDROCHLORIDE (Aldomet Ester HCl Injection) *(Continued)*

ACTIONS/ INDICATIONS	DOSAGE	PREPARATION AND STORAGE	DRUG INCOMPAT- IBILITIES	MODES OF IV ADMINISTRATION			CONTRAINDICATIONS; WARNINGS; PRECAUTIONS; ADVERSE REACTIONS
				INJECTION	INTERMITTENT INFUSION	CONTINUOUS INFUSION	

or any hypertensive situation where parenteral administration is needed, but where *rapid* reduction of blood pressure is not essential.[1]

Lowering of the blood pressure begins in 4–6 hours and lasts 10–16 hours.

Maximum recommended dose—1000 mg/day.

CHILDREN: IV route is reserved for hypertensive crises—20–40 mg/kg/day or 600–1200 mg/M² /day in divided doses every 6 hrs. (maximum total dose 65 mg/kg/day).

WARNINGS
1. Positive Coombs test, hemolytic anemia, and liver impairment may occur and have been fatal.
2. If positive Coombs occurs, it should be determined if hemolytic anemia exists.
3. CBC should be carried out before and during therapy to monitor for anemia.
4. Discontinue the drug if Coomb-positive hemolytic anemia occurs.
5. If patient needs a transfusion during therapy, obtain direct and indirect Coombs. If there is a positive *direct* test, there will be no problem typing and cross-matching. A *positive* indirect test will cause problems in correct matching.
6. Monitor hepatic function. If fever, abnormal liver function tests, or jaundice appears, discontinue the drug. Findings will revert to normal. This represents a hypersensitivity reaction. Do not use this drug in these patients again.
7. There may be reduction in WBC; that is reversible.
8. In pregnancy, the potential benefits for the mother must be weighed against possible risks to the fetus.

PRECAUTIONS
1. Use with caution in the presence of liver disease.
2. May interfere with the following lab studies:
   a. Uric acid (by phosphotungstate method)
   b. Creatinine (by alkaline picrate method)
   c. SGOT (by colorimeteric method)
   d. Urine catecholamine; will be falsely high (could interfere with the diagnosis of pheochromocytoma)
3. Paradoxical hypertensive response has been reported.
4. Do not use to manage hypertension in pheochromocytoma.
5. Urine may darken on exposure to air.
6. Chorealike movements have been reported in patients with known severe bilateral cerebrovascular disease. If it

occurs, discontinue the drug.

7. Patients on this drug will require lower dosage of anesthetics. Hypotension may occur during surgery and can be controlled with vasopressors.

8. Blood levels are reduced with hemodialysis.

9. Edema may occur; if it progresses or is associated with congestive heart failure, discontinue therapy.

ADVERSE REACTIONS

1. Sedation during initial period, may decrease with time. Headache and weakness may also be seen

2. Central nervous system: in addition to No. 1, dizziness, paresthesias, parkinsonism, Bell's palsy, mild psychoses, nightmares, depression

3. Cardiovascular: bradycardia, aggravation of angina pectoris, orthostatic hypotension, edema

4. Gastrointestinal: nausea, vomiting, constipation, diarrhea, sore tongue, dryness of mouth

5. Hepatic: see Warning No. 6

6. Hypersensitivity: rash, drug fever, anaphylaxis

7. Breast enlargement, gynecomastia

---

metries, nausea, vomiting, visual disturbances

b. Cerebrovascular accident

c. Myocardial ischemia or infarction—chest pain, ECG changes, arrhythmias

d. Left ventricular failure—shortness of breath, orthopnea, elevated central venous or pulmonary artery pressure, tachycardia, rales, third and/or fourth heart sound

e. Renal failure—oliguria, rising BUN and creatinine[2]
Excessive *reduction* in blood pressure can also precipitate these complications. Check the patient's blood pressure prior to each dose. The physician should set pressure limits for therapy.

10. Patients who are not in crisis can be ambulated after intermittent infusions; do so *with caution*. Measure lying and then standing pressures to detect postural hypotension. Instruct the patient to arise slowly from sitting and lying positions to prevent postural hypotension-induced dizziness and syncope. If sedation is pronounced, keep the patient on bed rest until the problem resolves.

11. Patients who will be receiving this drug in its oral form on a chronic basis must be instructed on hypertensive self-care.

REFERENCES

1. American Medical Association Committee on Hypertension: The Treatment of Malignant Hypertension and Hypertensive Emergencies. *JAMA* 228 (13):1675, June 24, 1974.

2. Ibid., p. 1675.

SUGGESTED READINGS

American Medical Association Committee on Hypertension: The Treatment of Malignant Hypertension and Hypertensive Emergencies. *JAMA*, 228:1673–

NURSING IMPLICATIONS

1. If the patient is in hypertensive crisis, be prepared to monitor arterial blood pressure preferably by direct arterial cannulation. Indirect measurements by sphygmomanometer can be used if direct measurement is not available, or if the patient is not in crisis.

2. If the patient is in a hypertensive crisis (this drug is used less often than more rapid-acting agents in these situations), monitor blood pressure every 15 minutes until stabilized, and then every 2–4 hours as the patient's condition dictates. Repeat the cycle with each dose. This drug's action is delayed for 3–5 hours after the infusion.

3. For noncrisis situations, check the blood pressure before the infusion and every 4–6 hours after. Be aware that the cumulative effects of this drug can produce severe hypotension after several doses. The physician should order blood pressure limits to govern administration, e.g., "Do not administer if blood pressure is less than xx."

4. Patients with coronary artery disease (history of myocardial infarction or angina) or history of arrhythmias should have continuous ECG monitoring during infusions.

5. Observe for jaundice, notify the physician.

6. Administer this drug after hemodialysis treatments (manufacturer's suggestion).

7. Report any unusual chorealike movements to the physician (See Precaution No. 6).

8. Weigh the patient daily; report unusual gains, or observable peripheral edema to the physician.

9. If the patient's blood pressure is severely elevated, monitor for the consequences:

a. Encephalopathy—confusion, stupor (the sedation produced by this drug may interfere with evaluation for this complication), reflex asym-

METHYLDOPATE HYDROCHLORIDE (Aldomet Ester HCl Injection) (Continued)

SUGGESTED READINGS (Continued)

Fleischmann, L. E.: Management of Hypertensive Crisis in Children. *Pediatric Annals*, 6(6):410–414, June 1977.

Jones, L. N.: Symposium on Teaching and Rehabilitation of the Cardiac Patient. Hypertension: Medical and Nursing Implications. *Nursing Clinics of North America*, 11:283–295, June 1976.

Keith, Thomas: Hypertensive Crisis. Recognition and Management. *JAMA*,

237(15):1570–1577, April 11,1977.

Koch-Weser, Jan: Hypertensive Emergencies. *New England Journal of Medicine*, 290:211–214, January 24, 1974.

Long, M. L., et al: Hypertension: What the Patient Needs to Know. *American Journal of Nursing*, 76:765–770, May 1976.

Romankiewicz, J. A.: Pharmacology and Clinical Use of Drugs in Hypertensive Emergencies. *American Journal of Hospital Pharmacy*, 34(2):185–193, February 1977 (references).

METHYLERGONOVINE MALEATE (Methergine)

ACTIONS/ INDICATIONS	DOSAGE	PREPARATION AND STORAGE	DRUG INCOMPAT- IBILITIES	MODES OF IV ADMINISTRATION			CONTRAINDICATIONS; WARNINGS; PRECAUTIONS; ADVERSE REACTIONS
				INJECTION	INTERMITTENT INFUSION	CONTINUOUS INFUSION	
Oxytocic agent induces rapid sustained effect which shortens the third stage of labor and reduces blood loss. Onset of action is immediate. Used also for postpartum atony, subinvolution, and hemorrhage.	May be given in the second stage of labor following delivery of the anterior shoulder.

Usual dose— 1 ml (0.2 mg); may be repeated in 2–4 hrs. | Supplied in 1-ml ampuls, 0.2 mg/ml.

Do not use if solution is not clear and odorless. Refrigerate. If stored at room temperature, discard after 60 days. | Do not mix with any other medication. | YES

IV injection should be reserved as a lifesaving measure. Give slowly over no less than 1 min. No need to dilute. May be given thru Y-injection site. | NO | NO | CONTRAINDICATIONS
1. Hypertension
2. Toxemia
3. During labor prior to the end of the second stage
4. Hypersensitivity to any ergotated derivative

WARNINGS
1. Intravenous route must be used *only* in emergencies as a lifesaving measure.
2. Can produce sudden severe hypertension that can result in cerebrovascular accidents.

PRECAUTIONS
1. Administer with caution in the presence of sepsis, obliterative vascular disease, hepatic or renal impairment.
2. Serum calcium must be within the normal range for desired effects to be produced.

ADVERSE REACTIONS
1. Nausea, vomiting
2. Hypertension (usually transient)
3. Dizziness, tinnitus
4. Headache
5. Diaphoresis
6. Palpitations, chest pain (transient)
7. Dyspnea
8. Shock, mental excitement, tremors may occur with overdosage |

NURSING IMPLICATIONS
1. Monitor blood pressure every 3–5 minutes after injection for 1–2 hours to detect possible secondary hypertension. Notify physician immediately if blood pressure rises. Chlorpromazine is sometimes prescribed to decrease the hypertensive reaction.
2. Be prepared to manage nausea and vomiting.
3. Monitor for fetal distress:
   a. Fetal heart rate changes:
      Type II bradycardia, beginning at or after peak of contraction; rate less than 120/minute
      Persistent fetal tachycardia (rate over 160/minute)
      Persistent bradycardia (rate less than 120/minute)
      Persistent irregularity
   b. Meconium in amniotic fluid
   c. Fetal hyperactivity
4. The postpartum patient receiving this drug should be kept on bed rest during therapy.
5. Maintain usual peripartum and postpartum care: monitoring location of fundus, lochea checks, presence of cramping.
6. Monitor volume of bleeding that this drug is being used to control.

METHYLPREDNISOLONE SODIUM SUCCINATE (Solu-Medrol)

ACTIONS/ INDICATIONS	DOSAGE	PREPARATION AND STORAGE	DRUG INCOMPATIBILITIES	MODES OF IV ADMINISTRATION			CONTRAINDICATIONS; WARNINGS; PRECAUTIONS; ADVERSE REACTIONS
				INJECTION	INTERMITTENT INFUSION	CONTINUOUS INFUSION	
Corticosteroid, anti-inflammatory agent. Indicated as effective in: • Endocrine disorders • Collagen diseases • Dermatologic disease • Allergic states • Gastrointestinal diseases May be effective in: • Generalized neurodermatitis • Acute rheumatic fever • Septic shock • Other forms of shock • Croup • Esophageal burns	ADULTS: Range— 10–500 mg every 6 hrs. Larger doses have been given in extreme cases of septic shock with other supportive care. Do not give massive doses for over 72 hrs. Usual dose— 10–40 mg repeated as needed. CHILDREN: Dosage must be according to condition of the patient and his response; no dosage less than 0.5 mg/ kg/day.	Use only Mix-o-Vial diluent or diluent accompanying the drug for reconstitution. Use within 48 hours. This is the only methylprednisolone preparation for intravenous use.	Do not combine in syringe with any other medication. Do not mix in solution or IV tubing with: Chlorpromazine (Thorazine) Digitoxin Diphenhydramine (Benadryl) Metaraminol (Aramine) Promethazine (Phenergan) Tetracycline Thiamylal (Surital) Sodium thiopental Tolazoline (Priscoline) Vitamins	YES To initiate therapy in emergencies, at a rate of 1 gm over 5 minutes.	YES Add prepared solution to D5W, NS or D5/NS in any volume. Infuse over 30–60 min.	YES Add prepared solution to D5W, NS or D5/NS in any volume.	CONTRAINDICATIONS 1. Systemic fungal infections 2. In long-term therapy: active or healed TB, ocular herpes, acute psychoses. 3. Considered by some groups to also be relatively contraindicated (in long-term and short-term therapy) in peptic ulcer disease, chickenpox, congestive heart failure, diabetes mellitus, diverticulitis, new intestinal anastomoses, hypertension, myasthenia gravis, osteoporosis, pregnancy, thromboembolism. WARNINGS 1. Dosage should be increased before and during unusual stress such as surgery. 2. May mask signs of infection. There may also be decreased ability to localize infection. 3. Prolonged use may produce cataracts, glaucoma, optic nerve damage, and enhance the establishment of viral or fungal infections. 4. Use in pregnancy should be after benefits are weighed against risks. Infants born of mothers who have received this drug during pregnancy should be observed for hypoadrenalism. 5. May cause elevation of blood pressure even in normal doses. Use with caution in patients with a history of or currently treated hypertension. 6. Will cause sodium and water reten-

METHYLPREDNISOLONE SODIUM SUCCINATE (Solu-Medrol) (Continued)

ACTIONS/ INDICATIONS	DOSAGE	PREPARATION AND STORAGE	DRUG INCOMPAT- IBILITIES	MODES OF IV ADMINISTRATION			CONTRAINDICATIONS; WARNINGS; PRECAUTIONS; ADVERSE REACTIONS
				INJECTION	INTERMITTENT INFUSION	CONTINUOUS INFUSION	
							tion, and potassium and calcium excretion. Use with caution in patients with renal insufficiency. 7. Do not vaccinate against smallpox or other diseases during therapy. 8. Use in TB should only be for fulminating or disseminated forms and when other supportive therapy is used. 9. Hypersensitivity has occured. 10. Circulatory collapse has occured following rapidly administered large doses. PRECAUTIONS 1. Drug-induced secondary adrenocortical insufficiency will be reduced by gradual reduction of dosage rather than abrupt cessation. This is probably not necessary following short-term therapy where adrenocortical suppression is minimal. 2. There is an enhanced response to steroids in hypothyroidism and cirrhosis. 3. Use lowest possible dosage. 4. Psychic disturbances of all forms occur. Pre-existing psychiatric problems, especially psychoses, may be exacerbated. 5. Use aspirin with caution, especially if there is hypoprothrombinemia. 6. Use with caution in the following gastrointestinal conditions: impending gastrointestinal perforation, abscess or other infection, diverticulitis, new intestinal anastomoses, peptic ulcer disease. 7. Use with caution in the presence of myasthenia gravis, osteoporosis. ADVERSE REACTIONS SEEN IN SHORT-TERM INTRAVENOUS THERAPY 1. Fluid and electrolyte imbalance: sodium and water retention with possible secondary hypertension, hypokalemia, hypocalcemia 2. Gastrointestinal: peptic ulcer with possible perforation, pancreatitis, ulcerative eosphagitis

3. Dermatologic: impaired wound healing.
4. Neurologic: increased intracranial pressure, seizures (increasing frequency in patients with pre-existing seizure disorder), vertigo, headaches, mental confusion, euphoria, excerbation of psychosis
5. Endocrine: decreased glucose tolerance, increased hypoglycemic agent and insulin requirements in diabetics.
6. Eye: increased intraocular pressure.
7. Metabolic: negative nitrogen balance secondary to rapid muscle catabolism.

9. Patients with a history of seizure activity may have an increasing number of seizures while on steroid therapy. Apply appropriate safety precautions.
10. Monitor for behavioral changes, which may range from simple euphoria to depression and psychosis. Apply appropriate safety precautions. A change in dosage may relieve such symptoms.
11. Turberculin testing should be carried out prior to initiation of steroid therapy if possible. The patient's reactivity to the tuberculin is altered by the drug, giving a false result.
12. Ambulate the patient with caution if vertigo occurs, and initiate the use of side rails to prevent patient injury. Report the onset to the physician.
13. Be alert to the signs of increasing intraocular pressure; eye pain, rainbow vision, blurred vision, nausea and vomiting.[3] Notify the physician immediately.

REFERENCES
1. Beeson, Paul, and McDermott, Walsh (editors): *Cecil-Loeb Textbook of Medicine* (14th ed.), Philadelphia: W. B. Saunders Company, 1975, p. 1587.
2. Ibid., p. 1815.
3. Newell, Frank W., and Ernest, J. Terry: *Ophthalmology—Principles and Concepts* (3rd ed.), St. Louis: C. V. Mosby Company, 1974, p. 329.

SUGGESTED READINGS
Glasser, Ronald J.: How the Body Works Against Itself: Autoimmune Disease. *Nursing '77*, September 1977, pp. 34–38.
Melick, M. E.: Nursing Intervention for Patients Receiving Corticosteroid Therapy. In *Advanced Concepts in Clinical Nursing* (2nd ed.), K. C. Kintzel, ed., Philadelphia, J. B. Lippincott Company, 1974, pp. 606–617.
Newton, David. Nichols, Arlene, and Newton, Marion: You Can Minimize the Hazards of Corticosteroids. *Nursing '77*, June 1977, pp. 26–33.
Reichgott, Michael J., and Melmon, Kenneth L.: The Role of Corticosteroids in Shock. In *Steroid Therapy*, Daniel Azarnoff, ed., Philadelphia, W. B. Saunders Company, 1975 pp. 118–133.

NURSING IMPLICATIONS
1. Take precautions to prevent infections in wounds by using strict aseptic technique in dressing changes, etc. Avoid traumatic procedures such as catheterizations. The skin may become more fragile because of the steroid therapy. Patients on bed rest and those with general body weakening secondary to an acute illness should be turned hourly (except during sleep, then every 2–3 hours) to prevent skin breakdown. Initiate the use of supportive measures such as flotation pads, water mattress, etc. Administer scrupulous skin care to prevent infection.
2. Monitor blood pressure every 2–4 hours, or as the patient's condition dictates. Monitor blood pressure before, during and immediately after intravenous injection; hypotension can occur.
3. Weigh the patient daily to detect for water and sodium retention. Dietary restriction in sodium may be prescribed by the physician. Examine daily for peripheral edema. Monitor for exacerbation of the congestive heart failure in susceptible patients (increasing dyspnea, increasing resting heart rate, fatigue, rales, etc.)
4. There may be delayed healing of wounds; take precautions to prevent dehiscence. Sutures may be left in longer than usual for this reason.
5. Monitor urine glucose in patients on high-dose therapy and with diabetes. Diabetic individuals may require a larger dosage of insulin or oral agent.
6. Administer antacid therapy as ordered to assist in preventing peptic ulcer. Monitor for signs of the development of an ulcer and/or acute intestinal bleeding; melena, positive stool guaiac, hematemesis, epigastric pain and/or distention, anemia or falling hematocrit.
7. Monitor for signs and symptoms of hypokalemia:[1] weakness, irritability, abdominal distention, poor feeding in infants, muscle cramps. Dietary or pharmacologic potassium supplements may be ordered, guided by serum potassium levels.
8. Monitor for signs and symptoms of hypocalcemia:[2] irritability, change in mental status, seizures, nausea, vomiting, diarrhea, muscle cramps, late effects—cardiac arrhythmias, laryngeal spasm and apnea. Dietary or pharmacologic supplements may be ordered, guided by serum calcium levels.

● METYRAPONE TARTRATE (Metopirone Tartrate)

ACTIONS/ INDICATIONS	DOSAGE	PREPARATION AND STORAGE	DRUG INCOMPATIBILITIES	MODES OF IV ADMINISTRATION			CONTRAINDICATIONS; WARNINGS; PRECAUTIONS; ADVERSE REACTIONS
				INJECTION	INTERMITTENT INFUSION	CONTINUOUS INFUSION	
Diagnostic agent to evaluate hypothalamicopituitary function.	ADULTS: *Day 1* — Collect 24-hr urine for 17-OHCS* and 17-KGS† *Day 2* — Carry out standard ACTH test (50 units ACTH over 8 hrs) and measure 24-hr urinary steroids. *Days 3–4* — rest. *Day 5* — metyrapone 30 mg/kg in 1000 ml NS or D5W, infuse over 4 hrs; starting at 8 A.M. Collect urine for 24 hrs for steroids, starting also at 8 A.M. See Interpretation under Contraindications column. *17-hydroxycorticosteroids †17-ketogenic steroids	Supplied in 10-ml ampuls, 100 mg/ml. Add only to D5W or NS.	Do not mix with any other medication in any manner.	NO	NO	YES Add 30 mg to 1000 ml D5W or NS. Infuse over 4 hrs (60 macro-drops/min). The drip rate must be accurate, use infusion pump.	CONTRAINDICATIONS 1. Adrenal cortical insufficiency 2. Hypersensitivity WARNINGS Safety for use in pregnancy has not been established. PRECAUTIONS 1. All corticosteroid therapy must be discontinued prior to and during the test. 2. The ability of the adrenals to respond to this agent must be determined by an ACTH test before use of this drug as a test. 3. May induce acute adrenocortical insufficiency in patients with compromised function. 4. Erroneous test results may be seen in patients concomitantly on phenytoin or estrogen therapy. Subnormal response can be seen in pregnancy. ADVERSE REACTIONS 1. Nausea 2. Abdominal pain 3. Dizziness 4. Headache 5. Sedation 6. Allergic rash 7. Thrombophlebitis at infusion site INTERPRETATION OF TESTS 1. ACTH: The normal 24-hour urinary excretion of 17-OHCS ranges from 3–12 mg. Following the infusion of 50 units of ACTH, the 17-OHCS excretion is increased to 15–45 mg/24 hours. 2. Metyrapone: In patients with normal pituitary function, metyrapone increases the 17-OHCS excretion by 2–4 times normal, and the 17-KGS by 2 times. 3. A subnormal or absent response in patients without adrenal insufficiency is indicative of some degree of impairment of pituitary function, either panhypopituitarism or partial hypopituitarism. 4. An excessive response (excretion of 17-OHCS or 17-KGS above normal range) is suggestive of Cushing's syn-

drome associated with adrenal hyperplasia.

b. Anorexia, nausea, vomiting, abdominal pain
c. Fever
d. Hypotension
e. Hyperkalemia (elevated serum potassium)
f. Irritability, anxiety
4. Be prepared to manage and administer comfort measures in the event of adverse reactions.

NURSING IMPLICATIONS
1. Be certain that corticosteroid drugs have been discontinued prior to the test.
2. Assist in administering an accurate test. Help to gain patient cooperation by providing clear instructions. Assist patients who have disabilities. Correct collection of the 24-hour urine is mandatory.
3. Monitor for acute adrenocortical insufficiency after infusion:
a. Extreme weakness, fatigue

● MINOCYCLINE HYDROCHLORIDE (Minocin, Vectrin)

ACTIONS/ INDICATIONS	DOSAGE	PREPARATION AND STORAGE	DRUG INCOMPATIBILITIES	MODES OF IV ADMINISTRATION			CONTRAINDICATIONS; WARNINGS; PRECAUTIONS; ADVERSE REACTIONS
				INJECTION	INTERMITTENT INFUSION	CONTINUOUS INFUSION	
Antibiotic, long-acting derivative of tetracycline.

Indicated in infections caused by:
• Rickettsiae
• *Mycoplasma pneumoniae*
• Agents of psittacosis and ornithosis
• Agents of lymphogranuloma venereum and granuloma inguinale
• Agent of relapsing fever

The following gram-negative organisms:
• *Hemophilus ducreyi*
• *Pasteurella pestis* and *tularensis*
• *Bartonella bacilliformis* | USUAL ADULT DOSE: 200 mg initially followed by 100 mg every 12 hrs. Do not exceed 400-mg in 24 hrs.

CHILDREN: 4 mg/kg initially followed by 2–4 mg/kg every 12 hrs. (See Warning No. 6.) | Supplied in vials of 100 mg.

Reconstitute dry powder with any volume of D5W, NS, D5/NS or RL. Solutions can be stored at room temperature for 24 hours only, then discard.

Further dilute reconstituted solutions as instructed in Continuous Infusion and Intermittent Infusion columns. | Do not mix with any magnesium- or calcium-containing solutions. | NO | YES | YES

In 12-hour infusions of 500 –1000 ml of NS, D5W, D5/ NS, or RL. | CONTRAINDICATIONS
Hypersensitivity to any tetracycline

WARNINGS
1. There may be a rise in BUN during therapy. This is not significant in normal renal function.
2. The drug should be avoided in patients with renal insufficiency. It may exacerbate renal dysfunction directly, indirectly causing an antianabolic state with acidosis and increasing azotemia.[1] Excessive systemic accumulation of the drug may also be seen, which can lead to liver toxicity.
3. Use in pregnant patients with renal dysfunction has been associated with death due to acute hepatic failure.
4. This drug is not readily hemodialyzable.[2]
5. May cause liver impairment secondary to fatty infiltration without necrosis, usually seen in intravenous doses over 2 gm/day or in normal doses in patient with renal failure.
6. The use of tetracycline during tooth development may cause permanent discoloration of the child's teeth. There may also be enamel hypoplasia.
7. This drug can affect bone growth in children (also see Warning No. 6).
8. Toxic effects have been seen in fetal development abnormalities.
9. This drug is secreted in breast milk. |

Add dose to 100 ml D5W, NS, D5/NS or RL for each 10 mg of drug. Infuse over 60 minutes.

405

● MINOCYCLINE HYDROCHLORIDE (Minocin, Vectrin) (Continued)

ACTIONS/ INDICATIONS	DOSAGE	PREPARATION AND STORAGE	DRUG INCOMPAT- IBILITIES	MODES OF IV ADMINISTRATION — INJECTION	INTERMITTENT INFUSION	CONTINUOUS INFUSION	CONTRAINDICATIONS; WARNINGS; PRECAUTIONS; ADVERSE REACTIONS
• Bacteroides • Brucella • Others as indicated in sensitivity tests. The following gram-positive organism: • Certain Streptococcus species, e.g., *Streptococcus pneumoniae* • *Staph. aureus* (for skin and soft tissues only) When penicillin is contraindicated, this drug can be used as an alternative in infections due to: • *Neisseria gonorrhoeae* • *Treponema pallidum and T. pertenue* • *Listeria monocytogenes* • *Clostridium* species • *Bacillus anthracis* • *Fusobacterium fusiformis* • *Actinomyces* species							PRECAUTIONS 1. There may be overgrowth of non-susceptible organisms including fungi. If a superinfection occurs, the drug should be discontinued and appropriate therapy instituted. 2. Patients who are on anticoagulant therapy may require lower dosage of that anticoagulant while on minocycline. 3. All infections secondary to Group A beta-hemolytic Streptococcus should be treated for at least 10 days. 4. Avoid using tetracyclines and penicillins together. The actions of penicillin can be reduced by this drug. ADVERSE REACTIONS 1. Gastrointestinal: anorexia, nausea, vomiting, diarrhea, glossitis, dysphagia, enterocolitis, monilial infections of the anogenital region 2. Skin: maculopapular and erythematous rashes, photosensitivity 3. Renal: rise in BUN (dose-related); see Warnings No. 1, 2, 3, 4 4. Hypersensitivity: urticaria, angioneurotic edema, anaphylaxis, exacerbation of lupus erythematosus 5. Blood: hemolytic anemia, thrombocytopenia, neutropenia, eosinophilia 6. Phlebitis at injection site 7. Vertigo 8. *In infants*: Bulging fontanels, papilledema (pseudotumor cerebri); usually disappears on discontinuation of the drug.

NURSING IMPLICATIONS
1. Take anaphylaxis precautions; see page 118.
2. If gastrointestinal disturbances occur, notify the physician. If disturbances such as nausea, vomiting and diarrhea are pronounced, the drug will probably be discontinued. Antiemetics, antacids, and constipating agents can be ordered to control symptoms. Monitor intake and output to assist the physician in planning for parenteral fluid replacement. Maintain hydration orally when possible.
3. If the patient will be taking the oral form of this drug as an outpatient, instruct him on the possibility of photosensitivity and the advisability of avoiding exposure to the sun (sun-block lotions may be of help if exposure cannot be avoided).
4. Women of childbearing age and potential and mothers of children who may receive this drug should be informed of Warnings No. 3, 6, 8, 9 and 10 by the physician. Assist in the interpretation of these warnings to the patient.
5. Even though blood dyscrasias are infrequently caused by this agent, be aware of the patient's complete blood cell count during therapy. If the platelet count begins to fall, the drug will probably be discontinued. Bleeding secondary to a low platelet count usually begins only after the count falls below 50,000/cu mm.
6. Monitor for signs and symptoms of overgrowth infections:
   a. Fever (take rectal temperature at least every 4–6 hours in all patients)
   b. Increasing malaise
   c. Newly appearing localized signs and symptoms: redness, soreness, pain, swelling, drainage (increased volume or change in character of pre-existing drainage)
   d. Monilial rash in perineal area (reddened areas with itching)
   e. Cough (change in pre-existing cough or sputum production)
   f. Diarrhea
7. Report the onset of any rash to the physician. Keep the patient's environment comfortably cool and the skin clean. Diphenhydramine (Benadryl) may be ordered to relieve itching.
8. Report the onset of jaundice to the physician.
9. Report the onset of bulging fontanels, and other signs of increasing intracranial pressure, to the physician.
10. Be aware of this drug's relationship with renal function. Most tetracyclines are usually not given to patients with renal impairment because:
    a. The drug accumulates in the body because of decreased excretion.
    b. The presence of the drug may cause further deterioration in renal function.
    c. It may cause a catabolic state with metabolic acidosis, increasing BUN, and possibly death due to uremia.[3]
    Know what the patient's pretreatment BUN and creatinine levels are. Report increases in these values with initiation of treatment. Monitor urine output in renal patients receiving the drug. Report increasing oliguria to the physician. Send urine for analysis at least every other day.

REFERENCES
1. Barza, Michael, and Schiefe, Richard T.: Antimicrobial Spectrum, Pharmacology and Therapeutic Use of Antibiotics. Part I: Tetracyclines. *American Journal of Hospital Pharmacy*, 34: 51, January 1977.
2. Ibid.
3. Ibid.

MITHRAMYCIN (Mithracin)

ACTIONS/INDICATIONS	DOSAGE	PREPARATION AND STORAGE	DRUG INCOMPATIBILITIES	MODES OF IV ADMINISTRATION			CONTRAINDICATIONS; WARNINGS; PRECAUTIONS; ADVERSE REACTIONS
				INJECTION	INTERMITTENT INFUSION	CONTINUOUS INFUSION	
Antineoplastic agent, cell-cycle specific. Used in the treatment of malignant tumors of the testes when surgery or radiation are impossible. Also used to treat symptomatic patients with hypercalcemia and hypercalciuria in advanced neoplasms. Not	TESTICULAR TUMORS: 25–30 mcg/kg (use actual body weight or *ideal* weight in the presence of edema)/day. Continue for 8–10 days unless significant toxic effects are seen. Do not exceed 10 daily doses. Do not exceed 30 mcg/kg. Courses of therapy can be	To reconstitute from powder add 4.9 ml sterile water for injection and shake to dissolve. Each ml = 500 mcg (0.5 mg). Discard unused portion. Prepare fresh on the day of use.	Do not mix with any other medication.	NO. Use of this mode has been associated with a higher incidence and greater severity of side effects.[2]	YES. Daily dose in 500–1000 ml D5W over 4–6 hours.	NO	CONTRAINDICATIONS 1. Thrombocytopenia, thrombocytopathy, coagulation disorder, or increased susceptibility to bleeding due to other causes 2. Impaired bone marrow function 3. The unhospitalized patient PRECAUTIONS 1. Severe thrombocytopenia, a hemorrhagic tendency and death may occur (this complication is usually seen following doses of 30 mcg/kg or duration longer than 10 days). 2. The following studies should be carried out before, during and after therapy: platelet count, prothrombin time, bleeding time. Thrombocytopenia or prolongation of prothrombin or

MITHRAMYCIN (Mithracin) (Continued)

ACTIONS/ INDICATIONS	DOSAGE	PREPARATION AND STORAGE	DRUG INCOMPAT- IBILITIES	MODES OF IV ADMINISTRATION			CONTRAINDICATIONS; WARNINGS; PRECAUTIONS; ADVERSE REACTIONS
				INJECTION	INTERMITTENT INFUSION	CONTINUOUS INFUSION	

recommended for any other neoplasm. Tumor regression is usually evident in 3–4 weeks.	HYPERCAL-CEMIA AND HYPER-CALCIURIA: 25 mcg/kg for 3–4 days. May use single weekly dose to control condition. Use *only* in hypercalcemia and hypercalciuria unresponsive to other therapy. Patients with renal impairment will require a 25–40% reduction in dosage based on dosage suggested above.[1]
	
	If desired effects are not seen with initial course, it can be repeated at intervals of 1 week.
							bleeding time must prompt discontinuation of the drug.
							3. Prior to treatment, electrolyte imbalance, such as hypocalcemia, hypokalemia, and hypophosphatemia, must be corrected.
							4. Use with extreme caution in the presence of renal or hepatic dysfunction. Abnormal liver function tests may occur, even in normal subjects. These changes are reversible on discontinuation of the drug.
							5. Facial flushing is an indication to discontinue therapy.[3]
							
							ADVERSE REACTIONS
							1. Blood:
							  a. Bleeding syndrome due to thrombocytopenia, elevation in prothrombin, clotting and bleeding times; seen in 5–12% of patients treated, usually heralded by an episode of epistaxis, advances to widespread GI bleeding
							  b. Leukopenia (seen in approximately 6% of patients treated)
							  c. Decreased hemoglobin
							2. Gastrointestinal: anorexia, nausea, vomiting, diarrhea, stomatitis
							3. Skin: facial erythema (see Precaution No. 5) or edema, increased pigmentation; rashes
							4. Fever (common)
							5. Hepatic: elevation in SGOT, SGPT, LDH, alkaline phosphatase, serum bilirubin.
							6. Renal: elevation in BUN and serum creatinine, proteinuria (secondary to drug-induced renal insufficiency)
							7. Electrolyte balance: decreased serum calcium, phosphorus, and potassium
							8. Miscellaneous: drowsiness, weakness, lethargy, mental depression

NURSING IMPLICATIONS

1. The patient receiving this medication will be experiencing the emotional and physical effects of malignancy. Knowledge of the patient's feelings about his disease and its implications will assist in helping him tolerate the chemotherapy. The incidence of uncomfortable side effects and adverse reactions is high. It is within the nurse's role to assist the patient in coping with the discomforts of the disease and its treatment, and to help

Replace dentures. This procedure should be carried out every 4 hours, and/or after meals.

(2) *Severe Inflammation:* Remove dentures, use soft gauze pads rather than a toothbrush. Use the peroxide solution as described above. Rinse with water using an asepto syringe and gentle suction until returns are clear. Do not replace dentures. It may be necessary to give this care every 2–4 hours.

him work through depression and anger toward acceptance of the disease at his own pace. Despite the unpleasantness this drug may bring, it can be a source of hope for the patient.

2. Management of hematologic effects:
   a. See Adverse Reaction No. 1.
   b. Be aware of the patient's platelet count, the prothrombin, clotting and bleeding times prior to each injection of this drug.
   c. Monitor for bleeding if the platelet count falls below 100,000/cu mm, if clotting (coagulation) time exceeds 6–17 minutes (Lee-White method using glass tubes), or if bleeding time exceeds 4 minutes (Ivy method). The bleeding syndrome this drug can precipitate is secondary to depression of hepatic synthesis of several coagulation factors.

   Signs of bleeding: petechiae, purpura, hematuria, melena, blood in the stools, gum bleeding, vaginal bleeding, epistaxis, hematemesis, shock, etc. Avoid traumatic procedures and patient injury. Transfusions of fresh whole blood may be ordered.
   d. Leukopenia occurs rarely. Be aware of the patient's white blood cell count prior to each injection of this drug. If the WBC falls below 2000/cu mm, take measures to protect the patient from infection such as protective (reversed) isolation, avoidance of traumatic procedures, maintaining bodily (especially perineal) cleanliness, carry out strict urinary catheter care when appropriate, etc. Monitor for infection by recording temperatures every 4 hours, examining for rashes, swellings, drainage and pain. Explain these measures to the patient.

3. Management of gastrointestinal symptoms:
   a. Administer antiemetics when they appear to be most effective, e.g., prior to the injection and/or 1 hour prior to meals, etc.
   b. Small frequent meals, timed with periods when the patient feels his best, are advisable. Bland foods are usually tolerated better than others. Carbohydrate and protein content should be high. If the patient is anorexic, encourage high nutrient liquids and water to maintain hydration.
   c. Keep accurate measurements of emesis volume and total intake and output to guide the physician in ordering parenteral fluids when necessary.
   d. Monitor for the onset of diarrhea and notify the physician. Administer antiperistaltics as ordered. Maintain hydration. Monitor for hypokalemia, e.g., muscle cramps and weakness.

4. Management of stomatitis:
   a. Administer preventive oral care every 4 hours and/or after meals.
   b. For preventive care, use a very soft toothbrush (child's) and toothpaste; avoid trauma to tissues.
   c. Examine oral membranes at least daily (instruct patient and/or family) to detect the onset of inflammation or ulceration.
   d. If stomatitis occurs, notify the physician and begin therapeutic oral care:[4]
      (1) *Mild Inflammation:* Remove dentures, use a soft toothbrush and a hydrogen peroxide solution (1 part peroxide and 4 parts saline). Do *not* use toothpaste. Rinse with the peroxide solution and then water.
   e. Order a bland, mechanical soft diet for patients with inflammation. If stomatitis is severe, the patient may be placed on NPO status by the physician.
   f. For the patients who can tolerate oral intake, administer Xylocaine Viscous or acetaminophen elixir as a mouthwash prior to meals to decrease pain (do not use aspirin rinses), as ordered by the physician.
   g. Patients with severe stomatitis may require parenteral analgesia.

5. Monitor for facial flushing. Notify the physician; this is an indication to discontinue the drug.
6. If rashes occur, administer cool compresses as ordered. If the patient is on bed rest, turn him frequently to prevent skin breakdown. Keep room temperature cool.
7. Monitor for fever (differentiation will have to be made between drug fever and temperature elevation secondary to infection).
8. Be aware of the patient's BUN and serum creatinine. If these values rise above normal, begin monitoring urine output every 8 hours. Report oliguria (urine output less than 240 ml in 8 hours) to the physician.
9. Monitor for signs and symptoms of hypocalcemia:[5] muscle cramps and aches, paresthesias, nausea and vomiting, diarrhea.
10. Monitor for hypokalemia (secondary to increased renal excretion of potassium):[6] muscle cramps, weakness, irritability, abdominal distention.
11. Observe for signs of mental depression. The patient should be informed that the drug is likely to cause such feelings. Give the patient time to express feelings and concerns. Elicit assistance from the family and/or significant others.

REFERENCES
1. Shinn, Arthur F., et al.: Dosage Modifications of Cancer Chemotherapeutic Agents in Renal Failure. *Drug Intelligence and Clinical Pharmacy,* 11:141, March 1977.
2. Trissel, Lawrence A.: *Handbook on Injectable Drugs,* Washington, DC: American Society of Hospital Pharmacists, 1977, p. 235.
3. Silver, Richard T., Lauper, R. David, and Jarwoski, Charles I.: *A Synopsis of Cancer Chemotherapy,* The York Medical Group, New York: Dun-Donnelley Publishing Company, 1977, p. 98.
4. Bruya, Margaret Auld, and Madeira, Nancy Powell: Stomatitis After Chemotherapy. *American Journal of Nursing,* 75(8):1351, August 1975.
5. Beeson, Paul, and McDermott, Walsh (editors): *Cecil-Loeb Textbook of Medicine* (14th ed.), Philadelphia: W. B. Saunders Company, 1975, p. 1815.
6. Ibid., p. 1587.

SUGGESTED READINGS
Bruya, Margaret Auld, and Madeira, Nancy Powell: Stomatitis After Chemotherapy. *American Journal of Nursing,* 75(8):1349–1352, August 1975.
Giadquinta, Barbara: Helping Families Face the Crisis of Cancer. *American Journal of Nursing,* 77:1583–1588, October 1977.
Gullo, Shirley: Chemotherapy—What to Do About Special Side Effects. *RN,* 40:30–32, April 1977.

MITOMYCIN (Mutamycin)

ACTIONS/INDICATIONS	DOSAGE	PREPARATION AND STORAGE	DRUG INCOMPATIBILITIES	MODES OF IV ADMINISTRATION			CONTRAINDICATIONS; WARNINGS; PRECAUTIONS; ADVERSE REACTIONS
				INJECTION	INTERMITTENT INFUSION	CONTINUOUS INFUSION	
Antineoplastic antibiotic that is cell-cycle nonspecific. Used in combination with other agents in disseminated adenocarcinoma of the stomach, breast or pancreas, carcinoma of the head or neck, and chronic myelogenous leukemia.	ADULTS: *Single dose*— 10–20 mg/M² every 6–8 weeks. *Multiple doses* —2 mg/M²/ day for 5 days; 2 days no dose; then 2 mg/M²/day for 5 days. If after two courses there is no improvement, discontinue. When used in combination, dosage must be individualized (see table below).	Supplied in vials of 5 mg and 20 mg of powder. Reconstitute by adding 10 ml or 40 ml of sterile water for injection, respectively. Shake to dissolve. If dissolution is not immediately seen, allow the vial to stand at room temperature for several minutes, shake again. The resulting solution contains 0.5 mg/ml.	Do not mix with any other medication except heparin.	YES Into the "Y" site of a running IV. No need to further dilute reconstituted solution. Flush vein with NS after injection.	YES Use D5W or NS, 100–200 ml, infused immediately after mixing, over 30–60 minutes.	NO	CONTRAINDICATIONS 1. Hypersensitivity 2. Thrombocytopenia or other coagulation disorders and increased bleeding tendency due to other causes

WARNINGS 1. There is a high incidence of bone marrow suppression—thrombocytopenia and leukopenia. Perform appropriate studies before, during and after therapy. 2. Discontinue if platelet count falls below 150,000/cu mm or if WBC is below 4000/cu mm. Death has resulted secondary to septicemia with low white count. 3. Monitor for renal toxicity. Discontinue if serum creatinine exceeds 1.7 mg/100 ml. 4. Safety for use in pregnancy has not been established. Fetal malformations have been seen in test animals. 5. Avoid extravasation.

ADVERSE REACTIONS 1. Bone marrow toxicity: usually reversible thrombocytopenia and leukopenia; suppression is cumulative. After a single dose, the peak suppression occurs in 3–4 weeks. Thrombocytopenia persists for 2–3 weeks and leukopenia for 1–2 weeks. Recovery after cessation of therapy is usually complete in 8 weeks.[1] Twenty-five percent do not recover. 2. Skin and mucous membranes: stomatitis and hair loss, cellulitis at injection or extravasation site. 3. Gastrointestinal: anorexia, nausea and vomiting (14% of patients). 4. Renal: rise in creatinine and BUN (toxicity is in the form of glomerular sclerosis) occurs several months after therapy (2% of patients) 5. Fever (rare) 6. Headache, blurred vision, fatigue, edema of the extremities, syncope (all rare) |

MANUFACTURER'S SUGGESTED DOSAGE GUIDE

Lowest cell count after prior dose		Percentage of prior dose to be given
Leukocytes	Platelets	
>4000	>100,000	100%
3000–3999	75,000–99,999	100%
2000–2999	25,000–74,000	70%
>2000	<25,000	50%

No repeat dosage should be given until the leukocyte count has returned to 3000 and the platelet count to 75,000.

The reconstituted solution is stable if refrigerated for 14 days; discard after that time (7 days if unrefrigerated).

If the drug is added to large volumes of solution, it will be stable for the following times

at room temper-
ature:
D5W—3 hours
NS—12 hours
Sod. Lactate—
24 hours

NURSING IMPLICATIONS

1. The patient receiving this medication will be experiencing the emotional and physical effects of the malignancy. Knowledge of the patient's feelings about his disease and its implications will assist in helping him tolerate the chemotherapy. The incidenc of uncomfortable side effects and adverse reactions is high. It is within the nurse's role to assist the patient in coping with the discomforts of the disease and its treatment, and to help him work through depression and anger toward acceptance of the disease at his own pace. Despite the unpleasantness this drug may bring, it can be a source of hope for the patient.
2. Management of Hematologic Effects:
   a. See Adverse Reaction No. 1, and Warnings Nos. 1 and 2.
   b. Be aware of the patient's white blood cell and platelet counts prior to each dose and daily if the patient is on daily doses of this drug.
   c. If WBC falls to 2000/cu mm, take measures to protect the patient from infection such as: protective (reverse) isolation, avoidance of traumatic procedures, maintain bodily (especially perineal) cleanliness, carry out strict urinary catheter care when appropriate. Monitor for infection by recording temperatures every 4 hours; examine for rashes, swellings, drainage and pain. Explain these measures to the patient.
   d. If the platelet count falls below 100,000/cu mm, monitor for thrombocytopenic bleeding: petechiae, purpura, hematuria, melena, blood in stools, gum bleeding, oozing from an incision, vaginal bleeding, epistaxis, hematuria, etc. Avoid trauma. Transfusions may be ordered.
   e. Instruct the patient and family on the importance of follow-up blood work if the drug is being administered on an outpatient basis.
3. Take all precautions to avoid extravasation; see page 96.
4. Management of Nausea and Vomiting:
   a. Usually occurs during the first 12–24 hours after an injection.
   b. Administer antiemetic 1 hour prior to injection and/or prior to meals, whichever schedule relieves the symptoms most efficiently.
   c. Small frequent meals, timed with periods when the patient feels his best, are advisable. Bland foods are usually tolerated more readily by a patient who is anorexic or nauseated. Carbohydrate and protein content should be high.
   d. If the patient is anorexic, encourage high nutrient liquids and water to maintain nutrition and hydration.
   e. Keep accurate measurements of emesis volume and total intake and output to guide the physician in ordering parenteral fluids when necessary.
5. Management of Hair Loss:
   a. Counsel the patient on the possibility of hair loss to enable him to prepare for this disfigurement.
   b. Reassure him of regrowth of hair following discontinuation of the drug.
   c. Provide privacy and time for the patient to discuss his feelings.
   d. The scalp tourniquet technique may be ineffective in preventing hair loss because of this drug's prolonged presence in the blood.
6. Management of Stomatitis:
   a. Administer preventive oral care every 4 hours and/or after meals.
   b. For preventive care, use a very soft toothbrush (child's) and toothpaste; avoid trauma to the tissues.
   c. Examine oral membranes at least once daily (instruct patient and/or family) to detect onset of inflammation and erythema.
   d. If stomatitis occurs, notify the physician and begin therapeutic oral care:[2]
      (1) *Mild Inflammation:* Remove dentures, use a soft toothbrush and a hydrogen peroxide solution (1 part peroxide and 4 parts saline). Do *not* use toothpaste. Rinse with the peroxide solution and then water. Replace dentures. This procedure should be carried out every 4 hours, and/or after meals.
      (2) *Severe Inflammation:* Remove dentures, use soft gauze pads rather than a toothbrush. Use the peroxide solution as described above. Rinse with water using an asepto syringe and gentle suction until returns are clear. Do not replace dentures. It may be necessary to give this care every 2–4 hours.
   e. Order a bland, mechanical soft diet for patients with inflammation. If severe stomatitis with ulceration is present, the patient may be placed on NPO status by the physician.
   f. For patients who can tolerate oral intake, administer Xylocaine Viscous or acetaminophen elixir as a mouthwash prior to meals to decrease pain (do not use aspirin rinses), as ordered by the physician.
   g. Patients with severe stomatitis may require parenteral analgesia.
7. Patients should be monitored for change in renal status for several months after discontinuation of therapy to detect the onset of renal insufficiency. Stress the importance of follow-up blood studies.

REFERENCES
1. Silver, Richard T., Lauper, R. David and Jarowski, Charles I.: *A Synopsis of Cancer Chemotherapy.* The York Medical Group, New York: Dun-Donnelly Publishing Company, 1977, p. 88.
2. Bruya, Margaret Auld, and Madeira, Nancy Powell: Stomatitis After Chemotherapy. *American Journal of Nursing,* 75(8):1351, August 1975.

SUGGESTED READINGS
Bruya, Margaret Auld, and Madeira, Nancy Powell: Stomatitis After Chemotherapy, *American Journal of Nursing,* 75(8):1349–1352, August 1975.
Giodquinta, Barbara: Helping Families Face the Crisis of Cancer. *American Journal of Nursing,* 77:1583–1588, October 1977.
Gullo, Shirley: Chemotherapy—What To Do About Special Side Effects. *RN,* 40:30–32, April 1977.

MORPHINE SULFATE

ACTIONS/ INDICATIONS	DOSAGE	PREPARATION AND STORAGE	DRUG INCOMPAT- IBILITIES	MODES OF IV ADMINISTRATION			CONTRAINDICATIONS; WARNINGS; PRECAUTIONS; ADVERSE REACTIONS
				INJECTION	INTERMITTENT INFUSION	CONTINUOUS INFUSION	
Narcotic analgesic. Affects psychic function, making the patient more tolerant of pain, and interferes centrally in the brain to decrease pain conduction. Depresses the respiratory center and cough reflex. For relief of severe pain and accompanying apprehension. In the treatment of pulmonary edema, this drug produces vasodilation (reduces venous return to the heart) and decreases anxiety. Maximum analgesic effect occurs in 20 minutes after IV injection, and lasts 4–7 hours.	*Range*— 5–20 mg. *Usual*— 10 mg for *adults*. May be repeated in 2–4 hrs. (Lower doses are required in patients concomitantly receiving other sedative or anesthetic drugs.) NOT ADMINISTERED INTRAVENOUSLY TO CHILDREN.	Supplied in ampuls of 8, 10, and 15 mg/ml, and disposable, prefilled syringes of the same concentrations. This is a Schedule II drug under the Controlled Substances Act of 1970. Maintain hospital or institutional regulations guiding its use.	Do not mix with any other medication. Do not inject into IV tubing containing: Aminophylline Heparin Methicillin Sodium bicarbonate Novobiocin Phenobarbital Sodium iodide Thiopental	YES Add dose to 10 ml sterile water for injection or NS. Administer through Y injection site or 3-way stopcock. Inject over 2–4 min.	NO Do not add to IV fluid.	NO Do not add to IV fluid.	CONTRAINDICATIONS 1. Bronchial asthma 2. Respiratory depression 3. Hypersensitivity WARNINGS 1. May be habit-forming, resulting in psychic and physical dependence. 2. Tolerance may develop after repeated doses. 3. Fatalities have occurred when this drug has been administered to patients with increased intracranial pressure, acute asthmatic attack, chronic obstructive lung disease, corpulmonale, pre-existing respiratory depression, hypoxia, or hypercapnia. 4. Severe hypotension may result in the presence of shock secondary to depleted blood volume; concomitant use of phenothiazines or certain anesthetics. 5. Syncope and orthostatic hypotension can occur in ambulatory patients. 6. Rapid IV injection or large doses will cause sudden respiratory depression. 7. Use in pregnancy requires consideration of the benefits versus the risks to mother and fetus. PRECAUTIONS 1. As an analgesic, this drug can mask important symptoms in head injuries (increasing intracranial pressure) and abdominal conditions (acute intestinal obstruction). 2. Caution is advised when administering the initial dose to elderly, debilitated patients, those with hepatic or renal dysfunction, history of asthma, hypothyroidism, toxic psychoses, Addison's disease, prostatic hypertrophy, or urethral stricture. These patients are more likely to exhibit severe adverse reactions. 3. In supraventricular tachyarrhythmias (atrial flutter, fibrillation or tachycardia), the ventricular rate may be increased by morphine. 4. There may be aggravation of convulsive disorders.

5. Reduce dosage when the patient is concomitantly receiving other narcotic analgesics, general anesthetics, phenothiazines, other tranquilizers, sedative-hypnotics, antidepressants, or any CNS depressant.
6. Nalorphine, narcotic antagonist, should be readily available to combat respiratory depression.

ADVERSE REACTIONS
1. Respiratory depression including respiratory arrest; bronchospasm
2. Circulatory depression (vasodilatation producing hypotension)
3. Minor effects: nausea, vomiting, light-headedness, sedation, diaphoresis (may be alleviated with a supine position)
4. Psychic changes: euphoria, agitation, hallucinations, confusion, visual changes
5. Constipation
6. Urinary retention, especially in the presence of prostatic hypertrophy or urethral stricture
7. Hypersensitivity: rash, urticaria, anaphylaxis

exacerbation of congestive heart failure secondary to rapid heart rate.
6. Seizure precaution in patients with a history of seizure.
7. Be prepared to manage hallucinations and disorientation.
8. Monitor for urinary retention in susceptible patients (see Adverse Reaction No. 6). Palpate bladder size every 4 hours; measure urinary output every 8 hours.
9. Patients on prolonged therapy may require laxatives or stool softeners to prevent constipation. Maintain hydration.
10. When scheduling doses, do not make the patient wait for total return of the pain before repeating a dose; to do so will reduce the effectiveness of the analgesic. Never withhold the drug when it is needed unless a contraindication arises, and then notify the physician for assistance.

SUGGESTED READINGS
Smith, Dorothy W., and Germain, Carol P. Hanley: *Care of the Adult Patient* (4th ed.), Philadelphia, J. B. Lippincott Company, 1975, Chapter 10, The Patient in Pain.
Mark, Lester C.: When to Use Narcotics Intravenously. *Drug Therapy* (Hospital Edition), June 1978, pp. 16–20.
McCaffery, Margo, and Hart, Linda: Undertreatment of Acute Pain with Narcotics. *American Journal of Nursing*, 76(10):1586–1591, October 1976.
Grad, Rae Krohn, and Woodside, Jack: Obstetrical Analgesics and Anesthesia: Methods of Relief for the Patient in Labor. *American Journal of Nursing*, 77(2):242–245, February 1977.
Vismara, Louis A., Mason, Dean T., and Amsterdam, Ezra A.: Cardiocirculatory Effects of Morphine Sulfate: Mechanisms of Action and Therapeutic Application. *Heart and Lung*, 3(3):495–499, May–June, 1974 (references).

NURSING IMPLICATIONS
1. Patient should be on bed rest with side rails up during, and for the first hour after, injection. Then ambulate with caution.
2. Respiratory support equipment must be readily available in the event of respiratory depression—narcotic antagonist agent: levallorphan tartrate (Lorfan, page 360), nalorphine HCl (Nalline, page 415), naloxone HCl (Narcan, page 417); airways, endotracheal tube and laryngoscope, suction, oxygen, manual breathing bag (Ambu, Hope, Puritan).
3. Monitor for respiratory depression: Count respiratory rate every 3–5 minutes during and after the injection for the first 15 minutes, then every 5–10 minutes for the next hour, then every 30 minutes for the next 2 hours. Repeat cycle for additional doses. If respiratory rate falls below 10/minute, notify physician and be prepared to assist ventilation. Observe for cyanosis (central: lips and tongue; peripheral: nailbeds), shallow respirations, change in mental status, and cardiac irregularities. Do not leave the patient unattended for the first 30 minutes. See Precaution No. 1.
   Take measures to prevent aspiration in the event of vomiting. Begin manual breathing assistance and use of airway if the patient cannot be aroused to increase his own respiratory rate and if the respiratory rate falls below 6 per minute or if cyanosis develops.
4. Monitor blood pressure and apical pulse before injection and every 3–5 minutes for the first 15 minutes, then every 5–10 minutes for the next hour, then every 30 minutes for the next 2 hours. The physician must determine acceptable blood pressure limits. Be prepared to treat hypotension with vasopressors.
5. Any patient with a supraventricular arrhythmia should be monitored with extreme care for an inordinate increase in ventricular rate. Notify physician if rate exceeds 110/minute. Such patients could develop or have an

NAFCILLIN, SODIUM (Nafcil, Unipen)

ACTIONS/ INDICATIONS	DOSAGE	PREPARATION AND STORAGE	DRUG INCOMPAT-IBILITIES	MODES OF IV ADMINISTRATION				CONTRAINDICATIONS; WARNINGS; PRECAUTIONS; ADVERSE REACTIONS
				INJECTION	INTERMITTENT INFUSION	CONTINUOUS INFUSION		
Semisynthetic penicillin. Antibiotic, penicillinase-resistant. Wide gram-positive spectrum. Used for infections due to: • *Staphylococcus aureus* • *Strep. pneumoniae* • Beta-hemolytic streptococcus • Alpha streptococcus. Susceptibility tests must be performed. (Usually used only in infections secondary to penicillinase-producing *Staph. aureus.*)	ADULTS: Dosage varies with severity of infection. 500–1000 mg every 4 hrs. (No need to adjust dosage in the presence of renal failure.) INFANTS AND CHILDREN: 60 mg/kg/24 hrs or 1.8 g/M²/24 hrs divided into 6 doses. For severe infections, double the above doses.[1]	To reconstitute powder, use sterile water for injection or bacteriostatic water for injection in the following volumes: 500 mg, add 1.7 ml, 1 gm, add 3.4 ml. 2 gm, add 6.8 ml. These solutions will contain 250 mg/ml. Solutions are stable for 3 days at room temperature or 7 days when refrigerated. May be frozen for up to 3 months. Available also in piggyback bottles for infusion. Dilute as follows: *1-gm bottle* — add 49 ml sterile water for injection or NS (concentration will be 20 mg/ml), or add 99 ml diluent to make a concentration of 10 mg/ml. *2-gm bottle* — add 49 ml sterile water for injection or NS (concentration will be 20 mg/ml), or add 99 ml diluent to	Do not mix in any manner with: Aminophylline Sodium bicarbonate Metaraminol Vitamins Gentamicin and other aminoglycosides Hydrocortisone	YES Into injection site of a running IV. Dilute dose in 15–30 ml sterile water for injection or NS. Administer over 5–10 min.	YES Use NS, D5W, D5/½ NS, RL, M/6 sodium lactate, in any appropriate amount, usually 100–200 ml. Infuse dose over 30–60 min.	YES Infusion must be completed in 24 hours. Use NS, D5W, D5/½ NS, RL, or M/6 sodium lactate, in an amount to make a concentration between 2–30 mg/ml.		CONTRAINDICATIONS Hypersensitivity to any penicillin WARNINGS 1. Anaphylaxis has been reported. 2. There may be cross-allergenicity with cephalosporins. PRECAUTIONS 1. Monitor renal, hepatic, and hematopoietic function before and during therapy, especially if therapy is prolonged. 2. Bacterial and fungal overgrowth of nonsusceptible organisms can occur. 3. Safety for use in pregnancy has not been established. 4. May cause thrombophlebitis at injection site. 5. Oral route should not be relied upon in patients with decreased gastrointestinal absorption, or who have gastrointestinal disturbances. ADVERSE REACTIONS 1. Hypersensitivity reactions: anaphylaxis, interstitial nephritis, neutropenia, rashes, serum sickness, cross-allergenicity with penicillin and cephalosporins[2] 2. Positive Coombs' test 3. Diarrhea 4. Glossitis and stomatitis (rare) 5. Overgrowth infections (1% of recipients)[3] 6. Thrombophlebitis at injection site.

make a concentration of 10 mg/ml.

4-gm bottle—add 97 ml diluent to make a concentration of 40 mg/ml.

NURSING IMPLICATIONS
1. Take anaphylaxis precautions; see page 118.
2. Management of glossitis and stomatitis:
   a. Therapeutic oral care:[4]
      (1) *Mild Inflammation:* Remove dentures; use a soft toothbrush and a hydrogen peroxide solution (1 part peroxide and 4 parts saline). Do not use toothpaste. Rinse with the peroxide solution and then water. Replace dentures. This procedure should be carried out every 4 hours, and/or after meals.
      (2) *Severe Inflammation and Ulceration:* Remove dentures; use soft gauze pads rather than a toothbrush. Use the peroxide solution as described above. Rinse with water using an asepto syringe and gentle suction until returns are clear. Do not replace dentures. Administer this care every 4 hours while the patient is awake.
   b. Order a bland, mechanical soft diet. The patient with severe inflammation and ulceration may be placed on NPO status.
   c. For patients who can tolerate oral intake, administer Xylocaine viscous or acetaminophen elixir as a mouthwash prior to meals to decrease pain (do not use aspirin rinses) as ordered by the physician.
   d. Maintain hydration with bland liquids (avoid fruit juices) and parenteral fluids if needed.

e. Severe inflammation and ulceration may require parenteral analgesia.
3. Monitor for overgrowth infections secondary to nonsusceptible organisms.
4. Monitor for signs and symptoms of overgrowth infections:
   a. Fever (take rectal temperature at least every 4–6 hours in all patients)
   b. Increasing malaise
   c. Newly appearing localized signs and symptoms: redness, soreness, pain, swelling, drainage (increased volume or change in character of pre-existing drainage)
   d. Monilial rash in perineal area (reddened areas with itching)
   e. Cough (change in pre-existing cough or sputum production)
   f. Diarrhea

REFERENCES
1. Shirkey, Harry C.: *Pediatric Drug Handbook,* Philadelphia: W. B. Saunders Company, 1977, p. 46.
2. Barza, Michael: Antimicrobial Spectrum, Pharmacology and Therapeutic Use of Antibiotics. Part 2: Penicillins. *American Journal of Pharmacy,* January 1977.
3. Ibid, p. 62.
4. Bruya, Margaret Auld, and Madeira, Nancy Powell: Stomatitis After Chemotherapy. *American Journal of Nursing,* 75(8):1351, August 1975.

NALORPHINE HYDROCHLORIDE (Nalline HCl Adult Concentration and Nalline HCl for Neonatal Use)

ACTIONS/ INDICATIONS	DOSAGE	PREPARATION AND STORAGE	DRUG INCOMPAT-IBILITIES	MODES OF IV ADMINISTRATION			CONTRAINDICATIONS; WARNINGS; PRECAUTIONS; ADVERSE REACTIONS
				INJECTION	INTERMITTENT INFUSION	CONTINUOUS INFUSION	
Narcotic antagonist; reverses respiratory depression caused by relative or absolute overdosage of morphine and narcotics related to morphine.

Used to prevent severe respiratory depression in | ADULTS: 5–10 mg repeated in 10–15 min as necessary. Effect lasts for 2–3 hrs. Doses as high as 40 mg may be given. Use adult concentration.

CHILDREN AND NEONATES: *Use neonatal* | If neonatal concentration is unavailable, dilute adult strength: 0.4 ml in 9.4 ml sterile water for injection. The resultant solution will be 0.2 mg/ml.

Discard all unused portions of ampuls.

(Adult concen- | Do not mix with any other medication in any manner. | YES

In adults, may be given undiluted into Y injection site or 3-way stopcock.

Inject over 30 seconds.

In neonates, dilute dose in 1 ml NS and inject into umbil- | NO | NO | CONTRAINDICATIONS
Respiratory depression not produced by narcotic agents. (See Precaution No. 3.)

WARNINGS
Do *not* use in asphyxia neonatorum due to conditions or agents other than the use of a morphine narcotic in the mother.

PRECAUTIONS
1. May induce violent withdrawal symptoms in morphine-addicted patients, and newborns of addicted mothers.
2. Will not counteract, but may *increase* respiratory depression due to non-nar- |

NALORPHINE HYDROCHLORIDE (Nalline HCl Adult Concentration and Nalline HCl for Neonatal Use) (Continued)

ACTIONS/ INDICATIONS	DOSAGE	PREPARATION AND STORAGE	DRUG INCOMPAT-IBILITIES	MODES OF IV ADMINISTRATION			CONTRAINDICATIONS; WARNINGS; PRECAUTIONS; ADVERSE REACTIONS
				INJECTION	INTERMITTENT INFUSION	CONTINUOUS INFUSION	
neonates resulting from narcotic use in the mother during labor and delivery; to prevent severe respiratory depression at the termination of IV narcotic anesthesia; to reverse narcosis in addicts; and to reverse significant respiratory depression caused by overdosage of or excessive response to a narcotic.	concentration — 0.1–0.2 mg/kg. (Inject into umbilical vein in neonates.) Repeat to a maximum of 0.5 mg.	tration: 5mg/ml; Neonatal concentration: 0.2 mg/ml) This is a Schedule III drug under the Controlled Substances Act of 1970. Maintain hospital or institutional regulations guiding its use.		ical vein over 15 seconds.			cotic agents or other causes. 3. In neonates, if first dose produces no effects, further use is contraindicated. 4. Overdose can result in respiratory depression. ADVERSE REACTIONS 1. Anxiety, lethargy, mild drowsiness, crying 2. Pseudoptosis (transient drooping of eyelid) 3. Diaphoresis, pallor 4. Hot and cold flushes

NURSING IMPLICATIONS

1. Respiratory depression can return if the duration of depressive effects of the narcotic last longer than the effects of nalorphine.
2. Place the following equipment at the bedside or nearby: oral-pharyngeal airways, endotracheal tubes and laryngoscope, suction, oxygen, manual breathing bag (Ambu, Hope, Puritan), arterial blood gas sampling equipment.
3. The patient should be under constant observation.
4. Monitor respiratory status; respiratory depression is the primary indication for the use of this drug and is diagnosed by the presence of hypercarbia (elevated pCO_2) and hypoxemia (reduced pO_2). Signs and symptoms of hypoxia include tachycardia, pallor, hypotension, confusion, restlessness.
5. Assist respirations until nalorphine is effective as indicated by an adequate spontaneous respiratory rate and return of gag, cough and swallow reflexes.
6. Examine frequently for signs of vomiting. Take precautions to prevent aspiration (position patient on one side, keep suction equipment ready to use, gastric intubation if abdominal distention is present).
7. Patients should be intubated if there is vomiting, if ventilation via airway and mask is ineffective (no improvement in arterial blood pO_2 or pCO_2) or if such support will be required for a prolonged period of time.
8. Monitor blood pressure and heart rate (apical or via ECG monitor) every 3–5 minutes until the patient has recovered and/or vital signs have reached desirable levels and stabilized (as determined by physician).
9. Patients with pre-existing ventricular irritability, secondary to pathology or drugs, should be placed on continuous ECG monitoring. Be prepared to treat ventricular tachycardia or fibrillation.
10. Be prepared to manage acute narcotic withdrawal symptoms in the narcotic addict. Use side rails at all times; restraints may be necessary.
11. Signs of acute withdrawal in the neonate:[1]
    a. Excessive irritability, crying, etc.
    b. Increased appetite, yet poor feeding ability
    c. Reduced sleeping periods
    d. Tremulousness
    e. Rarely seizures
    f. Diarrhea and vomiting
    g. Tachypnea
    h. Fever
    i. Sneezing
    Report the onset of any one of these signs to the physician.
12. Withdrawal of any form of support should be supervised by a physician.

REFERENCE

1. Kandall, Stephen R.: Managing Neonatal Withdrawal. *Drug Therapy*, May 1976, p. 48.

SUGGESTED READINGS

Kandall, Stephen R.: Managing Neonatal Withdrawal. *Drug Therapy*, May 1976, pp. 47–58.

McCaffery, Margo, and Hart, Linda: Undertreatment of Acute Pain With Narcotics. *American Journal of Nursing*, 76(10):1586–1591, October 1976.

Rogers, Robert M., and Juers, John A.: Physiologic Considerations in the Treatment of Acute Respiratory Failure. *Basics of Respiratory Disease*, 3(4), March 1975.

NALOXONE HYDROCHLORIDE (Narcan and Narcan Neonatal)

ACTIONS/ INDICATIONS	DOSAGE	PREPARATION AND STORAGE	DRUG INCOMPAT- IBILITIES	MODES OF IV ADMINISTRATION			CONTRAINDICATIONS; WARNINGS; PRECAUTIONS; ADVERSE REACTIONS
				INJECTION	INTERMITTENT INFUSION	CONTINUOUS INFUSION	
Narcotic antagonist. Does not produce respiratory depression seen in other narcotic antagonists. Exhibits no activity in the absence of a narcotic. Onset of action in 2 min. Used to reverse narcotic depression, including respiratory depression, induced by natural and synthetic narcotics, propoxyphene (Darvon) and pentazocine (Talwin).	ADULTS: *Narcotic overdosage*—0.4 mg (1 ml). Repeat at 2- to 3-min intervals as necessary. Failure after 2–3 doses indicates nonnarcotic source of depression. *Postoperative narcotic depression*—titrate with 0.1–0.2 mg at 2–3 min intervals. Objective is return of respiratory adequacy without loss of analgesia. CHILDREN AND NEONATES: *Narcotic overdosage*—0.01 mg/kg; repeat at 2- to 3-min intervals. Lack of response after 2–3 doses indicates nonnarcotic source of depression. Use only Neonatal Injection form.	*Adult strength solution*—0.4 mg/ml. *Neonatal strength*—0.02 mg/ml. Supplied in 1-ml vials. Do not add to fluids.	Do not mix with any other medication in any manner.	YES May be injected without further dilution directly into the vein (umbilical in neonates) or into the Y injection site of IV tubing.	NO Pharmacologically inappropriate.	NO Pharmacologically inappropriate.	CONTRAINDICATIONS Hypersensitivity WARNINGS 1. Administer with caution to any patient thought to be an opiate addict, including newborns. This drug will induce acute withdrawal. 2. Keep patients under constant surveillance. The duration of some narcotics may exceed that of naloxone. 3. This agent is not effective against respiratory depression secondary to nonopioid drugs or other conditions; can be used in respiratory depression secondary to pentazocine (Talwin), and propoxyphene (Darvon). 4. Safety for use in pregnancy has not been established; must be used only when benefits outweigh the potential risks. PRECAUTIONS 1. All other supportive measures for respiratory and circulatory depression must be applied. 2. Ventricular tachycardia and fibrillation have been reported in patients with pre-existing ventricular irritability, or who were on isoproterenal or epinephrine for hypotension. 3. In rare cases, rapid reversal of narcotic anesthesia in cardiac patients has resulted in pulmonary edema. ADVERSE REACTIONS 1. Nausea and vomiting (rarely seen) 2. Abrupt reversal of narcotic depression may result in diaphoresis, tachycardia, increased blood pressure, and tremulousness.

NURSING IMPLICATIONS
1. Respiratory depression can return if the duration of depressive effects of the narcotic last longer than the effects of naloxone.
2. Place the following equipment at the bedside or nearby: oral-pharyngeal airways, endotracheal tubes and laryngoscope, suction, oxygen, manual breathing bag (Ambu, Hope, Puritan), arterial blood gas sampling equipment.
3. The patient should be under constant observation.

417

NURSING IMPLICATIONS (Continued)

4. Monitor respiratory status; respiratory depression is the primary indication for the use of this drug and is diagnosed by the presence of hypercarbia (elevated pCO_2) and hypoxemia (reduced pO_2). Signs and symptoms of hypoxia include: tachycardia, pallor, hypotension, confusion, restlessness.
5. Assist respirations until naloxone is effective as indicated by an adequate spontaneous respiratory rate and return of gag, cough and swallow reflexes. (See no. 1 above.)
6. Examine frequently for signs of vomiting. Take precautions to prevent aspiration (position patient on one side, keep suction equipment ready to use, gastric intubation of abdominal distention is present).
7. Patients should be intubated if there is vomiting, if ventilation via airway and mask is ineffective (no improvement in arterial blood pO_2 or pCO_2) or if such support will be required for a prolonged period of time.
8. Monitor blood pressure and heart rate (apically or via ECG monitor) every 3–5 minutes until the patient has recovered and/or vital signs have reached desirable levels and stabilized (as determined by the physician).
9. Patients with pre-existing ventricular irritability, secondary to pathology or drugs, should be placed on continuous ECG monitoring. Be prepared to treat ventricular tachycardia or fibrillation.
10. Be prepared to manage acute narcotic withdrawal symptoms in the narcotic addict. Use side rails at all times; restraints may be necessary.
11. Signs of acute withdrawal in the neonate:[1]
    a. Excessive irritability, crying, etc.
    b. Increased appetite, yet poor feeding ability
    c. Reduced sleeping periods
    d. Tremulousness
    e. Rarely seizures
    f. Diarrhea and vomiting
    g. Tachypnea
    h. Fever
    i. Sneezing
    Report the onset of any one of these signs to the physician.
12. Withdrawal of any form of support should be supervised by a physician.

REFERENCE

1. Kandall, Stephen R.: Managing Neonatal Withdrawal. *Drug Therapy,* May 1976, p. 48.

SUGGESTED READINGS

Kandall, Stephen R.: Managing Neonatal Withdrawal. *Drug Therapy,* May 1976, pp. 47–58.

McCaffery, Margo, and Hart, Linda: Undertreatment of Acute Pain With Narcotics. *American Journal of Nursing,* 76(10):1586–1591, October 1976.

Rogers, Robert M., and Juers, John A.: Physiologic Considerations in the Treatment of Acute Respiratory Failure. *Basics of Respiratory Disease,* 3(4), March 1975.

● NEOSTIGMINE METHYLSULFATE (Prostigmin)

ACTIONS/INDICATIONS	DOSAGE	PREPARATION AND STORAGE	DRUG INCOMPATIBILITIES	MODES OF IV ADMINISTRATION			CONTRAINDICATIONS; WARNINGS; PRECAUTIONS; ADVERSE REACTIONS
				INJECTION	INTERMITTENT INFUSION	CONTINUOUS INFUSION	
Cholinesterase inhibitor; enhances transmission of impulses at nerve-muscle junction. *Intravenous route* is indicated as an antidote for tubocurarine or curarelike drugs, e.g., pancuronium. Also can be used in emergency management of myasthenia gravis.	ADULTS AND OLDER CHILDREN: 0.5–2.0 mg. Do not exceed 5 mg. SMALL CHILDREN, CARDIAC PATIENTS, SEVERELY ILL: Titrate an exact dose using 0.2–0.5 mg/kg increments and a nerve-stimulating device. The heart rate should be increased pharmaco-	Supplied in the following forms: 1-ml ampuls, 1:2000 (0.5 mg/ml) 1-ml ampuls, 1:4000 (0.25 mg/ml) 10-ml multi-dose vials, 1:1000 (1 mg/ml) 10-ml multi-dose vials, 1:2000 (0.5 mg/ml)	Do not mix with any other medication.	YES May give undiluted *slowly* 0.5 mg/min.	NO Pharmacologically inappropriate.	NO Pharmacologically inappropriate.	CONTRAINDICATIONS 1. Mechanical intestinal or urinary obstruction 2. Hypersensitivity PRECAUTIONS 1. Use with caution in asthmatics. 2. Atropine (1 mg) should be at the bedside. Some groups administer 0.5 mg of atropine prior to neostigmine. 3. Atropine may be used to abolish or decrease gastrointestinal side effects of this drug but can mask overdosage and lead to inadvertent induction of a cholinergic crisis, and should therefore be given in small doses, carefully titrated with patient response. 4. Overdose may result in a cholinergic crisis characterized by increasing muscular weakness involving respiratory muscles; apnea may result. This

logically (with atropine) to 80/min before neostigmine is administered (see Precaution No. 2).

Do not administer in the presence of high concentrations of halothane or cyclopropane.

Do not mix with fluids.

may be difficult to distinguish from a myasthenic crisis. Such distinction *must* be made to avoid grave consequences. Tension test (edrophonium) may be used to differentiate between cholinergic and myasthenic crises. See page 310.

ADVERSE REACTIONS
1. Usually due to overdosage: nausea, vomiting, diarrhea, cramps, increased salivation, increased bronchial secretions, diaphoresis. These can be counteracted by *careful* use of atropine 0.5 mg (see Precautions Nos. 2–4). Other symptoms of overdosage are muscle cramps, muscle twitching, and weakness.
2. Bradycardia may also occur, and can be treated with atropine if necessary.

Keep the patient in lateral decubitus position if possible; keep suction equipment ready for use.

SUGGESTED READINGS
Guyton, Arthur C.: *Textbook of Medical Physiology* (5th ed.), Philadelphia, W. B. Saunders Company, 1976; Chapter 12, Neuromuscular Transmission, Function of Smooth Muscle, pp. 147–157; Chapter 15, The Autonomic Nervous System; The Adrenal Medulla, pp. 768–781.
Jones, LeAnna: Myasthenia and Me. *RN*, June 1976, pp. 50–55.
Smith, Dorothy W., and Germain, Carol P. Hanley: *Care of the Adult Patient*, (4th ed.), Philadelphia, J. B. Lippincott Company, 1977, pp. 382–384.

NURSING IMPLICATIONS
1. Maintain an adequate airway and ventilation until recovery is complete and spontaneous respiration is obtained.
2. Respiratory support equipment (airways, oxygen, suction, endotracheal tubes and laryngoscope, manual breathing bag [Ambu, Hope, Puritan]) should be readily available or in use until respiratory effort, rate, and effectiveness are appropriate and gag, cough, swallow reflexes have returned. (See care of the patient receiving tubocurarine, p. 516.)
3. Atropine 1.0 mg should be at the bedside. (See administration of atropine, p. 194.)
4. Monitor for adverse effects (see above).
5. Be prepared to manage vomiting to maintain airway and prevent aspiration.

● NITROPRUSSIDE, SODIUM (Nipride)

ACTIONS/ INDICATIONS	DOSAGE	PREPARATION AND STORAGE	DRUG INCOMPAT- IBILITIES	MODES OF IV ADMINISTRATION			CONTRAINDICATIONS; WARNINGS; PRECAUTIONS; ADVERSE REACTIONS
				INJECTION	INTERMITTENT INFUSION	CONTINUOUS INFUSION	
Antihypertensive, potent and rapid-acting. Effect is immediate and ends on stopping infusion. Has direct action on blood vessel walls to produce vasodilatation.	ADULTS AND CHILDREN: Average dose in the absence of any other antihypertensive agent: 3 mcg/kg/min. *Range*—0.5–10.0 mcg/kg/min.	Reconstitute by adding 2–3 ml D5W to vial. Prepare for infusion by adding 50 mg of drug to 500 ml D5W *only*. This solution contains 100 mcg/ml (50 mg can also be added to 250 ml D5W	Do not mix with any other medication in bottle or line.	NO	NO	YES Use D5W only. See next column for preparation. USE INFUSION PUMP AND MICRODROP TUBING.	CONTRAINDICATIONS 1. Compensatory hypertension in A-V shunt or coarctation of the aorta 2. During surgery for controlled hypotension, in patients with known inadequate cerebral circulation WARNINGS 1. Use only dextrose 5% and water for reconstitution and infusion. 2. This drug is metabolized into thiocyanate. Excess infusion of nitroprusside can result in thiocyanate toxicity (tin-

● NITROPRUSSIDE, SODIUM (Nipride) (Continued)

ACTIONS/ INDICATIONS	DOSAGE	PREPARATION AND STORAGE	DRUG INCOMPAT- IBILITIES	MODES OF IV ADMINISTRATION			CONTRAINDICATIONS; WARNINGS; PRECAUTIONS; ADVERSE REACTIONS
				INJECTION	INTERMITTENT INFUSION	CONTINUOUS INFUSION	
Used to control hypertensive crisis in essential and malignant hypertension, acute glomerulonephritis, eclampsia, and dissecting aortic aneurysm. Also used by some groups for vasodilation in acute myocardial infarction and pump failure. (The use of this drug in this manner has not been approved by the FDA). Nitroprusside can also be used to produce controlled hypotension during surgery to decrease bleeding.	TITRATE WITH ARTERIAL BLOOD PRESSURE. Infusion rates greater than 10 mcg/kg/ min should not be used. If at this rate an adequate reduction of BP is not obtained in 10 min, STOP INFUSION. Infusion is usually continued for 24–48 hours while oral antihypertensive therapy is initiated.	to produce a solution of 200 mcg/ml). Promptly wrap IV bottle with aluminum wrap provided by manufacturer to protect the solution from light.* Use within 4 hours of preparation. Discard solution that is any color besides light brown. USE INFUSION PUMP AND MICRODROP TUBING. With the 100 mcg/ml solution, there is 1.5 mcg/ microdrop of solution. *It is not necessary to wrap the IV tubing because the time spent by the drug in the tubing is minimal.					nitus, blurred vision, delirium, muscle spasm). Gross overdosage can produce *cyanide* toxicity. 3. Thiocyanate inhibits uptake and binding of iodine. Use with caution in hypothyroidism. 4. Use with caution in severe renal impairment. Therapy should be guided by serum thiocyanate levels (not to exceed 10 mg/100 ml). 5. Chronically hypertensive patients and those receiving other antihypertensive agents are more sensitive to the action of this drug. Careful titration with blood pressure will prevent overdosage. 6. Safety for use in pregnancy has not been established. Benefits to the mother must outweigh potential hazards to the fetus. 7. Safety for use in children has not been established. 8. A rebound tachycardia may occur secondary to reduction in blood pressure. In patients where such a tachycardia could be detrimental (congestive heart failure, aortic aneurysm), pretreat with propranolol to reduce sinus rate (see page 473 for further information on propranolol). 9. Correct preexisting anemia and hypovolemia prior to administration of this drug. PRECAUTIONS 1. The patient must be under constant surveillance. Means by which to monitor direct arterial blood pressure (preferred) or indirect pressure (acceptable) must be employed. 2. Infusion rates greater than 10 mcg/ kg are rarely required. If adequate reduction in blood pressure is not seen at this rate, stop the infusion. 3. Avoid extravasation. ADVERSE REACTIONS 1. Nausea, vomiting, diaphoresis, abdominal pain, chest pain, anxiety, headache, restlessness, muscle twitching, dizziness, are usually due to

rapid infusion and disappear with decreased flow rate.
2. Cyanide toxicity; see Warning Nos. 2, 3, 4.
3. Irritation of vein at infusion site.

OVERDOSAGE
1. First sign is profound hypotension.
2. Metabolic acidosis may be an early indication of overdosage, and may be associated with dyspnea, headache, vomiting, dizziness, ataxia, loss of consciousness.
3. Infusion must be stopped with the appearance of any of the above.
4. Massive overdosage may produce signs similar to those of cyanide poisoning: coma, imperceptible peripheral pulses, absent reflexes, widely dilated pupils, pink skin color, hypotension and shallow breathing.
5. Treatment:
   a. Discontinue Nitroprusside.
   b. Administer amyl nitrite inhalations for 15–30 seconds each minute until a 3% sodium nitrite solution can be prepared for IV administration.
   c. Inject 3% sodium nitrite IV at a rate not to exceed 2.5–5.0 ml/minute up to a total dose of 10–15 ml with careful monitoring of blood pressure. Use vasopressors to correct hypotension.
   d. Following the above steps, inject sodium thiosulfate IV, 12.5 gm in 50 ml of D5W, over a 10-minute period.
   e. Signs of overdosage may reappear. If this occurs, repeat above therapy at 1/2 dosage.

to monitor serum thiocyanate levels. (Toxic signs and symptoms appear at serum levels of 5–10 mg/100 ml.; fatalities have occurred at levels of 20 mg/100 ml.[1]) Continue close monitoring of blood pressure. (See treatment of overdosage above.)
6. Monitor for the consequences of sudden severe elevation of blood pressure:
   a. Encephalopathy—confusion, stupor
   b. Cerebrovascular accident—muscle paralysis or weakness
   c. Myocardial ischemia and/or infarction—chest pain, ECG changes, arrhythmias
   d. Left ventricular failure—shortness of breath, orthopnea, elevated central venous pressure or pulmonary artery (wedge) pressure, tachycardia, rales, third and/or fourth heart sound
   e. Renal failure—oliguria, rising BUN and creatinine.[2]
   Prevent a sudden fall in blood pressure below normal levels for the patient. Hypotension can also produce the complications listed above. If the

NURSING IMPLICATIONS
1. Be prepared to accurately monitor arterial blood pressure, preferably by arterial cannulation. If this type of monitoring is unavailable, indirect readings using a sphygmomanometer can be used.
2. Monitor the ECG continuously during therapy.
3. Weigh the patient for dosage calculation.
4. Keeping in mind the patient's pretreatment blood pressure, begin the infusion at 0.5–1.0 mcg/kg/minute (approximately 1 microdrop/kg/minute using 100 mcg/ml solution). A lower dosage will be prescribed for renal patients. Obtain blood pressure readings every 1–2 minutes. The physician must determine the blood pressure goal to be reached by therapy. Increase the infusion every 5 minutes by 0.5–1.0 mcg/kg/min (or 5 microdrops) until the blood pressure goal has been reached.
5. Monitor for signs and symptoms of toxicity: ringing in the ears, blurring of vision, delirium, muscle spasms. If one or more of these effects occur, decrease the infusion rate immediately. Notify the physician, who may want

● NITROPRUSSIDE, SODIUM (Nipride) (Continued)

NURSING IMPLICATIONS (No. 6 continued)

patient is receiving nitroprusside for hypertension associated with an acute myocardial infarction, the physician must differentiate between chest pain caused by the pathology or by the drug, and then order adjustment in drug dosage.[3]

7. Keep the patient on bed rest.

8. After allowing the first dose of the oral antihypertensive agent to begin effects, the infusion to nitroprusside can be discontinued abruptly. Keep the infusion connected to the IV line, ready for reinitiation in the event the blood pressure has not been controlled by the oral agent.

9. Monitor urine output hourly. Excessive reduction of arterial pressure will decrease the urine output. If this occurs, reduce the infusion rate by 1 mcg every 5 minutes until urine output improves. Notify the physician.

10. Provide instruction on hypertension self-care prior to the patient's discharge from the hospital.

REFERENCES

1. Palmer, Roger F. and Lasseter, Kenneth C.: Sodium Nitroprusside. *New England Journal of Medicine*, 292(6):295, February 6, 1975.

2. Romankiewicz, J. A.: Pharmacology and Clinical Use of Drugs in Hypertensive Emergencies. *American Journal of Hospital Pharmacy*, 34(2):185, February 1977.

3. Ziesch, Susan and Franciosa, Joseph: Clinical Application of Sodium Nitroprusside. *Heart and Lung*, 6:102, January–February 1977.

SUGGESTED READINGS

American Medical Association Committee on Hypertension: The Treatment of Malignant Hypertension and Hypertensive Emergencies. *JAMA*, 228: 1673–1679, June 24, 1974.

Jones, L. N.: Symposium on Teaching and Rehabilitation of the Cardiac Patient. Hypertension: Medical and Nursing Implications. *Nursing Clinics of North America*, 11:283–295, June 1976 (references).

Keith, Thomas: Hypertension Crisis, Recognition and Management. *JAMA*, 237(15):1570–1577, April 11, 1977.

Koch-Wiser, Jan: Hypertensive Emergencies. *New England Journal of Medicine*, 290:211–214, January 24, 1974.

Kohli, R. K., et al.: Treating Acute Hypertensive Crisis With Sodium Nitroprusside. *American Family Physician*, 15(1):141–145, January 1977.

Long, M. L., et al.: Hypertension: What Patients Need to Know. *American Journal of Nursing*, 76:765–770, May 1976.

Moskowitz, Lani: Vasodilator Therapy in Acute Myocardial Infarction. *Heart and Lung*, 4(6):939–942, November–December 1975.

Palmer, Roger F. and Lasseter, Kenneth C.: Sodium Nitroprusside. *New England Journal of Medicine*, 292:294–296, February 6, 1975.

Romankiewicz, J. A.: Pharmacology and Clinical Use of Drugs in Hypertensive Emergencies. *American Journal of Hospital Pharmacy*, 34(2):185–193, February 1977 (references).

Ziesch, Susan, and Franciosa, Joseph: Clinical Application of Sodium Nitroprusside. *Heart and Lung*, 6:99–103, January–February 1977.

● NOVOBIOCIN (Albamycin)

ACTIONS/ INDICATIONS	DOSAGE	PREPARATION AND STORAGE	DRUG INCOMPATIBILITIES	MODES OF IV ADMINISTRATION			CONTRAINDICATIONS; WARNINGS; PRECAUTIONS; ADVERSE REACTIONS
				INJECTION	INTERMITTENT INFUSION	CONTINUOUS INFUSION	
Antibiotic used to treat infections due to Staphylococcus. Especially useful in infections resistant to other antibiotics. Used in Proteus urinary tract infections.	ADULTS: 500 mg. every 12 hours, depending on severity of infection. CHILDREN: *Newborns and premature* — 15 mg/kg/24 hrs in 2–3 divided doses. Severe infections may require 30 mg/kg daily (in divided 12-hr doses).	Supplied in a "Mix-O-Vial" (Upjohn), with diluent provided. Press rubber plunger stopper with a turning motion. Shake gently to mix. Use within 48 hours.	Do not mix with any other medications (many incompatibilities).	YES Dilute in 30–50 ml NS and inject over 5- to 10-minute period.	YES Add dose to 50–100 ml NS and infuse over 15–30 minutes.	YES Add 12-hr dose to 250–1000 ml NS and infuse over 12 hours.	CONTRAINDICATIONS Hypersensitivity WARNINGS 1. Use only for serious infections when less toxic agents cannot be employed or are ineffective. 2. There is a high incidence of allergy, hepatic dysfunction, and blood dyscrasias in the use of this drug. 3. Rapidly emerging resistant organisms, especially staphylococci, are frequently seen. 4. Safe use in pregnancy and lactation has not been established. 5. A high incidence of jaundice due to hyperbilirubinemia in infants has been reported. Avoid use in all children under 1 year of age unless no other agent can be used.

*Older infants
and children*—
15–30 mg/
kg/24 hrs in 2
divided doses.
Continue ther-
apy for at least
48 hrs after
patient is afe-
brile

NURSING IMPLICATIONS
1. Take anaphylaxis precautions; see page 118.
2. Be aware of the patient's complete blood count on a daily basis. This drug can reduce white cell and platelet counts. Notify the physician if changes in these values are seen on the CBC. If this occurs, the drug should be discontinued immediately.
3. Monitor for signs and symptoms of overgrowth infections:
   a. Fever (take rectal temperature at least every 4–6 hours in all patients)
   b. Increasing malaise
   c. Newly appearing localized signs and symptoms: redness, soreness, pain, swelling, drainage (increased volume or change in character of pre-existing drainage)
   d. Monilial rash in perineal area (reddened areas with itching)
   e. Cough (change in pre-existing cough or sputum production)
   f. Diarrhea
4. Monitor for the onset of jaundice. If hepatic toxicity occurs (indicated by jaundice and rise in serum bilirubin), the next dose of this drug should be held, and the physician notified.

PRECAUTIONS
1. Monitor total and differential blood cell counts and liver function test during therapy.
2. Discontinue if jaundice or hyperbilirubinemia occurs, unless no other agent can be used. Monitor hepatic function daily.
3. Monitor for overgrowth or superinfections. Discontinue novobiocin at that time and initiate appropriate therapy.
4. Discontinue if allergic reactions occur which cannot be eliminated with antihistamines.

ADVERSE REACTIONS
1. Hypersensitivity: rash, Stevens-Johnson syndrome (rare), anaphylaxis
2. Blood dyscrasias: pancytopenia, leukopenia, agranulocytosis, anemia, thrombocytopenia
3. Hepatic dysfunction indicated by jaundice and rise in serum bilirubin (especially common in newborns)
4. Hair loss
5. Pain at injection site
6. Gastrointestinal: nausea, vomiting, diarrhea
7. Overgrowth infections secondary to nonsusceptible organisms

5. Nausea and vomiting may be controlled with antiemetics. Administer these drugs prior to meals if necessary. Maintain hydration. Monitor intake and output if vomiting is uncontrolled by drugs. The physician will probably initiate parenteral fluid replacement and discontinue the novobiocin. Diarrhea should also be controlled with diphenoxylate hydrochloride (Lomotil) or a similar agent. Again, intake and ouput must be monitored to insure adequate fluid replacement. If symptoms are uncontrolled, the novobiocin should be discontinued. Monitor for signs of hypokalemia (weakness, muscle cramps) if diarrhea is present.
6. Hair loss is rare. However, if signs of this adverse effect are noted, inform the physician immediately. Reassure the patient that this is a transient effect of the drug. If hair loss is pronounced, provide privacy for the patient; allow him time to express concern about this disfigurement.
7. If infusions cause pain at the injection site, apply warm compresses over the affected vein. Monitor for signs of thrombophlebitis; e.g., redness and swelling along the vein tract. If this occurs, discontinue the infusion and use another vein. Follow dilution and infusion rate guidelines carefully.

ORPHENADRINE CITRATE (Norflex Injectable)

ACTIONS/ INDICATIONS	DOSAGE	PREPARATION AND STORAGE	DRUG INCOMPAT- IBILITIES	MODES OF IV ADMINISTRATION			CONTRAINDICATIONS; WARNINGS; PRECAUTIONS; ADVERSE REACTIONS
				INJECTION	INTERMITTENT INFUSION	CONTINUOUS INFUSION	
Centrally acting skeletal muscle relaxant and anti-cholinergic, sedative. Used as an adjunct to rest and physical therapy to relieve pain associated with acute, painful musculoskeletal conditions.	ADULTS: 60 mg (1 ampul) Repeat every 12 hrs. Use oral form for maintenance. CHILDREN: Not recommended.	Supplied in 2-ml ampuls, 30 mg/ml.	Do not mix with any other medication in any manner.	YES Undiluted at a rate of 30 mg/ min.	NO	NO	CONTRAINDICATIONS 1. Glaucoma 2. Pyloric or duodenal obstruction 3. Stenosing peptic ulcers 4. Obstruction of bladder neck 5. Cardiospasm (megaesophagus) 6. Myasthenia gravis 7. Hypersensitivity WARNINGS 1. Dizziness and syncope may occur following injection. 2. Safety for use in pregnancy, lactation, or children has not been established. 3. If prolonged use is planned, monitor hepatic and renal function. ADVERSE REACTIONS 1. Dryness of mouth 2. Larger doses: tachycardia, urinary retention, blurred vision, increased intraocular pressure, nausea, weakness, vomiting, headache 3. Hallucinations, anxiety, agitation 4. Hypersensitivity 5. Rarely—aplastic anemia

NURSING IMPLICATIONS
1. Monitor for signs of increased intraocular pressure: severe ocular pain, nausea and vomiting, decreasing vision, patient sees rainbows around lights.[1]
2. Palpate bladder size every 4 hours and measure urine output every 8 hours to detect urinary retention.
3. Observe for mental confusion and hallucinations. Reassurance and safety precautions such as restraints and side rails may be needed.
4. Ambulate with caution; there may be mild dizziness, blurred vision and weakness.
5. Take anaphylaxis precautions, see page 118.

REFERENCE
1. Newell, Frank W., and Ernest, J. Terry: *Ophthalmology—Principles and Concepts* (3rd ed.), St. Louis: C. V. Mosby Company, 1974, p. 337.

OUABAIN (Strophanthin-G)

ACTIONS/ INDICATIONS	DOSAGE	PREPARATION AND STORAGE	DRUG INCOMPAT- IBILITIES	MODES OF IV ADMINISTRATION			CONTRAINDICATIONS; WARNINGS; PRECAUTIONS; ADVERSE REACTIONS
				INJECTION	INTERMITTENT INFUSION	CONTINUOUS INFUSION	
Short-acting cardiac glycoside, with the same effects as digitalis.	ADULTS: *Initial*—0.25 mg. *Full digitalizing*	Supplied in 2-ml ampuls, 0.25 mg/ml. Do not add to	Do not mix with any other medication in syringe.	YES Over 1–2 minutes.	NO Cannot be mixed with flu-ids.	NO Cannot be mixed with flu-ids.	CONTRAINDICATIONS Digitalis toxicity WARNINGS Administration should be discontinued if

Used to produce rapid digitalization in acute congestive heart failure and in the management of atrial tachyarrhythmias.

This is the most rapid-acting digitalis preparation available. Full effect is seen within 2 hours of injection.

dose—0.50 mg can be given initially, then 0.1-mg increments hourly until digitalization is reached at 1.0 mg.

Maintenance is obtained with digoxin or digitoxin.

CHILDREN: 0.3 mg/M²/ dose (0.01 mg/kg/dose), one-half dose immediately then fractions of the dose every 30 min. until response is seen or total dose given.[1]

IV fluids; this drug is unstable when diluted.

nausea, vomiting, or arrhythmia occurs. These are signs of digitalis toxicity.

PRECAUTIONS
1. The patient must be monitored electrocardiographically during therapy to detect the onset of arrhythmias due to toxicity (usually premature ventricular contractions, conduction defects, and sinus bradycardia).
2. Administer with caution to patients who have received digitalis preparations in the past 2–3 weeks. These patients will require lower dosage of ouabain.
3. Arrhythmias that this drug is used to treat may be produced by digitalis toxicity. Discontinue injections if arrhythmias become more severe.

TREATMENT OF DIGITALIS TOXICITY
1. Discontinue the drug at the first suspicion of toxicity, and do not reinitiate until signs and symptoms of toxicity subside.
2. Initiate continuous ECG monitoring if not already present.
3. Maintain a normal serum potassium (3.5–5.5 mEq/liter), but do *not* administer intravenous potassium in the presence of advanced or complete heart block secondary to digitalis toxicity; the block may increase.[2]
4. Pharmacologic treatment of toxicity should be guided by the arrhythmia produced. Phenytoin (Dilantin) is usually the drug of choice. Quinidine, lidocaine, procainamide, and propranolol can also be used depending on the clinical situation. (If propranolol is used, monitor atrioventricular conduction closely. This drug may cause increasing A-V block.) Atropine can be used to treat bradyarrhythmias. See entries for each drug for further details on their use.
5. If profound bradycardia and/or complete A-V block occur, transvenous temporary pacing may be necessary until toxicity resolves.

NURSING IMPLICATIONS
1. Patients receiving this medication intravenously should, in most instances, be observed for arrhythmias via continuous ECG monitoring. Observe for improvement if the drug is given to treat an arrhythmia, and observe for arrhythmias which may be produced by the drug (see Precaution No. 1). Some of the more common arrhythmias produced by toxic levels of ouabain are sinus bradycardia, premature ventricular and atrial contractions, atrioventricular block of all degrees, paroxysmal atrial tachycardia. Notify the physician of improvement in the arrhythmia being treated and document with an ECG tracing. If arrhythmias of toxicity appear, notify the physician, document with an ECG tracing, and hold the next dose of ouabain until the physician decides what course of action is appropriate.
2. Be prepared to administer immediate care in the event of arrhythmias due to toxicity. (See Treatment of Digitalis Toxicity above.) Atropine 0.5–1.0 mg can be given for a heart rate less than 50–60/minute. (In units where registered nurses are expected to administer drugs in such an event, the unit

OUABAIN (Strophanthin-G) (Continued)

NURSING IMPLICATIONS (No. 2 continued)
physician should decide at what heart rate the atropine should be administered and in what amount.) See page 194 for details on atropine.

For premature ventricular contractions or ventricular tachycardia, lidocaine 50–100 mg can be given by intravenous injection. Again, unit policy should dictate when and how much drug is given. See page 365 for details on lidocaine.

3. Observe for noncardiac symptoms of digitalis toxicity: anorexia; nausea; vomiting and diarrhea; visual disturbances, e.g., rainbow vision or yellow vision (rare); in children, poor feeding and irritability; headache (rare); confusion (rare); severe fatigue.[3]

4. Monitor for signs of improvement if the patient is being treated for congestive heart failure:
   a. Reduction in weight (weigh the patient daily)
   b. Reduction in peripheral edema
   c. Increased urine output (measure every 8 hours)
   d. Decreased resting heart rate to normal limits (record every 4–8 hours)
   e. Decreased respiratory rate, disappearance of rales
   f. Increased exercise tolerance
   Note that worsening congestive failure despite digitalis administration may be a sign of digitalis toxicity.

5. Be aware of the patient's serum potassium. Hypokalemia can precipitate digitalis toxicity. Administer potassium supplements as ordered. These may produce nausea and vomiting (liquid preparations especially) usually soon after administration. The nurse's observations will be needed to differentiate between potassium-induced nausea and vomiting and that due to digitalis toxicity. (Normal serum potassium: 3.5–55 mEq/liter).

6. Rarely, elderly patients experience hallucinations, anxiety, and delusions secondary to toxic levels of digitalis preparations. Monitor for onset of this complication; notify the physician and initiate safety measures.

7. Patients who will require a digitalis preparation on a chronic basis must be instructed on safe self-administration of the digitalis. Points that must be presented are:
   a. The actions of the drug, what it can and cannot do for the patient
   b. Correct daily dosage
   c. Pulse-taking (if possible, not absolutely required), and what to do if arrhythmias occur
   d. Signs and symptoms of toxicity and what to do if they appear
   e. Need for follow-up care
   f. Potassium intake
   g. Diet, activity, etc., necessary for general care of congestive heart failure
   The patient and/or family should be able to demonstrate and verbalize knowledge of these areas.

REFERENCES
1. Shirkey, Harry C.: Pediatric Drug Handbook, Philadelphia: W. B. Saunders Company, 1977, p. 135.
2. Davis, Richard H., and Risch, Charles: Potassium and Arrhythmias. *Geriatrics*, November 1970, p. 110.
3. Lely, A. H., and van Enter, C. H. J.: Noncardiac Symptoms of Digitalis Intoxication. *American Heart Journal*, 83(2):150, February 1972.

SUGGESTED READINGS
Amsterdam, Ezra A., et al.: Systemic Approach to the Management of Cardiac Arrhythmias. *Heart and Lung*, 2(5):747–753, September–October 1973 (references).
Arbeit, Sidney, et al.: Recognizing Digitalis Toxicity. *American Journal of Nursing*, 77(12):1936–1945, December 1977 (references).
Isacson, Lauren Marie, and Schultz, Klaus: Treating Pulmonary Edema. *Nursing 78*, February 1978, pp. 42–46.
Lely, A. H., and vanEnter, C. G. J.: Noncardiac Symptoms of Digitalis Intoxication. *American Heart Journal*, 83(2):149–152, February 1972.
Rosen, Michael R., Wit, Andrew, and Hoffman, Brian F.: Electrophysiology and Pharmacology of Cardiac Arrhythmias. IV Cardiac Antiarrhythmic and Toxic Effects of Digitalis. *American Heart Journal*, 89(3):391–399, March 1975 (references).
Treatment of Cardiac Arrhythmias. *Medical Letter on Drugs and Therapeutics*, 16(25):101–108, December 6, 1974.
Tanner, Gloria: Heart Failure in the MI Patient. *American Journal of Nursing*, 77:230–234, February 1977.

OXACILLIN SODIUM (Prostaphlin, Bactocil)

ACTIONS/ INDICATIONS	DOSAGE	PREPARATION AND STORAGE	DRUG INCOMPATIBILITIES	MODES OF IV ADMINISTRATION			CONTRAINDICATIONS; WARNINGS; PRECAUTIONS; ADVERSE REACTIONS
				INJECTION	INTERMITTENT INFUSION	CONTINUOUS INFUSION	
Antibiotic, penicillinase-resistant penicillin. Used to treat infections due to penicillinase-producing staphylococci. Sen-	ADULTS AND CHILDREN OVER 40 KG: *Mild to moderate infections of upper respiratory tract, skin, and soft tissue* — 250–500 mg every	Reconstitute with: sterile water for injection or sodium chloride injection as follows:	Do not mix with any other medication in an IV bottle and do not inject into an IV line containing: Penicillin Aminoglyco-	YES Dilute the reconstituted solution further with an equal amount of NS. Inject over 10 min.	YES Dilute each gm of dose with 50 ml. Infuse over 20 min. Use any fluid listed in Continuous Infusion column.	YES Add 6-hr dose to any of the following IV solutions: NS D5W D5/NS 10% fructose	CONTRAINDICATIONS Hypersensitivity to any penicillin WARNINGS There may be cross-allergenicity to cephalosporins. Use with caution in patients with this hypersensitivity. PRECAUTIONS 1. There can be bacterial or fungal over-

sitivity tests must be performed. Also may be effective in infections caused by *Strep. pneumonae,* Group A beta-hemolytic streptococci, pneumococci, and nonpenicillinase-producing staphylococci.

4–6 hrs.

Severe infections of lower respiratory tract or disseminated infections—1 gm or more every 4–6 hrs.

CHILDREN LESS THAN 40 KG, OVER 2 WEEKS OF AGE:
Mild to moderate infections—50 mg/kg/24 hrs in equally divided doses every 6 hrs.

Severe infections—100 mg/kg/day given in equally divided doses every 6 hrs. Infections due to Group A beta-hemolytic streptococci must be treated for at least 10 days to prevent rheumatic fever.

NEONATES UNDER 2 WEEKS OF AGE:
50 mg/kg/24 hrs in equally divided doses every 6 hrs.

RENAL IMPAIRMENT:
In mild impairment, no change in dosage is necessary. In uremia the dosage should be reduced to 1 gm every 6 hours for *adults.* Administer after dialysis.[1]

---

side antibiotics
Tetracycline

Vial Size	Vol. Diluent
250 mg	5 ml
500 mg	5 ml
1 gm	10 ml
2 gm	20 ml
4 gm	40 ml

(Piggyback bottles of 1, 2 and 4 gm are also available. See directions on bottles for dilution.) Shake well until a clear solution is obtained.

Discard reconstituted solutions after 3 days if unrefrigerated, 7 days if refrigerated.

---

in water
10% fructose in saline
LR
10% invert sugar in water
10% invert sugar in saline
Travert 10%
#1, #2, and #3

Use enough volume to produce a drug concentration of 0.5–2.0 mg/ml and infuse over 6 hrs.

---

growth secondary to organisms resistant to this drug.

2. Renal, hepatic, and hematopoietic systems should be monitored during therapy.
3. Use with caution in premature and newborn infants.
4. Safety for use in pregnancy has not been established.
5. This drug contains 3.1 mEq. of sodium per gram.[2] This should be considered when giving this drug to patients with congestive heart failure or any patient where sodium intake is limited.
6. Can cause acute interstitial nephritis which is preceded by fever, eosinophilia and a rash. Urinalysis will show white cells, casts and proteinuria. There may also be oliguria and azotemia. If this occurs, the drug should be discontinued. Some groups then treat with steroids.

ADVERSE REACTIONS
1. Hypersensitivity reactions ranging from rash to anaphylaxis have been reported; increased SGOT and SGPT may also be manifestations of hypersensitivity
2. Oral lesions: glossitis (inflammation of the tongue) and stomatitis (inflammation of oral membranes)
3. Fever
4. Oral (thrush) and perineal (monilia) *Candida albicans* infections
5. Blood dyscrasias
6. Nephrotoxicity (oliguria, albuminuria, hematuria, pyuria) especially in infants

427

OXACILLIN SODIUM (Prostaphlin, Bactocil) (Continued)

NURSING IMPLICATIONS
1. Take anaphylaxis precautions; see page 118.
2. Monitor for signs and symptoms of overgrowth infections:
   a. Fever (take rectal temperature at least every 4–6 hours in all patients)
   b. Increasing malaise
   c. Newly appearing localized signs and symptoms: redness, soreness, pain, swelling, drainage (increased volume or change in character of pre-existing drainage)
   d. Monilial rash in perineal area (reddened areas with itching), or reddened areas on oral membranes (thrush)
   e. Cough (change in pre-existing cough or sputum production)
   f. Diarrhea
3. Monitor renal status for onset of nephrotoxicity:
   a. Measure urine output every 8 hours (or more frequently if the patient's condition warrants). Notify the physician as to the onset of oliguria (urine output less than 240 ml in 8 hours for adults; see chart on page 546 for normal urine outputs in children).
   b. Observe for hematuria.
   c. Collect urine for analysis at least every other day to be examined for white cells, casts, proteinuria.
4. Examine oral membranes and tongue daily for signs of stomatitis and glossitis. Notify the physician of findings and begin therapeutic oral care:[3]

a. *Mild Inflammation:* Remove dentures. Use a soft toothbrush and a hydrogen peroxide solution (1 part peroxide and 4 parts saline). Do not use toothpaste. Rinse with peroxide solution and then water. Replace dentures. Repeat every 4 hours and/or after meals.
b. *Severe Inflammation and Ulceration:* Remove dentures. Use soft gauze pads rather than a toothbrush. Use the peroxide solution as described above. Rinse with water using an asepto syringe and gentle suction until returns are clear. Do not replace dentures. Repeat every 4 hours while patient is awake.
c. Place the patient on a bland, soft diet. Patients with severe reactions may be placed on NPO status by the physician. Those who can tolerate oral intake may benefit from the use of Xylocaine Viscous or acetaminophen elixir mouthwashes before meals.
d. Keep the patient hydrated.
e. Administer parenteral analgesics as needed.

REFERENCES
1. Appel, Geral B. and Neu, Harold C.: The Nephrotoxicity of Antimicrobial Agents. *New England Journal of Medicine*, 296(12):667, March 24, 1977.
2. Ibid, p. 664.
3. Bruya, Margaret Auld, and Madeira, Nancy Powell: Stomatitis After Chemotherapy. *American Journal of Nursing*, 75(5):1351, August 1975.

OXYTETRACYCLINE HYDROCHLORIDE (Terramycin Intravenous)

ACTIONS/ INDICATIONS	DOSAGE	PREPARATION AND STORAGE	DRUG INCOMPATIBILITIES	MODES OF IV ADMINISTRATION			CONTRAINDICATIONS; WARNINGS; PRECAUTIONS; ADVERSE REACTIONS
				INJECTION	INTERMITTENT INFUSION	CONTINUOUS INFUSION	
Antibiotic used to treat infections caused by the following organisms: • Rickettsiae • *Mycoplasma pneumoniae* • Agents of psittacosis and ornithosis • Agents of lymphogranuloma venereum and granuloma inguinale • Agent of relapsing fever • Other gram-positive, gram-nega-	ADULTS: 250–500 mg every 12 hrs. Do not exceed 500 mg. every 6 hrs. CHILDREN (over 8 years of age): 10–15 mg/ kg/day divided into 2 doses. Up to 20 mg/ kg/day can be given in severe infections. See Warning No. 1. Not recommended for newborn in-	There are separate oxytetracycline preparations for IM and IV use. Be certain to use *IV form.* IV form should not be used for IM. Reconstitute from powder by adding 10 ml of sterile water for injection to both 250-mg and 500-mg vials. Concentrations produced are 25 mg/ml and 50 mg/ml, respectively.	Do not mix with any other medication.	NO	YES Preferred mode. Use D5W, NS or RL, at least 100 ml. Infuse over 1 hour.	YES Use D5W, NS or RL in desired volume. Infuse over 6– 12 hours.	CONTRAINDICATIONS Hypersensitivity to any tetracycline WARNINGS 1. Use during tooth development may cause permanent discoloration of the child's teeth. Enamel hypoplasia has also been reported. Use should be limited to situations where no other drug may be effective. 2. If renal impairment exists, even at normal doses, accumulation may occur and lead to liver toxicity. Avoid use of this drug in such patients, and in postpartum patients with pyelonephritis. 3. Monitor liver function. Do not use other hepatotoxic drugs concomitantly. Liver failure and death has been reported in the presence of renal failure especially during pregnancy, when daily doses exceeded 2 gm. 4. Exposure to ultraviolet radiation may

tive and anaerobic organisms as determined by sensitivity testing

In patients with renal impairment, dosage should be decreased or time interval between doses increased.

Store in refrigerator and discard after 48 hours.

5. There may be an increase in BUN secondary to an anabolic effect. This is not a problem in the presence of normal renal function, but may lead to azotemia, hyperphosphatemia and acidosis in the presence of renal impairment.

6. Use in pregnancy can cause retardation in fetal bone development.

7. This drug is secreted in breast milk.

PRECAUTIONS

1. Overgrowth of nonsusceptible organisms, including fungi, may occur. If a significant superinfection develops, discontinue oxytetracycline and initiate appropriate therapy.

2. Patients concomitantly receiving anticoagulants may require lower doses of the anticoagulant.

3. All infections secondary to Group A beta-hemolytic Streptococcus must be treated for at least 10 days to prevent rheumatic fever.

4. Do not administer concomitantly with penicillin. Penicillin activity may be reduced by this drug.

ADVERSE REACTIONS

1. Gastrointestinal: anorexia, nausea, vomiting, diarrhea, glossitis (inflammation of the tongue — rare).

2. Skin: rashes, photosensitivity

3. Renal toxicity: rise in BUN secondary to an anabolic effect

4. Hypersensitivity: urticaria and anaphylaxis, exacerbation of lupus erythematosus. Bulging fontanels have been reported in young infants with full therapeutic dosage. This disappeared on discontinuation of the drug. (See Contraindications.)

5. Hematologic: hemolytic anemia, thrombocytopenia, neutropenia, eosinophilia.

6. Overgrowth infection secondary to nonsusceptible organisms.

NURSING IMPLICATIONS

1. Take anaphylaxis precautions; see page 118.

2. If gastrointestinal disturbances occur, notify the physician. If disturbances such as nausea, vomiting and diarrhea are pronounced, the drug will probably be discontinued. Antiemetics, antacids, and constipating agents can be ordered to control symptoms. Monitor intake and output to assist the physician in planning for parenteral fluid replacement. Maintain hydration orally when possible.

3. If the patient will be taking the oral form of this drug as an outpatient, instruct him/her on the possibility of photosensitivity and the advisability of avoiding exposure to the sun (sun-block lotions may be of help if exposure cannot be avoided).

4. Women of childbearing age and potential and mothers of children who may receive this drug should be informed of Warning Nos. 1, 2, 3, 6 and 7 by the physician. Assist in the interpretation of these warnings to the patient.

5. Even though blood dyscrasias are infrequently caused by this agent, be aware of the patient's complete blood cell count during therapy. If the platelet count begins to fall, the drug will probably be discontinued. Bleeding secondary to a low platelet count usually begins only after the count

produce exaggerated sunburn.

OXYTETRACYCLINE HYDROCHLORIDE (Terramycin Intravenous) (Continued)

NURSING IMPLICATIONS (No. 5 continued)

6. Monitor for signs and symptoms of overgrowth infections:
   a. Fever (take rectal temperature at least every 4–6 hours in all patients)
   b. Increasing malaise
   c. Newly appearing localized signs and symptoms: redness, soreness, pain, swelling, drainage (increased volume or change of pre-existing drainage)
   d. Monilial rash in perineal area (reddened areas with itching)
   e. Cough (change in pre-existing cough or sputum production)
   f. Diarrhea
7. Report the onset of any rash to the physician. Keep the patient's environment comfortably cool and the skin clean. Diphenhydramine (Benadryl) may be ordered to relieve itching.
8. Report the onset of jaundice to the physician.
9. Report the onset of bulging fontanels and other signs of increasing intracranial pressure to the physician.
10. Be aware of this drug's relationship with renal function. Tetracyclines are usually not given to patients with renal impairment because:
    a. The drug accumulates in the body because of decreased excretion.
    b. The presence of the drug may cause further deterioration in renal function.
    c. It may cause a catabolic state with metabolic acidosis, increasing BUN and possibly death due to uremia.[1] If it is given, know what the patient's pretreatment BUN and creatinine levels are. Monitor for change in these values with initiation of treatment. Monitor urine output in renal patients receiving this drug. Report increasing oliguria to the physician. Send urine for analysis at least every other day.

REFERENCE

1. Barza, Michael, and Schiefe, Richard T.: Antimicrobial Spectrum, Pharmacology and Therapeutic Use of Antibiotics. Part I: Tetracyclines. *American Journal of Hospital Pharmacy*, 34:51, January 1977.

OXYTOCIN CITRATE (Pitocin, Syntocinon)

ACTIONS/INDICATIONS	DOSAGE	PREPARATION AND STORAGE	DRUG INCOMPATIBILITIES	MODES OF IV ADMINISTRATION			CONTRAINDICATIONS; WARNINGS; PRECAUTIONS; ADVERSE REACTIONS
				INJECTION	INTERMITTENT INFUSION	CONTINUOUS INFUSION	
Synthetic oxytocic hormone. Increases uterine contractility. Used to initiate or improve uterine contractions. Can also be used to control postpartum uterine bleeding.	INDUCTION OR STIMULATION OF LABOR: Dosage is determined by uterine response titration, using a solution of 10 units/ml. *Initial dose—* 1–2 milliunits/min. At 15- to 30-min intervals, increase dose by 1–2 milliunits/min until desired contraction pattern is seen. CONTROL OF UTERINE BLEEDING: 10–40 units	Availability: 0.5-ml ampul containing 5 units. 1-ml ampul containing 10 units. 10-ml vial containing 100 units. Disposable syringe containing 10 units in 1 ml. For infusion add 1 (1-ml) ampul to 1000 ml D5W. The final solution contains 10 milliunits/ml. Mix well. More concen-	Do not mix with any other medication in IV bottle, and do not mix in an IV line with warfarin.	YES. Only for *extreme* emergencies. Dilute dose in 5 ml NS and inject slowly.	NO	YES. Use infusion pump. Attach as a secondary bottle to enable infusion to be discontinued when necessary. Titrate with desired uterine response.	CONTRAINDICATIONS 1. Significant cephalopelvic disproportion 2. Unfavorable fetal positions 3. In emergencies where the benefit-to-risk ratio for fetus or mother favors surgical intervention 4. In fetal distress where delivery is not imminent 5. Prolonged use in uterine inertia or severe toxemia 6. Hypertonic uterine patterns 7. Allergic and functional hypersensitivity 8. In cases where vaginal delivery is contraindicated such as cervical carcinoma, cord presentation or prolapse, placenta previa, and vasa praevia WARNINGS 1. Must be used only in a hospital under adequate medical supervision. 2. Use only one route at a time to administer. PRECAUTIONS 1. When properly administered, the drug should stimulate normal contractions.

in 1000 ml D5W titrated with uterine firmness and bleeding rate.

trated solutions can be used if the patient requires fluid restriction. Solutions (i.e. units/ml) should be made for easy dose calculation.

2. Overstimulation can endanger the mother and the fetus. Hypertonic contractions can occur, leading to fetal distress and possible uterine rupture.

3. Probably should not be administered in fetal distress, prematurity, placenta previa, abruptio placentae, borderline disproportion, any situation with predisposition for uterine rupture (previous C-section or uterine surgery, overdistention of the uterus, grand multiparity, traumatic delivery, or sepsis).

4. Hypertensive episodes have been reported and have led to cerebrovascular accident.

5. This drug increases water reabsorption; water intoxication may occur.

ADVERSE REACTIONS

Mother:
1. Tetanic uterine contractions
2. Uterine rupture, pelvic hematomas
3. Hypotension
4. Arrhythmias (sinus tachycardia, premature ventricular contractions)
5. Water intoxication
6. Hypertensive episodes leading to CVA or subarachnoid hemorrhage
7. Rarely—chest pain, anxiety, dyspnea
8. Hypersensitivity

Fetus:
1. Death
2. Arrhythmias (premature ventricular contractions, bradycardia, tachycardia)
3. Hypoxia
4. Intracranial hemorrhage.

NURSING IMPLICATIONS
1. Physician should be in attendance or readily available during the administration of this drug.
2. Monitor uterine contractions constantly: number per minute, strength (use contraction meter if available; report if exceeds 50 mm Hg), duration, and resting tone. In the event of overstimulation, *stop infusion;* report to the physician. Administer oxygen to the mother as ordered.
3. Monitor maternal vital signs every 15 minutes or according to hospital policy. Report rising blood pressure, cardiac irregularities. Patients with a history of arrhythmia or other cardiac problems should be connected to a cardiac monitor to detect arrhythmias.
4. Monitor the mother for signs of water intoxication: fall in urine output, rise in weight, edema (lower extremities, sacral area, face).
5. Monitor fetal heart rate every 5 to 10 minutes or use continuous fetal ECG. Report arrhythmias immediately and discontinue infusion.

431

● **PANCURONIUM BROMIDE** (Pavulon)

ACTIONS/ INDICATIONS	DOSAGE	PREPARATION AND STORAGE	DRUG INCOMPAT- IBILITIES	MODES OF IV ADMINISTRATION			CONTRAINDICATIONS; WARNINGS; PRECAUTIONS; ADVERSE REACTIONS
				INJECTION	INTERMITTENT INFUSION	CONTINUOUS INFUSION	
Nondepolarizing (competitive) neuromuscular blocking agent.

Used as an adjunct to anesthesia to induce skeletal muscle relaxation and paralysis. Also used to control patients on mechanical ventilation; to increase muscle relaxation during electroconvulsive therapy, tetanus and status epilepticus.

Onset and duration of action are dose-dependent. With an average adult or pediatric dose, onset will be within 30 seconds, with the peak effect after 3 minutes. Recovery is nearly complete after 1 hour with a single dose. Repeated doses will prolong recovery time. | Dosage must be individualized in relation to anesthetic used and patient's condition. See Nursing Implication No. 6 and Precaution No. 1 for situations which require reduction in dosage.

ADULTS:
Initial dose range—0.04–0.10 mg/kg followed by 0.01 mg/kg titrations based on patient response, at 25- to 60-minute intervals.

CHILDREN OVER 1 MONTH OF AGE:
0.04–0.10 mg/kg, with 0.01 mg increments titrated with patient response (same as adult).

NEONATES:
Test dose of 0.02 mg/kg; evaluate responsiveness (infants are sensitive to this type of neuromuscular blocking agent), then titrate as with adult. | Supplied in 2-ml and 5-ml ampuls (2 mg/ml) and in 10-ml vials (1 mg/ml).

Refrigerate unopened and opened vials. | Do not mix with any other medication in any manner. | YES
Over 1–2 minutes. No further dilution needed. | NO | NO | CONTRAINDICATIONS
Hypersensitivity to this drug or the bromide ion contained in the compound

WARNINGS
1. Must be administered only by clinicians thoroughly experienced in its use (usually an anesthiologist or anesthetist).
2. Should not be administered unless facilities for endotracheal intubation, assisted ventilation, oxygen and reversal agents are immediately available. Be prepared to assist and control ventilation.
3. Use with caution in patients with myasthenia gravis.
4. May have adverse effects on fetal development. Benefits must be weighed against risks to the fetus.
5. May be used during cesarean section. Reversal may be unsatisfactory in patients receiving magnesium sulfate for toxemia (magnesium salts enhance the blockade produced by this drug). Reduce the dosage in these cases. Pancuronium does not cross the placental barrier.

PRECAUTIONS
1. Use with caution in patients with pre-existing pulmonary, hepatic or renal disease. This is particularly true of patients with renal disease since the drug is partially excreted in the urine. These patients can experience a prolongation of the neuromuscular blockade (20–40 minutes longer than normal, after a single dose).[1]
2. Neostigmine 0.5–2.0 mg reverses the actions of this drug. Atropine 0.5–1.0 mg should be administered a few minutes prior to neostigmine. See page 418 for detailed information on neostigmine.
3. Histamine release and resultant bronchospasm is rarely seen.
4. Prior administration of succinylcholine should warrant that the dose of pancuronium be delayed until the effects of succinylcholine have worn off.
5. See Nursing Implications for informa- |

tion on elements which alter the duration and intensity of this drug's effects.

1. Neuromuscular: extension and intensification of the drug's effects beyond the usual times
2. Cardiovascular: slight increase in heart rate
3. Gastrointestinal: increased salivation especially if an anticholinergic agent has not been given prior to pancuronium or anesthesia
4. Skin: transient rash

A reversal agent is administered at the end of surgery or at any time when the effects of this drug are no longer needed or are undesirable. See Precaution No. 2.

A peripheral nerve stimulator can be used for dosage titration, especially in patients who require a reduction in dosage.

NURSING IMPLICATIONS
Postanesthesia Care:
1. Equipment that should be readily available: suction, manual breathing bag, endotracheal tubes and laryngoscope, oxygen.
2. Patients receiving this agent must be intubated to assist in maintaining an adequate airway and ventilation. Monitor for adequacy of ventilation by presence or absence of cyanosis and arterial blood gases.
3. Be aware of the onset and duration of action of this drug (see Actions/Indications column), and when the patient received the last dose.
4. Beware of the sequence of progression of the paralytic effects as they will occur after an injection of this drug:
   a. Loss of eye movement
   b. Eyelid droop
   c. Stiffness of jaw muscles
   d. Paralysis of trunk muscles
   e. Paralysis of pharyngeal muscles (tongue, swallowing, etc.)
   f. Respiratory paralysis, intercostal muscles and finally diaphragm
   Recovery will be a complete reverse of this sequence.[2]
5. During recovery, observe for rebound of the paralytic effects and for incomplete reversal of the paralytic effects by the antagonist agent (neostigmine). Keep reversal agent and atropine at the bedside or readily available (see Precaution No. 2).
6. Be aware of elements which may *prolong* the effects of this drug:
   a. Decreased circulation time, e.g., as in the presence of congestive heart failure or shock
   b. Decreased body temperature
   c. Dehydration
   d. Low blood pH[3]
   e. Hepatic or renal insufficiency (drug is excreted in bile and urine)
   f. Concomitant use of aminoglycoside antibiotics, polymyxin B, or bacitracin
   g. Other drugs, e.g., diazepam, halothane, quinidine, quinine, enflurane, methoxyflurane, magnesium salts, other neuromuscular blocking agents
   h. Age, e.g., the elderly
   i. The presence of myasthenia gravis
   j. Hypokalemia
   Patients under the influence of any one of these elements will require reduced dosage (in some cases), monitoring as described in Nursing Implication No. 7, and possibly prolonged respiratory support.
7. Discharge from the recovery room will depend on the following criteria:
   a. Grip strength
   b. Ability to lift the head
   c. Ability to open the eyes
   d. Respiratory status, e.g., vital capacity and tidal volume (preoperative values of these parameters are useful for comparison)

Maintenance Care for Ventilatory Control:
1. This drug is usually administered on a p.r.n. basis for control of ventilation. The criteria for when to administer the drug (by the anesthesiologist, qualified physician, or in some institutions, registered nurse) are determined by the physician. The criteria will include:
   a. A respiratory rate greater than ___ per minute
   b. When the patient's respiratory effort is out of phase with the respirator
   c. When the patient is struggling against the respirator
   d. When positive end-expiratory pressure (P.E.E.P.) is in use
   Monitor for the onset of any of the criteria and administer (or have administered) the prescribed amount of the drug.
2. Make certain that the endotracheal or tracheostomy tube is securely and correctly inserted. Check the connection between the tube and the respirator; it must be tight. KEEP RESPIRATOR ALARM SYSTEMS FUNCTIONING AT ALL TIMES.
3. This drug paralyzes skeletal muscles; it does not alter consciousness or relieve pain and anxiety. Therefore, the patient must be adequately sedated and given analgesics as needed to relieve anxiety and pain. He will not be able to make his needs known to those caring for him; needs must be anticipated. Many institutions assign one or more RNs to stay in constant attendance with these patients. Explain the paralysis to the patient and family as indicated.

PANCURONIUM BROMIDE (Pavulon) (Continued)

NURSING IMPLICATIONS (Continued)
4. Monitor vital signs before administration and every 5 minutes after until stabilization is seen, then every 15–30 minutes. Repeat the cycle with each dose. A slight increase in heart rate may be seen. Patients with a history of cardiac arrhythmias should be observed for exacerbation of those arrhythmias via a continuous ECG monitor.
5. Because this agent produces muscle paralysis, handle the patient with care to prevent trauma to joints and muscles during turning and positioning. The patient's position should be changed hourly to prevent skin breakdown. Use water-mattresses, floatation pads and similar devices as needed.
6. When this drug is discontinued, proceed with the nursing management as described under *Postanesthesia Care.*

REFERENCES
1. Miller, Ronald D., Stevens, Wendell C., and Way, Walter L.: The Effect of Renal Failure and Hyperkalemia on the Duration of Pancuronium Neuromuscular Blockade in Man. *Anesthesia and Analgesia,* 52(4):663, July–August 1973.
2. Wylie, W. D., and Churchill-Davidson, H. C. (editors): *A Practice of Anesthesia* (3rd ed.), Chicago: Year Book Medical Publishers, 1972, p. 816.
3. Ibid, p. 833.

SUGGESTED READING
Hartridge, Virginia: Pancuronium Bromide (Pavulon). *American Association of Nurse Anesthetists Journal,* 42(4):301–310, August 1974, (references).

PAPAVERINE HYDROCHLORIDE

ACTIONS/ INDICATIONS	DOSAGE	PREPARATION AND STORAGE	DRUG INCOMPATIBILITIES	MODES OF IV ADMINISTRATION			CONTRAINDICATIONS; WARNINGS; PRECAUTIONS; ADVERSE REACTIONS
				INJECTION	INTERMITTENT INFUSION	CONTINUOUS INFUSION	
Smooth muscle relaxant and anti-spasmodic, causes vasodilatation and depresses speed of conductivity in myocardial conduction system. Used in the following conditions: Vascular spasm in • Acute myocardial infarction • Angina pectoris • Peripheral and pulmonary embolism • Peripheral vascular disease with spasm • Cerebral angiospastic	ADULTS: 1–4 ml (30–120 mg) repeated every 3 hours as needed. *Management of premature ventricular contractions —30 mg every 10 min for 2 doses.* CHILDREN: 6 mg/kg day, given in 4 divided doses, as needed.	Supplied in ampuls of 30 mg/ml. Do not add to Ringer's lactate; a precipitate will form.	Do not mix with any other medication.	YES *Slowly over 1–2 min.*	YES In any fluid, except Ringer's lactate. Titrate with patient response.	NO	CONTRAINDICATIONS IV injection, in presence of complete (third degree) atrioventricular heart block ADVERSE REACTIONS 1. Intensive flushing of the face 2. Diaphoresis 3. Increased depth of respirations 4. Increased heart rate 5. Slight rise in blood pressure 6. Sedation

tinuous ECG monitoring. Atropine 1.0 mg will be used to treat bradycardia or increasing heart block.

conditions
• Visceral spasm: ureteral colic, biliary colic, gastrointestinal colic
• Premature ventricular contractions

NURSING IMPLICATIONS
1. Monitor vital signs at least hourly.
2. Patients with first or second-degree atrioventricular heart block should be observed for intensification of the block and for other arrhythmias via continuous ECG monitoring. Atropine 1.0 mg will be used to treat bradycardia or increasing heart block.
3. Keep patient on bed rest during administration.

● PENICILLIN G, POTASSIUM AND SODIUM

ACTIONS/ INDICATIONS	DOSAGE	PREPARATION AND STORAGE	DRUG INCOMPAT- IBILITIES	MODES OF IV ADMINISTRATION			CONTRAINDICATIONS; WARNINGS; PRECAUTIONS; ADVERSE REACTIONS
				INJECTION	INTERMITTENT INFUSION	CONTINUOUS INFUSION	
Antibiotic. Used to treat infections caused by susceptible strains of the following organisms or conditions: • Streptococcus • *Strep. pneumoniae* • Susceptible Staphylococcus • Anthrax • Actinomycosis • Clostridium • Diphtheria • Erysipelothrix • Fusospirochetosis (Vincent's gingivitis) • Gram-negative organisms, if sensitive (many	Dosage varies greatly with organism, general condition of the patient, the severity of the infection. *Ranges:* ADULTS 0.3–100 million units/day in 2–4 divided doses. In the presence of renal failure, increase the time interval between usual doses as follows based on glomerular filtration rate (GFR):	To reconstitute, loosen powder by shaking vial. Using sterile water for injection, NS or D5W, add the amounts shown in the table below to make required concentrations (vial contains 5 million units). Hold vial horizontally and rotate while slowly directing stream of diluent against vial wall. Shake vigorously. Dry powder may be stored at room temperature. Prepared solutions should be refrigerated; discard after 1 week. (Lilly	Do not mix in any manner with: Metaraminol Ascorbic acid Tetracyclines Aminophylline Sodium Bicarbonate THAM Vancomycin Cephalosporins Heparin Lincomycin Phenothiazines Thiopental Vitamins Aminoglycoside antibiotics	NO	YES Use D5W or NS for infusion, at least 100 ml.	YES Use D5W or NS for infusion, at least 100 ml. Entire daily dose can be given in two 12-hour infusions.	CONTRAINDICATIONS Hypersensitivity to any penicillin WARNINGS 1. Anaphylaxis can occur. 2. There may be cross-allergenicity with cephalosporins. PRECAUTIONS 1. Use with caution in patients with significant allergy history. 2. Monitor renal and hematopoietic systems during therapy. 3. Streptococcal infections must be treated for at least 10 days. Follow-up cultures must be obtained. 4. Reduction of dosage may be required in patients with renal or cardiac dysfunction because of sodium or potassium content of the drug and systemic accumulation of the drug (sodium or potassium content: 1.7 mEq/1 million units). See Dosage column. 5. Overgrowth of nonsusceptible organisms may occur. Discontinue this drug if possible and initiate appropriate therapy in this situation. ADVERSE REACTIONS 1. Most frequent is hypersensitivity ranging from rash or drug fever to anaphylaxis

435

PENICILLIN G, POTASSIUM AND SODIUM (Continued)

ACTIONS/ INDICATIONS	DOSAGE	PREPARATION AND STORAGE	DRUG INCOMPATIBILITIES	MODES OF IV ADMINISTRATION			CONTRAINDICATIONS; WARNINGS; PRECAUTIONS; ADVERSE REACTIONS
				INJECTION	INTERMITTENT INFUSION	CONTINUOUS INFUSION	
are not): *E. coli, A. aerogenes, A. faecalis, Salmonella, P. mirabilis* • *Pasteurella* infections • *N. gonorrhoeae* • Syphilis (*T. pallidum*) • Meningococcus	*GFR (ml/min)* *Time Interval for Doses* 80–50 every 8 hours 50–10 every 8 hours <10 every 12 hours No dosage adjustment is needed with dialysis.[1] CHILDREN: 50,000–400,000 units/kg/day (Follow above schedule in the presence of renal failure.) NEONATES AND CHILDREN: *0–7 days of age*—50,000 units/kg/day, 100,000–150,000 units/kg/day in meningitis. *Over 7 days of age*—75,000 units/kg/day, 150,000–250,000 units/kg/day in meningitis. (Larger doses for group B streptococcal meningitis than for pneumococcal meningitis are	preparation without buffer must be discarded after 3 days.)	*Amount of Diluent* *Resulting Concentration* (to 5 million Unit vial) 23 ml 200,000 U/ml 18 ml 250,000 U/ml 8 ml 500,000 U/ml 3 ml 1,000,000 U/ml				2. Congestive heart failure secondary to high sodium content (See Precaution No. 4, page 435.) 3. Minor hypersensitivity reactions may be controlled by antihistamines and corticosteroids if continued use of the penicillin cannot be avoided 4. Jarisch-Herxheimer reaction has been reported in patients being treated for syphilis 5. Hyperkalemia (elevated serum potassium) in patients with compromised renal function 6. Positive Coombs' test 7. Diarrhea 8. Seizures, usually seen in patients with renal impairment who are on high doses of penicillin 9. Overgrowth infections

appropriate.)
Avoid doses
over 250,000
units/kg/day
because of
likelihood of
CNS toxicity.
Administer at
12-hour inter-
vals for neo-
nates 0–7
days of age;
every 8 hours
for children
over 7 days of
age, and every
6 hours in
meningitis re-
gardless of
age.[2]

NURSING IMPLICATIONS
1. Take anaphylaxis precautions; see page 118.
2. Monitor for signs of fluid overload and congestive heart failure:
   a. Increased weight (weigh daily)
   b. Peripheral edema
   c. Increased heart rate, CVP (engorged external jugular veins), and respira-
      tory rate
   d. Rales in lung bases
   e. Decreased exercise tolerance
3. Monitor for nonsusceptible organism overgrowth infection:
   a. Fever (take rectal temperature at least every 4–6 hours)
   b. Increasing malaise
   c. Localized signs and symptoms of an infection: redness, soreness, pain,
      swelling, drainage
   d. Cough
   e. Diarrhea
   f. Infection due to *Candida albicans*, oral (thrush) or perineal (monilia).

REFERENCES
1. Bennett, William M., et al.: Guidelines for Drug Therapy in Renal Failure. *An-nals of Internal Medicine*, 86:759, 1977.
2. McCracken, George H. and Nelson, John D.: *Antimicrobial Therapy for New-borns: Practical Application of Pharmacology to Clinical Usage.* New York: Grune and Stratton, 1977, p. 9.

PENTAZOCINE LACTATE (Talwin)

ACTIONS/ INDICATIONS	DOSAGE	PREPARATION AND STORAGE	DRUG INCOMPAT-IBILITIES	MODES OF IV ADMINISTRATION			CONTRAINDICATIONS; WARNINGS; PRECAUTIONS; ADVERSE REACTIONS
				INJECTION	INTERMITTENT INFUSION	CONTINUOUS INFUSION	
Analgesic, with pain-re-lieving quali-ties similar to morphine and meperidine. Also has seda-tive activity. Use to relieve moderate to severe pain; preoperative analgesic-sed-ative. Analgesia usu-	ADULTS: *Pain*—30 mg repeated every 3–4 hrs. Do not exceed 30 mg in a single dose and 360 mg in 24 hrs. *Labor*—20 mg at 2- to 3-hr intervals. CHILDREN UN-DER 12: Intravenous	Supplied in sev-eral forms: Ampuls of 1.0, 1.5, and 2.0 ml with a concen-tration of 30 mg/ml. Multidose vials of 10 ml, with a concentration of 30 mg/ml. Follow hospital or institutional	Can be mixed in syringe with: Scopolamine Atropine Promethazine Do not inject into an IV line containing: Aminophylline Sodium bicar-bonate Any barbitu-rate	YES Dilute dose in 1 ml sterile water for injec-tion; adminis-ter at a rate of 5 mg/min.	NO	NO	CONTRAINDICATIONS Hypersensitivity WARNINGS 1. Drug dependence does occur (psycho-logical and physiological). 2. This drug may increase cerebrospinal fluid pressure. Use with caution in pa-tients with head injuries or increased intracranial pressure. This drug may also mask symptoms and indirectly in-crease intracranial pressure. 3. Safety for use in pregnancy, other than labor, has not been established. Use with caution during delivery of premature infants. May decrease

437

● **PENTAZOCINE LACTATE** (Talwin) (*Continued*)

ACTIONS/ INDICATIONS	DOSAGE	PREPARATION AND STORAGE	DRUG INCOMPAT- IBILITIES	MODES OF IV ADMINISTRATION			CONTRAINDICATIONS; WARNINGS; PRECAUTIONS; ADVERSE REACTIONS
				INJECTION	INTERMITTENT INFUSION	CONTINUOUS INFUSION	
ally occurs within 2–3 min. after IV injection.	administration not recom- mended	regulations on the control and accounting of this drug. See Warning No. 1.					strength of uterine contractions. 4. Hallucinations and disorientation have been reported (especially in the elderly). 5. Use in children under 12 years of age is not recommended.

PRECAUTIONS

1. May cause respiratory depression. Administer with caution to patients with any respiratory problem, especially when respiratory depression is present. If respiratory depression occurs, methylphenidate (Ritalin), or naloxone (Narcan), page 417 can be administered to counteract the effects.
2. Administer with caution to patients with hepatic or renal impairment. These patients may have more intense adverse reactions because of decreased metabolism and excretion. Smaller doses are required.
3. Use with caution in the presence of acute myocardial infarction when nausea and vomiting are present.
4. Use with caution in patients who are about to undergo surgery of the biliary tract since it may cause spasm of the sphincter of Oddi.
5. This drug is a mild narcotic antagonist; patients who are addicted to narcotics or who are on methadone may experience withdrawal symptoms after a dose of pentazocine.
6. May cause seizures in patients who are prone to them.

ADVERSE REACTIONS

1. Most common: nausea, vomiting, dizziness, euphoria
2. Infrequent: respiratory depression, apnea in newborns whose mothers has received pentazocine during labor, shock, hypertension, sedation, depression, constipation, rashes, urinary retention
3. Rare: Hallucinations, taste alteration, blurred vision, diplopia, blood dyscrasias, allergic reactions

NURSING IMPLICATIONS

1. Patient should be on bed rest with side rails up during and for the first hour after injection. Then ambulate with caution.
2. Respiratory support equipment be readily available in the event of respira-

to increase his own respiratory rate and if the respiratory rate falls below 6/minute or if cyanosis develops.

4. Monitor blood pressure and apical pulse before injection and every 3–5 minutes for the first 15 minutes, then every 5–10 minutes for the next

hour, then every 30 minutes for the next 2 hours. The physician must determine acceptable blood pressure limits. Be prepared to treat hypotension with vasopressors.

tory depression:

a. Narcotic antagonist agent: naloxone HCL (Narcan, see page 417). Do not use levallorphan (Lorfan) or nalorphine (Nalline) to counteract the respiratory depression caused by this drug. These agents may intensify the respiratory problem rather than eliminate it.

b. Airways, endotracheal tube and laryngoscope, suction, oxygen, manual breathing bag (Ambu, Hope, Puritan)

3. Monitor for respiratory depression: Count respiratory rate every 3–5 minutes during and after the injection for the first 15 minutes, then every 5–10 minutes for the next hour, then every 30 minutes for the next 2 hours. Repeat cycle for additional doses. If respiratory rate falls below 10/minute, notify physician and be prepared to assist ventilation. Observe for cyanosis (central: lips and tongue; peripheral: nail-beds), shallow respirations, change in mental status, and cardiac irregularities. Do not leave the patient unattended for first 30 minutes. See Precaution No. 1.

Take measures to prevent aspiration in the event of vomiting. Begin manual breathing assistance and use of airway if the patient cannot be aroused

5. Be prepared to manage hallucinations and disorientation.

6. Monitor for urinary retention in susceptible patients (see Adverse Reaction No. 6). Palpate bladder size every 4 hours; measure urinary output every 4 hours.

7. Patients on prolonged therapy may require laxatives or stool softeners to prevent constipation. Maintain hydration.

8. When scheduling doses, do not make the patient wait for total return of the pain before repeating a dose; to do so will reduce the effectiveness of the analgesic. Never withhold the drug when it is needed unless a contraindication arises, and then notify the physician for assistance.

9. Monitor for withdrawal signs and symptoms in patients who have been addicted to narcotics, e.g., tremulousness, tachycardia, muscle cramps, diaphoresis. Notify the physician at the onset.

PENTOBARBITAL, SODIUM (Nembutal)

ACTIONS/INDICATIONS	DOSAGE	PREPARATION AND STORAGE	DRUG INCOMPATIBILITIES	MODES OF IV ADMINISTRATION			CONTRAINDICATIONS; WARNINGS; PRECAUTIONS; ADVERSE REACTIONS
				INJECTION	INTERMITTENT INFUSION	CONTINUOUS INFUSION	
Short-acting barbiturate, CNS depressant. Used as a sedative and hypnotic; for preoperative sedation and to control seizures.	ADULTS: *Average dose* —100 mg (70-kg patient). *Titrate in small increments to obtain desired effect.* A total dose of 200–500 mg may be used. Keep dose at a minimum in convulsive states to prevent over-depression. CHILDREN: Inject at a rate of 30 mg/M²/min. Titrate with response.* *At least 1 minute is necessary to determine the full effect.	Available in ampuls and multi-dose vials of 50 mg/ml; multi-dose vials of 12 mg/ml; and prefilled syringes of 1 and 2 ml of a 50 mg/ml solution. Do not use a solution that is not clear and colorless. Do not mix with fluids except to inject into the tubing of a running IV. This is a Schedule II drug under the Controlled Substances Act of 1970. Maintain hospital or institutional regulations guiding its use.	Do not mix with other medications in any manner.	YES Dilute every 50-mg of drug in 9 cc NS. Inject at a rate of 50 mg/min. (In children, inject at a rate of 1 mg/min or 30 mg/M²/min).	NO	NO	CONTRAINDICATIONS 1. Hypersensitivity to any barbiturate 2. Porphyria (confirmed or familial history) WARNINGS 1. May antagonize some drugs by increasing liver enzyme activity, especially narcotic drugs. 2. Decreases potency of coumarin anticoagulants. 3. May produce psychic dependence with prolonged use. 4. May cause respiratory and circulatory depression, especially after rapid injection. 5. Safety for use in pregnancy has not been established insofar as the effects on fetal development. 6. May cause respiratory depression in newborn infants when it is used during labor and delivery. Premature infants are more susceptible to this. PRECAUTIONS 1. Use with caution in patients with impaired liver function. This drug is detoxified in the liver. 2. Administer with extreme caution in the presence of status asthmaticus, any respiratory depression, shock, uremia or after other respiratory de-

PENTOBARBITAL, SODIUM (Nembutal) (Continued)

ACTIONS/ INDICATIONS	DOSAGE	PREPARATION AND STORAGE	DRUG INCOMPAT- IBILITIES	MODES OF IV ADMINISTRATION			CONTRAINDICATIONS; WARNINGS; PRECAUTIONS; ADVERSE REACTIONS
				INJECTION	INTERMITTENT INFUSION	CONTINUOUS INFUSION	

CONTRAINDICATIONS; WARNINGS; PRECAUTIONS; ADVERSE REACTIONS

pressants have been given. Be prepared to provide artificial ventilation.

3. Avoid extravasation and intra-arterial injection. Extravasation can lead to tissue necrosis. Intra-arterial injection can cause pain in the extremity and possibly gangrene. Signs and symptoms of accidental intra-arterial injection.
   a. Pain in extremity
   b. Delayed onset of sedation
   c. Pallor and cyanosis of the extremity
   d. Patchy discoloration of the skin
   Any IV injection causing pain in the limb must be stopped

4. Hypotension can occur, especially in hypertensive patients. Slow injection can prevent this.

ADVERSE REACTIONS
1. Respiratory depression, apnea
2. Circulatory collapse (hypotension)
3. Hypersensitivity; rashes and anaphylaxis
4. Central nervous system depression (excessive)
5. Residual sedation
6. Nausea, vomiting
7. Paradoxical excitement
8. Coughing, hiccups, laryngospasm, chest wall spasm
9. Most reactions can be avoided by slow injection.

NURSING IMPLICATIONS
1. Strictly adhere to maximum injection rate suggestions and maximum limits. Patients with liver impairment should receive smaller doses and should be monitored more closely and for a longer period of time than usual.
2. Keep the patient supine during and after injection. Monitor blood pressure, heart rate and respiratory rate every 5 minutes for 1 hour following an injection. This includes fetal heart rate monitoring. Do not leave the patient unattended. See Implication No. 7 for management of overdosage.
3. Patients with porphyria are sensitive to barbiturates in that they may experience an acute attack of the disease secondary to the administration of a barbiturate (see Contraindications). The onset of an acute attack is indicated by severe colicky abdominal pain radiating to the back. There is usually severe vomiting, fever and leukocytosis in addition.[1]
4. Avoid extravasation; see page 96. Extravascular or intra-arterial injection of this drug can cause tissue necrosis and gangrene of the affected extremity,

Stop the injection immediately upon noting one of these symptoms. Notify the physician.
7. Management of acute overdosage:
   a. Continue to stay with the patient and monitor vital signs
   b. Maintain an open airway and adequate ventilation
   c. Keep the patient as alert as possible by verbal and physical stimuli. Encourage the patient to breathe at an adequate rate (12–14 breaths/minute for an adult). If necessary, initiate artificial ventilation with a manual breathing bag (Puritan, Hope, Ambu, etc.) or mouth-to-mouth breathing at a rate of 12–14 breaths/minute
   d. Circulatory support in the form of fluids and drugs may be ordered
8. The sedation produced by this drug may be preceded by transient changes in mental status, such as feelings of euphoria and confusion. If this occurs, attempt to calm the patient and take measures to prevent injury until the patient returns to his normal status.

respectively. Thrombophlebitis can also occur. Examine for redness and pain along the vein tract. See Precaution No. 3.
5. Take anaphylaxis precautions; see page 118.
6. Monitor for symptoms of acute overdosage (listed in order of progression):
   a. Respiratory depression, i.e., decreased respiratory rate and depth
   b. Peripheral vascular collapse, i.e., fall in blood pressure, pallor, diaphoresis, tachycardia
   c. Pulmonary edema (rare)
   d. Decreased or absent reflexes, pupillary constriction
   e. Stupor
   f. Coma

9. If a patient is to be ambulatory following an injection, ambulate with assistance; there may be transient dizziness. Obtain lying, then sitting and standing blood pressures to detect postural hypotension. If this drug has been used for an outpatient procedure, a responsible adult should accompany the patient home. The patient should not drive for at least the next 8 hours.

REFERENCE
1. Beeson, Paul B., and McDermott, Walsh (editors): *Cecil-Loeb Textbook of Medicine* (14th ed.). Philadelphia: W. B. Saunders Company, 1975, p. 1873.

PERPHENAZINE (Trilafon)

ACTIONS/ INDICATIONS	DOSAGE	PREPARATION AND STORAGE	DRUG INCOMPATIBILITIES	MODES OF IV ADMINISTRATION			CONTRAINDICATIONS; WARNINGS; PRECAUTIONS: ADVERSE REACTIONS
				INJECTION	INTERMITTENT INFUSION	CONTINUOUS INFUSION	
Major tranquilizer of the phenothiazine group. Used in the management of psychotic disorders and for control of nausea and vomiting in adults and for hiccups unrelieved by other methods. Many times more potent than chlorpromazine.	ADULTS AND CHILDREN OVER 12 YEARS OF AGE: Dosage must be individualized. Do not exceed 5 mg. Must be administered intravenously *only* in recumbent hospitalized patients. See Precautions for indications for reduced dosage. CHILDREN 12 YEARS AND UNDER: Use is not recommended.	Available in 5 mg/ml ampuls. Keep in package until use; protect from light. Slight yellow color will not alter potency; do not use if markedly discolored. Be certain to use ampul labeled for IV use.	Do not mix with any other medication.	YES. Dilute 5 mg (1 ml) or fraction of, in 9 ml NS. Inject only 1 mg (2 ml) at a time over 2–3 minutes' time, at 2- to 3-minute intervals until symptoms are controlled.	YES. Add to NS and titrate with relief of symptoms. Drip rate should be 0.5 mg/min or less. (convenient solution is 250 ml NS with 125 mg of drug added, the concentration will be 0.5 mg/ml) Use an infusion pump.	YES. Add to NS and titrate with relief of symptoms. Drip rate should be 0.5 mg/min or less. When this drug will be given over a prolonged period, use a solution of 250 mg of drug in 500 ml of NS. Concentration will be 0.5 mg/ml. Use an infusion pump.	CONTRAINDICATIONS 1. Drug-associated central nervous system depression 2. Blood dyscrasias 3. Bone marrow depression 4. Pre-existing liver impairment 5. Hypersensitivity 6. Coma or severely depressed states WARNINGS 1. Use in pregnant women *only* when possible benefits outweigh potential risks to the fetus. 2. May lower convulsive threshold in susceptible individuals. An increase in the patient's anticonvulsant agent may be necessary. 3. Use with caution in psychotic depressive states. 4. Do not use in children under 12. PRECAUTIONS 1. Administer with caution in reduced dosage to patients who have had any severe reaction to phenothiazines or to imipramine. 2. Hypotension can occur, and is treatable with levarterenol drip (do not use epinephrine). 3. If fever occurs, discontinue use. 4. Antiemetic effects may mask nausea and vomiting symptoms of other conditions such as gastrointestinal obstruction and increasing intracranial pressure.

PERPHENAZINE (Trilafon) (Continued)

ACTIONS/ INDICATIONS	DOSAGE	PREPARATION AND STORAGE	DRUG INCOMPAT- IBILITIES	MODES OF IV ADMINISTRATION			CONTRAINDICATIONS; WARNINGS; PRECAUTIONS; ADVERSE REACTIONS
				INJECTION	INTERMITTENT INFUSION	CONTINUOUS INFUSION	
							5. Avoid solution contact with skin; can cause staining.
							6. This drug can potentiate central nervous system depressant actions of opiates, antihistamines, barbiturates, alcohol, etc. Lower dosage of all agents will be necessary.
							7. The action of atropine is potentiated by this agent.
							ADVERSE REACTIONS SEEN IN SHORT-TERM INTRAVENOUS USE
							1. Neurologic:
							a. Sedation, drowsiness and deep sleep
							b. Blurred vision
							c. Extrapyramidal reactions such as motor restlessness resembling Parkinson's disease, drooling, tremors, muscle spasms, shuffling gait, dystonias (involuntary movement), difficulty swallowing
							d. Agitation and nervousness
							If these occur, dosage must be reduced or the drug discontinued. Symptoms will subside in 24–48 hours.
							2. Rashes usually due to hypersensitivity
							3. Hypotension (especially immediately after injection); may be postural type
							4. Palpitations, especially immediately after an injection
							5. Liver damage producing jaundice (cholestatic hepatitis)
							6. Anticholinergic reactions such as:
							a. Dryness of mouth
							b. Tachycardia
							c. Blurred vision
							d. Increased salivation
							e. Nasal congestion
							7. Exacerbation of seizure disorders
							OVERDOSAGE
							1. Evidenced by stupor or coma, following muscle spasms, tremors and motor restlessness.
							2. Treatment is symptomatic and supportive. There is no specific antidote. Maintain an open airway, ECG monitoring, hydration, adequate body temperature.

3. If shock or metabolic acidosis occurs, use corticosteroids, fluids, oxygen, etc., as indicated.
4. Cardiac arrhythmias may occur. Manufacturer suggests treatment with neostigmine, pyridostigmine, or propranolol. Digitalis may be used if needed for cardiac failure.
5. Seizures may also occur, use diazepam for control.
6. If acute symptoms of Parkinsonism result, benztropine mesylate or diphenhydramine (Benadryl) may be used.

NURSING IMPLICATIONS
1. Monitor for neurologic disturbances following an injection, or during an infusion; see Adverse Reaction No. 1. Report any of these reactions to the physician immediately. If the patient experiences difficulty in swallowing, discontinue infusion immediately and remain with the patient until the severity of the reaction is determined. The patient may need parenteral hydration and nutrition until ability to swallow returns.
2. Examine for rashes; report them to the physician.
3. Keep the patient supine during injection or infusion.
4. Monitor blood pressure before, during and after injection or infusion. If hypotension occurs during an infusion, discontinue administration and continue to take the blood pressure until stabilization occurs. Hypotension can usually be avoided with slow injection. If a patient is to be ambulated after an injection, obtain lying and standing blood pressure. If postural hypotension is significant, report the fact to the physician and keep the patient at rest. As postural effects decrease over time, begin to ambulate the patient if desirable. Do so cautiously to prevent injury. Warn the patient not to stand up suddenly until the effects of the drug have disappeared. Ambulate the patient with caution if he is experiencing sedation or blurred vision. Initiate safety precautions, such as side rails, to prevent injury.
5. Monitor for jaundice; notify the physician.
6. The patient may experience anticholinergic side effects; see Adverse Reaction No. 6. Inform patient of the origin of the symptoms and its transient nature.
7. Initiate seizure precautions if not already in effect.
8. This drug can cause the urine to darken or turn orange for 24 hours after administration. Inform the patient of the harmlessness of this effect.
9. Monitor temperature every 8 hours; notify physician of any elevation. The drug may be discontinued if this occurs.

PHENOBARBITAL SODIUM (Sodium Luminal)

ACTIONS/ INDICATIONS	DOSAGE	PREPARATION AND STORAGE	DRUG INCOMPAT-IBILITIES	MODES OF IV ADMINISTRATION			CONTRAINDICATIONS; WARNINGS; PRECAUTIONS; ADVERSE REACTIONS
				INJECTION	INTERMITTENT INFUSION	CONTINUOUS INFUSION	
Sedative, anticonvulsant, hypnotic, long-acting barbiturate.

Used in the intravenous mode for relief of severe anxiety, as an anticonvulsant, and as an antispasmotic, alone or in | ADULTS: *Sedative*— 16–32 mg 2–4 times a day.

Hypnotic— 100–300 mg.

Seizures—30–120 mg repeated as needed depending on patient response. | Protect vials from light.

Reconstitute powder form with sterile water for injection in an amount to make dose calculation simple. Vials contain 120 mg or 130 mg. Discard unused portions of reconstituted | Do not mix with any other medication. | YES

Slowly, at a rate not to exceed 50 mg/minute, into the tubing of a running IV. | NO | NO | CONTRAINDICATIONS
1. Hypersensitivity to any barbiturate
2. Porphyria (confirmed or familial history)
3. In children: renal or hepatic dysfunction

WARNINGS
1. Physical and psychological dependence can occur as can withdrawal symptoms.
2. Signs of intoxication are: ataxia, slurred speech, vertigo, excessive sedation.
3. Safety for use in pregnancy has not |

● PHENOBARBITAL SODIUM (Sodium Luminal) (Continued)

ACTIONS/ INDICATIONS	DOSAGE	PREPARATION AND STORAGE	DRUG INCOMPAT- IBILITIES	MODES OF IV ADMINISTRATION			CONTRAINDICATIONS: WARNINGS: PRECAUTIONS: ADVERSE REACTIONS
				INJECTION	INTERMITTENT INFUSION	CONTINUOUS INFUSION	
combination with other drugs.	*Status epilepticus, delirium tremens*—up to 600 mg may be needed depending on patient response. CHILDREN: *Status epilepticus*—5 mg/kg followed by 2.5 mg/kg every 5 min until seizures stop.	solutions. Also available in a premixed form in 1-ml vials of 130 mg/ml, and prefilled syringes of 60 and 130 mg/ml. This is a Schedule IV drug under the Controlled Substances Act of 1970. Maintain hospital or institutional regulations guiding its use.					been established. 4. Withdrawal symptoms can occur in newborns when the mother has received this drug (even in low doses as used for anticonvulsant therapy). 5. Status epilepticus has occurred with withdrawal of this drug from epileptic patients, after prolonged use. 6. Concomitant use with other central nervous system depressants will result in additive effects. 7. May lower blood levels of coumarin anticoagulants, dosage may need to be increased to maintain therapeutic prothrombin time. Conversely, phenobarbital withdrawal may lead to rise in prothrombin time and possible bleeding. 8. Accelerates metabolism of antihistamines, steroids and anticonvulsants. 9. May increase vitamin-D requirements, usually only in long-term oral therapy. PRECAUTIONS 1. Careful adjustment of dosage (usually lower doses) is needed in patients with hepatic, renal, cardiac and respiratory impairment, and in patients with myasthenia gravis and myxedema. 2. Lower doses are also required in elderly and debilitated patients to prevent oversedation. ADVERSE REACTIONS 1. Central nervous system: dizziness, headache, confusion (especially in elderly), paradoxical excitation 2. Gastrointestinal: nausea, vomiting, epigastric pain 3. Allergy: facial edema, rashes, purpura, rarely exfoliative dermatitis, liver degeneration, anaphylaxis

NURSING IMPLICATIONS
1. Strictly adhere to maximum injection rate suggestions and maximum dosage limits to insure maximum benefit from the drug and to prevent overdosage. Patients with liver impairment should receive smaller doses and should be monitored more closely and for a longer period of time than usual.
2. Keep the patient supine during and after injection. Monitor blood pres-

The injection should be stopped immediately upon noting one of these symptoms.
7. Management of acute overdosage:
   a. Continue to stay with the patient and monitor vital signs
   b. Maintain an open airway and adequate ventilation
   c. Keep the patient as alert as possible by verbal and physical stimuli. Encourage the patient to breathe at an adequate rate (12–14 breaths/

sure, heart rate and respiratory rate every 5 minutes for 1 hour following injection. This includes fetal heart rate monitoring. Do not leave the patient unattended.

3. Patients with porphyria are sensitive to barbiturates in that they may experience an acute attack of the disease secondary to the administration of a barbiturate (see Contraindications). The onset of an acute attack is indicated by severe colicky abdominal pain radiating to the back. There is usually severe vomiting, fever and leukocytosis in addition.[1]

4. Avoid extravasation; see page 96. Extravascular or intra-arterial injection of this drug can cause tissue necrosis and gangrene of the affected extremity, respectively. Thrombophlebitis can also occur. Examine for redness and pain along the vein tract.

5. Take anaphylaxis precautions; see page 118.

6. Monitor for symptoms of acute overdosage (listed in order of progression):
   a. Respiratory depression, i.e., decreased respiratory rate and depth
   b. Ataxia, slurred speech, vertigo, excessive sedation
   c. Peripheral vascular collapse, i.e., fall in blood pressure, pallor, diaphoresis, tachycardia
   d. Pulmonary edema (rare)
   e. Decreased or absent reflexes, pupillary constriction
   f. Stupor
   g. Coma

minute for an adult). If necessary, initiate artificial ventilation with a manual breathing bag (Puritan, Hope, Ambu, etc.) or mouth-to-mouth breathing at a rate of 12–14 breaths/minute

   d. Circulatory support in the form of fluids and drugs may be ordered

8. The sedation produced by this drug may be preceded by transient changes in mental status, such as feelings of euphoria and confusion. If this occurs, attempt to calm the patient and take measures to prevent injury until the patient returns to his normal status.

9. If a patient is to be ambulatory following an injection, ambulate with assistance; there may be transient dizziness. Obtain lying, then sitting and standing blood pressures to detect postural hypotension. If this drug has been used for an outpatient procedure, a responsible adult should accompany the patient home. The patient should not drive for at least the next 8 hours.

10. If this drug is given for seizures, monitor effectiveness and initiate seizure precautions if not already in effect.

REFERENCE
1. Beeson, Paul B., and McDermott, Walsh (editors): *Cecil-Loeb Textbook of Medicine* (14th ed.). Philadelphia: W. B. Saunders Company, 1975, p. 1873.

● PHENTOLAMINE MESYLATE (Regitine)

ACTIONS/ INDICATIONS	DOSAGE	PREPARATION AND STORAGE	DRUG INCOMPAT- IBILITIES	MODES OF IV ADMINISTRATION			CONTRAINDICATIONS; WARNINGS; PRECAUTIONS; ADVERSE REACTIONS
				INJECTION	INTERMITTENT INFUSION	CONTINUOUS INFUSION	
Alpha adrenergic blocking agent. Produces vasodilation. Used to prevent or control hypertensive episodes in pheochromocytoma; prevention and treatment of tissue necrosis and sloughing caused by extravasation of sympathomimetic agents that produce vasoconstriction. Diagnostic agent for pheochromocytoma.	ADULTS: *Prevention and control of hypertensive crises in pheochromocytoma*—5 mg every 6 hrs. *Diagnosis of pheochromocytoma*—5 mg. See Nursing Implications No. 1 for test procedure. *Prevention of dermal necrosis*—10 mg added to each 1000 ml levarterenol.	Supplied in ampuls of 5 mg accompanied by an ampul of 1 ml sterile water for injection for reconstitution of the drug powder. Resulting solution will contain 5 mg/ml. Discard unused portions of solution; do not store.	Do not mix with any other medications, except levarterenol.	YES Dilute 5 mg in 1 ml sterile water for injection.	NO	YES 5 mg can be added to each liter of levarterenol solution, for prevention of dermal necrosis.	CONTRAINDICATIONS 1. Acute myocardial infarction 2. History of myocardial infarction, coronary insufficiency, angina 3. Hypersensitivity WARNINGS 1. Myocardial infarction, cerebrovascular spasm, and occlusion have occurred after an injection of phentolamine in association with marked lowering of blood pressure. 2. The phentolamine test for pheochromocytoma should be done only when other simpler tests have been positive. 3. Safety for use during pregnancy and lactation has not been established. ADVERSE REACTIONS 1. Acute prolonged hypotensive episodes, with tachycardia and other arrhythmias after IV injection 2. Weakness 3. Dizziness

445

ACTIONS/ INDICATIONS	DOSAGE	PREPARATION AND STORAGE	DRUG INCOMPAT- IBILITIES	MODES OF IV ADMINISTRATION			CONTRAINDICATIONS; WARNINGS; PRECAUTIONS; ADVERSE REACTIONS
				INJECTION	INTERMITTENT INFUSION	CONTINUOUS INFUSION	
	Treatment of dermal necrosis—5–10 mg diluted in 10–15 ml NS for subcutaneous injection. See Nursing Implications No. 3 for procedure.						4. Flushing 5. Orthostatic hypotension 6. Nasal stuffiness 7. Nausea, vomiting, diarrhea
	CHILDREN: *Prevention and control of hypertensive crises in pheochromocytoma* —1 mg every 6 hrs.						
	Diagnosis of pheochromocytoma—1 mg/kg. See Nursing Implications No. 1 for test procedure.						
	Prevention and treatment of dermal necrosis is the same as for adults.						

NURSING IMPLICATIONS
1. Phentolamine test for pheochromocytoma:
   a. Discontinue all nonessential medications at least 24 hours before the test, especially antihypertensives.
   b. This test is usually not performed on normotensive patients.
   c. Place the patient on bed rest in a quiet, dark room, and begin taking his blood pressure every 10 minutes.
   d. When the blood pressure has stabilized, notify the physician and prepare the phentolamine. Combine 5 mg of drug (1 mg/kg in children) with 1 ml sterile water for injection.
   e. The needle should then be inserted into the vein, and after a waiting period of 2 to 3 minutes, the phentolamine is injected rapidly.
   f. Monitor blood pressure immediately after the injection and every 30 seconds for the first 3 minutes, and at 60-second intervals for the next 7 minutes.
   g. A positive test consists in a drop in blood pressure more than 35 mm

readily available.
   c. After one hour of bed rest, the patient can be ambulated, but with caution. Evaluate for postural hypotension by taking lying and standing blood pressures. If there is a significant drop in blood pressure on standing, notify the physician and keep the patient at rest.
   d. Assist in interpreting the test to the patient.
3. Infiltration therapy for extravasation of vasoconstrictor agents (e.g., dopamine, levarterenol):
   a. The affected area should be infiltrated with phentolamine as soon after the extravasation has occurred as possible. The affected area will be blanched and cool to touch.
   b. Follow hospital policy as to who performs the treatment, i.e., nurse or physician.
   c. A 25- or 26-gauge needle should be used with a 20 ml syringe. A solution of 5–10 mg of phentolamine in 10–15 ml of normal saline is recommended.

d. Infiltrate the area thoroughly. Monitor for hypotension secondary to the phentolamine for the next 2 hours. See No. 2 above for aftercare.
e. The affected area will become reddened secondary to the vasodilatation produced by the phentolamine.
f. Protect the area from further trauma, and examine daily for the onset of tissue necrosis and sloughing. If these occur, the area should be cared for as a burn, to prevent infection and further damage.
g. Do not use the affected extremity for injections or blood pressure readings until healing has occurred.

Hg systolic and 25 mm Hg diastolic. Maximal fall in pressure should occur in 2 minutes after the injection. The suspicion of pheochromocytoma should be confirmed by other diagnostic techniques.
2. Care of the patient receiving and phentolamine test:
a. Be prepared to manage hypotension; vasopressors should be readily available.
b. Monitor for cardiac arrhythmias either by frequent pulse readings in patients without a history of cardiac disease, or by continuous ECG monitoring in patients with cardiac disease. Lidocaine and atropine should be

PHENYLEPHRINE HYDROCHLORIDE (Neo-synephrine Injection)

ACTIONS/ INDICATIONS	DOSAGE	PREPARATION AND STORAGE	DRUG INCOMPAT- IBILITIES	MODES OF IV ADMINISTRATION			CONTRAINDICATIONS; WARNINGS; PRECAUTIONS; ADVERSE REACTIONS
				INJECTION	INTERMITTENT INFUSION	CONTINUOUS INFUSION	
Vasopressor, sympathomimetic amine.	ADULTS: *Mild to moderate hypotension*— injection of 0.2 mg (range: 0.1–0.5 mg). Repeat no more frequently than every 10–15 min as needed; do not exceed 0.5 mg in one injection. Duration of action of one dose is 15 min.	Available in 1-ml ampuls, 10 mg/ml (1% solution): *DOSAGE CALCULATIONS:* *Vol. of 1% Solu-* *Dose Requir- tion to* *ed Use* 10 mg 1.0 ml 5 mg 0.5 ml 1 mg 0.1 ml	Do not add any other agent to IV bottle. Do not inject into an IV line containing: Sodium bicarbonate or Aminophylline.	YES Using a 1% or 0.1% solution as stated in Dosage column.	YES Using a 1:50,000 solution as stated in Dosage and Preparation columns. Use an infusion pump.	YES Using a 1:50,000 solution as stated in Dosage and Preparation columns. Use an infusion pump.	CONTRAINDICATIONS 1. Uncontrolled hypertension 2. Ventricular tachycardia PRECAUTIONS 1. Use with extreme caution in: a. The elderly b. Hyperthyroidism c. Bradycardia d. Heart block of any degree e. Myocardial disease (coronary insufficiency, myocardial fibrosis, etc.) f. Severe arteriosclerosis g. Halothane anesthesia (can produce *severe* arrhythmias) h. In labor and delivery if an oxytocic drug has also been used (the combination can produce *severe* hypertension)
This agent stimulates alpha receptors and produces the following effects either directly or indirectly through reflex action: • Decreased heart rate (indirect) • Increased cardiac output (direct) • Vasoconstriction (direct) • Does not usually produce arrhythmias	*Severe hypotension and shock*—By infusion, start with 0.1–0.2 mg/min using a 1:50,000 solution (0.02 mg/ml). Titrate with blood pressure. Average maintenance dosage is 0.05–0.08 mg/min.	To prepare an 0.1% solution, dilute 1 ml of a 1% solution (10 mg) in 9 ml sterile water for injection. *Vol. of 0.1% Solu-* *Dose Requir- tion to* *ed Use* 0.1 mg 0.1 ml 0.2 mg 0.2 ml 0.5 mg 0.5 ml					2. The pressor effect of this drug is potentiated by MAO inhibitor agents. If the patient has been receiving an MAO inhibitor, the initial dose of phenylephrine should be reduced. 3. If excessive hypertension occurs with this drug, phenotolamine (Regitine) can be used. See page 445 for further information on phentolamine. 4. In hypotension secondary to hypovolemia, blood volume depletion must always be corrected before or during use of this drug. 5. When used to treat paroxysmal supraventricular tachycardia, a large dose of this drug (greater than 1 mg) can precipitate premature ventricular contraction, ventricular tachycardia, a sensation of fullness in the head and
Indicated in: • Maintenance of blood pressure during spinal or general anesthesia • Treatment of shock due to vascular collapse, ana-	See Preparation column for solutions.	For continuous infusion use a					

447

PHENYLEPHRINE HYDROCHLORIDE (Neo-synephrine Injection) (Continued)

ACTIONS/ INDICATIONS	DOSAGE	PREPARATION AND STORAGE	DRUG INCOMPAT- IBILITIES	MODES OF IV ADMINISTRATION			CONTRAINDICATIONS; WARNINGS; PRECAUTIONS; ADVERSE REACTIONS
				INJECTION	INTERMITTENT INFUSION	CONTINUOUS INFUSION	
phylaxis or drug-in- duced hypo- tension • Conversion of paroxys- mal supra- ventricular tachycardia to normal si- nus rhythm.	Higher doses may be re- quired for hy- potension pro- duced by powerful pe- ripheral adren- ergic blocking agents or chlorpro- mazine. *Paroxysmal su- praventricular tachycardia— rapid* injection (over 20–30 seconds) ini- tially of 0.5 mg (0.5 ml of a 1% solution). Subsequent doses which are deter- mined by the initial blood pressure re- sponse should not exceed the preceding dose by more than 0.1–0.2 mg. DO NOT EXCEED A DOSE OF 1 MG. CHILDREN: Intravenous administration in any mode is not recom- mended. Use subcutaneous or intramuscu- lar routes.	1:50,000 solu- tion. Prepare by adding 10 mg of drug to 500 ml of D5W or NS. This solu- tion will contain 0.02 mg/ml.					tingling of the extremities. The effects of the drug last 15–20 minutes. ADVERSE REACTIONS 1. Excessive elevation in blood pressure 2. Ventricular irritability producing pre- mature ventricular contractions, sinus tachycardia, ventricular tachycardia and fibrillation 3. A feeling of fullness in the head 4. Tingling in the extremities

NURSING IMPLICATIONS
1. Monitor blood pressure (direct arterial pressure is the preferred method) continuously during push injection and for 15 minutes following, followed by determinations every 5 minutes for 30 minutes, and every 10–15 min- utes thereafter until pressure has stabilized at a desirable level (as deter- mined by the physician). An 0.5 mg injection will elevate systemic blood

2. Administer supportive care such as replacement of fluids, maintenance of body warmth, and use of Trendelenberg position (unless contraindicated) for the patient in shock.
3. Monitor urine output hourly in the shock patient; report oliguria (output less than 30 ml in 2 consecutive hours) to the physician.
4. All patients should be observed for cardiac arrhythmias via a continuous

pressure for approximately 15 minutes.

During infusions, monitor blood pressure every 2 minutes until a desirable level is reached (as determined by the physician) and every 15–30 minutes thereafter. As blood pressure is rising toward desired level, slow infusion. When level is reached, stop infusion. Continue to monitor blood pressure and heart rate for return of hypotension. See No. 5 below.

ECG monitor. Be prepared to treat premature ventriculation contractions and ventricular tachycardia (lidocaine and defibrillator should be readily available).

5. Use an infusion pump. If unavailable, use microdrop IV tubing and do not leave the patient unattended.

PHENYTOIN SODIUM (Dilantin)

ACTIONS/ INDICATIONS	DOSAGE	PREPARATION AND STORAGE	DRUG INCOMPATIBILITIES	MODES OF IV ADMINISTRATION: INJECTION	MODES OF IV ADMINISTRATION: INTERMITTENT INFUSION	MODES OF IV ADMINISTRATION: CONTINUOUS INFUSION	CONTRAINDICATIONS; WARNINGS; PRECAUTIONS; ADVERSE REACTIONS
Anticonvulsant, antiarrhythmic agent. Used to prevent and control seizures of grand mal variety. Also used to control arrhythmias such as: • Supraventricular tachycardia • Premature ventricular contractions • Ventricular tachycardia especially those arrhythmias secondary to digitalis toxicity. Exerts little effect on atrial flutter or fibrillation or recurrent ventricular tachycardia. Plasma concentrations between 10 and 18 mcg/ml produce therapeutic effects.[1] Plasma drug concentration is the most re-	ADULTS: *Status epilepticus*—150–250 mg followed by 100–150 mg 30 min later; repeat until seizures are controlled. Do not exceed 750 mg in 1 hr. *Seizure prophylaxis, postsurgery or trauma*—100–200 mg every 4 hrs. *Arrhythmias*—50–100 mg every 5 min until toxicity (nystagmus) occurs, the arrhythmia is controlled, or 1000 mg has been given. Follow with 500 mg in 24 hrs. Place patient on oral antiarrhythmic therapy as soon as possible. See Warning No. 2.	Available in a premixed form, 50 mg/ml. Discard unused portions of ampuls. Do not add to IV fluids of any kind.	Do not mix with any other medication in any manner.	YES *Slowly. Do not exceed an injection rate of 50 mg/min* (25 mg/min in patients with coronary artery disease). Inject either directly into the vein or cannula, or into an injection site in the IV tubing that is *immediately* above the junction between the tubing and cannula. This prevents mixing of the drug with the fluid. Flush IV line or vein with 10 ml NS after injection. It is not necessary to further dilute ready-mixed solution prior to injection.	NO This drug precipitates in *all* solutions. Effects such precipitation may have on the patient are not known.[2]	NO See Intermittent column.	CONTRAINDICATIONS 1. Hypersensitivity to hycantoin products 2. Sinus bradycardia 3. Sinus node exit block (sinoatrial block) 4. Second and third degree A-V block 5. Stokes-Adams syndrome WARNINGS 1. This agent is not indicated for seizures secondary to hypoglycemia. 2. There are many drug interactions associated with this agent: *DRUGS THAT MAY AFFECT THE PHARMACOKINETICS OF PHENYTOIN (DIPHENYLHYDANTOIN) IN MAN*[3] *Drugs That May Increase Phenytoin Levels in the Blood* Bishydroxycoumarin, Chloramphenicol, Chlordiazepoxide, Chlorpromazine, Diazepam, Disulfiram, Estrogens, Ethyl alcohol, Isoniazid, Methylphenidate, Phenyramidol, Phenobarbital, Prochlorperazine, Propoxyphene, Sulthiame *Drugs That May Decrease Phenytoin Levels in The Blood* Carbamazepine, Ethyl alcohol, Phenobarbital *Drugs That May Alter Plasma Protein Binding of Phenytoin* Phenylbutazone, Salicylic acid, Sulfafurazole Dosage requirements of phenytoin will be altered in the presence of

PHENYTOIN SODIUM (Dilantin) (Continued)

ACTIONS/ INDICATIONS	DOSAGE	PREPARATION AND STORAGE	DRUG INCOMPAT- IBILITIES	MODES OF IV ADMINISTRATION			CONTRAINDICATIONS; WARNINGS; PRECAUTIONS; ADVERSE REACTIONS
				INJECTION	INTERMITTENT INFUSION	CONTINUOUS INFUSION	
liable guide for adequate dosage.	Patients with renal impairment and uremia may require reduced dosage according to the severity of impairment. CHILDREN: *Seizures and status epilepticus*—3–8 mg/kg/24 hrs or 250 mg/ M²/24 hrs in divided doses.						these agents, to prevent toxicity or underdosage. 3. Use with caution in patients with coronary artery disease or hypotension. Injections may cause further lowering of pressure and possibly reduced myocardial perfusion. See injection rate in Injection column. 4. The effects of this drug in pregnancy and nursing infants are unknown. Some studies suggest the possibility of drug-related birth defects. However, anticonvulsant drugs should not be withheld in patients likely to have major seizures because of the possibility of precipitating status epilepticus. PRECAUTIONS 1. Patients with liver impairment, or the elderly may need dosage modification. Serum levels must be closely followed. 2. This drug may cause hyperglycemia in normal individuals and further elevation of serum glucose in diabetics. ADVERSE REACTIONS 1. During injection at a rate greater than 50 mg/min—respiratory arrest, hypotension, idioventricular rhythm, asystole, ventricular fibrillation 2. This drug usually improves A-V conduction, but can also cause slowing of atrial and A-V conduction, precipitating heart block 3. Vertigo, nausea and drowsiness are side effects 4. Toxic blood levels can cause: nystagmus or lateral gaze, ataxia, lethargy 5. Can also precipitate megaloblastic anemia (responsive to folate), thrombocytopenia, leukopenia, granulocytopenia and agranulocytosis 6. Peripheral neuropathy 7. Rashes, mild and severe 8. Hyperglycemia 9. Vomiting and constipation OVERDOSAGE AND MANAGEMENT Initial signs of toxicity: nystagmus, ataxia, dysarthria. Signs of advancing toxicity

are coma, unresponsive pupils, hypotension. Death can occur secondary to apnea. Treatment:
1. Prevent by following serum drug levels frequently (range of therapeutic level: 10–18 mcg/ml).
2. No antidote known. Discontinue the drug with appearance of earliest signs.
3. In advanced toxicity, support respirations with airway or endotracheal tube, oxygen and respirator as needed.
4. Vasopressors to support blood pressure (dopamine).
5. Hemodialysis if necessary to clear drug from the serum.

pare it for immediate use: airways, suction, oxygen, endotracheal tubes and laryngoscope, manual breathing bag (Ambu, Hope, Puritan) with mask. Begin ventilatory support via airway and manual bag if respiratory rate falls below 8–10/minute despite verbal stimuli. Continue ventilation until patient regains an appropriate respiratory rate and arterial blood gases return to normal. Patient may require endotracheal intubation.

REFERENCES
1. Winkle, Roger A., Glantz, Stanton A., and Harrison, Donald C.: Pharmacologic Therapy of Ventricular Arrhythmias. *American Journal of Cardiology,* 36:643, October 31, 1975.
2. Trissel, Lawrence A: *Handbook on Injectable Drugs,* American Society of Hospital Pharmacists, Washington, D.C., 1977, p. 297.
3. Winkle, p. 643.

SUGGESTED READINGS
Amsterdam, Ezra, et al.: Systemic Approach to the Management of Cardiac Arrhythmias. *Heart and Lung,* 2:747–753, September–October 1973 (references).
Levitt, Barrie, Borer, Jeffrey, and Sarapa, Arleen: The Clinical Pharmacology of Antiarrhythmic Drugs. Part II: Quinidine, Propranolol, Diphenylhydantoin, and Bretylium. *Cardiovascular Nursing,* November–December, 1974, pp. 27–32.
————: Treatment of Cardiac Arrhythmias. *Medical Letter on Drugs and Therapeutics,* 16 (25):101–108, December 6, 1974.

NURSING IMPLICATIONS
1. Follow hospital policy as to who can administer this drug intravenously, physician or nurse.
2. This medication should not be added to IV fluid for infusion.
3. Closely observe all patients receiving this drug intravenously, using continuous ECG monitoring during the injection. The injection should be stopped if the P-R interval becomes prolonged beyond 0.12 second. Maximal effect of the drug is seen in 5 minutes after IV injection. Monitor for drug effectiveness at this time. Do not leave the patient unattended for the first 10 minutes following injection.
4. Obtain a blood pressure reading just prior to and immediately following injection of the drug. Monitor every 5 minutes for the following 30 minutes. The injection should be slowed or momentarily stopped if the patient complains of dizziness or diaphoresis. Take the blood pressure at this time. Monitor closely until return to the preinjection level and stabilization are seen.
5. Ambulate the patient with caution, after 1 hour of bed rest following an injection.
6. Observe for signs of toxicity. It is important to discontinue injections at the earliest sign: ataxia, nystagmus (constant involuntary eye movements), dysarthria (difficulty or slurring of speech), change in mental status. Notify the physician immediately on appearance of any of these signs.
7. If early signs of toxicity are present, monitor for advancing signs: hypotension, depressed mental activity, decreasing respiratory rate. Be prepared to support ventilation. Place the following equipment at the bedside and pre-

PHYSOSTIGMINE SALICYLATE (Antilirium)

ACTIONS/ INDICATIONS	DOSAGE	PREPARATION AND STORAGE	DRUG INCOMPAT- IBILITIES	MODES OF IV ADMINISTRATION			CONTRAINDICATIONS; WARNINGS; PRECAUTIONS; ADVERSE REACTIONS
				INJECTION	INTERMITTENT INFUSION	CONTINUOUS INFUSION	
Cholinesterase inhibitor, prolongs and exaggerates the effect of ace-	ADULTS: 0.05–2.0 mg. Repeat 1 mg doses as	Discard unused portions of vials. Supplied in 2	Do not mix with fluids or any other medication.	YES Inject undiluted over 1–2 minutes.	NO	NO	CONTRAINDICATIONS 1. Asthma 2. Gangrene 3. Diabetes mellitus 4. Cardiovascular disease

PHYSOSTIGMINE SALICYLATE (Antilirium) (Continued)

ACTIONS/INDICATIONS	DOSAGE	PREPARATION AND STORAGE	DRUG INCOMPATIBILITIES	MODES OF IV ADMINISTRATION			CONTRAINDICATIONS; WARNINGS; PRECAUTIONS; ADVERSE REACTIONS
				INJECTION	INTERMITTENT INFUSION	CONTINUOUS INFUSION	
tylcholine at the myoneural junction. Produces: • Constriction of pupil • Increased tone of gastrointestinal muscles • Constriction of bronchi • Stimulation of salivary and sweat glands Used to reverse toxic effects on the central nervous system caused by anticholinergic drugs (atropine, scopolamine, benztropine, and tricyclic antidepressants). Toxic effects of these drugs are: hallucinations, disorientation, hyperactivity, coma, medullary paralysis. This is the only cholinesterase inhibitor that can effectively cross the blood-brain barrier.	needed To reverse the toxic or clinical effects of anticholinergic drugs, the dose of physostigmine is twice that of the drug in milligrams. For example, if the dose of atropine had been 2 mg, the dose of physostigmine could be 4 mg. CHILDREN: No data available.	ml ampuls, 1 mg/ml.					5. Mechanical obstruction of the intestinal or urinary tract 6. In patients receiving choline esters or neuromuscular blocking agents (succinylcholine or decamethonium) PRECAUTIONS 1. Patients may exhibit hyperreactivity to this agent. Keep atropine readily available as an antidote. 2. If excessive symptoms of salivation, emesis, urination and defecation occur, injection and use of this drug should be terminated. 3. If excessive sweating or nausea occurs, the dosage should be reduced. 4. Rapid administration can cause bradycardia, hypersalivation leading to respiratory difficulties and possible convulsions. 5. An overdose of this drug will cause a cholinergic crisis.

NURSING IMPLICATIONS
1. Monitor for signs of cholinergic crises following injection of this drug; see Precautions.
2. Keep atropine at the bedside. Do not leave the patient alone for the first agent: mental confusion, stupor, nausea and diaphoresis. Notify the physician of these effects and be prepared to administer additional doses of physostigmine.

SUGGESTED READING

Guyton, Arthur C.: *Textbook of Medical Physiology*, Chapter 57 — The Autonomic Nervous System: The Adrenal Medulla, Philadelphia: W. B. Saunders Company, 1976, pp. 768–780.

15–30 minutes after injection.

3. This drug is rapidly metabolized by the body, and additional doses may be required if the duration of the anticholinergic agent's action exceeds that of the physostigmine. Monitor for signs of the effects of the anticholinergic

● PHYTONADIONE (Vitamin K-1, Aqua Mephyton, Konakion)

ACTIONS/ INDICATIONS	DOSAGE	PREPARATION AND STORAGE	DRUG INCOMPAT- IBILITIES	MODES OF IV ADMINISTRATION			CONTRAINDICATIONS; WARNINGS; PRECAUTIONS; ADVERSE REACTIONS
				INJECTION	INTERMITTENT INFUSION	CONTINUOUS INFUSION	
Vitamin necessary for the production of active prothrombin, and clotting factors VII, IX and X, in the liver. After IV administration hemorrhage can be controlled in 3–6 hrs. Used to treat coagulation disorders caused by vitamin K deficiency or interference with vitamin K activity; as an antidote for coumarin drugs.	IV administration should be used *only* when subcutaneous or intramuscular routes cannot be used. See Adverse Reactions No. 1. *Anticoagulant-induced prothrombin deficiency and hypoprothrombinema due to other causes*— 2.5–10 mg or up to 25 mg. Repeat if prothrombin level has not been shortened satisfactorily in 8 hrs. Use smallest dose for effectiveness without lowering prothrombin level too far below an effective level. Short-acting anticoagulants will require lower dose than long-acting.	Supplied in 1-ml ampuls and multidose vials of 10 mg/ ml. Use immediately after adding to fluids. Do not use if, when mixed with fluid, an oily layer or droplets appear. Discard all unused portions. Protect solution from light. Keep vials in box; place a paper bag around IV bottle during infusion	Do not mix with any other medication in any manner.	YES In emergency, 5–25 mg over 5–10 min into the tubing of a running IV. No more than 1 mg/min. Dilution prior to injection is not required.	YES Use only NS, D5/NS, or D5W, 5.0 ml. *Preferred route.* Infuse no more rapidly than 1 mg/min. Dilute dose in enough fluid to make drip rate calculation easy. Use an infusion pump.	NO	CONTRAINDICATIONS Hypersensitivity WARNINGS 1. An immediate coagulant effect cannot be expected even after IV push administration. Measurable effect will not be seen before 1–2 hrs. Whole blood or component therapy must be used in hypotension and hemorrhage. 2. This drug will not counteract the effects of heparin. 3. In anticoagulant-induced hypoprothrombinemia, overzealous therapy with vitamin K may restore conditions which originally permitted thromboembolic phenomena. Keep vitamin K dose as low as possible to prevent under-anticoagulation. 4. Monitor prothrombin time during therapy. 5. Repeated large doses of vitamin K are not warranted in liver disease if response to initial dose is unsatisfactory. 6. It is not known whether this drug affects fertility or fetal development. PRECAUTIONS 1. A temporary resistance to prothrombin-depressing anticoagulants (coumarin) may result, especially in larger doses. Increased doses of the anticoagulant may be required when reinitiated, or another agent such as heparin may be used. 2. Follow injection-rate limitations *absolutely.* ADVERSE REACTIONS 1. Deaths have occurred after IV administration.

453

PHYTONADIONE (Vitamin K-1, Aqua Mephyton, Konakion) (Continued)

ACTIONS/INDICATIONS	DOSAGE	PREPARATION AND STORAGE	DRUG INCOMPATIBILITIES	MODES OF IV ADMINISTRATION			CONTRAINDICATIONS; WARNINGS; PRECAUTIONS; ADVERSE REACTIONS
				INJECTION	INTERMITTENT INFUSION	CONTINUOUS INFUSION	
	Newborn hemorrhagic disease—IV route not recommended.						2. Transient flushing sensations and alterations of taste have been reported. 3. Dizziness, rapid weak pulse, profuse sweating, brief hypotension, dyspnea and cyanosis. 4. Anaphylaxis, shock and cardiac arrest.

NURSING IMPLICATIONS
1. Signs and symptoms of too-rapid injection are chills and fever, chest tightness, hypotension, seizures, cyanosis.
2. Monitor blood pressure frequently during injection and infusion, every 2–5 minutes. If any of the above signs or symptoms appear, slow or stop infusion or injection. Do not leave the patient unattended.
3. Be aware of the patient's prothrombin times.
4. Monitor for bleeding until an effect is seen from the drug. Administer supportive measures as prescribed.
5. Monitor for adverse reactions and initiate appropriate care. Notify physician if tachycardia, diaphoresis, hypotension, dyspnea or cyanosis occur.
6. Take anaphylaxis precautions; see p. 118.

POLYMYXIN-B SULFATE (Aerosporin)

ACTIONS/INDICATIONS	DOSAGE	PREPARATION AND STORAGE	DRUG INCOMPATIBILITIES	MODES OF IV ADMINISTRATION			CONTRAINDICATIONS; WARNINGS; PRECAUTIONS; ADVERSE REACTIONS
				INJECTION	INTERMITTENT INFUSION	CONTINUOUS INFUSION	
Antibiotic; used to treat infections caused by susceptible strains of: • Pseudomonas aeruginosa • H. influenzae • E. coli • Aerobacter aerogenes • Klebsiella pneumoniae The intravenous route is indicated in infections in all locations except meningeal infections.	ADULTS AND CHILDREN: 15,000–25,000 units/kg/day in the presence of normal kidney function. (Do not exceed 25,000 units/kg/day.) ADULTS AND CHILDREN WITH RENAL FAILURE:[1] Mild impairment—25,000 units/kg the first day and then 10,000 units/kg every 3 days.	Reconstitute 500,000-unit vial with 2 ml sterile water for injection, D5W or NS. Store under refrigeration; discard any unused portions after 72 hrs. Use only D5W or NS for infusion fluid.	Do not mix in any manner with: Penicillins Cephalothin Cefazolin Amphotericin Chloramphenicol Chlorothiazide Chlortetracycline Heparin Magnesium sulfate Prednisolone Tetracycline	NO	NO	YES 500,000 units in 500 cc D5W or NS with drip rate set to deliver ½ daily dose over 12 hrs.	CONTRAINDICATIONS Hypersensitivity to polymyxin or colistin. WARNINGS 1. Renal function must be monitored during therapy. 2. Patients with renal impairment must have a reduced dosage. 3. Nephrotoxicity due to this drug is evidenced by albuminuria, cellular casts in the urine and increased BUN. Diminishing urine output and rising BUN are indications for discontinuation of the drug. 4. Neurotoxicity may be manifested by irritability, weakness, drowsiness, ataxia, numbness of the extremities, blurring of vision. This is usually seen in high doses or in patients with renal failure. The drug should be discontinued with the onset of these signs and symptoms. 5. Concurrent use of other neurotoxic antibiotics (kanamycin, streptomycin polymyxin E, neomycin, gentamicin

Uremia—
25,000 units/kg the first day and then 10,000 units/kg every 5–7 *days*.

INFANTS:
Up to 40,000 units/kg/day. Depending on condition of the patient, organism being treated, response to the drug.

PREMATURE AND NEW-BORN IN-FANTS:
25,000–40,000 units/kg/day via infusion.

NURSING IMPLICATIONS
1. Take anaphylaxis precautions; see page 118.
2. Monitor for the onset of renal damage:
   a. Measure urine output at least every 8 hours. A urine output less than 30 ml/hour for 2–3 consecutive hours in an adult (see chart on page 546 for normal urine output in children) should be reported to the physician.
   b. Send urine for analysis daily or on alternate days.
   c. Be aware of the patient's pretreatment BUN and any changes during therapy.
3. Monitor for the onset of signs and symptoms of neurotoxicity as listed in Warning No. 4. Notify the physician of positive findings.
4. If neurotoxicity occurs, begin monitoring for respiratory depression:
   a. Count respiratory rate and depth hourly
   b. Notify the physician if the respiratory rate falls below 8–10/minute
   c. Monitor arterial blood gases as indicated

and viomycin) should be avoided.
6. Neurotoxicity can result in respiratory paralysis, especially when the drug is given soon after anesthesia and/or muscle relaxants.
7. Safety for use in pregnancy has not been established.

PRECAUTIONS
1. Obtain baseline renal function prior to use.
2. Avoid concurrent use of a curariform muscle relaxant: ether, tubocurarine, succinylcholine, gallamine, decamethonium, or sodium citrate, which may precipitate respiratory depression (see Warning No. 6).
3. If respiratory depression occurs, drug must be discontinued.
4. Overgrowth of nonsusceptible organism can occur; if so, this drug must be discontinued.

ADVERSE REACTIONS
1. Renal: albuminuria, cylindruria, azotemia, rising polymyxin blood levels without increase in dose.
2. Neurologic: dizziness, ataxia, drowsiness, circumoral numbness, respiratory paralysis.
3. Rash, drug fever, anaphylaxis
4. Thrombophlebitis at injection site.

   d. Be prepared to support ventilation
5. Monitor for signs and symptoms of nonsusceptible organism overgrowth infection:
   a. Fever (take rectal temperature at least every 4–6 hours)
   b. Increasing malaise
   c. Localized signs and symptoms of infection—redness, soreness, pain, swelling, drainage (change in volume or character of pre-existing drainage)
   d. Cough (change in volume or character of pre-existing sputum)
   e. Diarrhea
   f. Rash (monilial) in the perineal area or mouth (thrush) (*Candida albicans*)

REFERENCE
1. Appel, Gerald B. and Neu, Harold C.: The Nephrotoxicity of Antimicrobial Agents. *New England Journal of Medicine*, 296(12):667, March 24, 1977.

POTASSIUM CHLORIDE and POTASSIUM LACTATE

ACTIONS/ INDICATIONS	DOSAGE	PREPARATION AND STORAGE	DRUG INCOMPAT- IBILITIES	MODES OF IV ADMINISTRATION			CONTRAINDICATIONS; WARNINGS; PRECAUTIONS; ADVERSE REACTIONS
				INJECTION	INTERMITTENT INFUSION	CONTINUOUS INFUSION	
Electrolyte solution to provide potassium ions to intra-cellular and extra-cellular fluids, to maintain osmotic balance and cell membrane electrical potential.\n\nUsed to maintain serum potassium at normal levels during parenteral fluid therapy and to correct hypokalemic states.	Dosage and rate of infusion are dependent on serum potassium (K+) levels:\n\nADULTS:\nIf serum K+ is greater than 2.5 mEq/liter, administer at a rate no greater than 10 mEq/hour in an infusion concentration less than 30 mEq/liter. The total 24-hour dose should not exceed 200 mEq.	Use any IV solution except mannitol (see reference to indications for the use of NS, in Dosage column).\n\nMix all preparations well after adding potassium by inverting bottle several times to avoid concentrated accumulation of the potassium at the bottom of the container. Mixing is especially important in the use of plastic IV bags.	Do not add to mannitol.	NO\n\nPOTASSIUM SHOULD NEVER BE ADMINISTERED BY THIS MODE OR IN AN UNDILUTED FORM.	YES\n\nIn emergency treatment of hypokalemia—Add 40–60 mEq to 500 ml NS.\n\nUse cardiac monitoring during use of this mode for emergency treatment.\n\nSee Dosage column for infusion rates.	YES\n\nUsually 20–40 mEq in 1000 ml. See Dosage column for rate of infusion.	CONTRAINDICATIONS\nIn conditions where high serum potassium levels are likely to develop, such as renal failure and shock.\n\nWARNINGS\n1. To avoid potassium intoxication, follow infusion rate recommendations in dosage column.\n2. In patients with renal or adrenal insufficiency, serum potassium levels may already be elevated.\n3. Monitor serum potassium and ECG changes frequently during therapy.
	If serum K+ is equal to or less than 2.0 mEq/liter with ECG changes or paralysis present, infuse at a rate of 40 mEq/hour. As much as 400 mEq can be given in 24 hours. (Use saline for infusion in this situation; dextrose solutions may lower serum K+.)	Use only clear solutions.\n\nSupplied in several forms and concentrations.			FOR CHILDREN —add 10–20 mEq to 500 ml D5W or NS. See Dosage column for infusion rates.\n\nUse infusion pump.		PRECAUTIONS\n1. Plasma potassium levels do not necessarily correlate to cell potassium levels.\n2. A high serum potassium level may precipitate death due to cardiac depression or arrhythmias (such as conduction defects).\n3. The patient should be well hydrated and should demonstrate adequate renal function prior to the parenteral administration of potassium.
	CARDIAC MONITORING IS MANDATORY DURING THIS THERAPY.						ADVERSE REACTIONS\n1. Gastrointestinal: nausea, vomiting, diarrhea, abdominal pains\n2. Hyperkalemia:\n a. Numbness and tingling in the extremities\n b. Flaccid muscle paralysis\n c. Listlessness\n d. Confusion\n e. Hypotension\n f. Cardiac arrhythmias: atrioventricular block, loss of P-waves, widening QRS, peaked T-waves, bradycardia\n\nMANAGEMENT OF OVERDOSAGE (serum potassium greater than 6 mEq/liter)[1]\n1. Discontinue the infusion immediately; keep the vein open.\n2. Reduce serum potassium:\n a. If there are ECG changes, administer 5–10 ml of calcium gluceptate intravenously until ECG appears

normal. See entry on calcium gluceptate, page 215. (Calcium gluconate or chloride, 10% solutions, can be used in place of calcium gluceptate.) Administration of the calcium preparation should continue until definitive measures are successful in reducing serum potassium.

b. A rapid injection of 44 mEq of sodium bicarbonate over 5-10 minutes will lower the serum potassium level by increasing blood pH and subsequently moving the potassium intracellularly. This initial sodium bicarbonate should be followed by 88-132 mEq in a continuous infusion each hour.

c. Another method for reducing serum potassium is with glucose and insulin administration. Usually 500-1000 ml of 10% dextrose and water is given over 1 hour with 10-15 units of regular insulin. As with the use of sodium bicarbonate, this technique only moves the potassium into the intracellular space.

d. To remove potassium from the body, cation exchange resins such as polystyrene sodium sulfonate (Kayexalate) should be given as a retention enema. Usually 30 gm of the polystyrene is added to 100-200 ml of water. See specific instructions accompanying the drug. Keep in mind that sodium is exchanged for the potassium. This may be a problem in patients with congestive heart failure. Sorbitol solution can also be administered to induce diarrhea and thus increase potassium loss.

e. In severe cases of hyperkalemia, hemo- or peritoneal dialysis may be indicated to rapidly reduce serum potassium.

f. In all therapy, care must be taken to closely monitor serum potassium and to prevent hypokalemia.

during therapy.
4. Monitor for signs and symptoms of hyperkalemia. See Adverse Reaction No. 2.
5. Avoid extravasation. Thrombophlebitis is common following potassium infusions, especially if the infusion rate is rapid or concentrated. To prevent this complication, use a large central vein, such as the subclavian, if possible. Discontinue if phlebitis is suspected; apply warm compresses until signs and symptoms subside.

Do not administer in a concentration greater than 80 mEq/liter or infusion rate greater than 40 mEq/hour, under any circumstances.

CHILDREN:
Do not administer over 5 mEq/kg in 24 hours except in severe cases. Base replacement on daily need vs. deficit. Use a solution of 20-40 mEq/L.

Do not administer until patient is excreting adequate amounts of urine.

Do not give:
(1) until patient is out of shock;
(2) to patients with oliguria, anuria;
(3) in chronic nephritis;
(4) in the presence of potassium retention.

May take several days of therapy to correct a marked deficit.

NURSING IMPLICATIONS
1. Monitor the patient's ECG continuously if:
a. The potassium infusion must be rapid in the presence of severe hypokalemia.
b. There are ECG changes secondary to the hypokalemia.
c. The patient has pre-existing arrhythmias.
2. Use an infusion pump for rapid infusions to prevent overdosage.
3. Be aware of the patient's serum potassium (normal is 3.5-4.5 mEq/liter)

NURSING IMPLICATIONS (Continued)
6. The signs and symptoms of hypokalemia: weakness, muscle cramps, irritability, abdominal distention, cardiac arrhythmias.

REFERENCE
1. Newmark, Stephen R., and Dluhy, Robert G.: Hyperkalemia and Hypokalemia. *JAMA*, 231(6):632, February 10, 1975.

● **PRALIDOXIME CHLORIDE** (PAM, Protopam Chloride)

ACTIONS/ INDICATIONS	DOSAGE	PREPARATION AND STORAGE	DRUG INCOMPAT- IBILITIES	MODES OF IV ADMINISTRATION			CONTRAINDICATIONS; WARNINGS; PRECAUTIONS; ADVERSE REACTIONS
				INJECTION	INTERMITTENT INFUSION	CONTINUOUS INFUSION	
Anticholines- terase antago- nist, reacti- vates cholines- terase which has been inactivated by an organo- phosphate (in- secticides*). Used to relieve respiratory pa- ralysis in such poisoning. Also relieves the salivation, broncho- spasm, etc. Also weakly antagonizes the effect of: neostigmine, pyridostig- mine, and am- benonium used in the treatment of myasthenia gravis, where one of these agents has precipitated a cholinergic cri- sis. *Parathion, sairin, tetraum, TEPP, and Diazi- non.	In poisoning; while main- taining respira- tory support in the absence of cyanosis, give *atropine* IV, 2– 4 mg. If cyano- sis is present, atropine should be giv- en IM, admin- ister every 5– 10 minutes un- til signs of at- ropine toxicity appear (tachy- cardia, mental confusion). Maintain atro- pine effects for at least 48 hours. Start prali- doxime at the same time as atropine. ADULTS (for all indications): *Initially*— 1–2 gm as an infu- sion in 100 ml NS over 15– 30 minutes. If pulmonary edema is pres- ent, give as an injection over not less than 5 minutes.	To reconstitute, add 20 ml of sterile water for injection to each 1-gm vial to be used. Shake until powder cake is dissolved. Add to NS for infu- sion.	Do not mix with any other medication in syringe or in- fusion fluid.	YES Inject undi- luted over not less than 5 minutes. See Dosage col- umn for indica- tions for this mode.	YES Add dose to 100 ml NS. In- fuse over 15– 30 minutes. See Dosage column for in- dications for this mode. PREFERRED MODE.	NO Administer doses via short-term infu- sions or injec- tions.	WARNINGS 1. Not effective in the treatment of poi- soning due to phosphorus, inorganic phosphates, or organophosphates not having anticholinesterase activity. Consult local poison control center for this information. 2. No recommendation is made as to the use of this drug in the management of poisoning by pesticides of the car- bamate class (Sevin). Pralidoxime can intensify the signs of toxicity. PRECAUTIONS 1. Poisoning symptoms may mask side effects of this drug. 2. Rapid infusion may cause tachycardia, laryngospasm, and muscle rigidity; follow infusion recommendations. 3. Renal insufficiency will contribute to accumulation of the drug; a reduced dosage is recommended. 4. Use with great caution in the manage- ment reversal of therapeutic drug overdose in myasthenia gravis since it may precipitate a myasthenic crisis. 5. Barbiturates are potentiated by the poisons being treated by this drug. Use them with caution to treat sei- zures produced by the poisoning. 6. Morphine, theophylline, aminophyl- line, succinylcholine, reserpine, and phenothiazine-type tranquilizers should be avoided in the presence of this type of poisoning. ADVERSE REACTIONS 1. It is difficult to differentiate drug side effects from the effects of the poison or atropine 2. Central nervous system: excitement, manic behavior following recovery of consciousness, dizziness, blurred vi-

After 1 hour, give a second dose of 1–2 gm if muscle weakness has not been relieved. Additional doses may be needed if muscle weakness persists.

In Cholinergic crisis produced by neostigmine, pyridostigmine, or ambenonium —1–2 gm followed by 250 mg every 5 min up to 1–2 gm as needed.

CHILDREN: 20–40 mg/kg as 5% solution most effective when given within a few hours after poisoning. Little effect is seen if given after 48 hours; but in severe poisoning, the therapy should be initiated regardless. Repeat doses, titrate with recurring signs of poisoning.

3. Gastrointestinal: nausea, vomiting
4. Cardiac: tachycardias
5. Hyperventilation

NURSING IMPLICATIONS
Management of Organophosphate Poisoning:
1. Signs and symptoms of organophosphate poisoning appear at varying times and in varying degrees after exposure; depending on the route of administration and degree of exposure, but always appear at least within 24 hours. In *mild* poisoning, signs and symptoms can be—fatigue, headache, dizziness, numbness of extremities, nausea and vomiting, excessive sweating, and salivation, tightness in the chest, abdominal cramps, and a serum cholinesterase activity of 20–50% above normal.
   Severe poisoning can result in unconsciousness, seizures, loss of pupillary reaction to light, muscle fasciculations, flaccid paralysis, heavy secretions from the mouth and nose, rales, cyanosis, respiratory distress, and a serum cholinesterase activity of less than 10% below normal. This degree of poisoning, if untreated, can be fatal.[1]
2. Patient must be in an ICU while receiving this drug.
3. Maintain respiratory support as indicated.
4. Monitor vital signs, including ECG, continuously during therapy in the acute states. Be prepared to treat any arrhythmia. Keep lidocaine 100 mg and atropine 1 mg at the bedside.
5. Confirm nature of poisoning and recommended treatment by the local poison control center.
6. Wear rubber gloves and use good handwashing techniques when handling patient to avoid contamination by the poison. Remove and rinse contaminated clothing and place in plastic bags for disposal. Bathe skin thoroughly with a water-baking soda solution. Rinse well. *Discard* bath linen in plastic bags; do not launder. Flush eyes well with saline. Gastric lavage will be performed if ingestion of the poison is suspected.
7. Monitor urine output hourly during the first 24 hours and every 8 hours for the next 48 hours. Notify the physician if the urine output falls below 30 ml/hours for 2–3 successive hours in adults. See chart on page 546 for normal output in children. Monitor urine glucose and acetone every 4 hours.

459

● **PRALIDOXIME CHLORIDE** (PAM, Protopam Chloride) (Continued)

NURSING IMPLICATIONS (Continued)

8. Take precautions to prevent patient injury in the event of excitement or manic behavior on return of consciousness. Use seizure precautions.

In Myasthenia Gravis:

1. If this drug is being administered to antagonize an anticholinesterase drug in the patient with myasthenia gravis, monitor for the signs of a myasthenia crisis: drooping eyelids, slurring of speech, generalized muscle weakness, difficulty swallowing, decreasing respiratory rate.

The patient can pass quickly from a cholinergic crisis (for which the pralidoxime is being given) to a myasthenic crisis. Keep neostigmine or pyr-

idostigmine readily available, as well as respiratory support equipment. See neostigmine, page 418, and pyridostigmine, page 479.

REFERENCE

1. Namba, Tatsuji, *et al*.: Poisoning Due to Organophosphate Insecticides. *The American Journal of Medicine*, 50:481, April, 1971.

SUGGESTED READING

Namba, Tatsuji, *et al*.: Poisoning Due to Organophosphate Insecticides. *The American Journal of Medicine*, 68(3):335–339, March, 1975.

● **PREDNISOLONE, SODIUM PHOSPHATE** (Hydeltrasol) and **SODIUM SUCCINATE** (Meticortelone)

ACTIONS/INDICATIONS	DOSAGE	PREPARATION AND STORAGE	DRUG INCOMPATIBILITIES	MODES OF IV ADMINISTRATION				CONTRAINDICATIONS; WARNINGS; PRECAUTIONS; ADVERSE REACTIONS
				INJECTION	INTERMITTENT INFUSION	CONTINUOUS INFUSION		
Synthetic glucocorticoid (analog of hydrocortisone) that has salt-retaining anti-inflammatory properties and other profound and varied effects on metabolism. The following is a partial list of the major indications for the use of this drug: • Endocrine disorders, such as adrinocortical insufficiency • Rheumatic disorders • Collagen diseases • Dermatologic disorders • Allergic states • Ophthalmic diseases • Gastroin-	ADULTS AND CHILDREN: *Range*—4–60 mg/day depending on condition and response. Dosage must be individualized. (In life-threatening conditions, dosage may exceed 60 mg/day.)	*Prednisolone Sodium Succinate:* To reconstitute, add 2 ml sterile water for injection or NS to the 50-mg vial. Use only clear colorless solutions. Refrigerate unused portions and discard after 24 hours. Do not autoclave or store near heat. *Prednisolone Sodium Phosphate:* Supplied in 2- and 5-ml vials, 20 mg/ml.	Do not mix with any other medication in solution. Do not inject into an IV line containing Calcium Metaraminol Polymyxin B	YES At a rate of 10 mg/minute. Decrease rate if patient complains of burning or tingling at injection site.	YES Use D5W or NS for infusion; infuse over 15–30 minutes.	YES Use D5W or NS for infusion. Usually in a 12-hour infusion of ½ the daily dose.		CONTRAINDICATIONS 1. Systemic fungal infections. 2. In the absence of a life-threatening condition, this glucocorticoid should be avoided in: active peptic ulcer disease, systemic or ophthalmic viral disease, infections without antibiotic treatment, active and healed TB, myasthenia gravis, psychoses. 3. Hypersensitivity. WARNINGS 1. Increase dosage before and during stress, such as surgery, which increases need for glucocorticoids. 2. There may be a decreased resistance to infection and inability to localize infection during therapy. Signs of infection may be masked by steroids. 3. In pregnancy and lactation, benefits must be weighed against the risks. Observe infants born of mothers receiving this drug for signs of hypoadrenalism. 4. Can cause elevation in blood pressure, salt and water retention and increased excretion of potassium. Dietary salt restriction and potassium supplementation may be needed, along with the use of a mild diuretic. 5. Do not vaccinate during therapy. 6. Use in active TB should be limited to fulminating, disseminated cases where antituberculosis drugs are be-

testinal dis-
eases
• Respiratory
disorders
• Hematologic
disorders
• Neoplastic
diseases

ing used.
7. Patients with positive TB reactivity, administer chemoprophylaxis and monitor for activation of disease.

PRECAUTIONS

1. Gradual reduction of doses prior to discontinuation may prevent secondary adrenocortical insufficiency (may not be necessary with short-term intravenous therapy).
2. Effects of this drug are enhanced in hypothyroidism and cirrhosis; dosage should be reduced in these cases.
3. Use the lowest possible effective dose.
4. Psychic disturbances may occur ranging from euphoria to psychoses.
5. Use aspirin cautiously during use of this drug in the presence of hypothrombinemia to prevent aggravation of bleeding problems, and to prevent gastric irritation.
6. Use with caution if there is a possibility of perforation in ulcerative colitis, or diverticulitis, fresh intestinal anastomoses, active or latent peptic ulcer disease.
7. Use with caution in renal disease and congestive heart failure because of enhanced salt and water retention.
8. Use with caution in the presence of osteoporosis; this drug increases calcium loss from bones and excretion via the kidney.
9. May precipitate a crisis in myasthenia gravis.
10. Initiate antiulcer therapy during use of this drug.
11. This drug should be used with caution in patients with glaucoma because it can increase the intraocular pressure.

ADVERSE REACTIONS SEEN IN SHORT-TERM INTRAVENOUS THERAPY

1. Fluid and electrolyte imbalance: sodium and water retention with possible secondary hypertension, hypokalemia, hypocalcemia
2. Gastrointestinal: peptic ulcer with possible perforation, pancreatitis, ulcerative eosophagitis
3. Dermatologic: impaired wound healing
4. Neurologic: increased intracranial pressure, seizures (increasing fre-

461

PREDNISOLONE, SODIUM PHOSPHATE (Hydeltrasol) and SODIUM SUCCINATE (Meticortelone) (Continued)

| | | PREPARATION | DRUG | MODES OF IV ADMINISTRATION | | | |
ACTIONS/ INDICATIONS	DOSAGE	AND STORAGE	INCOMPAT- IBILITIES	INJECTION	INTERMITTENT INFUSION	CONTINUOUS INFUSION	CONTRAINDICATIONS: WARNINGS: PRECAUTIONS: ADVERSE REACTIONS
							quency in patients with pre-existing seizure disorder), vertigo, headaches, mental confusion, euphoria, exacerbation of psychosis. 5. Endocrine: decreased glucose tolerance, increased hypoglycemic agent and insulin requirements in diabetics. 6. Eye: increased intraocular pressure. 7. Metabolic: negative nitrogen balance secondary to rapid muscle catabolism.

NURSING IMPLICATIONS

1. Take precautions to prevent infections in wounds by using strict aseptic technique in dressing changes, etc. Avoid traumatic procedures such as catheterizations. The skin may become more fragile because of the steroid therapy. Patients on bed rest and those with general body weakening secondary to acute illness should be turned hourly (except during sleep, then every 2–3 hours) to prevent skin breakdown. Initiate the use of supportive measures, such as flotation pads, water mattress, etc. Administer scrupulous skin care to prevent infection.

2. Monitor blood pressure every 2–4 hours, or as the patient's condition dictates. Monitor blood pressure before, during and immediately after intravenous injection; hypotension can occur.

3. Weigh the patient daily to detect for water and sodium retention. Dietary restriction in sodium may be prescribed by the physician. Examine daily for peripheral edema.

4. There may be delayed healing of wounds; take precautions to prevent dehiscence. Sutures may be left in longer than usual for this reason.

5. Monitor urine glucose in patients on high-dose therapy and with diabetes. Diabetic individuals may require a larger dosage of insulin or oral agent.

6. Administer antacid therapy as ordered to assist in preventing peptic ulcer. Monitor for signs of the development of an ulcer and/or acute intestinal bleeding: melena, positive stool guaiac, hematemesis, epigastric pain and/ or distention, anemia or falling hematocrit.

7. Monitor for signs and symptoms of hypokalemia: weakness, irritability, abdominal distention, poor feeding in infants, muscle cramps.[1] Dietary or pharmacologic potassium supplements may be ordered, guided by serum potassium levels.

8. Monitor for signs and symptoms of hypocalcemia (a serum calcium of 6 mg%): irritability, change in mental status, seizures, nausea, vomiting, diarrhea, muscle cramps, carpopedal spasm, late effects—cardiac arrhythmias, laryngeal spasm and apnea.[2,3] Dietary or pharmacologic supplements may be ordered, guided by serum calcium levels.

9. Patients with a history of seizure activity may have an increasing number of seizures while on steroid therapy. Apply appropriate safety precautions.

10. Monitor for behavioral changes, which may range from simple euphoria to depression and psychosis. Apply appropriate safety precautions. A change in dosage may relieve such symptoms.

11. Tuberculin testing should be carried out prior to initiation of steroid therapy, if possible. The patient's reactivity to the tuberculin is altered by the drug, giving a false result.

12. Ambulate the patient with caution if vertigo occurs, and initiate the use of side rails to prevent injury. Report the onset to the physician.

13. Be alert to the signs of increasing intraocular pressure: eye pain, rainbow vision, blurred vision, nausea and vomiting.[4] Notify the physician immediately.

REFERENCES

1. Beeson, Paul, and McDermott, Walsh (editors): *Cecil-Loeb Textbook of Medicine* (14th ed.), Philadelphia: W. B. Saunders Company, 1975, p. 1587.
2. Ibid., p. 1815.
3. Guyton, Arthur C.: *Textbook of Medical Physiology* (5th ed.), Philadelphia: W. B. Saunders Company, 1976, p. 1056.
4. Newell, Frank W., and Ernest, J. Terry: *Ophthalmology—Principles and Concepts* (3rd ed.), St. Louis: C. V. Mosby Company, 1974, p. 329.

SUGGESTED READINGS

Glasser, Ronald J.: How the Body Works Against Itself: Autoimmune Disease. *Nursing '77,* September 1977, pp. 38–39.
Melick, M. E.: Nursing Intervention for Patients Receiving Corticosteroid Therapy. In *Advanced Concepts in Clinical Nursing* (2nd ed.), K. D. Kintzel, ed., Philadelphia: J. B. Lippincott Company, 1977, pp. 606–617.
Newton, David W., Nichols, Arlene, and Newton, Marion: You Can Minimize the Hazards of Corticosteroids. *Nursing '77,* June 1977, pp. 26–33.
Reichgott, Michael J., and Melmon, Kenneth L.: The Role of Corticosteroids in Shock. In *Steroid Therapy,* Daniel Azarnoff, ed., Philadelphia, W. B. Saunders Company, 1975, pp. 118–133.

PROCAINAMIDE HYDROCHLORIDE (Pronestyl)

ACTIONS/ INDICATIONS	DOSAGE	PREPARATION AND STORAGE	DRUG INCOMPATIBILITIES	MODES OF IV ADMINISTRATION			CONTRAINDICATIONS; WARNINGS; PRECAUTIONS; ADVERSE REACTIONS
				INJECTION	INTERMITTENT INFUSION	CONTINUOUS INFUSION	
Antiarrhythmic. Depresses the excitability of cardiac muscle to stimulation; slows conduction in the atrium, bundle of His, and ventricles. Contractility is usually not affected. Used to treat: • Premature ventricular contractions • Ventricular tachycardia • Atrial fibrillation • Paroxysmal atrial tachycardia • Supraventricular tachyarrhythmias unresponsive to digitalis Action begins almost immediately after intravenous injection. Therapeutic plasma levels have been reported to be 3–10 mcg/ml. This drug is excreted primarily in the urine.	The intravenous mode should be used only in extreme emergencies. ADULTS: 100 mg at 5-min intervals. Stop injections when desired effect is achieved or when a total dose of 1 gm is reached. Begin an infusion at a rate of 2–6 mg/min simultaneously with the first injection dose. Titrate with patient response. CHILDREN: 2 mg/kg/dose (maximum dose is 100 mg). Administer by slow infusion over 5 min, repeat every 10–30 min until desired effect is seen or the maximal dose is reached. Titrate with patient response.	Available in 10-ml vials with a concentration of 100 mg/ml, and 2-ml vials with a concentration of 500 mg/ml. Protect vials from light (keep in original package) and store in refrigerator. Solution should be clear and colorless; discard if yellow.	Do not mix in infusion bottle with any other medication. Do not combine in IV line with: Diazepam (Valium) Phenytoin (Dilantin) Chlordiazepoxide (Librium) Narcotics Barbiturates	YES Dilute 500 mg/ml solution with an equal amount of D5W or sterile water. Inject at a rate no greater than 25–50 mg/min.	YES Use a 4 mg/ml solution (2 gm in 500 ml D5W or NS). Infuse as a secondary line and use an infusion pump. Infuse at a rate no greater than 25–50 mg/min.	YES Use a 4 mg/ml solution (2 gm in 500 ml D5W or NS). Infuse as a secondary line and use an infusion pump. Infuse at a rate no greater than 25–50 mg/min.	CONTRAINDICATIONS 1. Myasthenia gravis (not an absolute contraindication) 2. Hypersensitivity to this drug or any procaine-related drugs 3. Complete atrioventricular heart block or second degree heart block in the absence of a pacemaker PRECAUTIONS 1. Monitor for changes in cardiac function (blood pressure, cardiac output). 2. This drug produces peripheral vasodilatation. 3. In atrial fibrillation or flutter the ventricular rate may increase as the atrial rate is slowed, due to a transient anticholinergic effect. Digitalis may decrease this, but not entirely. 4. Use with caution for ventricular tachycardia in acute myocardial infarction. 5. In the presence of first, second or third degree block, this drug may precipitate complete heart block, ventricular asystole or fibrillation. 6. ECG monitoring must be carried out during administration in any mode. Discontinue drug if A-V conduction is compromised to prevent asystole. Widening of the QRS complex or prolongation of the P-R interval suggest myocardial toxicity, and administration of this drug should be temporarily discontinued. 7. Renal or hepatic impairment will cause accumulation of this drug. Reduce dosage and monitor closely for symptoms of overdosage. 8. A syndrome resembling systemic lupus erythematosus may occur with high-dose chronic therapy, producing polyarthralgias, arthritis, and pleuritic pain. There may also be fever, myalgia, rashes, pleural effusion. Rarely, thrombocytopenia, or Coombs-positive hemolytic anemia, may also be seen. Discontinue the drug if there is a rising antinuclear antibody titer, or if symptoms of the syndrome appear. This syndrome

DILUTIONS AND RATES FOR INFUSIONS

Approximate Final Concentration	Infusion Bottle Size (ml.)	ml. of Pronestyl (100 mg./ml. solution) to be added	ml. of Pronestyl (500 mg./ml. solution) to be added	Infusion Rate
0.2% (2mg./ml.)	500	10	2	1–3 ml./min. (2–6 mg./min.)
	250	5	1	
0.4% (4 mg./ml.)	500	20	4	0.5–1.5 ml./min. (2–6 mg./min.)
	250	10	2	

CAUTION: The flow rate of all intravenous infusion solutions must be closely monitored. These dilutions are calculated to deliver 2 to 6 mg. per minute at the infusion rates listed.

Courtesy of E. R. Squibb and Sons, P.O. Box 4000, Princeton, N.J. 08540

PROCAINAMIDE HYDROCHLORIDE (Pronestyl) (Continued)

ACTIONS/ INDICATIONS	DOSAGE	PREPARATION AND STORAGE	DRUG INCOMPATIBILITIES	MODES OF IV ADMINISTRATION			CONTRAINDICATIONS; WARNINGS; PRECAUTIONS; ADVERSE REACTIONS
				INJECTION	INTERMITTENT INFUSION	CONTINUOUS INFUSION	
							may be reversible. Steroids may relieve symptoms.
							9. In the emergency treatment of ventricular arrhythmias, lidocaine is the drug of choice.
							10. When initiating oral therapy, give the first oral dose 3–4 hrs after discontinuing the intravenous infusion.

ADVERSE REACTIONS
1. May produce transient but severe hypotension
2. Ventricular asystole or fibrillation
3. Lupuslike syndrome (see Precaution No. 8 above)
4. Nausea, vomiting, abdominal pain, diarrhea, bitter taste
5. Hepatomegaly, rise in SGOT
6. Weakness, mental depression, hallucinations, seizures
7. Hypersensitivity: eosinophilia, urticaria
8. Agranulocytosis with oral lesions, fever, infection

NURSING IMPLICATIONS
1. Close ECG monitoring must be maintained during intravenous therapy. Monitor for onset of:
   a. Increasing A-V block (e.g., prolongation of PR interval, second degree block)
   b. Signs of toxicity (e.g., widening of QRS complex, prolongation of PR interval). If any of these signs appear, stop the infusion and notify the physician.
   c. Ineffective control of arrhythmia being treated; another agent may be needed.
2. Keep atropine, defibrillator and temporary transvenous pacemaker equipment readily available.
3. Keep patient supine during drug administration; monitor blood pressure continuously during infusion (direct arterial pressure preferred). Do not leave the patient unattended. If fall in blood pressure exceeds 15 mm Hg, discontinue infusion. Phenylephrine hydrochloride (Neo-Synephrine) or levarterenol bitartrate (Levophed) can be used to correct hypotension.
4. Be prepared to manage vomiting to prevent aspiration.
5. Be prepared to manage hallucinations to protect patient from injury.
6. Use an infusion pump, or at least microdrop tubing to control drip rate.

SUGGESTED READINGS
Cardiac Drugs Today—Part Four: Antiarrhythmics. *Nursing '73*, August 1973, pp. 29–34.
Treatment of Cardiac Arrhythmias—Part I: The Arrhythmias. *The Medical Letter*, 16:101–108, December 6, 1974.
Amsterdam, Ezra A., et al.: Systematic Approach to the Management of Cardiac Arrhythmias. *Heart and Lung*, 2:747–753, September–October 1973 (references).
Levitt, Barrie, Borer, Jeffrey, and Saropa, Arleen: The Clinical Pharmacology of Antiarrhythmic Drugs. Part II: Quinidine, Propranolol, Diphenylhydantion, and Bretylium. *Cardiovascular Nursing*, 10:27–32, November–December 1974 (references).
Pamintuan, Jose C., Dreifus, Leonard S., and Watanabe, Yoshio: Comparative Mechanisms of Antiarrhythmic Agents. *American Journal of Cardiology*, 26:512–523, November 1970 (references).
Hoffman, Brian F., Rosen, Michael R., and Wit, Andrew L.: Electrophysiology and Pharmacology of Cardiac Arrhythmias. VII. Cardiac Effects of Quinidine and Procainamide. *American Heart Journal*, 89(6):804–808, June 1975.

PROCHLORPERAZINE EDISYLATE (Compazine)

ACTIONS/ INDICATIONS	DOSAGE	PREPARATION AND STORAGE	DRUG INCOMPATIBILITIES	MODES OF IV ADMINISTRATION				CONTRAINDICATIONS; WARNINGS; PRECAUTIONS; ADVERSE REACTIONS
				INJECTION	INTERMITTENT INFUSION	CONTINUOUS INFUSION		

ACTIONS/ INDICATIONS	DOSAGE	PREPARATION AND STORAGE	DRUG INCOMPATIBILITIES	INJECTION	INTERMITTENT INFUSION	CONTINUOUS INFUSION	CONTRAINDICATIONS; WARNINGS; PRECAUTIONS; ADVERSE REACTIONS
Phenothiazine tranquilizer, antiemetic. Used to control • Severe nausea and vomiting • Psychoses • Anxiety, tension, agitation	ADULTS: *Nausea and vomiting*—5–10 mg; repeat if necessary. (do not exceed 40 mg/day.) *Preoperative*— IV injection: 5–10 mg 15–30 minutes before induction of anesthesia, or by infusion during surgery. IV infusion: 20 mg/liter of an isotonic solution; add to IV 15–30 min before induction. CHILDREN: Intravenous administration not recommended in children.	Protect vials from light. Slight yellow discoloration will not alter potency. Discard if markedly discolored. Supplied in 2-ml ampuls (5 mg/ml; and 10-ml multiple dose vials (5 mg/ml)	Do not mix with any other medication in solution, IV line, or syringe.	YES Dilute each 5 mg in 9 ml NS; inject over 1–2 min.	YES Usually 5–10 mg in 100 ml NS or D5W. Titrate with patient response.	YES Usually 20 mg to 1000 ml of any IV fluid. Titrate with patient response.	CONTRAINDICATIONS 1. CNS depression 2. Bone marrow depression 3. Pediatric surgery 4. Hypersensitivity to any phenothiazine WARNINGS 1. May impair mental/physical alertness. 2. May intensify or prolong the actions of CNS depressants (alcohol, anesthetics, narcotics, sedatives). 3. Safety for use in pregnancy has not been established. 4. Use lower range of suggested dosages for the elderly, debilitated or emaciated patient. PRECAUTIONS 1. Antiemetic effects may mask signs of overdosage of toxic drugs, of intestinal obstruction or increased intracranial pressure. 2. Use of the drug does not preclude adequate postanesthesia care to prevent aspiration of vomitus. 3. Administer at the lowest dosage to produce desired results. 4. This drug may depress gag and cough reflexes. ADVERSE REACTIONS SEEN IN SHORT-TERM INTRAVENOUS USE 1. Neurologic: a. Sedation, drowsiness and deep sleep b. Blurred vision c. Extrapyramidal reactions, such as motor restlessness resembling Parkinson's disease, drooling, tremors, muscle spasms, shuffling gait, dystonias (involuntary movements), difficulty swallowing d. Agitation and nervousness. If these occur, dosage must be reduced or the drug discontinued. Symptoms will subside in 24–48 hours. 2. Rashes usually due to hypersensitivity 3. Hypotension (especially immediately after injection); may be postural type 4. Palpitations, especially immediately after an injection

PROCHLORPERAZINE EDISYLATE (Compazine) (Continued)

ACTIONS/ INDICATIONS	DOSAGE	PREPARATION AND STORAGE	DRUG INCOMPAT- IBILITIES	MODES OF IV ADMINISTRATION			CONTRAINDICATIONS; WARNINGS; PRECAUTIONS; ADVERSE REACTIONS
				INJECTION	INTERMITTENT INFUSION	CONTINUOUS INFUSION	
							5. Liver damage producing jaundice (cholestatic hepatitis)
							6. Anticholinergic reactions such as: dryness of the mouth, tachycardia, blurred vision, increased salivation, nasal congestion.
							7. Exacerbation of seizure disorders.

NURSING IMPLICATIONS
1. Monitor for neurologic disturbances following an injection or during an infusion; see Adverse Reaction No. 1. Report any of these reactions to the physician immediately. If the patient experiences difficulty in swallowing, discontinue infusion immediately, and remain with the patient until the severity of the reaction is determined. The patient may need parenteral hydration and nutrition until swallowing returns. Initiate safety measures such as side rails and close observation, to prevent patient injury.
2. Examine for rashes; report them to the physician.
3. Keep the patient supine during injection or infusion.
4. Monitor blood pressure before, during and after injection or infusion. If hypotension occurs during an infusion, discontinue administration and continue to take the blood pressure until stabilization occurs. Hypotension

can usually be avoided with slow injection. If a patient is to be ambulated after an injection, obtain lying and standing blood pressure. If postural hypotension is significant, report the fact to the physician and keep the patient at rest. As postural effects decrease over time, begin to ambulate the patient if desirable; do so cautiously to prevent injury. Warn the patient not to stand up suddenly until the effects of the drug have disappeared.
5. Monitor for jaundice; notify the physician.
6. The patient may experience anticholinergic side effects; see Adverse Reaction No. 6. Inform him of the origin of the symptoms and their transient nature.
7. Initiate seizure precautions if not already in effect.
8. This drug can cause the urine to darken or turn orange for 24 hours after administration. Inform the patient of the harmlessness of this effect.

PROMAZINE HYDROCHLORIDE (Sparine)

ACTIONS/ INDICATIONS	DOSAGE	PREPARATION AND STORAGE	DRUG INCOMPAT- IBILITIES	MODES OF IV ADMINISTRATION			CONTRAINDICATIONS; WARNINGS; PRECAUTIONS; ADVERSE REACTIONS
				INJECTION	INTERMITTENT INFUSION	CONTINUOUS INFUSION	
A major tranquilizer (a phenothiazine), antiemetic. Used in the management of psychoses and alcohol withdrawal, for sedation prior to surgery; for control of nausea and vomiting.	ADULTS: 50–100 mg every 4–6 hours. DO NOT EXCEED 1 gm/ DAY. CHILDREN 12–16 YEARS OF AGE: 10–25 mg every 4–6 hours. (The dosage of analgesics and sedatives may be reduced by	Supplied in 25 mg/ml and 50 mg/ml concentrations. Use 25 mg/ml concentration, for IV injection. (If only 50 mg/ ml concentration is available, dilute each ml in 9 ml NS before injection.)	Do not mix with: Aminophylline Chlorothiazide Chlortetracycline Nafcillin Penicillin G Phenobarbital Sodium bicarbonate Thiopental Warfarin Heparin Hydrocortisone Vitamin B complex	YES May be given undiluted. Use 25 mg/ml concentration ONLY. Inject at a rate of 25 mg/min.	NO	NO	CONTRAINDICATIONS 1. Intra-arterial injection 2. Hypersensitivity to this and any other phenathiazine 3. Bone marrow depression 4. Children under 12 5. Lactation 6. Pregnancy, except during labor and delivery PRECAUTIONS 1. Avoid extravasation. 2. Intra-arterial injection can cause gangrene of the extremity. 3. Avoid contact with skin, eyes, and clothing; can cause staining or burns. 4. Antiemetic effects may mask symptoms of increased intracranial pressure, drug intoxication, and intestinal

obstruction.

5. Potentiates central nervous system depressants (narcotics, barbiturates, alcohol, anesthetics).
6. Potentiated by MAO inhibitors.
7. Potentiates oral hypoglycemic agents and insulin, anticholinergics, antihistamines, antihypertensives, hypnotics, muscle relaxants.
8. Reduce dosage of any medication potentiated by this drug by one-half or one-fourth.

ADVERSE REACTIONS SEEN IN SHORT-TERM INTRAVENOUS USE
1. Neurologic:
   a. Sedation, drowsiness and deep sleep
   b. Blurred vision
   c. Extrapyramidal reactions such as motor restlessness resembling Parkinson's disease, drooling, tremors, muscle spasms, shuffling gait, dystonias (involuntary movements) and difficulty swallowing
   d. Agitation and nervousness
   If these occur, dosage must be reduced or the drug discontinued. Symptoms will subside in 24–48 hours.
2. Rashes usually due to hypersensitivity
3. Hypotension (especially immediately after injection); may be postural type
4. Palpitations, especially immediately after an injection
5. Liver damage producing jaundice (cholestatic hepatitis)
6. Anticholinergic reactions such as: dryness of the mouth, tachycardia, blurred vision, increased salivation, nasal congestion
7. Exacerbation of seizure disorders

stand up suddenly until the effects of the drug have disappeared. Ambulate the patient with caution if he is experiencing sedation or blurred vision. Initiate safety precautions, such as side rails, to prevent injury.
5. Monitor for jaundice; notify the physician.
6. The patient may experience anticholinergic side effects; see Adverse Reaction No. 6. Inform him of the origin of the symptom and its transient nature.
7. Initiate seizure precautions if not already in effect.
8. This drug can cause the urine to darken or turn orange for 24 hours after administration. Inform the patient of the harmlessness of this effect.
9. Take all precautions to avoid intra-arterial injection and extravasation. Inject into IV tubing of an IV system known to be working satisfactorily. If the patient complains of pain during an injection, stop administration immediately and evaluate for the possibility of intra-arterial injection or perivascular extravasation. Signs and symptoms are severe pain in the affected area, edema along the vessel tract and possibly blanching of the extremity. Notify the physician immediately.

⅓ to ½ when this drug is used.)

Intramuscular route is preferred.

CHILDREN UNDER 12 YEARS OF AGE:
IV administration not recommended.

NURSING IMPLICATIONS
1. Monitor for neurologic disturbances following an injection, or during an infusion; see Adverse Reaction No. 1. Report any of these reactions to the physician immediately. If the patient experiences difficulty in swallowing, discontinue infusion immediately, and remain with the patient until the severity of the reaction is determined. The patient may need parenteral hydration and nutrition until swallowing returns.
2. Examine for rashes; report them to the physician.
3. Keep the patient supine during injection or infusion.
4. Monitor blood pressure before, during and after injection or infusion. If hypotension occurs during an infusion, discontinue administration and continue to take the blood pressure until stabilization occurs. Hypotension can usually be avoided with slow injection. If a patient is to be ambulated after an injection, obtain lying and standing blood pressure. If postural hypotension is significant, report the fact to the physician and keep the patient at rest. As postural effects decrease over time, begin to ambulate the patient if desirable; do so cautiously to prevent injury. Warn the patient not to

PROMETHAZINE HYDROCHLORIDE (Phenergan)

ACTIONS/ INDICATIONS	DOSAGE	PREPARATION AND STORAGE	DRUG INCOMPAT- IBILITIES	MODES OF IV ADMINISTRATION				CONTRAINDICATIONS; WARNINGS; PRECAUTIONS; ADVERSE REACTIONS
				INJECTION	INTERMITTENT INFUSION	CONTINUOUS INFUSION		
Antihistamine, antiemetic, sedative (a phenothiazine derivative). Used to manage • Allergic reactions to blood and plasma • Anaphylaxis • Preoperative, postoperative, obstetric sedation • Nausea and vomiting • Motion sickness Also used to potentiate analgesics, induce sedation.	ALLERGY: *Adults*—25 mg every 2–4 hours. *Children*— 6.25–12.5 mg every 3–4 hours.* NAUSEA AND VOMITING: *Adults*—12.5–25 mg every 4–6 hours. *Children*—0.5–1.1 mg/kg every 4–6 hours as needed.* SEDATION: *Adults*—25–50 mg. *Children*—12.5–25 mg (or 0.5 mg/kg)* *OBSTETRICS:* 25–75 mg as needed. *Intramuscular route is preferred.	Supplied in ampuls and disposable syringes of 25/ml and 50 mg/ml solutions. Refrigerate and protect from light (keep in individual box). Do not use if discolored darker than light yellow. Avoid contact with skin, eyes, clothing.	Do not mix with any other medication in solution; and do not inject into an IV line containing the following drugs: Aminophylline Chloramphenicol Chlorothiazide Heparin Hydrocortisone Methicillin Methohexital Penicillin G	YES Use a 25 mg/ ml concentration, further dilute with 9 ml NS. Inject at a rate of 25 mg/ min. If administering via a heparinized intermittent scalp vein or heparin-lock set, flush system with NS before and after injecting the drug.	YES Use any IV fluid at a rate no greater than 25 mg/minute. Flush system with NS before and after infusion if heparin is present.	YES Use any IV fluid; infuse at a rate to produce desired response, no more rapid than 25 mg/ min.		**CONTRAINDICATIONS** 1. Hypersensitivity to this or any other phenothiazine 2. Intra-arterial injection (can cause gangrene of the extremity) 3. Comatose states, and when the patient has received large amounts of CNS depressants. **WARNINGS** 1. Potentiates other central nervous system depressants. Reduce dosage of narcotics, barbiturates, hypnotics and sedatives. 2. Safety for use in pregnancy has not been established. 3. Avoid extravasation. 4. Use with caution in children; large doses can cause hallucinations, convulsions and sudden death, especially in children who are acutely ill and dehydrated. Do not administer for uncomplicated vomiting. The extrapyramidal symptoms which can occur secondary to this drug may be confused with the CNS signs of encephalopathy or Reye's syndrome. 5. Reduce dosage in the elderly. 6. Because of this drug's anticholinergic effects, use with caution in patients with an acute asthmatic attack, narrow-angle glaucoma, prostatic hypertrophy, stenosis, peptic ulcer, or bladder-neck obstruction. 7. Use with caution in the presence of bone marrow depression; leukopenia and agranulocytosis have been reported. 8. Do not use concomitantly with epinephrine. **PRECAUTIONS** 1. The antiemetic actions can mask the symptoms of increased intracranial pressure, intestinal obstruction, drug toxicity. 2. Can cause dizziness and hypotension. 3. Use with caution in the presence of liver dysfunction.

ADVERSE REACTIONS SEEN IN SHORT-TERM INTRAVENOUS USE

1. Neurologic:
   a. Sedation, drowsiness and deep sleep
   b. Blurred vision
   c. Extrapyramidal reactions such as motor restlessness resembling Parkinson's disease, drooling, tremors, muscle spasms, shuffling gait, dystonias (involuntary movements), difficulty swallowing
   d. Agitation and nervousness
   If these occur, dosage must be reduced or the drug discontinued. Symptoms will subside in 24–48 hours.
2. Rashes usually due to hypersensitivity
3. Hypotension (especially immediately after injection); may be postural type
4. Palpitations, especially immediately after an injection
5. Liver damage producing jaundice (cholestatic hepatitis)
6. Anticholinergic reactions such as: dryness of the mouth, tachycardia, blurred vision, increased salivation, nasal congestion.
7. Exacerbation of seizure disorders.

NURSING IMPLICATIONS

1. Monitor for neurologic disturbances following an injection, or during an infusion; see Adverse Reaction No. 1. Report any of these reactions to the physician immediately. If the patient experiences difficulty in swallowing, discontinue infusion immediately, and remain with the patient until the severity of the reaction is determined. The patient may need parenteral hydration and nutrition until swallowing returns. Monitor children for change in mental status, hallucinations and seizures. See Warning No. 4.
2. Examine for rashes; report them to the physician.
3. Keep the patient supine during injection of infusion.
4. Monitor blood pressure before, during and after injection or infusion. If hypotension occurs during an infusion, discontinue administration and continue to take the blood pressure until stabilization occurs. Hypotension can usually be avoided with slow injection. If a patient is to be ambulated after an injection, obtain lying and standing blood pressure. If postural hypotension is significant, report the fact the physician and keep the patient at rest. As postural effects decrease over time, begin to ambulate the patient if de-

sirable; do so cautiously to prevent injury. Warn the patient not to stand up suddenly until the effects of the drug have disappeared. Ambulate the patient with caution if he is experiencing sedation or blurred vision. Initiate safety precautions, such as side rails, to prevent injury.
5. Monitor for jaundice; notify the physician.
6. The patient may experience anticholinergic side effects; see Adverse Reaction No. 6. Inform him of the origin of the symptom and its transient nature.
7. Initiate seizure precautions if not already in effect.
8. This drug can cause the urine to darken or turn orange for 24 hours after administration. Inform the patient of the harmlessness of this effect.
9. Intra-arterial injection and extravasation must be avoided. Inject into IV tubing of an IV system known to be working when possible. Do not inject or infuse into a scalp vein in children. If the patient complains of pain during an injection, stop administration immediately and evaluate for the possibility of intra-arterial injection or perivascular extravasation. Notify the physician. Signs and symptoms are severe pain in the affected area, edema along the vessel tract, and possibly blanching of the extremity.

PROPANTHELINE BROMIDE (Pro-Banthine)

ACTIONS/ INDICATIONS	DOSAGE	PREPARATION AND STORAGE	DRUG INCOMPAT- IBILITIES	MODES OF IV ADMINISTRATION			CONTRAINDICATIONS; WARNINGS; PRECAUTIONS; ADVERSE REACTIONS
				INJECTION	INTERMITTENT INFUSION	CONTINUOUS INFUSION	
Antispasmotic, anticholinergic. Inhibits gastrointestinal motility; decreases gastric acid secretion. Used in: • Acute pancreatitis • Peptic ulcer disease • Intestinal hypermotility • Pylorospasm • Ureteral and bladder spasm • Spastic colon • Radiology, to reduce duodenal motility, e.g., for hypotonic duodenography.	ADULTS: *Initial*—30 mg. *Maintenance* —15 mg every 6 hrs, depending on patient response. *Hypotonic duodenography*— 30–60 mg just prior to the procedure, at a rate of 6 mg/min.	Available in 30-mg vials. To reconstitute powder add 10 ml NS, and shake. Store reconstituted solution in refrigerator; discard reconstituted solution after 2 weeks.	Do not mix with any other medication in any manner.	YES Dilute each reconstituted 30 mg with an additional 10 ml NS. Inject at a rate of 30 mg/min.	NO	NO	CONTRAINDICATIONS 1. Glaucoma 2. Gastrointestinal obstruction of any form 3. Obstructive uropathy 4. Intestinal atony 5. Toxic megacolon complicating ulcerative colitis 6. Hiatal hernia with reflux esophagitis 7. Unstable cardiovascular adjustment in acute hemorrhage WARNINGS 1. Use with caution if an increase in heart rate is undesirable. 2. Anhidrosis (decreased perspiration) may occur. 3. Overdosage may produce curarelike effects (muscle paralysis, especially respiratory muscles). PRECAUTIONS 1. Urinary hesitancy or obstruction may occur in patients with prostatic enlargement. 2. Use with caution in patients with ulcerative colitis. ADVERSE REACTIONS 1. Dryness of mouth 2. Blurred vision, dilation of pupils, headache 3. Nervousness 4. Drowsiness or insomnia 5. Dizziness 6. Nausea, vomiting, constipation 7. Impotence 8. Tachycardia MANAGEMENT OF OVERDOSAGE 1. Manifestations of overdosage progress from an intensification of the usual side effects (see Adverse Reactions) to central nervous system disturbances such as restlessness, excitement and psychotic behavior; circulatory changes such as fall in blood pressure, flushing and circulatory failures; respiratory failure and paralysis; coma; fever. 2. To counteract drug effects give physostigmine 0.5 to 2.0 mg intravenous-

ly, repeated up to a total of 5 mg as needed. (See page 451 for details on this drug.)

3. Fever should be controlled with a hypothermia blanket.
4. If excitement or psychotic behavior is severe, sodium thiopental 2% can be given intravenously, or chloral hydrate, 100–200 ml of a 2% solution, can be given as a rectal infusion.
5. If the curarelike effect progresses to a paralysis of the respiratory muscles, assisted ventilation must be initiated and maintained until effective ventilation, cough, gag and swallow reflexes return.

(physostigmine 2.0 mg).

3. Have patient void prior to injection. Examine for bladder distention hourly. Measure urinary output every 4 hours.
4. Monitor for signs and symptoms of acute glaucoma (increased intraocular pressure): ocular pain, blurred vision, rainbow vision, nausea and vomiting.[1] Notify the physician. This drug can precipitate such an attack in a previously asymptomatic patient.

REFERENCE
1. Newell, Frank W. and Ernest, J. Terry: Ophthalmology—Principles and Concepts. (3rd ed.), St. Louis: C. V. Mosby Company, 1974, p. 329.

NURSING IMPLICATIONS
1. Monitor heart rate before, during, and every 5–10 minutes after injection, for 1 hour. If patient has cardiac problems, continuous ECG monitoring may be advisable. If heart rate is accelerated, monitor for cardiac decompensation, e.g., shortness of breath, orthopnea, engorgement of external jugular veins, rales. Notify physician at the onset of tachycardia.
2. Monitor for loss of voluntary muscle control, especially pharyngeal and respiratory muscles. Check respiratory rate frequently during the first hour after injection. Be prepared to manage respiratory depression or difficulty in maintaining an open airway. Equipment: airways, oxygen, suction, endotracheal tubes and laryngoscope, manual breathing bag (Ambu, Puritan, Hope). See Management of Overdosage section; keep antidotes at the bedside

● PROPIOMAZINE HYDROCHLORIDE (Largon)

ACTIONS/ INDICATIONS	DOSAGE	PREPARATION AND STORAGE	DRUG INCOMPATIBILITIES	MODES OF IV ADMINISTRATION			CONTRAINDICATIONS; WARNINGS; PRECAUTIONS; ADVERSE REACTIONS
				INJECTION	INTERMITTENT INFUSION	CONTINUOUS INFUSION	
Sedative and antiemetic, phenothiazine derivative. Used to sedate and to treat nausea and vomiting in surgery and obstetrics.	ADULTS: *Preoperative sedation and during labor*— 20–40 mg. *Sedation during surgery*— 10–20 mg. *Postoperative sedation and antiemetic*— 10–20 mg.	Supplied in ampuls and disposable syringes in a 20 mg/ml solution. Protect vials from light. Do not use if cloudy or contains a precipitate.	May combine in syringe with atropine or pentazocine.	YES. Use a solution of 20 mg/ml, at a rate of 10 mg/min.	NO	NO	CONTRAINDICATIONS 1. Intra-arterial injection; may impair local circulation. 2. Allergy to any phenothiazine. WARNINGS 1. Other CNS depressant drugs will be potentiated by this drug. 2. Use with caution in patients with glaucoma or obstructive uropathy. 3. Safety for use in pregnancy has not been established. PRECAUTIONS 1. When used concurrently with certain

471

PROPIOMAZINE HYDROCHLORIDE (Largon) (Continued)

ACTIONS/ INDICATIONS	DOSAGE	PREPARATION AND STORAGE	DRUG INCOMPAT- IBILITIES	MODES OF IV ADMINISTRATION			CONTRAINDICATIONS; WARNINGS; PRECAUTIONS; ADVERSE REACTIONS
				INJECTION	INTERMITTENT INFUSION	CONTINUOUS INFUSION	
	May repeat every 3 hours. CHILDREN (under 60 lbs): *Any indication* —0.25–0.5 mg/lb, *or* 2–4 years: 10 mg 4–6 years: 15 mg 6–12 years: 25 mg						drugs, dosage of these drugs should be reduced: barbiturates: reduce by one-half; meperidine: reduce by one-quarter to one-half; morphine: reduce by one-quarter to one-half. 2. Avoid extravasation. 3. Will cause dizziness or drowsiness. ADVERSE REACTIONS SEEN IN SHORT-TERM INTRAVENOUS USE 1. Neurologic: a. Sedation, drowsiness and deep sleep b. Blurred vision c. Extrapyramidal reactions such as motor restlessness resembling Parkinson's disease, drooling, tremors, muscle spasms, shuffling gait, dystonias (involuntary movement); difficulty swallowing d. Agitation and nervousness If these occur, dosage must be reduced or the drug discontinued. Symptoms will subside in 24–48 hours. 2. Rashes, usually due to hypersensitivity 3. Hypotension (especially immediately after injection), may be postural type 4. Palpitations, especially immediately after an injection 5. Liver damage producing jaundice (cholestatic hepatitis) 6. Anticholinergic reactions such as: dryness of the mouth, tachycardia, blurred vision, increased salivation, nasal congestion 7. Exacerbation of seizure disorders

NURSING IMPLICATIONS

1. Monitor for neurologic disturbances following an injection, or during an infusion; see Adverse Reaction No. 1. Report any of these reactions to the physician immediately. If the patient experiences difficulty in swallowing, discontinue infusion immediately, and remain with the patient until the severity of the reaction is determined. The patient may need parenteral hydration and nutrition until swallowing returns.
2. Examine for rashes, report them to the physician.
3. Keep the patient supine during the injection or infusion.
4. Monitor blood pressure before, during and after injection or infusion. If hypotension occurs during an infusion, discontinue administration and

6. The patient may experience anticholinergic side effects; see Adverse Reaction No. 6. Inform him of the origin of the symptom and its transient nature.
7. Initiate seizure precautions if not already in effect.
8. This drug can cause the urine to darken or turn orange for 24 hours after administration. Inform the patient of the harmlessness of this effect.
9. Intra-arterial injection and extravasation must be avoided. Inject into IV tubing of an IV system known to be working satisfactorily. Do not inject or infuse into a scalp vein in children. If the patient complains of pain during an injection, stop administration immediately and evaluate for the possibility of intra-arterial injection or perivascular extravasation. Signs and symp-

continue to take the blood pressure until stabilization occurs. Hypotension can usually be avoided with slow injection. If a patient is to be ambulated after an injection, obtain lying and standing blood pressure. If postural hypotension is significant, report the fact to the physician and keep the patient at rest. As postural effects decrease over time, begin to ambulate the patient if desirable. Do so cautiously to prevent injury. Warn the patient not to stand up suddenly until the effects of the drug have disappeared. Ambulate the patient with caution if he is experiencing sedation or blurred vision. Initiate safety precautions such as side rails to prevent injury.

5. Monitor for jaundice; notify the physician.

toms are severe pain in the affected area, edema along the vessel tract, and possibly blanching of the extremity. Notify the physician.

10. Monitor for signs and symptoms of increased intraocular pressure, *i.e.* acute glaucoma—ocular pain, blurred vision, rainbows around lights, nausea and vomiting.[1] Notify the physician.

REFERENCE
1. Newell, Frank W. and Ernest, J. Terry: *Ophthalmology—Principles and Concepts* (3rd ed.), St. Louis: C. V. Mosby Company, 1974, p. 329.

PROPRANOLOL HYDROCHLORIDE (Inderal)

ACTIONS/ INDICATIONS	DOSAGE	PREPARATION AND STORAGE	DRUG INCOMPATIBILITIES	MODES OF IV ADMINISTRATION			CONTRAINDICATIONS; WARNINGS; PRECAUTIONS; ADVERSE REACTIONS
				INJECTION	INTERMITTENT INFUSION	CONTINUOUS INFUSION	
Beta adrenergic blocking agent. Blocks beta receptor sites, most importantly in the heart and blood vessels, to the effects of epinephrine and norepinephrine. The major effects produced are: 1. Decreased heart rate (decreased sinus node rate, prolongation of the A-V node refractory period, decreased ventricular automaticity) 2. Decreased cardiac contractility 3. Decreased blood pressure (secondary to decreased	ADULTS: 1–3 mg may be followed by a second dose in 2 min. Subsequent doses should *not* be given in less than 4 hrs. CHILDREN: Dosage has not been established There is no simple correlation between dose or plasma level and therapeutic effect. This is probably because sympathetic tone varies widely between individuals. Proper dosage, then requires titration.	Available in solution with a concentration of 1 mg/ml. Do not dilute in fluids.	Do not mix with any other medication in any manner.	YES Rate of injection should not exceed 1 mg/ min. Titrate injections with antiarrhythmic response. May be injected into Y injection site of IV tubing.	NO Do not add to fluids.	NO Do not add to fluids.	CONTRAINDICATIONS 1. Bronchial asthma (can cause bronchial constriction) 2. Allergic rhinitis during the pollen season 3. Sinus bradycardia 4. Heart block greater than first degree 5. Cardiogenic shock 6. Right ventricular failure secondary to pulmonary hypertension 7. Congestive heart failure, unless it is secondary to propranolol-treatable arrhythmia (see Warning No. 2) 8. In the presence of adrenergic-augmenting psychotropic drugs (MAO inhibitors) and within 2 weeks of their discontinuation WARNINGS 1. This drug is not currently indicated in the management of hypertensive crisis. 2. Propranolol can further depress myocardial contractility and precipitate pulmonary edema in patients with congestive heart failure. This drug may also reduce the positive inotropic effects of digitalis. 3. The effects of propranolol and digitalis are additive in depressing A-V conduction. Use propranolol with great caution in the presence of atrioventricular block secondary to digitalis. 4. At the first sign of heart failure the patient should be digitalized. If the

473

PROPRANOLOL HYDROCHLORIDE (Inderal) (Continued)

ACTIONS/ INDICATIONS	DOSAGE	PREPARATION AND STORAGE	DRUG INCOMPAT- IBILITIES	MODES OF IV ADMINISTRATION			CONTRAINDICATIONS; WARNINGS; PRECAUTIONS: ADVERSE REACTIONS
				INJECTION	INTERMITTENT INFUSION	CONTINUOUS INFUSION	
cardiac output. inhibition of renin release, decreased tonic sympathetic nerve outflow from the vasomotor center) INTRAVENOUS ADMINISTRA- TION is indicated *only* for the emergency management of life-threatening arrhythmias, or arrhythmias occurring during general anesthesia such as: • Paroxysmal atrial tachycardias secondary to increased catecholamines, digitalis, or Wolff-Parkinson-White syndrome • Persistent sinus tachycardia which is non-compensatory and is a hazard to the patient • Tachycardias or other arrhythmias due to thyrotoxicosis (as an adjunct to specific							progression of failure continues, propranolol must be discontinued. 5. Use in hyperthyroidism may mask continuing hyperactivity of the thyroid and its complications. 6. May cause severe bradycardia when used in Wolff-Parkinson-White syndrome. 7. Use with caution in anesthesia; hazardous myocardial depression can occur precipitating pulmonary edema or shock. 8. This drug should be discontinued 48 hours prior to surgery, except when used in pheochromocytoma. In emergency surgery, isoproterenol or levarterenol may be used to counteract the hypotensive effects of propranolol. 9. May cause bronchoconstriction in susceptible patients (chronic lung disease, asthmatics). 10. May depress early signs and symptoms of hypoglycemia. 11. Safety for use in pregnancy has not been established. 12. This is not the first drug of choice in the management of ventricular arrhythmias. 13. Patients with angina pectoris may experience an exacerbation of the condition with abrupt withdrawal of propranolol therapy; gradually reduce dosage prior to discontinuation in these patients. PRECAUTIONS 1. Use with caution in patients receiving catecholamine-depleting drugs such as reserpine. 2. May produce hypotension, marked bradycardia, dizziness, syncopal attacks, or orthostatic hypotension due to its relaxing effect on vascular smooth muscle. 3. Use with caution in patients with hepatic or renal impairment; decreased dosage is advisable. 4. Monitor ECG continuously during intravenous use, to observe for bradycardia and for effectiveness in abolishing arrhythmias.

- thyroid therapy)
- Persistent atrial extrasystoles which are a hazard to the patient and unresponsive to other therapies
- Atrial flutter and fibrillation, to control ventricular rate, when digitalis cannot be used or is ineffective alone
- Ventricular tachycardias induced by excessive serum catecholamines and digitalis; in other situations propranolol is not the drug of first choice (lidocaine should be used)
- Persistent premature ventricular contractions which do not respond to conventional drugs
- Tachyarrhythmias during surgery for pheochromocytoma

This is only a brief outline of the uses and effects of this drug in the intravenous mode. The cli-

ADVERSE REACTIONS
1. Cardiovascular: bradycardia, congestive heart failure, intensification of A-V block, hypotension, numbness of hands, arterial insufficiency (Raynaud type)
2. Central nervous system: lightheadedness, mental depression, insomnia, weakness, catatonia, visual disturbances, hallucinations, acute reversible syndrome of confusion, memory loss, emotional lability
3. Gastrointestinal: nausea, vomiting, diarrhea or constipation
4. Allergic: pharyngitis, agranulocytosis, rash, fever, laryngospasm, respiratory distress
5. Respiratory: bronchospasm
6. Hematologic: thrombocytopenic purpura, nonthrombocytopenic purpura
7. Reversible hair loss (rare)
8. In patients with heart disease: elevated SGOT, alkaline phosphatose, LDH, BUN

MANAGEMENT OF OVERDOSAGE OR UNTOWARD RESPONSE
1. Bradycardia: atropine 0.25–1.0 mg; if no response, isoproterenol drip titrated cautiously; initiate temporary transvenous pacing if necessary
2. Cardiac failure: digitalization and diuretics
3. Hypotension: levarterenol or epinephrine via transfusion, titrate with blood pressure
4. Bronchospasm: isoproterenol via infusion, aminophylline via intermittent infusion, intubation and mechanical ventilation if necessary

ACTIONS/ INDICATIONS	DOSAGE	PREPARATION AND STORAGE	DRUG INCOMPAT- IBILITIES	MODES OF IV ADMINISTRATION			CONTRAINDICATIONS; WARNINGS; PRECAUTIONS; ADVERSE REACTIONS
				INJECTION	INTERMITTENT INFUSION	CONTINUOUS INFUSION	
nician is en- couraged to do additional reading in the current litera- ture.							

NURSING IMPLICATIONS

1. Monitor for signs and symptoms of cardiac failure:
   a. Elevation of CVP (or pulmonary artery wedge pressure); measure every 15 minutes after injection for 1 hour, then hourly.
   b. Shortness of breath, orthopnea, coughing; count respirations every 15 minutes after injection for 1 hour, then hourly.
   c. Rales; auscultate lungs every half hour for the first 2 hours after injec- tion.
   d. Be prepared to treat as outlined above. Notify physician immediately.
2. Monitor PR interval for prolongation. Monitor the patient continuously via cardiac monitor during and after injection. Be prepared to treat bradycardia or A-V block; see above.
3. If used to supress supraventricular tachycardia in Wolff-Parkinson-White syndrome, be prepared to treat severe bradycardia with atropine, isoproter- enol and temporary pacing.
4. Monitor for respiratory distress secondary to bronchospasm. Signs and symptoms: wheezing, tightness in the chest, increased respiratory rate. Be prepared to treat with isoproterenol and aminophylline, and assisted venti- lation.
5. Monitor for hypoglycemia when appropriate. This drug may mask the onset of diaphoresis and tachycardia. Observe for visual changes, dizziness, and changes in mental status. Be prepared to treat with glucose.
6. Keep patient supine during injection and monitor blood pressure continu- ously. Following injection monitor blood pressure every 5 minutes for ½ hour, then every 15 minutes for ½ hour, then hourly until stable. Ambulate

with caution 1 hour postinjection. Check lying and standing blood pressure.
7. Hypotensive effects, cardiac failure, bradycardia, A-V block, and other ad- verse effects may occur in a more severe form, with greater duration in pa- tients with hepatic or renal impairment.
8. Be prepared to manage mental confusion and hallucinations, to prevent pa- tient injury.

SUGGESTED READINGS

Cardiac Drugs Today—Part Four: Antiarrhythmics. *Nursing '73*, August 1973, pp. 29–34.

Treatment of Cardiac Arrhythmias—Part I: The Arrhythmias. *The Medical Letter*, 16:101–108, December 6, 1974.

Amsterdam, Ezra A., et al.: Systematic Approach to the Management of Car- diac Arrhythmia. *Heart and Lung*. 2:747–753, September-October, 1973 (ref- erences).

Levitt, Barrie, Borer, Jeffrey, and Saropa, Arleen: The Clinical Pharmacology of Antiarrhythmic Drugs. Part I: Quinidine, Propranolol, Diphenylhydantoin, and Bretylium. *Cardiovascular Nursing*, 10:27–32, November-December 1974 (references).

Pamintuan, Jose C., Dreifus, Leonard S., and Watanabe, Yoshio: Comparative Mechanisms of Antiarrhythmic Agents. *American Journal of Cardiology*, 26:512–523, November 1970 (references).

Guyton, Arthur C.: *Textbook of Medical Physiology* (5th ed.) Philadelphia, W. B. Saunders Company, 1976, Chapter 57, The Autonomic Nervous System; The Adrenal Medulla, pp. 768–781.

ACTIONS/ INDICATIONS	DOSAGE	PREPARATION AND STORAGE	DRUG INCOMPAT- IBILITIES	MODES OF IV ADMINISTRATION			CONTRAINDICATIONS; WARNINGS; PRECAUTIONS; ADVERSE REACTIONS
				INJECTION	INTERMITTENT INFUSION	CONTINUOUS INFUSION	
Heparin neu- tralizer (when given in the presence of heparin). A ba- sic protein car- rying a posi- tive charge that will neu-	ADULTS AND CHILDREN: Dosage is de- termined by the amount and kind of heparin that has been ad- ministered in	Refrigerate; avoid freezing. Discard unused portions of vials. Supplied in am- puls: 5 ml con- taining 50 mg	Do not mix with any other medication in any manner.	YES Dilute in an equal volume of NS prior to injection. In- ject over 1-3- minute period.	YES Use NS as in- fusion fluid; add to at least an equal vol- ume of NS. Ti- trate drip rate with clotting	YES Use NS as in- fusion fluid; add to at least an equal vol- ume of NS. Ti- trate drip rate with clotting	CONTRAINDICATIONS None when used as indicated. WARNINGS 1. Administer additional doses titrated with anticoagulation studies (clotting time and plasma thrombin time). 2. Be prepared to treat hypotension. 3. Safety for use in pregnancy has not

tralize the negatively charged heparin molecule. This drug has anticoagulant effects when given in the absence of heparin. Used to treat heparin overdosage or to counteract the effects of heparin on clotting time during extracorporeal circulation (hemodialysis, cardiopulmonary bypass).

the last 3–4 hours.

Each 1 mg of protamine neutralizes 90 units of heparin activity when the heparin has been derived from *lung tissue* and 115 units of heparin when the heparin has been derived from *intestinal mucosa.*

Do not exceed the equivalent of 50 mg of protamine activity in a 10-minute period.

Do not exceed a dose of 100 mg in a short period unless guided by coagulation studies.

Dosage required decreases rapidly with time elapsed following the injection of the heparin. If protamine is injected 30 minutes after heparin, one-half a dose of protamine should be given. Use anticoagulation studies to guide subsequent doses.

of active drug; and 25 ml containing 250 mg of active drug.

Use caution; note the difference in dosage contained in the two ampuls available.

time or plasma thrombin time.

been established.

4. Hyperheparinemia and bleeding have occurred after cardiopulmonary bypass despite adequate doses of protamine.

PRECAUTIONS
1. Do not exceed a dose of 100 mg in a short period of time unless guided by coagulation studies.
2. Patients with an allergy to fish may develop hypersensitivity to protamine.

ADVERSE REACTIONS
1. Hypotension
2. Bradycardia
3. Dyspnea
4. Transient flushing of the face
These reactions usually occur after rapid administration.

NURSING IMPLICATIONS
1. Assist in monitoring thrombin time or clotting time during therapy. Observe for signs of overanticoagulation; e.g., oozing around vascular access or other surgical incisions.

2. Monitor blood pressure every 2–3 minutes during and immediately following a direct intravenous injection. Vasopressors may be used in the event of hypotension. Keep the patient supine during injection. Take blood pressure every 30 minutes during an infusion.

PROTAMINE SULFATE (Continued)

NURSING IMPLICATIONS (Continued)

3. Monitor heart rate during and immediately after a direct intravenous injection and every 30 minutes during an infusion.
4. Heparin rebound can occur 8–9 hours after protamine neutralization. This is due to the more rapid metabolism of protamine in relation to that of heparin; i.e., heparin activity may exist after the protamine effects have diminished.[1] Monitor for sudden bleeding tendency during the first 24 hours after neutralization.

Signs of bleeding: epistaxis, gum bleeding, hemoptysis, hematemesis, melena and bright red blood in stools, vaginal bleeding, hematuria, bruising, oozing of blood at incisions, sudden appearance of blood in drainage tubes (chest, abdominal, etc.)

REFERENCE
1. Ellison, Norig, et al.: Heparin Rebound. *Journal of Thoracic and Cardiovascular Surgery,* 67(5):724, May 1974.

PROTIRELIN (Thypinone)

ACTIONS/ INDICATIONS	DOSAGE	PREPARATION AND STORAGE	DRUG INCOMPATIBILITIES	MODES OF IV ADMINISTRATION			CONTRAINDICATIONS; WARNINGS; PRECAUTIONS; ADVERSE REACTIONS
				INJECTION	INTERMITTENT INFUSION	CONTINUOUS INFUSION	
Synthetic thyrotropin-releasing hormone. Increases the release of the thyroid stimulating hormone (TSH) from the anterior pituitary. Used in the assessment of thyroid function to distinguish between pituitary and thyroid gland dysfunction.	ADULTS: 500 mcg (range 200–500 mcg). CHILDREN (6–16 years): 7 mcg/kg, up to a dose of 500 mcg. INFANTS AND CHILDREN UP TO 6 YEARS: 7 mcg/kg. TEST PROCEDURE: Keep the patient supine during and for 15 minutes after the injection. Inject a dose as a bolus over 15–30 seconds. Obtain one blood sample for TSH assay before and 30 minutes after the injection.	Supplied in 1-ml ampuls, 500 mcg/ml.	Do not mix with any other medication in any manner.	YES As bolus over 15–30 seconds.	NO Pharmacologically inappropriate.	NO Pharmacologically inappropriate.	WARNINGS 1. There may be transient blood pressure changes during administration. Keep the patient supine during and for at least 15 minutes after injection. Blood pressure changes usually stabilize within 15 minutes. 2. Use with caution in patients with hypo- or hypertension. PRECAUTIONS 1. The administration of triiodothyronine (T_3) should be discontinued at least 7 days prior to the test. 2. Thyroid medications containing levothyroxine (T_4) should be discontinued 14 days prior to the test. 3. Levodopa may inhibit the TSH response to protirelin. 4. Prolonged treatment with physiologic levels of glucocorticoids, as in hypopituitarism, does not alter this test. However, larger doses may reduce the thyroid stimulating hormone (TSH) response. 5. Therapeutic doses of aspirin can inhibit the TSH response to this drug. 6. Use in pregnancy only when clearly needed. ADVERSE REACTIONS 1. Most side effects are mild and transient. The most common are: nausea, urge to urinate, flushed sensation, light-headedness, bad taste in mouth,

abdominal discomfort, headache, dry mouth
2. Less frequent: anxiety, sweating, tightness in the throat and chest, tingling sensation in the extremities, drowsiness
3. May cause breast engorgement and leakage in lactating women for up to 2 to 3 days after administration.

NURSING IMPLICATIONS
1. Be certain that thyroid-containing drugs have been correctly discontinued prior to the test. (See Precautions above.)
2. Monitor blood pressure every 2–3 minutes before and during the injection and for 15 minutes after. Keep patient supine during this time.
3. Reassure the patient if adverse reactions occur. Be prepared to manage nausea and vomiting.

● PYRIDOSTIGMINE BROMIDE (Mestinon Injectable, Regonol)

ACTIONS/ INDICATIONS	DOSAGE	PREPARATION AND STORAGE	DRUG INCOMPATIBILITIES	MODES OF IV ADMINISTRATION			CONTRAINDICATIONS; WARNINGS; PRECAUTIONS; ADVERSE REACTIONS
				INJECTION	INTERMITTENT INFUSION	CONTINUOUS INFUSION	
Cholinesterase inhibitor, facilitates the transmission of impulses across the myoneural junction by inhibiting the destruction of acetylcholine by cholinesterase. Used to treat myasthenia gravis when oral agents cannot be given, and also used as a reversal agent for curariform neuromuscular blocking agents, and gallamine triethiodide.	MYASTHENIA GRAVIS: *Adults*—1/3 of previous oral dose (approximately 200 mg, average oral dose is 600 mg/day). *In labor and delivery*— Give 1 hr before completion of the second stage of labor. *Neonates of myasthenic mothers*—IM or oral route only, 0.05– 0.15 mg/kg. See Warning No. 2. REVERSAL OF NONDEPOLARIZING MUSCLE RELAXANTS: *Adults*—give atropine sul-	Discard unused portions of vials. Supplied in 2-ml ampuls of a 5 mg/ml solution.	Do not mix with any other medications in any manner.	YES *Very* slowly over 2–4 min into the tubing of a running IV.	NO	NO	CONTRAINDICATIONS 1. Hypersensitivity to any anticholinesterase drug 2. Mechanical intestinal or urinary obstruction WARNINGS 1. Use with caution in patients with bronchial asthma or cardiac arrhythmias. Transient bradycardia may occur. 2. Overdosage may result in a cholinergic crisis—increasing muscle weakness involving muscles or respiration. This may be impossible to distinguish from worsening of myasthenia gravis itself. Crisis secondary to drugs requires immediate withdrawal of the drugs. Crisis secondary to the disease requires more drugs. An edrophonium test should be employed to distinguish them. Keep atropine available when giving this drug. (See Adverse Reaction No. 3.) This applies also to neonates of myasthenic mothers. See page 310, on edrophonium. 3. Maintain respiratory support until there is full recovery from muscle relaxant drugs (curare). Recovery may be prolonged. 4. Safety for use in pregnancy and lactation has not been established. 5. Failure of this drug to provide reversal

479

PYRIDOSTIGMINE BROMIDE (Mestinon Injectable, Regonol) (Continued)

ACTIONS/INDICATIONS	DOSAGE	PREPARATION AND STORAGE	DRUG INCOMPATIBILITIES	MODES OF IV ADMINISTRATION			CONTRAINDICATIONS; WARNINGS; PRECAUTIONS; ADVERSE REACTIONS
				INJECTION	INTERMITTENT INFUSION	CONTINUOUS INFUSION	
	fate (0.5 – 1.2 mg) prior to dose of pyridostigmine. Then give the pyridostigmine 10 –20 mg. Full recovery is usually seen in 15 min. (See detailed information in this book on muscle relaxant being used.)						of neuromuscular blocking agents within 30 minutes may be seen in extreme debilitation, carcinomatosis, with concomitant use of certain antibiotics or anesthetic agents. ADVERSE REACTIONS 1. Side effects are most often due to overdosage. 2. Muscarinic effects: nausea, vomiting, diarrhea, abdominal cramps, increased salivation, increased bronchial secretions, constricted pupils, diaphoresis. 3. Muscarinic effects can be counteracted with atropine, but this can mask the signs of overdosage and lead to the iatrogenic induction of a cholinergic crisis. 4. Thrombophlebitis at injection site. 5. Rashes.

NURSING IMPLICATIONS
1. In patients with a history of bronchial asthma, monitor for respiratory distress, wheezing, increased respiratory effort, increased rate, restlessness.
2. Monitor ECG in patients with a history of cardiac arrhythmias during and for 2 hours following injection. Be prepared to treat bradycardia with atropine.
3. In myasthenia gravis patients, notify physician immediately if signs of increasing muscle weakness occur. Be prepared to support respiration with airways, a manual breathing bag (Hope, Ambu, Puritan), suction, oxygen, endotracheal tube, and laryngoscope. Have atropine 1.0 mg and edrophonium at the bedside. Do not leave the patient alone. Begin ventilatory support if respiratory rate falls below 8–10/minute if there is cyanosis or restlessness. Continue until physician determines that spontaneous ventilation is adequate. Monitor neonates of myasthenic mothers, for respiratory weakness.
4. In patients recovering from curare muscle blockade, keep respiratory support intact until full recovery has been made from the drug, evidenced by full spontaneous respirations of adequate rate and depth and adequate arterial blood gases. A physician should discontinue respiratory support. Monitor vital signs according to recovery room policy. See detailed information in this book on the muscle relaxant being used.
5. Monitor for signs of overdosage (see Adverse Reactions above). Be prepared to manage vomiting to prevent aspiration. Keep patient in a lateral position if there is a threat of vomiting. Suction equipment must be at the bedside. Do not leave the patient alone if there is nausea, vomiting, or abdominal cramping.
6. Patients with myasthenia gravis and their families will require self-care instruction and close nursing follow-up.

SUGGESTED READINGS
Guyton, Arthur C.: *Textbook of Medical Physiology* (5th ed.). Philadelphia: W. B. Saunders Company, 1976, Chapter 12, Neuromuscular Transmission, Function of Smooth Muscle, pp. 147–157; Chapter 15, The Autonomic Nervous System; The Adrenal Medulla, pp. 768–781.
Jones, LeAnna: Myasthenia and Me. *RN*, June 1976, pp. 50–55.
Smith, Dorothy W., and Germain, Carol P. Hanley: *Care of the Adult Patient* (4th ed.). Philadelphia: J. B. Lippincott Company, 1977, pp. 382–384.

PYRIDOXINE HYDROCHLORIDE (Vitamin B$_6$, Hexa-Betalin)

ACTIONS/ INDICATIONS	DOSAGE	PREPARATION AND STORAGE	DRUG INCOMPAT- IBILITIES	MODES OF IV ADMINISTRATION			CONTRAINDICATIONS; WARNINGS; PRECAUTIONS; ADVERSE REACTIONS
				INJECTION	INTERMITTENT INFUSION	CONTINUOUS INFUSION	
Vitamin. Coenzyme in the metabolism of protein, carbohydrate and fat. Need for this vitamin increases in dietary protein, treatment with INH or oral contraceptives. The adult minimum daily requirement is 1.25 mg (2.5 mg in pregnancy and lactation). Used to treat: • Pyridoxine deficiency • Vitamin B$_6$ dependent convulsions • Vitamin B$_6$ responsive anemia Also used when gastrointestinal absorption is impaired. Used in some instances to reduce the severity of the gastrointestinal symptoms of nitrogen mustard therapy and irradiation sickness.	*Dietary deficiency*— 10– 20 mg daily for 3 weeks. *Vitamin B$_6$ dependency syndrome*—up to 600 mg/day and a daily intake of 30 mg for life (orally). *INH poisoning* —if more than 10 gm of INH has been ingested, an equal amount of pyridoxine should be given in the following manner: 4 gm IV injection, followed by 1 gm IM every 30 minutes until the symptoms subside (nausea, vomiting, slurred speech, visual hallucinations, stupor, coma, seizures). *Gastrointestinal symptoms of nitrogen mustard or radiation therapy*— 25 – 100 mg/day.	Protect solution from light when in storage.	Do not mix with: Ascorbic acid Sodium bicarbonate Aminophylline Any agent containing iron salts	YES Undiluted at a rate of 50 mg/ minute.	YES In any IV fluid at a rate of 50 mg/minute.	YES In any IV fluid at a rate to meet fluid requirements	CONTRAINDICATONS Hypersensitivity WARNING Protect solution from light while in storage. PRECAUTIONS 1. Single deficiency of this vitamin alone is rare. 2. Patients on levodopa should not take supplemental vitamins that contain more than 5 mg of pyridoxine in a daily dose. ADVERSE REACTIONS 1. Paresthesia (numbness or tingling) 2. Somnolence 3. Low serum folic acid

NURSING IMPLICATIONS
1. Vitamin B$_6$ deficient patients must receive dietary counseling and follow-up to improve intake.
2. Slight feeling of warmth may occur during administration; inform the patient that this is a normal response.

481

QUINIDINE GLUCONATE

ACTIONS/ INDICATIONS	DOSAGE	PREPARATION AND STORAGE	DRUG INCOMPAT- IBILITIES	MODES OF IV ADMINISTRATION			CONTRAINDICATIONS; WARNINGS; PRECAUTIONS; ADVERSE REACTIONS
				INJECTION	INTERMITTENT INFUSION	CONTINUOUS INFUSION	
Antiarrhythmic agent that has several actions: increases the effective refractory period of the atrial and ventricular myocardium thereby depressing automaticity and thus ectopic rhythms. Atrioventricular conduction velocity can be increased or decreased depending on several factors.

Used to treat the following arrhythmias:
• Premature atrial and ventricular contractions
• Paroxysmal supraventricular tachycardia
• Paroxysmal atrial fibrillation
• Atrial fibrillation (established)
• Atrial flutter
• Paroxysmal ventricular tachycardia not associated with complete heart block

Effect after IV injection | Use IV route for emergency management of arrhythmias; and except in these emergencies, it is recommended that an IM test dose be given before IV administration, if time permits.

ADULTS:
Initial IM dose —200 mg.

Subsequent or emergency IV dose :
Usual—330 mg. Range— 500–750 mg.

CHILDREN: Test dose of 2 mg/kg; (60 mg/M²)

Therapeutic dose—30 mg/ kg/24 hrs (900 mg/M² 24 hrs) divided into 5 equal doses.[1]

Effective dosage must be determined for each patient to abolish the ectopic rhythm without disturbing normal cardiac mechanisms. | Use D5W or NS for infusion.

Supplied in ampuls and vials of 50 mg/ml. | Do not mix with any other medication. | NO | YES

Add 800 mg of drug to 40 ml D5W or NS, making a solution of 20 mg/ ml. Begin with a rate of 20 mg/min. (1 ml/ min.)

Dose must then be titrated with patient response and guided by suggested doses in Dosage column.

Use an infusion pump. | YES

Use a solution of approximately 20 mg/ ml, add 800 mg to every 40 ml of D5W or NS. Begin at a rate of 20 mg/min. (1 ml/ min.)

Dose must then be titrated with patient response and guided by suggested doses in Dosage column.

Use an infusion pump. | CONTRAINDICATIONS
1. Abnormal rhythms due to escape mechanisms
2. Hypersensitivity to this drug or any cinchona derivative (quinine, etc.)

WARNINGS
1. In the treatment of atrial fibrillation or atrial flutter, reversion to sinus rhythm may be preceded by progressive reduction in A-V block to a 1:1 ratio of conduction and rapid ventricular rate. Use with caution when a rapid rate may precipitate cardiac decompensation. Such patients should be pretreated with digitalis.
2. Use with caution in the presence of any degree of A-V block or absence of atrial activity since complete A-V block or cardiac standstill could occur.
3. Use with caution in the presence of extensive myocardial damage; adverse reactions are more likely.
4. Use with *extreme* caution in the presence of an arrhythmia that could be secondary to digitalis intoxication; impairment in A-V conduction is more likely to occur.
5. Discontinue infusion if widening of the QRS occurs and exceeds a 25% increase over pretreatment duration, if PVC's, or ventricular tachycardia begins, if sinus rhythm is restored, if pre-existing P-waves disappear.

ADVERSE REACTIONS
1. Nausea, vomiting, abdominal cramps, urge to defecate or urinate, diaphoresis, apprehension (unrelated to size of dosage)
2. *Signs of overdosage*: vertigo, tinnitus, headache, fever, visual disturbances, widening of the QRS complex
3. Rapid infusion may cause hypotension
4. Large doses can cause complete A-V block and cardiac standstill
5. Quinidine fever |

should be seen in 4–6 min.

NURSING IMPLICATIONS

1. All patients must be under close observation during infusion; use continuous ECG monitoring. Observe for:
   a. Abolition of arrhythmia being treated for; drug dosage is usually titrated with response of the arrhythmia to the drug
   b. Increasing ventricular rate
   c. Increasing A-V block as evidenced by increasing P-R interval and dropped beats
   d. Widening of QRS complex.
   Slow the drip rate if any of the above occur; notify physician immediately for further instructions.
2. Atropine and isoproterenol may be used in the event of complete A-V block. Temporary transvenous pacing equipment should be readily available.
3. Monitor blood pressure every 3–5 minutes during the first half-hour of the infusion; then if stable, every half-hour to hour until infusion is terminated.
4. Be prepared to manage vomiting to prevent aspiration in the critically ill, weakened, or lethargic patient. Suction equipment must be at the bedside ready for use.
5. If adverse reactions occur, such as apprehension, urge to defecate or urinate, reassure the patient, administer supportive care, and stay at the bedside.
6. If possible, instruct the patient to report tinnitus, headache, visual disturbances, or dizziness. These are symptoms of overdosage.
7. Dosage and excretion are not affected by renal impairment.
8. Use infusion pump to prevent rapid infusion or overdosage.

REFERENCE

1. Shirkey, Harry C.: *Pediatric Drug Handbook.* Philadelphia: W. B. Saunders Company, 1977, p. 123.

SUGGESTED READINGS

Amsterdam, Ezra, et al.: Systemic Approach to the Management of Cardiac Arrhythmias. *Heart and Lung.* 2:747–753, September–October 1973 (references).

Levitt, Barrie, Borer, Jeffrey, and Sarapa, Arleen: The Clinical Pharmacology of Antiarrhythmic Drugs. Part II: Quinidine, Propranolol, Diphenylhydantoin, and Bretylium. *Cardiovascular Nursing,* November–December 1974, pp. 27–31 (references).

Selzer, Arthur: The Use and Abuse of Quinidine. *Heart and Lung,* November–December 1972, pp. 755–761 (references).

———: Treatment of Cardiac Arrhythmias. *The Medical Letter on Drugs and Therapeutics,* 16(25):101–108, December 6, 1974 (references).

SCOPOLAMINE HYDROBROMIDE (Hyoscine Hydrobromide)

ACTIONS/INDICATIONS	DOSAGE	PREPARATION AND STORAGE	DRUG INCOMPATIBILITIES	MODES OF IV ADMINISTRATION			CONTRAINDICATIONS; WARNINGS; PRECAUTIONS; ADVERSE REACTIONS
				INJECTION	INTERMITTENT INFUSION	CONTINUOUS INFUSION	
Anticholinergic, central nervous system depressant, sedative, tranquilizer, potent mydriatic (causes dilation of pupils), and cycloplegic. Used as preanesthetic sedation; to treat some forms of parkinsonism and paralysis agitans.	ADULTS: 0.32–0.65 mg. CHILDREN: 6 mo.–3 yrs. —0.10–0.15 mg. 3–6 yrs.— 0.15–0.2 mg. 6–12 yrs.— 0.2–0.3 mg.	Available in 1-ml vials and 1-ml disposable prefilled syringes, in concentrations of: 0.3 mg/ml 0.4 mg/ml 0.43 mg/ml 0.5 mg/ml 0.6 mg/ml from various manufacturers.	Do not mix with any medication other than: Atropine Meperidine Morphine Pentazocine. *When mixed with these agents, use immediately.*	YES Dilute in 10 ml sterile water for injection, inject over 1 min.	NO	NO	CONTRAINDICATIONS 1. Glaucoma (all forms) 2. Prostatic hypertrophy 3. Hypersensitivity to scopolamine 4. Pyloric stenosis PRECAUTIONS 1. Use with caution in patients with any form of cardiac disease or those who are over 40 years of age. 2. Acute delirium can occur if analgesics are not given during a painful procedure. ADVERSE REACTIONS 1. At therapeutic doses: blurred vision, flushing, tachycardia, urinary retention, mental confusion. 2. Large doses: fever, stupor, coma, respiratory failure. 3. Use with caution in the presence of respiratory disease. Neostigmine or

● SCOPOLAMINE HYDROBROMIDE (Hyoscine Hydrobromide) (*Continued*)

ACTIONS/ INDICATIONS	DOSAGE	PREPARATION AND STORAGE	DRUG INCOMPATIBILITIES	MODES OF IV ADMINISTRATION			CONTRAINDICATIONS; WARNINGS; PRECAUTIONS; ADVERSE REACTIONS
				INJECTION	INTERMITTENT INFUSION	CONTINUOUS INFUSION	
							physostigmine may be used to treat overdosage (see pages 418 and 451).

NURSING IMPLICATIONS
1. Keep patient oriented and reassured; take precautions to prevent patient injury. Use bed rails and restraints as indicated.
2. Monitor for cardiac decompensation if tachycardia occurs. Signs of decompensation:
   a. Dyspnea, orthopnea, increasing tachypnea
   b. Rales
   c. Distended external jugular veins
   d. Fall in blood pressure.
3. Observe for urinary retention, especially in elderly males. Have the patient void prior to administration. Palpate bladder size every 4 hours for the next 24 hours after administration of this drug. Measure urinary output every 8 hours (or as patient's condition dictates).

● SECOBARBITAL SODIUM (Seconal Sodium)

ACTIONS/ INDICATIONS	DOSAGE	PREPARATION AND STORAGE	DRUG INCOMPATIBILITIES	MODES OF IV ADMINISTRATION			CONTRAINDICATIONS; WARNINGS; PRECAUTIONS; ADVERSE REACTIONS
				INJECTION	INTERMITTENT INFUSION	CONTINUOUS INFUSION	
CNS depressant, barbiturate, short-acting. Response depends on dose, and ranges from mild sedation to profound hypnosis.

Used as a sedative, anticonvulsant in:
• Status epilepticus
• Toxic reactions to strychnine or local anesthetics
• Tetanus
• Adjunct to anesthesia | ADULTS: *Anesthesia*—Inject at a rate not to exceed 50 mg/15 seconds; discontinue when desired effects are seen. Do not exceed 250 mg.

In dentistry for heavy sedation when nerve blocks are also used—100–150 mg.

Convulsions and tetanus—5.5 mg/kg every 3–4 hours as needed or via continuous infusion.

Total IV dose should not ex- | Available in 1-ml ampuls and 50-ml multidose vials; both contain 50 mg/ml.

Also supplied in ampuls of dry powder to be reconstituted with sterile water for injection. Add 2 ml of diluent to the 100 mg vial, and 5 ml to the 250 mg vial. The resulting concentration is 50 mg/ml.

Use only clear, colorless solutions.

This is a Schedule II drug under the Con- | Do not mix with any other medication in any manner. | YES

Rate not to exceed 50 mg/ 15 seconds.

May be given undiluted or diluted 2:1 in sterile water for injection or NS. | YES

Use NS or RL in any amount.

Use an infusion pump. | YES

Use NS or RL in any amount.

Use an infusion pump. | CONTRAINDICATIONS:
1. Hypersensitivity to any barbiturate
2. Porphyria (confirmed or familial history)
3. Respiratory depression
4. Severe cardiac disease
5. During labor and delivery

WARNINGS:
1. Do not exceed an injection rate of 50 mg/15 seconds; respiratory depression, apnea, laryngospasm, or hypotension may result.
2. Use with caution in any patient with impaired hepatic function.
3. Use with caution in patients concomitantly receiving analgesics, other sedatives or hypnotics, or tranquilizers. There is a greater chance of respiratory depression.
4. The polyethylene glycol vehicle contained in this drug may be irritating to the kidneys when renal disease is present.
5. Safety for use in pregnancy has not been established. If benefits outweigh risks, fetal heart rate must be monitored during administration. |

ceed 500 mg. Doses of 1.1–1.7 mg/kg produce moderate to heavy sedation. A dose of 2.2 mg/kg will produce hypnosis. In extreme agitation, 3.3–4.4 mg/kg may be required but should be administered with caution.[1]

trolled Substances Act of 1970. Maintain hospital or institutional regulations guiding its use.

PRECAUTIONS:
1. When used on an outpatient basis, the patient should only be discharged after full recovery has been made, and then only in the company of a responsible adult.
2. This drug decreases responsiveness to coumarin anticoagulants, i.e., there is less suppression of prothrombin time; adjust anticoagulant dose accordingly.
3. Patient must be warned against operating hazardous machinery, or participating in hazardous activities, e.g., walking in traffic or on stairs, until there is full recovery from drowsiness, etc.

ADVERSE REACTIONS:
1. Respiratory depression
2. Idiosyncrasy in the form of excitement, "hangover" or pain
3. Hypersensitivity: rashes to anaphylaxis
4. Laryngospasm with large, rapidly administered doses
5. Hypotension with rapid administration

e. Stupor
f. Coma
Stop the injection or infusion immediately upon noting one of these symptoms. Notify the physician. Discontinuation of the infusion is usually all that is necessary to prevent further problems. If not, see No. 7 below.
7. Management of acute overdosage:
   a. Continue to stay with the patient and monitor vital signs
   b. Maintain an open airway and adequate ventilation
   c. Keep the patient as alert as possible by verbal and physical stimuli. Encourage the patient to breathe at an adequate rate (12–14 breaths/minute for an adult). If necessary, initiate artificial ventilation with a manual breathing bag (Puritan, Hope, Ambu, etc.) or mouth-to-mouth breathing at a rate of 12–14 breaths/minute
   d. Circulatory support in the form of fluids and drugs may be ordered.
8. The sedation produced by this drug may be preceded by transient changes in mental status, such as feelings of euphoria and confusion. If this occurs, attempt to calm the patient and take measures to prevent injury until the patient returns to his normal status.
9. If a patient is to be ambulatory following an injection, ambulate with assistance; there may be transient dizziness. Obtain lying, then sitting and standing blood pressures to detect postural hypotension. If this drug has been used for an outpatient procedure, a responsible adult should accompany the patient home. The patient should not drive for at least the next 8 hours.

REFERENCES
1. Formulary 28:24. American Hospital Formulary Service, American Society of Hospital Pharmacists, Washington, D.C., 1979.
2. Beeson, Paul B., and McDermott, Walsh (editors): Cecil-Loeb Textbook of Medicine (14th ed.) Philadelphia: W. B. Saunders Company, 1975, p. 1873.

NURSING IMPLICATIONS
1. Strictly adhere to maximum injection and infusion rate suggestions and maximum limits. Use an infusion pump to assist with rate control, to insure maximum benefit from the drug and to prevent overdosage. Patients with liver impairment should receive smaller doses and should be monitored more closely and for a longer period of time than usual.
2. Keep the patient supine during and after injection or infusion. Monitor blood pressure, heart rate and respiratory rate every 5 minutes for 1 hour following an injection, or every 5 minutes through the duration of an infusion. This includes fetal heart rate monitoring. (See Warning No. 5.) Do not leave the patient unattended.
3. Patients with porphyria are sensitive to barbiturates in that they may experience an acute attack of the disease secondary to the administration of a barbiturate (see Contraindications). The onset of an acute attack is indicated by severe colicky abdominal pain radiating to the back. There is usually severe vomiting, fever and leukocytosis in addition.[2]
4. Avoid extravasation: see page 96. Extravascular or intra-arterial injection of this drug can cause tissue necrosis and gangrene of the affected extremity, respectively. Thrombophlebitis can also occur during the course of an infusion. Examine for redness and pain along the vein tract, and discontinue the infusion if signs and symptoms appear; notify the physician immediately.
5. Take anaphylaxis precautions; see page 118.
6. Monitor for symptoms of acute overdosage (listed in order of progression):
   a. Respiratory depression, i.e., decreased respiratory rate and depth
   b. Peripheral vascular collapse, i.e., fall in blood pressure, pallor, diaphoresis, tachycardia
   c. Pulmonary edema (rare)
   d. Decreased or absent reflexes, pupillary constriction

SODIUM LACTATE (5.0 mEq/ml)

ACTIONS/ INDICATIONS	DOSAGE	PREPARATION AND STORAGE	DRUG INCOMPAT-IBILITIES	MODES OF IV ADMINISTRATION			CONTRAINDICATIONS; WARNINGS; PRECAUTIONS; ADVERSE REACTIONS
				INJECTION	INTERMITTENT INFUSION	CONTINUOUS INFUSION	
Buffering agent to contribute material for the body to regenerate bicarbonate (HCO_3) from lactate. Used for prevention and treatment of mild to moderate metabolic acidosis in patients with restricted oral intake whose ability to convert lactate to bicarbonate has not been impaired.	Dosage must be individualized according to the patient's electrolyte requirements. Usually administered in units of 50 mEq.	Solution contains 50 mEq of sodium and 50 mEq of lactate in 10 ml. Discard unused portions of vials. An approximately isotonic (1/6 molar) solution can be made by the addition of 50 mEq (10 ml) sodium lactate to 290 ml sterile water for injection.	Do not mix with: Novobiocin Oxytetracycline Sodium bicarbonate Sulfadiazine.	NO	NO	YES Use the following solutions: • Dextran (any form) • D5/NS • Any dextrose solution • Fructose solution • Invert sugar solutions • Ionosol products • Protein hydrolysate • Ringer's solutions • NS Infuse each 1000 ml over at least 4 hours.	CONTRAINDICATIONS 1. Hypernatremia 2. Fluid retention PRECAUTIONS: 1. Must be used in diluted form. 2. Avoid rapid infusion. 3. Administer with caution to patients who may not tolerate a large amount of sodium; e.g., congestive heart failure, edematous or sodium-retaining states, and patients with oliguria or anuria. 4. This drug is not intended nor effective for correcting severe acidotic states which require immediate restoration of serum bicarbonate levels. Sodium lactate has no advantage over sodium bicarbonate and may be detrimental in the management of lactic acidosis.

NURSING IMPLICATIONS
1. Monitor cardiac status in patients likely to decompensate (those known to have congestive heart failure; the elderly; etc.):
   a. Increasing heart rate > 110/minute in adults (for children, see page 545 for normal values)
   b. Elevation of central venous pressure or external jugular venous distention
   c. Increasing respiratory rate, orthopnea, rales, cough
   d. Onset of third and/or fourth heart sounds
   e. Peripheral edema (see Contraindications). Notify physician of the onset of any of these signs.
2. Weigh patients before and after therapy and thereafter as needed.
3. Monitor intake and output every 8 hours to detect fluid retention.
4. Be aware of the patient's serum sodium concentration, arterial blood gas values (pH, $pHCO_3$, pO_2, pCO_2). Do not administer this drug in the presence of hypernatremia or alkalosis (pH greater than 7.3).

STREPTOKINASE (Streptase)

ACTIONS/ INDICATIONS	DOSAGE	PREPARATION AND STORAGE	DRUG INCOMPAT-IBILITIES	MODES OF IV ADMINISTRATION			CONTRAINDICATIONS; WARNINGS; PRECAUTIONS; ADVERSE REACTIONS
				INJECTION	INTERMITTENT INFUSION	CONTINUOUS INFUSION	
An enzyme, indirect plasminogen activator, to stimulate production of a proteolytic enzyme plas-	ADULTS ONLY: Obtain 10–15 ml clotted blood for Streptokinase Resis-	Reconstitute each vial needed with 5 ml sodium chloride for injection. Add diluent slowly and roll	Do not mix with any other medication in any manner.	NO	NO	YES Use an infusion pump and administer at a rate as determined by	CONTRAINDICATIONS This drug, through its thrombolytic activity, increases the risk of bleeding and is contraindicated because of that effect in the following situations: 1. Surgery within 10 days 2. Liver or kidney biopsy within 10

min. Plasmin hydrolyses fibrin to dissolve blood clots. Activity begins immediately upon injection and can persist for up to 12 hours after discontinuation.

Indicated in the treatment of:

• Acute massive pulmonary emboli (defined as obstruction or significant filling defects of two or more lobar pulmonary arteries or an equivalent amount of emboli in other vessels);

• Pulmonary embolism producing unstable hemodynamics (inability to maintain blood pressure without supportive measures)

The diagnosis of these two situations must be made by pulmonary arteriography. Treatment should be instituted as soon as possible after onset of symptoms, and no later than 5 days after onset.

tance Test

Loading dose —250,000 units over 30 minutes. Rinse the 250,000-unit vial with 50 ml NS and add this solution to piggyback container and infuse into the patient.

Maintenance dose— 100,000 units/hour for 72 hours. Adjust rate according to the results of the Streptokinase Resistance Test:

1. If results are greater than 1,000,000 units, discontinue administration.

2. If between 250,000 and 1,000,000 units, increase infusion to 200,000 units/hour

3. If less than 250,000 units, decrease dosage to 50,000 units/hour

After the maintenance infusion has been initiated, obtain a thrombin time and a fibrinogen level at 3, 12, and 24 hours, and then twice

the vial gently until contents are mixed, then further dilute to 45 ml according to the table below.

*SUGGESTED DILUTIONS AND INFUSION RATES**

Streptase® (streptokinase) Dosage/Infusion Rate	*Streptase®* (streptokinase) Vial Content Needed	Total Volume of Solution (ml)	Pump Infusion Rate (ml/hr)
A. Loading Dose			
250,000 IU/30 min	1 vial, 250,000 IU	45	90
B. Maintenance Dose			
50,000 IU/hr	1 vial, 750,000 IU	45	3
100,000 IU/hr	1 vial, 750,000 IU	45	6
200,000 IU/hr	1 vial, 750,000 IU	45	12

(Depending on the type of infusion pump available, dosage rate may have to be adjusted with corresponding adjustment of total volume of the solution.)

For use in arteriovenous cannula occlusion, reconstitute the contents of 250,000 IU/Streptase® (streptokinase) vial with 2 ml Sodium Chloride Injection USP or 5% Dextrose Injection USP.

*Courtesy of Hoechst-Roussel Pharmaceuticals, Inc., Sommerville, N.J. 08876, 1977.

Use solutions within 24 hours.

Supplied in 100,000-, 250,000-, and 750,000-unit vials. Store at room temperature.

thrombin time. See Dosage column.

Use NS or D5W for infusion fluid.

days
3. Intra-arterial diagnostic procedure within 10 days
4. Ulcerative wound
5. Recent trauma
6. Visceral carcinoma
7. Pregnancy; the first 10 days of the postpartum period
8. Ulcerative colitis or diverticulosis
9. Hypertension
10. Liver or kidney disease
11. Thrombocytopenia or other evidence of defective hemostasis
12. Active tuberculosis
13. Subacute bacterial endocarditis
14. Gastrointestinal bleeding within 6 months
15. Known hypersensitivity to streptokinase
16. Cerebral embolism, thrombosis, or hemorrhage within 2 months
17. Use of this drug in septic thrombophlebitis or in an occluded arteriovenous cannula at a seriously infected site may induce systemic infection.

WARNINGS
1. Bleeding:
   a. This agent causes more profound alteration of the hemostatic status than does heparin or coumarin drugs. In its action of stimulating the production of plasmin for lysis of intravascular fibrin deposits, such deposits that provide control of bleeding at needle puncture sites and other trauma will also be subject to lysis, and bleeding may occur. There is great possibility of bruising or hematoma formation, especially with intramuscular injections. These injections must be avoided during streptokinase therapy, as should arterial punctures and venipunctures. If an arterial puncture is absolutely necessary, the femoral artery must be avoided in preference to the radial or brachial. Following the procedure, pressure must be applied to the site for at least *15 minutes,* a pressure dressing applied, and the site checked frequently for bleeding for the next 24 hours.
   b. Spontaneous bleeding from internal sites can occur. The risk is greater in patients with pre-existing hemostatic defects such as abnormalities in platelet count, prothrombin time, partial thromboplastin time, or

STREPTOKINASE (Streptase) (Continued)

ACTIONS/INDICATIONS	DOSAGE	PREPARATION AND STORAGE	DRUG INCOMPATIBILITIES	MODES OF IV ADMINISTRATION			CONTRAINDICATIONS; WARNINGS; PRECAUTIONS; ADVERSE REACTIONS
				INJECTION	INTERMITTENT INFUSION	CONTINUOUS INFUSION	
• Deep vein thrombosis, acute extensive thrombi confirmed by ascending venography or other objective methods. Treatment should be initiated as soon after onset of symptoms as possible • Arteriovenous shunt occlusion	a day (7 AM and 3 PM) for 2 more days and adjust dosage on the basis of the thrombin time: 1. If thrombin time is 2–5 times control keep infusion at 100,000 units/hour 2. If thrombin time is greater than 5 times normal, *increase* the infusion to 150,000 units/hour for 6–8 hours 3. If thrombin time is less than 2 times normal, *decrease* the infusion to 50,000 units/hour. Treatment is continued for 72 hours, thrombin time permitting, and then stopped. Thrombin time must then fall below 2 times normal at which time a heparin infusion is initiated at a rate of 1,000 units/						bleeding time. c. Besides its fibrinolytic action, plasmin also degrades fibrinogin, Factor V, Factor VII and other proteins. Products of plasmin degradation of fibrinogen and fibrin possess an anticoagulant effect, making bleeding difficult to control. If serious spontaneous bleeding occurs, the streptokinase infusion should be terminated immediately and treatment instituted as described under Adverse Reactions. 2. In patients with a predisposition to cerebral embolism, such as in cases of atrial fibrillation, the use of streptokinase may be hazardous because of the possibility of bleeding into the infarcted area. 3. Concurrent use of anticoagulants is not recommended and may be hazardous. If the patient has been on heparin, its effects must be allowed to diminish until the thrombin time is less than twice the normal control value. Rethrombosis has occurred after termination of streptokinase treatment. To lessen this risk, heparin followed by oral anticoagulants (warfarin) should be part of therapy. 4. Safety and effectiveness of this therapy in children has not been established and is not recommended. PRECAUTIONS 1. If the patient's history indicates an elevated resistance to streptokinase because of recent streptococcal infection, or recent treatment with streptokinase, a streptokinase resistance test is advisable (see Dosage column). Do not administer this drug if the resistance level is in excess of 1,000,000 units, for it will be ineffective due to the high level of streptococcal antibodies in the patient. 2. This drug may alter platelet function.

Concurrent use of any other agent that may potentiate this effect, such as aspirin, indomethacin, or phenylbutazone, should be avoided.

ADVERSE REACTIONS

1. Bleeding—The incidence of severe bleeding was between 4 and 6% in clinical trials. Fatalities have occurred due to cerebral hemorrhage during streptokinase therapy. Less severe bleeding has occurred at approximately twice the frequency as that occurring with heparin therapy. Oozing of blood from sites of percutaneous trauma is frequent. There may be a moderate fall in hematocrit without detectable bleeding.

   Management of severe bleeding: Discontinue the streptokinase infusion. If blood loss is large, packed red cell transfusions are indicated. Plasma volume expanders and fluids (other than dextran) should also be used, along with whole blood. If the hemorrhage is unresponsive to blood replacement, aminocaproic acid can be used as an antidote; see page 175 for details on this drug.

2. Allergic reactions are not unusual because of the high frequency of exposure to the streptococcal organism. These reactions range from rashes to anaphylaxis.

3. Fever can occur and should be controlled with acetaminophen.

hour for 7 days. On the fifth day of the heparin therapy, begin warfarin 10 mg/day. On the eighth day obtain a prothrombin time, having stopped the heparin 12 hours earlier; continue warfarin as indicated. See summary table below.

VARIABLE DOSAGE SCHEME FOR STREPTOKINASE (SK) IN THE TREATMENT OF PULMONARY EMBOLISM (24–72 HRS) AND DEEP VENOUS THROMBOSIS (72 HOURS)*

Time	Thrombin Clotting Time (TCT)	Streptokinase Dosage	Streptokinase Resistance	Streptokinase Dosage Based on SK Resistance
0 hr.	Determine TCT. Should be within normal limits	Loading dosage 250,000 IU in 30 minutes.	Determine if necessary	Loading dose may be higher based on SK resistance level.
30 min.		Maintenance dosage. Continue with 100,000 IU/hr for 3½ hrs.		
4 hrs.	Determine TCT If ≥ 2 Normal → Continue with 100,000 IU/hr.		Or if SK resistance → Increase SK data unavailable dosage to 200,000 IU/hr.*	
	If < 2 Normal ——————————————→		If SK resistance is: a) > 1,000,000 IU b) > 250,000 IU to } → 1,000,000 IU } c) ≤ 250,000 IU →	Discontinue SK Increase SK dosage to 200,000 IU/hr.* Decrease SK dosage to 50,000 IU/hr.*
			*Determine TCT 4 hours later. If < 2 Normal, discontinue SK; if ≥ 2 Normal, revert to 100,000 IU/hr. Repeat TCT at 12 hours.	
12 hrs.	Determine TCT 2–5 Normal < 2 Normal > 5 Normal	Continue 100,000 IU/hr. Decrease dosage to 50,000 IU/hr. Double dosage to 200,000 IU/hr.		

ACTIONS/ INDICATIONS	DOSAGE	PREPARATION AND STORAGE	DRUG INCOMPATIBILITIES	MODES OF IV ADMINISTRATION			CONTRAINDICATIONS; WARNINGS; PRECAUTIONS; ADVERSE REACTIONS
				INJECTION	INTERMITTENT INFUSION	CONTINUOUS INFUSION	

*VARIABLE DOSAGE SCHEME FOR STREPTOKINASE (SK) IN THE TREATMENT OF PULMONARY EMBOLISM (24–72 HRS) AND DEEP VENOUS THROMBOSIS (72 HOURS)** (Continued)*

DOSAGE	PREPARATION AND STORAGE	DRUG INCOMPATIBILITIES
Up to 72 hrs.	Determine TCT every 12 hrs.	Adjust dosage as recommended for 12 hrs. After any change in dosage determine TCT 4 hrs. later and readjust dosage.
After 72 hrs.	Determine TCT. Should be <2 Normal	Commence Heparin by I.V. infusion and an oral anticoagulant. Adjust Heparin dose to maintain TCT at 2–5 times normal.
After 120–144 hrs. (5–6 days)		Continue therapy with oral anticoagulant alone. Adjust dosage to maintain prothrombin time at 2–3 times control.

**Courtesy of Hoechst-Roussel Pharmaceuticals, Inc., Sommerville, N.J. 08876, 1977.

For arteriovenous shunt occlusion:
1. Before treatment, attempt to clear the cannula by careful syringe technique, using heparinized saline. If this does not reestablish adequate flow, streptokinase can be used. Allow heparin effects to diminish.
2. Administer streptokinase via infusion pump at a constant rate. Give 250,000

units in 2 ml of solution into each limb of the cannula over a 25–35 minute period. Clamp off the limbs for 2 hours.
3. Aspirate the contents of the infused cannula limbs, flush with saline, reconnect cannula.

NURSING IMPLICATIONS
1. Be aware of contraindications and clinical situations in which the risk of bleeding is great. Monitor even more cautiously than patients without these risks.
2. Monitor for all signs of bleeding:
   a. Intracerebral bleeding, as indicated by change in mental status, change in neurologic signs (pupil size, hand grip, extremity motion), headache, or change in vision. Check neurologic signs every 2–4 hours.
   b. Gastrointestinal bleeding, as indicated by hematemesis, abdominal pain or tenderness, fall in blood pressure, melena or red blood in the stools.
   c. Respiratory tract bleeding (hemoptysis may already be present secondary to pulmonary embolus) as indicated by hemoptysis, increase in amount of hemoptysis, respiratory distress, chest pain, hypotension.
   d. Bleeding from the urinary tract as indicated by hematuria (micro- and macroscopic) or dark brown urine.
   e. Vaginal bleeding.
   f. Ecchymosis or petechiae.
   Oozing from venipuncture, arterial puncture and intramuscular injections is to be expected. It is advisable to avoid these procedures during streptokinase therapy when possible. Pressure should be applied to all venipuncture and arterial puncture sites for 15 minutes followed by the application of a pressure dressing. These sites should be inspected hourly for continued bleeding for the duration of therapy.
3. Avoid other traumatic procedures such as nasogastric intubation and uri-

nary catheterization when possible. When performing endotracheal suctioning, use low vacuum settings (below 110 mm Hg) and keep the frequency and duration of suctioning at a minimum. Watch for blood in the aspirate.
4. Handle the patient carefully to prevent bruising and hematoma formation. Use adequate numbers of personnel when turning to prevent tissue trauma. Use protective devices on the bed (flotation pad, water mattress or air mattress) when possible to lessen trauma to the skin. If a hematoma does occur, notify the physician. Pressure dressings (Ace bandage) and ice packs may be ordered.
5. Monitor blood pressure and pulse indirectly every 1–4 hours depending on the patient's overall condition. If there is an increased risk of bleeding, vital signs should be taken hourly to detect the onset of bleeding.
6. Monitor temperature every 4–6 hours. Fever can occur; acetaminophen will be ordered to control it.
7. The clinician is encouraged to read further on this drug and the conditions for which it is indicated.

SUGGESTED READINGS
Cudkowicz, Leon, and Sherry, Sol: The Venous System and the Lung. *Heart and Lung.* 7(1):91–96, January/February 1978.
————: Current Status of Thrombolytic Therapy. *Heart and Lung.* 7(1): 97–100, January/February 1978.

● **SUCCINYLCHOLINE CHLORIDE** (Anectine, Quelicin, Sucostrin)

ACTIONS/ INDICATIONS	DOSAGE	PREPARATION AND STORAGE	DRUG INCOMPAT- IBILITIES	MODES OF IV ADMINISTRATION			CONTRAINDICATIONS; WARNINGS; PRECAUTIONS; ADVERSE REACTIONS
				INJECTION	INTERMITTENT INFUSION	CONTINUOUS INFUSION	
Neuromuscular blocking agent of the depo-	Administer only after un- consciousness	Many preparations are available from the	Do not mix with any other medication in	YES May be given	YES Use a 0.1% so-	YES Use a 0.1% so-	CONTRAINDICATIONS Known hypersensitivity

491

SUCCINYLCHOLINE CHLORIDE (Anectine, Quelicin, Sucostrin) (Continued)

ACTIONS/ INDICATIONS	DOSAGE	PREPARATION AND STORAGE	DRUG INCOMPAT- IBILITIES	MODES OF IV ADMINISTRATION			CONTRAINDICATIONS; WARNINGS; PRECAUTIONS; ADVERSE REACTIONS
				INJECTION	INTERMITTENT INFUSION	CONTINUOUS INFUSION	
larizing type, ultra-short-acting. Produces flaccid paralysis of skeletal muscles. A single paralyzing dose produces effects within one minute of injection, that last up to 8 minutes.* Used as an adjunct to anesthesia to facilitate intubation and manipulation of abdominal wall or other skeletal muscles, usually for short surgical procedures. Also used to reduce the intensity of muscle contractions induced pharmacologically, electrically (electroconvulsive therapy) or by disease states. Can also be used in certain situations to control respirations when artificial ventilation is required. *Nondepolarizing* neuromuscular blocking agents (pan-	or a sedated state has been induced. ADULTS: A test dose of 10 mg can be given to evaluate the patient's sensitivity to the drug. *Short procedures*— 40 mg initially (after test dose) then titrate with response and to reaction to the test dose. (Dose range: 25–80 mg) *Long procedures or for prolonged control of respiration.*— by small intermittent doses or by infusion: 2.5 mg/minute, titrate with patient response. (Dose range: 0.5–5.0 mg/minute) INFANTS AND CHILDREN: 1.0–2.0 mg/kg, titrated with patient responses, for all indications. Note: When administering this drug during electroshock therapy administer it approximately 1 minute be-	manufacturers. Use appropriate preparation for infusion modes.	any manner.	undiluted.	lution (1 mg/ ml) to make calculation of dose simple. (A 0.2% solution, 2 mg/ml, can be used for patients requiring fluid restriction.) Use D5W, NS or RL. Use of an infusion pump is advisable.	lution (1 mg/ ml) to make calculation of dose simple. (A 0.2% solution, 2 mg/ml, can be used for patients requiring fluid restriction.) Use D5W, NS or RL. Use of an infusion pump advisable.	WARNINGS 1. Intubation must be performed concomitantly with the administration of this drug. Adequate artificial ventilation, oxygen under positive pressure and the elimination of carbon dioxide must be maintained throughout the administration of this drug and the duration of its effects. 2. Safety for use in pregnancy has not been established. Effects on fetal development are not known. This drug does not cross the placental barrier in amounts sufficient to affect the fetus, as far as the drug's effects on skeletal muscles. PRECAUTIONS 1. Administer with caution, i.e., closely monitor reaction to test dose, in patients with cardiovascular, hepatic, pulmonary, metabolic, or renal disorders. 2. Administer with caution to patients with severe burns, those who are digitalized or who have been severely traumatized; severe electrolyte disturbances can result, leading to cardiac arrhythmias and possibly arrest. 3. Severe hyperkalemia can occur in patients with pre-existing elevations in serum potassium, in paraplegics, spinal cord injuries, or in patients with dystrophic neuromuscular disease. 4. Myoglobinemia and myoglobinuria can occur, especially in children. Small doses of nondepolarizing neuromuscular blocking agents given before succinylcholine can decrease the incidence of myoglobinuria. 5. A low level of plasma pseudocholinesterase may be associated with prolongation of respiratory paralysis following succinylcholine. Such low plasma levels are seen in patients with severe liver impairment, anemia, malnutrition, dehydration, recent exposure to neurotoxic insecticides (organophosphates), those receiving quinine, and those with a hereditary trait.[1] Such patients should be monitored carefully during administration of the test dose. Administration of succinylcho-

curonium, tubocurarine) are usually preferred for controlling ventilation because they do not cause muscle fasciculations.

*Respirations usually return within 30 seconds to 3 minutes after discontinuation of an infusion.

fore the shock, usually in a dose of 10–30 mg. (Atropine and a tranquilizer [barbiturate] are usually given prior to the succinylcholine.)

See precaution No. 5 for dosage modifications.

line should be via a slow 0.1% infusion. Drugs which either inhibit plasma pseudocholinesterase (neostigmine) or compete with succinylcholine for the enzyme (intravenous procaine) should not be given concomitantly with succinylcholine, to avoid prolongation of the paralyzing effects of this drug.

6. When administered over a prolonged period of time, the block produced by this drug can assume the characteristics of a nondepolarizing block. This can result in prolonged respiratory depression or apnea. The usual nondepolarizing agent antagonists, e.g., neostigmine, plus atropine can be used to counteract the paralysis. A nerve stimulator can be used to determine if the block is a depolarizing or nondepolarizing type.

7. This drug can increase intraocular pressure during the initial stages of administration. Use with caution during eye surgery or in patients with glaucoma.

8. Caution should be observed when this drug is used in patients with fractures where the muscle fasciculations produced may aggravate the trauma. Fasciculations and hyperkalemia can be reduced by the administration of a small dose of a nondepolarizing type of neuromuscular blocking agent prior to succinylcholine.

9. MAO inhibitor drugs can increase and prolong the effects of this drug.

ADVERSE REACTIONS
1. Prolongation of effects producing respiratory depression and apnea (see Precautions and Nursing Implications for agents and conditions that can cause prolongation)
2. Hypersensitivity, rare
3. Cardiovascular: tachycardia, elevation in blood pressure, lowering of blood pressure, arrythmias and cardiac arrest; in children, bradycardia, hypotension, arrhythmias including sinus arrest can occur during intubation following a second dose of succinylcholine; this may be due to increased vagal tone. These effects are enhanced by the presence of cyclopropane and halothane anesthetics
4. Respiratory: prolonged respiratory depression, apnea
5. Malignant hyperthermia in patients with personal or family history of the disease

SUCCINYLCHOLINE CHLORIDE (Anectine, Quelicin, Sucostrin) (Continued)

ACTIONS/ INDICATIONS	DOSAGE	PREPARATION AND STORAGE	DRUG INCOMPAT- IBILITIES	MODES OF IV ADMINISTRATION			CONTRAINDICATIONS; WARNINGS; PRECAUTIONS: ADVERSE REACTIONS
				INJECTION	INTERMITTENT INFUSION	CONTINUOUS INFUSION	

NURSING IMPLICATIONS

Postanesthesia Care:

1. Equipment that should be readily available: suction, manual breathing bag, airways, endotracheal tubes and laryngoscope, oxygen.
2. Patients receiving this agent must be intubated to assist in maintaining an adequate airway and ventilation.
3. Be aware of the duration of action of this drug (See Actions/Indications column), and when the patient received the last dose.
4. Be aware of the sequence of progression of the paralytic effects as they will occur after an injection of succinylcholine:
   a. Loss of eye movement
   b. Eye lid droop
   c. Stiffness of jaw muscles
   d. Fasciculations and then paralysis of upper trunk muscles spreading to lower trunk and then extremities
   e. Paralysis of pharyngeal muscles (tongue, muscles of swallowing, etc.)
   f. Respiratory paralysis, i.e., paralysis of intercostal muscles and finally the diaphragm

   Recovery will occur as a complete reverse of this sequence,[2] and usually occurs rapidly.
5. Be aware of elements which may prolong the effects of this drug according to the manufacturer:
   a. Decreased circulation time, e.g., congestive heart failure or shock
   b. Decreased body temperature (especially in infants)[3]
   c. Dehydration
   d. Decreased renal function
   e. Decreased hepatic function
   f. Concomitant use of neurotoxic antibiotics such as the aminoglycosides (gentamicin, amikacin, etc.) polymyxin B or bacitracin
   g. Other drugs that effect the central nervous system, e.g., diazepam, quinine, quinidine, MAO inhibitors, magnesium salts (magnesium sulfate), procaine
   h. Extremes in age
   i. Hypokalemia and hypocalcemia
   j. Anticholinesterase agents and other depolarizing or nondepolarizing neuromuscular blocking agents
   k. Low serum pseudocholinesterase (see Precaution No. 5)
6. Discharge from the recovery room will depend on the following criteria:
   a. Grip strength
   b. Ability to lift the head
   c. Ability to open the eyes
   d. Respiratory status, e.g., vital capacity and tidal volume (it is helpful to obtain these values preoperatively for comparison)

   Patients under the effects of any one of these elements will require prolonged monitoring as described in No. 5 above, for recovery from the succinylcholine.

Maintenance Care for Ventilatory Control:

1. Nondepolarizing agents are usually given for controlling ventilation because they do not cause fasciculations of the muscles.
2. When used, this drug is usually administered on a p.r.n. basis for control of ventilation. The criteria for when to administer succinylcholine are determined by the physician. The criteria will include such situations as:
   a. A respiratory rate greater than _____ respirations/minute (a limit set by the physician)
   b. When the patient's respiratory effort is out of phase with the respirator
   c. When the patient is struggling against the respirator
   d. When positive-end expiratory pressure (P.E.E.P.) is in use

   Monitor for the onset of any of these situations and administer the drug or have the drug given. Who administers neuromuscular blocking agents is usually governed by hospital policy.
3. Make certain that the endotracheal tube is securely and correctly inserted. Check the connection between the endotracheal tube and the respirator; it must be tight. *Keep respirator alarm systems functioning at all times.* The patient is totally dependent on the respirator for ventilation.
4. This drug paralyzes skeletal muscles, it does not alter consciousness or relieve pain and anxiety. Therefore, the patient must be adequately sedated and given analgesics as indicated by his condition. These agents will also decrease discomfort caused by fasciculations. He will not be able to make his needs known; the persons caring for him must anticipate those needs. Many institutions assign one or more nurses to be in constant attendance with these patients.
5. Monitor vital signs before administration and every 5 minutes after until stabilization is seen, then every 15–30 minutes. Repeat the cycle with each dose. Succinylcholine can cause bradycardia or tachycardia, elevation of temperature and increased salivation. Monitor accordingly. Patients with cardiac disease should be observed via continuous ECG monitoring.
6. Monitor for the signs and symptoms of increased intraocular pressure, i.e., dilation of pupils, and vomiting.
7. Because this agent produces muscle paralysis, handle the patient with care to prevent trauma to joints and muscles during turning and positioning. Turn frequently to prevent skin breakdown.
8. When the patient is taken off this medication and the respirator, proceed with the nursing management as described under Postanesthesia Care.

REFERENCES

1. Melmon, Kenneth L., and Morrelli, Howard F. (editors): *Clinical Pharmacology, Basic Principles in Therapeutics*, New York: Macmillan Publishing Company, 1972, p. 539.
2. Wylie, W. D., and Churchill-Davidson, H. C. (editors): *A Practice of Anesthesia* (3rd ed.), Chicago: Year Book Medical Publishers, 1972, p. 816.
3. Ibid., p. 833.

6. Increased intraocular pressure
7. Postoperative muscle pain (secondary to fasciculations)
8. Excessive salivation (when atropine or scopolamine has not been given prior to surgery)

SULFOBROMOPHTHALEIN SODIUM (BSP, Bromsulphalein)

ACTIONS/ INDICATIONS	DOSAGE	PREPARATION AND STORAGE	DRUG INCOMPATIBILITIES	MODES OF IV ADMINISTRATION			CONTRAINDICATIONS; WARNINGS; PRECAUTIONS; ADVERSE REACTIONS
				INJECTION	INTERMITTENT INFUSION	CONTINUOUS INFUSION	
Diagnostic agent to determine liver function. When injected into the blood, BSP is removed by the liver and excreted into the bile within a short time. The amount of dye retained by the blood is a measure of liver function.	ADULTS: With patient fasting and at rest, 5 mg/kg of BSP is injected slowly into an arm vein. Forty-five minutes after injection, 4–5 ml of blood is drawn from the opposite arm. A retention of less than 5% of the BSP dose is normal. CHILDREN: Not recommended.	Store in a warm (room temperature) place to prevent crystallization. Should crystals form, warm vial to body temperature. NEVER ADMINISTER IF CRYSTALS HAVE NOT REDISSOLVED. Do not mix with fluids.	Do not mix with fluids.	YES Slowly over a period of 5 minutes, undiluted as directed in dosage column.	NO	NO	PRECAUTIONS 1. Administer with extreme caution, if at all, to patients with asthma or known allergic disease. Anaphylaxis has been reported. Patients with an allergy history should be given an intradermal test (0.1 ml of a 1:100 solution) before full injection. 2. Do not inject into an artery. 3. Avoid extravasation. If it occurs, elevate the extremity, and apply ice immediately for 1 hour. Anaphylaxis occurs more frequently following extravasation. 4. Patient should remain under close observation for 1 hour after injection. 5. Anabolic steroids, certain estrogens, androgens, B vitamins, and oral contraceptives alter with BSP excretion in nearly all patients. Discontinue these drugs at least 1 week before the BSP test when possible. 6. Morphine, meperidine, amidone, and MAO inhibitors may elevate the amount of BSP left in the serum. Discontinue these drugs at least 1 week before BSP test if possible. 7. Avoid injecting into the same vein where gallbladder study dye has been injected within the last week to prevent thrombophlebitis. These dyes may also interfere with the BSP test. Schedule at least 1 week apart. ADVERSE REACTIONS 1. Nausea 2. Thrombophlebitis at injection site

NURSING IMPLICATIONS
1. Prepare the patient for the test:
   a. Explanation of purpose and procedure
   b. Make patient NPO after midnight (or at least 8 hours before the test)
   c. Patient should be at rest at least 1 hour before test
   d. Keep patient supine during injection and for ½ hour afterward.
2. Be prepared for an anaphylactic reaction. A properly equipped emergency

cart should be readily available. Keep a syringe of 1 mg of epinephrine (1:10,000 solution) at the bedside to administer intravenously at the earliest sign of anaphylaxis. Notify physician. (See page 118 for management of anaphylaxis.)
3. Stay with the patient for 1 hour after test.
4. Follow hospital policy on administration of this drug (in most institutions this drug is only administered by the physician).

TETRACYCLINE HYDROCHLORIDE (Achromycin, Panmycin, Tetracyn, Bristacycline, Steclin)

ACTIONS/ INDICATIONS	DOSAGE	PREPARATION AND STORAGE	DRUG INCOMPATIBILITIES	MODES OF IV ADMINISTRATION			CONTRAINDICATIONS; WARNINGS; PRECAUTIONS; ADVERSE REACTIONS
				INJECTION	INTERMITTENT INFUSION	CONTINUOUS INFUSION	
Antibiotic; broad spectrum, active against a wide range of organisms: • Gram-positive bacteria • Gram-negative bacteria • Rickettsiae (Rocky Mountain spotted fever, typhus, Q fever) • Chlamydia • Actinomycetes • *Mycoplasma pneumoniae* Use must be guided by sensitivity testing.	ADULTS: 250–500 mg every 12 hours. Do not exceed 500 mg every 6 hours. CHILDREN (over 40 kg): 10–20 mg/kg/day in equally divided doses every 12 hrs (See Warning No. 6.) INFANTS AND CHILDREN (under 40 kg): 10–15 mg/kg/day in equally divided doses every 12 hrs (See Warning No. 6.) NEONATES: Not recommended. Therapy should be continued for at least 24–48 hours after symptoms and fever have subsided.	To reconstitute from powder, add 5 ml sterile water for injection to 250-mg vial, 10 ml to the 500-mg vial. Store at room temperature; discard after 12 hours. Use only the following fluids for infusion: • D5/NS • D5W • Protein hydrolysate 5%, plain with dextrose 5% or with invert sugar 10% • RL • Ringer's Injection Infuse immediately after preparation of solution. Darkening solution indicates deterioration of the drug. Discontinue and use a different infusion fluid. Discontinue if a haze or crystals appear in solution or IV tubing.	Do not mix with any other medication in the IV bottle. Do not add as a secondary line to tubing containing: Calcium compounds Cephalosporins Chloramphenicol Chlorothiazide Phenytoin Erythromycin Heparin Hydrocortisone Methicillin Novobiocin Oxacillin Penicillin Polymyxin B Sodium Bicarbonate Thiopental	NO	YES Dilute to 10 mg/ml infuse over at least 1–2 hours (20 mg/minute). See Preparation column for acceptable fluids to use for infusion.	YES Preferred mode of administration. Use a concentration of 2 mg/ml of fluid, or add a 12-hour dose to 1000 ml of any fluid listed in Preparation column. Infuse at a rate of 1.5 ml/minute.	CONTRAINDICATIONS Hypersensitivity to any tetracycline WARNINGS 1. Tetracycline should be avoided in patients with renal insufficiency. This drug may exacerbate renal dysfunction directly and indirectly by causing a catabolic state with acidosis and increasing azotemia.[1] 2. The use of tetracycline in pregnant patients with renal dysfunction has been associated with death due to acute hepatic failure. 3. This drug is not readily hemodialyzable.[2] 4. May cause an elevation in BUN in normal individuals. This is not harmful and will decrease on discontinuation of the drug. 5. Tetracycline may cause liver damage in the form of fatty infiltration in previously normal individuals. Do not use other potentially hepatotoxic agents concomitantly. Avoid use in patients with liver disease.[3] 6. Use of this drug during the years of tooth development can cause permanent discoloration of the teeth. Enamel hypoplasia has also been reported. Do not use tetracyclines in this age group (last half of pregnancy, infancy, childhood up to 8 years of age) unless other drugs are ineffective or contraindicated. 7. This drug can cause fetal malformations (skeletal development) in animals; therefore, safety in pregnancy has not been established. Also, see No. 6 above. 8. May cause bone growth retardation in premature infants receiving large doses. This is reversible on discontinuation. 9. This drug is secreted in breast milk. Nursing should be discontinued when this drug is being used. PRECAUTIONS 1. Overgrowth of nonsusceptible organisms may occur. If a superinfection occurs, discontinue the drug and initi-

ate appropriate therapy.
2. Patients on anticoagulants may require lower doses of those drugs while on tetracycline.
3. Monitor hepatic, renal and hematopoietic systems during therapy.
4. Treat all group A beta hemolytic streptococcus infections for at least 10 days.
5. Avoid concomitant use of this drug and penicillin. Penicillin activity may be decreased.

ADVERSE REACTIONS
1. Gastrointestinal: anorexia, nausea, vomiting, diarrhea, glossitis, dysphagia, enterocolitis, Candida albicans overgrowth in the perineal area (monilia) and mouth (thrush)
2. Skin: rashes, exfoliative dermatitis
3. Renal toxicity: rise in BUN; see Warning Nos. 1, 2, and 4.
4. Hypersensitivity: rashes, anaphylaxis
5. In infants: bulging fontanels, papilledema (pseudotumor cerebri); usually disappears on discontinuation of the drug
6. Hematopoietic: hemolytic anemia, thrombocytopenia (rare)
7. Discoloration of teeth and enamel hypoplasia if administered during tooth development.

d. Monilial rash in perineal area (reddened areas with itching); red lesions on oral mucosa (thrush)
e. Cough (change in pre-existing cough or sputum production)
f. Diarrhea
7. Report the onset of any rash to the physician. Keep the patient's environment comfortably cool and the skin clean. Diphenhydramine (Benadryl) may be ordered to relieve itching.
8. Report the onset of jaundice to the physician.
9. Report the onset of bulging fontanels and other signs of increasing intracranial pressure to the physician.
10. Be aware of this drug's relationship with renal function. Most tetracyclines are usually not given to patients with renal impairment because:
a. The drug accumulates in the body because of decreased excretion
b. The presence of the drug may cause further deterioration in renal function
c. It may cause a catabolic state with metabolic acidosis, increasing BUN, and possibly death due to uremia [4]
Know what the patient's pretreatment BUN and creatinine levels are. Monitor for change in these values with initiation of treatment. Monitor urine output in renal patients receiving the drug. Report increasing oliguria to the physician. Send urine for analysis at least every other day.

REFERENCES
1. Barza, Michael and Schiefe, Richard: Antimicrobial Spectrum, Pharmacology and Therapeutic Use of Antibiotics. Part I: Tetracyclines. American

NURSING IMPLICATIONS
1. Take anaphylaxis precautions; see page 118.
2. If gastrointestinal disturbances occur, notify the physician. If disturbances such as nausea, vomiting and diarrhea are pronounced, the drug will probably be discontinued. Antiemetics, antacids, and constipating agents can be ordered to control symptoms. Monitor intake and output to assist the physician in planning for parenteral fluid replacement. Maintain hydration orally when possible.
3. If the patient will be taking the oral form of this drug as an outpatient, instruct him on the possibility of photosensitivity and the advisability of avoiding exposure to the sun (sun-block lotions may be of help if exposure cannot be avoided).
4. Women of child-bearing age and potential, and mothers of children who may receive this drug, should be informed of Warning Nos. 2, 6, and 7 by the physician. Assist in the interpretation of these warnings to the patient.
5. Even though blood dyscrasias are infrequently caused by this agent, be aware of the patient's complete blood cell count during therapy. If the platelet count begins to fall, the drug will probably be discontinued. Bleeding secondary to a lower platelet count usually begins only after the count falls below 100,000/cu.mm.
6. Monitor for signs and symptoms of overgrowth infections:
a. Fever (take rectal temperature at least every 4–6 hours in all patients)
b. Increasing malaise
c. Newly appearing localized signs and symptoms: redness, soreness, pain, swelling, drainage (increasing volume or change in character of pre-existing drainage)

● **TETRACYCLINE HYDROCHLORIDE** (Achromycin, Panmycin, Tetracyn, Bristacycline, Steclin) (*Continued*)

REFERENCES (Continued)
2. Ibid.
3. Ibid., p. 53.
4. Ibid., p. 51.
Journal of Hospital Pharmacists, 34(1):51, January 1977.

● **TETRADECYL SULFATE, SODIUM** (Sotradecol Injection)

ACTIONS/ INDICATIONS	DOSAGE	PREPARATION AND STORAGE	DRUG INCOMPAT- IBILITIES	MODES OF IV ADMINISTRATION			CONTRAINDICATIONS; WARNINGS; PRECAUTIONS; ADVERSE REACTIONS
				INJECTION	INTERMITTENT INFUSION	CONTINUOUS INFUSION	
Mild sclerosing agent for treating uncomplicated varicose veins of the lower extremities in patients where surgery is a risk.	0.5 – 2.0 ml for each vessel; use a 1% – 3% solution. Do not exceed 10 ml for a single treatment.	Do not use if solution has a precipitate. Supplied in 1, 2, and 3% solutions.	Do not mix with any other medication.	YES 1% for small veins; 2% and 3% for larger veins. Slow injection.	NO	NO	CONTRAINDICATIONS 1. Acute superficial thrombophlebitis 2. Underlying arterial disease 3. Varicosities caused by abdominal or pelvic tumors 4. Uncontrolled diabetes mellitus 5. Thyrotoxicosis 6. Tuberculosis 7. Neoplasms 8. Asthma 9. Sepsis 10. Blood dyscrasias 11. Acute respiratory or skin diseases 12. Bedridden patients PRECAUTIONS 1. This therapy should not be undertaken if tests show significant valvular or deep vein incompetence. 2. Necrosis can result from injection of this agent. 3. Deep venous patency must be determined by angiography before the drug is used. 4. Use with caution in patients on birth control pills who may be more susceptible to thrombophlebitis. 5. Safety for use in pregnancy has not been established. ADVERSE REACTIONS 1. There may be tissue sloughing along the vein tract following injection. 2. Permanent discoloration, though very slight, may occur. 3. Allergic reactions can occur. It is advisable to give a test dose of 0.5 ml and observe the patient for 2–3 hours before full treatment is given. Be prepared for anaphylaxis.

NURSING IMPLICATIONS
1. Take anaphylaxis precautions; See page 118.
2. Monitor for tissue sloghing along the vein tract. Instruct the patient to avoid trauma to affected areas. Use aseptic technique in caring for affected areas.

● THIAMINE HYDROCHLORIDE (Vitamin B$_1$)

ACTIONS/ INDICATIONS	DOSAGE	PREPARATION AND STORAGE	DRUG INCOMPAT- IBILITIES	MODES OF IV ADMINISTRATION			CONTRAINDICATIONS; WARNINGS; PRECAUTIONS; ADVERSE REACTIONS
				INJECTION	INTERMITTENT INFUSION	CONTINUOUS INFUSION	
Vitamin necessary for carbohydrate metabolism. Used therapeutically to treat severe vitamin B$_1$ depletion or beriberi.

Intravenous route is approved only for emergency treatment of wet beriberi with cardiac failure.

Thiamine is also contained in vitamin B complex preparations for intravenous administration. These agents are used to prevent vitamin B deficiencies such as beriberi during chronic illness and during prolonged periods of abstinence from food intake. See pages 529 and 530 for details on vitamin B complex. | ADULTS: 10–20 mg every 8 hrs until cardiac symptoms begin to subside. | May be infused in plastic IV bags. | Do not mix with aminophilline.

Do not mix with alkaline solutions of barbiturates, carbonates, sodium bicarbonate, citrates, and acetates. | YES

Slowly. | YES

Use any IV fluid, in any amount. | YES

Use any IV fluid, in any amount. | CONTRAINDICATIONS
Hypersensitivity to thiamine.

WARNINGS
Serious sensitivity reactions, such as anaphylaxis, have occurred. Deaths have occurred from the intravenous route. An intradermal test dose is recommended prior to administration.

PRECAUTIONS
Multiple vitamin deficiencies should be observed for in any patient with thiamine deficiency.

ADVERSE REACTIONS
1. Feeling of warmth
2. Pruritus, urticaria
3. Weakness
4. Diaphoresis
5. Nausea
6. Tightness in the throat
7. Angioneurotic edema
8. Cyanosis
9. Pulmonary edema
10. Gastrointestinal hemorrhage
11. Circulatory collapse and death |

NURSING IMPLICATIONS
1. Take anaphylaxis precautions; see page 118.
2. Stop infusion if any adverse reaction occurs; it may be the first sign of anaphylaxis.
3. Signs of thiamine deficiency will begin to appear when the dietary intake is less than 0.2 mg. per 1000 calories of food intake. (See Recommended Daily Dietary Allowances pages 541–542.)
4. Signs and symptoms of wet beriberi (cardiac failure secondary to thiamine deficiency):
   a. Persistent tachycardia
   b. Severe dyspnea, rales
   c. Violent palpitations of the heart
   d. Intense chest pain (substernal)
   e. Heaviness, constrictive, oppressive feelings in the chest

● **THIAMINE HYDROCHLORIDE** (Vitamin B₁) (*Continued*)

NURSING IMPLICATIONS (No. 4 continued)
  f. Cardiomegaly, hepatomegaly
  g. Cyanosis
  h. Insomnia
  i. Vomiting
  j. Peripheral edema.
  These signs should disappear within a few days with therapy.[1]
5. Administer supportive care for cardiac failure:
  a. Monitor heart rate, respiratory rate, blood pressure, C.V.P. as needed
  b. Place patient in a semi-Fowler's position (patient will probably be or-thopnic)
  c. Administer oxygen and supportive medications as ordered
  d. Monitor weight daily
6. Patients with beriberi must receive dietary counseling and follow-up to prevent recurrence of the condition.

REFERENCE
1. Beeson, Paul B., and McDermott, Walsh (editors): *Cecil-Loeb Textbook of Medicine* (15th ed.). Philadelphia: W. B. Saunders Company, 1975, p. 1373.

● **THIAMYLAL SODIUM** (Surital)

ACTIONS/INDICATIONS	DOSAGE	PREPARATION AND STORAGE	DRUG INCOMPATIBILITIES	MODES OF IV ADMINISTRATION			CONTRAINDICATIONS; WARNINGS; PRECAUTIONS; ADVERSE REACTIONS
				INJECTION	INTERMITTENT INFUSION	CONTINUOUS INFUSION	
Anesthetic, ultra-short-acting barbiturate. Used for anesthesia induction or to induce a hypnotic state. Following an injection, anesthesia usually occurs within 20–60 seconds. Recovery occurs within 10–30 minutes after the last injection, depending on the amount administered.	ADULTS: Individualize according to patient response. *Induction:* Push injection —1 ml of a 2.5% solution every 5 seconds until desired effects are obtained (3–6 ml is usually sufficient). Maintenance can be obtained by continuous infusion (see Intermittent and Continuous Infusion columns.) CHILDREN: No recommendations available.	Supplied in 1, 5, and 10 gm vials. To prepare a 2.5% solution for *injection,* add the contents of the vials to the following amounts of sterile water for injection: 1 gm to 40 ml 5 gm to 200 ml 10 gm to 400 ml To prepare a 0.3% solution for *infusion,* add the contents of the vials to the following amounts of NS or D5W: 1 gm to 333 ml 5 gm to 1,670 ml 10 gm to 3,333 ml Some solutions of D5W are acidic enough to cause drug	Do not mix with other medications in solution. Atropine, succinylcholine and other anesthetic agents can be injected into thiamylal line or vice versa.	YES Use a 2.5% solution.	YES Use a 0.3% solution. Titrate with patient response. See Preparation column for solutions.	YES Use a 0.3% solution. Titrate with patient response. See Preparation column for solutions.	CONTRAINDICATIONS 1. When general anesthesia is contraindicated 2. Latent or manifest porphyria 3. Known hypersensitivity to any barbiturate WARNINGS 1. Repeated and continuous infusion may cause cumulative effects producing prolonged somnolence, respiratory and circulatory depression. 2. Safety for use in pregnancy has not been established. PRECAUTIONS 1. Use with caution in debilitated patients, those with respiratory impairment, circulatory, renal, hepatic and endocrine disorders. These patients will require lower dosage and more careful monitoring to prevent overdosage and respiratory depression, and hypotension. 2. Use with extreme caution in the presence of status asthmaticus; respiratory arrest can result from the sedative effects and bronchospasm produced by this drug. The patient should be intubated prior to administration. 3. Avoid extravasation. 4. Intra-arterial injection may produce gangrene of the extremity.

1. Circulatory depression, hypotension
2. Thrombophlebitis at the injection site
3. Respiratory depression, apnea, laryngospasm, bronchospasm
4. Headache
5. Emergence delirium
6. Hypersensitivity: rashes, urticaria and anaphylaxis
7. Nausea and vomiting

f. Coma

Stop the injection or infusion immediately upon noting one of these symptoms. Notify the physician. Discontinuation of the infusion is usually all that is necessary to prevent further problems. If not, see No. 8 below.

8. Management of acute overdosage:
   a. Continue to stay with the patient and monitor vital signs
   b. Maintain an open airway and adequate ventilation
   c. Keep the patient as alert as possible by verbal and physical stimuli. Encourage the patient to breathe at an adequate rate (12–14 breaths/minute for an adult). If necessary, initiate artificial ventilation with a manual breathing bag (Puritan, Hope, Ambu, etc.)
   d. Circulatory support in the form of fluids and drugs may be ordered
   e. Because of the drug's short duration of action, recovery should be prompt
9. Thiamylal can produce bronchospasm and laryngospasm. Monitor for the onset of laryngeal stridor, wheezing and respiratory distress. Bronchodilator agents and discontinuation of infusion may be required. Be prepared to intubate, if the patient has not already been intubated.
10. The sedation produced by this drug may be preceded by transient changes in mental status, such as feelings of euphoria and confusion. If this occurs, attempt to calm the patient and take measures to prevent injury until the patient returns to his normal status.
11. If the patient is to be ambulatory following an injection, ambulate with assistance; there may be transient dizziness. Obtain lying, then sitting and standing blood pressures to detect postural hypotension. If this drug has been used for an outpatient procedure, a responsible adult should accompany the patient home. The patient should not drive for at least the next 8 hours.
12. Postanesthesia Care:
    a. Maintain a patent airway with the endotracheal tube, or an oral-pharyngeal airway as required, until the patient is able to swallow and has a

precipitation. If this occurs, make a new solution using NS.

Cloudiness is a sign of solution aging; discard if this occurs. Store in refrigerator. Discard after 6 days.

Protect from excessive exposure to light.

This is a Schedule III drug under the Controlled Substances Act of 1970. Maintain hospital or institutional regulations controlling its use.

NURSING IMPLICATIONS

1. This drug is usually administered only by or under the direct supervision of an anesthesiologist. Follow individual hospital regulations.
2. Strictly adhere to maximum injection and infusion rate suggestions and maximum limits. Use an infusion pump to assist with rate control, to insure maximum benefit from the drug and to prevent overdosage. Patients with liver impairment should receive smaller doses and should be monitored more closely and for a longer period of time than usual.
3. Monitor blood pressure, heart rate and respiratory rate every 5 minutes for 1 hour following an injection, or every 5 minutes through the duration of an infusion. This includes fetal heart rate monitoring if the drug is used during pregnancy or delivery. Do not leave the patient unattended.
4. Patients with porphyria are sensitive to barbiturates in that they may experience an acute attack of the disease secondary to the administration of a barbiturate (see Contraindications). The onset of an acute attack is indicated by severe colicky abdominal pain radiating to the back. There is usually severe vomiting, fever and leukocytosis in addition.[1]
5. Avoid extravasation: see page 96. Extravascular or intra-arterial injection of this drug can cause tissue necrosis and gangrene of the affected extremity, respectively. Thrombophlebitis can also occur during the course of an infusion. Examine for redness and pain along the vein tract, and discontinue the infusion if signs and symptoms appear. Notify the physician immediately.
6. Take anaphylaxis precautions; see page 118.
7. Monitor for symptoms of acute overdosage (listed in order of progression):
   a. Respiratory depression, i.e., decreased respiratory rate and depth
   b. Peripheral vascular collapse, i.e., fall in blood pressure, pallor, diaphoresis, tachycardia
   c. Pulmonary edema (rare)
   d. Decreased or absent reflexes, pupillary constriction
   e. Stupor

NURSING IMPLICATIONS (No. 12 continued)

    return of the gag reflex.

  b. Monitor the respiratory rate continuously until an adequate spontaneous rate has been reached and has stabilized. (Standard respiratory support equipment should be readily available, such as: manual breathing bag, suction, oxygen, airways and intubation equipment.)

  c. Monitor heart rate and blood pressure at a schedule dictated by recovery room or institutional policy, usually every 15 minutes for the duration of the stay of an uncomplicated patient.

  d. Be prepared to treat hypotension; pressor agents and/or fluids are usually prescribed.

  e. Be prepared to manage emergence delirium. Take precautions to prevent injury with the use of side rails, etc.

  f. Take precautions to prevent aspiration, by patient positioning.

  g. Administer supportive care as indicated for drugs used concomitantly with this anesthetic agent such as neuromuscular blocking agents (succinylcholine, tubocurarine, etc.) and analgesics.

  h. An anesthesiologist usually decides when a patient can be discharged from the recovery area; follow institutional policy.

REFERENCE

1. Beeson, Paul B., and McDermott, Walsh (editors): *Cecil-Loeb Textbook of Medicine* (14th ed.), Philadelphia: W. B. Saunders Company, 1977, p. 1873.

● THIOPENTAL SODIUM (Sodium Pentothal)

ACTIONS/ INDICATIONS	DOSAGE	PREPARATION AND STORAGE	DRUG INCOMPAT- IBILITIES	MODES OF IV ADMINISTRATION			CONTRAINDICATIONS; WARNINGS; PRECAUTIONS; ADVERSE REACTIONS
				INJECTION	INTERMITTENT INFUSION	CONTINUOUS INFUSION	
Anesthetic, ultra-short-acting barbiturate. Depresses the CNS to the point of hypnosis and anesthesia 30–40 seconds after IV injection. Used in anesthesia: • Sole agent of anesthesia • Induction • Adjunct to other agents • Anticonvulsant • Narcoanalysis Recovery is rapid after one small dose, with some residual somnolence and retrograde amnesia. Howev-	ADULTS: Individualized according to patient's response, usually proportional to body weight. *Test dose—* 25–75 mg injected with 60-second observation of the patient for unusual response. *Induction—* adult: average, 50–75 mg at intervals of 20–40 seconds titrated to patient's reaction. As an initial dose, 210–280 mg (3–4 mg/kg) is required for rapid induction in the average 70 kg	To reconstitute, use only sterile water for injection, NS, or D5W, or Abbott Pentothal Diluent. (see table below). This drug contains no bacteriostatic agents. Use extreme caution to prevent contamination; use only fresh solutions; discard all stock solutions after 24 hours.	Do not mix in solution with other agents. Succinyl-choline, atropine, etc., may be injected into IV tubing containing thiopental and vice versa.	YES Use a 2.5% solution, slowly.	YES Use 0.2–0.4% solution; titrate with patient response. Use D5W, NS, or Normosol-R for infusion when volumes over 100 ml are required; do not use sterile water for injection.	YES Use 0.2–0.4% solution; titrate with patient response. Use D5W, NS or Normosol-R for infusion when volumes over 100 ml are required; do not use sterile water for injection.	CONTRAINDICATIONS *Absolute:* 1. Absence of suitable veins 2. Hypersensitivity to any barbiturate 3. Status asthmaticus 4. Porphyria (confirmed or familial history) *Relative:* 1. Severe cardiovascular disease 2. Hypotension and shock 3. Conditions in which effects may be prolonged: Addison's disease, excessive premedication, hepatic or renal dysfunction, myxedema, increased BUN, severe anemia (dosage must be adjusted accordingly, if the drug is given at all) 4. Increased intracranial pressure 5. Asthma 6. Myasthenia gravis WARNINGS May be habit-forming. PRECAUTIONS 1. Respiratory support equipment must be readily available to maintain a patent airway and ventilation. Momentary apnea following each injection is typical, and requires assisted ventilation. 2. Avoid extravasation. Intra-arterial in-

er, repeated doses lead to prolonged anesthesia because fatty tissues in the body act as a reservoir to the drug, they accumulate thiopental in concentrations 6–12 times greater than the plasma, and then release the drug slowly to produce prolonged anesthesia.

adult.

Maintenance of anesthesia—25–50 mg whenever the patient moves. Use minimal dose to achieve desirable level.

Continuous drip can be used throughout procedure.

Convulsive states—75–125 mg, up to 250 mg over a 10-minute period. Also by infusion.

To decrease intracranial pressure during surgery—1.5–3.5 mg/kg via intermittent bolus.

Psychiatry—use a test dose (see above), then 100 mg/min injection. Patient should be instructed to count backward from 100. When confused counting occurs, injection is stopped. Infusion may also be used.

CHILDREN: Recommendations not available.

| CONCENTRATION DESIRED | | AMOUNTS TO USE | |
%	mg/ml	Thiopental gm	Diluent ml
0.2	2	1	500*
0.4	4	2	500*
		5	250*
2.0	20	10	500*
		1	40
2.5	25	5	200*
		1	20

Never use a solution with visible precipitate.

Follow directions for dilution and transfer techniques accompanying the equipment and container.

This is a Schedule III drug under the Controlled Substances Act of 1970. Maintain hospital or institutional regulations guiding the use of this drug.

*For volume over 100 ml, do not use sterile water for injection, to prevent hemolysis. Use D5W, NS, or Normosol-R for large volume infusion, or Abbott Pentothal diluent.

jection can cause gangrene of the extremity.
3. If used in the presence of relative contraindications, reduce dosage and administer slowly.

ADVERSE REACTIONS
1. Respiratory depression, laryngospasm, bronchospasm
2. Myocardial depression
3. Cardiac arrhythmias
4. Prolonged somnolence and recovery
5. Sneezing, coughing, shivering
6. Hypersensitivity

NURSING IMPLICATIONS
1. Strictly adhere to maximum injection and infusion rate suggestions and maximum limits. Use an infusion pump to assist with rate control, to insure maximum benefit from the drug and to prevent overdosage. Patients with liver impairment, severe cardiovascular disease, hypotension, Addison's disease, renal impairment, myxedema, or severe anemia should receive smaller doses and should be monitored more closely and for a longer period of time than usual.

503

THIOPENTAL SODIUM (Pentothal) (Continued)

NURSING IMPLICATIONS (Continued)

2. Keep the patient supine during and after injection or infusion. Monitor blood pressure, heart rate and respiratory rate every 5 minutes for 1 hour following an injection, or every 5 minutes through the duration of an infusion. This includes fetal heart rate monitoring. Do not leave the patient unattended.

3. Patients with porphyria are sensitive to barbiturates in that they may experience an acute attack of the disease secondary to the administration of a barbiturate (see Contraindications). The onset of an acute attack is indicated by severe colicky abdominal pain radiating to the back. There is usually severe vomiting, fever and leukocytosis in addition.[1]

4. Avoid extravasation; see page 96. Extravascular or intra-arterial injection of this drug can cause tissue necrosis and gangrene of the affected extremity, respectively. Thrombophlebitis can also occur during the course of an infusion. Examine for redness and pain along the vein tract, and discontinue the infusion if signs and symptoms appear. Notify the physician immediately.

5. Take anaphylactic precautions; see page 118.

6. Monitor for symptoms of acute overdosage (listed in order of progression):
   a. Respiratory depression, i.e., decreased respiratory rate and depth, apnea (intermittent apnea is expected after each injection and during induction. Respiratory depression is termed as prolonged insufficient ventilation or apnea.)
   b. Peripheral vascular collapse, i.e., fall in blood pressure, pallor, diaphoresis, tachycardia
   c. Pulmonary edema (rare)
   d. Decreased or absent reflexes, pupillary constriction
   e. Stupor
   f. Coma

Stop the injection or infusion immediately upon noting one of these symptoms. Support ventilation. Notify the physician. Discontinuation of the infusion is usually all that is necessary to prevent further problems. If not, see No. 7 below.

7. Management of acute overdosage:
   a. Continue to stay with the patient, and monitor vital signs
   b. Maintain an open airway and adequate ventilation
   c. Keep the patient as alert as possible by verbal and physical stimuli. Encourage the patient to breathe at an adequate rate (12–14 breaths/minute for an adult). If necessary, initiate artificial ventilation with a manual breathing bag (Puritan, Hope, Ambu, etc.) or mouth-to-mouth breathing at a rate of 12–14 breaths/minute
   d. Circulatory support in the form of fluids and drugs may be ordered

8. The sedation produced by this drug may be preceded by transient changes in mental status, such as feelings of euphoria and confusion. If this occurs, attempt to calm the patient and take measures to prevent injury until the patient returns to his normal status.

9. If a patient is to be ambulatory following an injection, ambulate with assistance. There may be transient dizziness. Obtain lying, then sitting and standing blood pressures to detect postural hypotension. If this drug has been used for an outpatient procedure, a responsible adult should accompany the patient home. The patient should not drive for at least the next 8 hours.

REFERENCE
1. Beeson, Paul B., and McDermott, Walsh (editors): *Cecil-Loeb Textbook of Medicine* (14th ed.). Philadelphia: W. B. Saunders Company, 1975, p. 1873.

THIOPHOSPHORAMIDE (Thiotepa)

ACTIONS/ INDICATIONS	DOSAGE	PREPARATION AND STORAGE	DRUG INCOMPAT-IBILITIES	MODES OF IV ADMINISTRATION			CONTRAINDICATIONS: WARNINGS: PRECAUTIONS: ADVERSE REACTIONS
				INJECTION	INTERMITTENT INFUSION	CONTINUOUS INFUSION	
Antineoplastic agent, of the alkylating type, related to nitrogen mustard. Excreted unchanged in the urine.

Used for palliation of many types of cancers, including:
• Adenocarcinoma | ADULTS: *Initial*—30 mg (20 mg in the presence of marked debilitation, chronic cardiovascular or renal disease or shock).

Maintenance —45–60 mg/ dose, adjusted on basis of blood counts, at 1- to 4-week | To reconstitute from powder, use sterile water for injection. Add 1.5 ml. This produces a concentration of 10 mg/ml. Add to NS, D5W, D5/NS, RL, Ringer's injection for infusion.

Solution should | Do not mix with any other medication in any manner. | YES

Further dilution is not necessary.

Inject over 1– 3 minutes. | YES

Add dose to 50–100 ml D5W, NS, D5/NS, RL or Ringer's injection.

Infuse over 30 minutes. | NO

Injection and intermittent infusion are the preferred modes of administration. | CONTRAINDICATIONS
1. Hepatic, renal or bone marrow dysfunction. If need outweighs risks, use lower dosage and monitor organ function.
2. Hypersensitivity.

WARNINGS
1. This drug is actively teratogenic (causes fetal abnormalities).
2. Highly toxic to hematopoietic system (blood cell production). Rapidly falling WBC should prompt discontinuation of the drug.
3. Weekly CBC and platelet counts should be performed before, during |

Malignant lymphomas stages III and IV (lymphosarcoma, reticulum cell sarcoma, Hodgkin's disease and giant follicular lymphoma).
- Bronchogenic carcinoma

Also used to control intracavitary effusions secondary to neoplastic disease, and is administered directly into tumor masses and affected body cavities (e.g., abdominal, chest).

intervals (bronchogenic carcinoma — one dose is given every 5 days).

CHILDREN: 0.8–1.0 mg/kg/dose repeated at 2-week intervals.

be clear to slightly opaque. Grossly opaque solutions, or those with a precipitate, should not be used. Refrigerate reconstituted solution and discard after 5 days.

and for 3 weeks after therapy.

PRECAUTIONS

1. Bone marrow depression, if not checked by discontinuation of therapy, can lead to death. Fall in white cell count may occur from 2–3 weeks after therapy has been discontinued. Therapy should be stopped when white cell count is less than 3000/cu.mm. or when the platelet count falls below 150,000/cu.mm.
2. This drug should not be administered after a course of x-ray therapy or after therapy with other radiomimetic drugs until the full effects (leukocyte count) of such treatments have been observed and the leukocyte count has returned to normal.
3. In the presence of infection, use with caution and with antimicrobial agents.
4. Prophylactic antibiotics may be used if WBC falls below 3000/cu.mm.
5. Avoid concomitant use with other bone marrow depressing drugs.
6. There is no known antidote to overdosage.

ADVERSE REACTIONS

1. Pain and thrombophlebitis at injection site
2. Nausea, vomiting, anorexia, stomatitis
3. Tightness in throat
4. Dizziness
5. Headache
6. Amenorrhea
7. Allergic reactions: rash, urticaria, anaphylaxis
8. Depression of spermatogenesis and ovarian function
9. Hyperuricemia with uric acid nephropathy
10. Fever
11. Blood dyscrasias: thrombocytopenia (may result in hemorrhage), leukopenia (may result in infection)

NURSING IMPLICATIONS

1. The patient receiving this medication will be experiencing the emotional and physical effects of the malignancy. Knowledge of the patient's feelings about his disease and its implications will assist in helping him to tolerate the chemotherapy. The incidence of uncomfortable side effects and adverse reactions is high. It is within the nurse's role to assist the patient in coping with the discomforts of the disease and its treatment, and to help him work through depression and anger toward acceptance of the disease at his own pace. Despite the unpleasantness this drug may bring, it can be a source of hope for the patient.
2. Many patients experience fewer injection side effects when they are placed in a reclining position during the administration of this drug.
3. *Management of nausea and vomiting*
   a. Usually occurs 1–3 hours after injection. Vomiting may subside after 8 hours, but nausea can persist for 24 hours.
   b. Administer this drug at night if possible to correlate with normal sleep pattern, accompanied by sedation and an antiemetic drug to combat these side effects.

THIOPHOSPHORAMIDE (Thiotepa) (Continued)

NURSING IMPLICATIONS (No. 3 continued)

c. To be effective, antiemetics should be administered 1 hour prior to the injection of the drug.

d. Small frequent meals, timed with periods when the patient feels his best, are advisable. Bland foods are usually better tolerated. Carbohydrate and protein content should be high.

e. If the patient is anorexic, encourage high nutrient liquids and water to maintain hydration. Hydration will help prevent uric acid nephropathy.

f. Keep accurate measurements of emesis volume and total intake and output to guide the physician in ordering parenteral fluids when necessary.

4. *Management of hematologic effects*

a. Be aware of the patient's white blood cell and platelet counts prior to each injection.

b. If the WBC falls to 2000/cu.mm., take measures to protect the patient from infection such as protective (reverse) isolation, avoidance of traumatic procedures, maintenance of bodily (especially perineal) cleanliness, carrying out strict urinary catheter care when appropriate, etc. Monitor for infection by recording temperatures every 4 hours, examining for rashes, swellings, drainage and pain. Explain these measures to the patient.

c. If the platelet count falls below 100,000/cu.mm., monitor for thrombocytopenic bleeding: petechiae, purpura, hematuria, melena, blood in stools, gum bleeding, vaginal bleeding, epistaxis, hematemesis, etc. Avoid trauma. Transfusions may be ordered.

d. Instruct the patient and family on the importance of follow-up blood studies if the drug is being administered on an outpatient basis.

5. Thrombophlebitis can occur at the injection site. Notify the physician at onset; apply warm compresses as ordered; elevate the extremity. Protect the area from trauma. Avoid extravasation. If it occurs, apply warm compresses until symptoms subside. Monitor for tissue sloughing.

6. *Management of stomatitis*

a. Administer preventive oral care every 4 hours and/or after meals.

b. For preventive care use a very soft toothbrush (child's) and toothpaste; avoid trauma to tissues.

c. Examine oral membranes at least once daily (instruct patient and/or family) to detect the onset of inflammation or ulceration.

d. If stomatitis occurs, notify the physician and begin therapeutic oral care:[1]

(1) *Mild Inflammation:* Remove dentures; use a soft toothbrush and a hydrogen peroxide solution (1 part peroxide and 4 parts saline). Do *not* use toothpaste. Rinse with the peroxide solution and then water. Replace dentures. This procedure should be carried out every 4 hours and/or after meals.

(2) *Severe Inflammation:* Remove dentures; use soft gauze pads rather than a toothbrush. Use the peroxide solution as described above. Rinse with water using an asepto syringe and gentle suction until returns are clear. Do not replace dentures. It may be necessary to give this care every 2–4 hours.

e. Order a bland mechanical soft diet for patients with mild inflammation. If stomatitis is severe, the patient may be placed on NPO status by the physician.

f. For patients who can tolerate oral intake, administer Xylocaine Viscous or acetaminophen elixir as a mouthwash prior to meals to decrease pain (do not use aspirin rinses) as ordered by the physician.

g. Patients with severe stomatitis may require parenteral analgesia.

7. If rashes occur, administer cool compresses as ordered. Turn the patient frequently to prevent skin breakdown.

8. Patients can experience a sensation of tightness in the throat while on this drug. Reassure them as to the origin of this reaction; notify the physician.

REFERENCE

1. Bruya, Margaret Auld, and Madeira, Nancy Powell: Stomatitis After Chemotherapy. *American Journal of Nursing,* 75(8):1351, August 1975.

SUGGESTED READINGS

Bolin, Rose Homan, and Auld, Margaret E.: Hodgkin's Disease. *American Journal of Nursing,* 74:1982–1986, November 1974.

Bruya, Margaret Auld, and Madeira, Nancy Powell: Stomatitis After Chemotherapy. *American Journal of Nursing,* 75(8):1349–1352, August 1975.

Foley, Genevieve, and McCarthy, Ann Marie: The Disease (Hodgkin's) and Its Treatment. *American Journal of Nursing,* 76:1109–1114, July 1976 (references).

Giadquinta, Barbara: Helping Families Face the Crisis of Cancer. *American Journal of Nursing,* 77:1583–1588, October 1977.

Gullo, Shirley: Chemotherapy—What To Do About Special Side Effects. *RN,* 40:30–32, April 1977.

Hannan, Jeanne Ferguson: Talking Is Treatment, Too. *American Journal of Nursing,* 74:1991–1992, November 1974.

Showfety, Mary Patricia: The Ordeal of Hodgkin's Disease. *American Journal of Nursing,* 74:1987–1991, November 1974.

Vietti, Teresa J., and Valeriote, Frederick: Conceptual Basis for The Use of Chemotherapeutic Agents and Their Pharmacology. *Pediatric Clinics of North America,* 23:67–92, February 1976.

TICARCILLIN DISODIUM (Ticar)

ACTIONS/ INDICATIONS	DOSAGE	PREPARATION AND STORAGE	DRUG INCOMPATIBILITIES	MODES OF IV ADMINISTRATION			CONTRAINDICATIONS; WARNINGS; PRECAUTIONS; ADVERSE REACTIONS
				INJECTION	INTERMITTENT INFUSION	CONTINUOUS INFUSION	
Antibiotic, synthetic penicillin. Used for infections due to a	ADULTS: *Bacterial septicemia, pulmonary infections, skin and soft tissue in-*	Reconstitute vials with 4 ml. of sterile water for injection for each *gram* of drug.	Do not mix in solution with any other medication, and do not add to an IV	YES Slowly, over at least 3–5 minutes.	YES Use D5W or NS. Infuse over 30 min to 2 hrs time.	YES Use D5W, NS, Invert sugar 10% in water, Ringer's Injec-	CONTRAINDICATIONS Hypersensitivity to any penicillin. WARNINGS In the presence of impaired renal function and high doses of this drug, patients

may develop hemorrhagic conditions associated with abnormal clotting and prothrombin times. This disappears on withdrawal of the drug.

PRECAUTIONS

1. Because of this drug's high sodium content, 6.5 mEq/Gm, monitor cardiac status carefully for the onset of decompensation in susceptible patients.
2. Hypokalemia may occur.
3. Monitor renal hepatic and hematopoietic function blood studies during therapy, as with any antibiotic.
4. Overgrowth of nonsusceptible organisms can occur.
5. This drug has not been shown to produce fetal abnormalities in laboratory animals, but should be used in pregnant women only when clearly indicated.
6. Gentamicin or tobramycin are usually administered with this drug until specific sensitivity tests are available.

ADVERSE REACTIONS

1. Hypersensitivity: skin rashes, pruritis, urticaria, anaphylaxis, drug fever
2. Gastrointestinal: nausea, vomiting
3. Blood dyscrasias: anemia, thrombocytopenia, leukopenia: inhibition of platelet aggregation
4. Hepatic: elevated SGOT, SGPT
5. Central nervous system: convulsions, neuromuscular irritability (especially in patients with impaired renal function)
6. Phlebitis at injection site
7. Hypokalemia

tion, RL, or similar fluids.

This drug is stable in these fluids for at least 48 hrs.

---

variety of gram-positive or gram-negative organisms, including *Pseudomonas aeruginosa* and Proteus.

Use with an aminoglycoside antibiotic (gentamicin) for *Pseudomonas* infections.

fections—200 –300 mg/kg/ day by intermittent infusions, every 3, 4 or 6 hrs divided doses.

Urinary tract infections—150–200 mg/ kg/day by push injections or intermittent infusions every 3, 4, or 6 hrs divided doses. (See Table below.)

CHILDREN: Under 40 kg of body weight, do not exceed adult dose.

Range—50– 300 mg/kg/ day divided into 4–6 equal doses.

NEONATES (less than 1 week of age): *Infants under 2000 gm*— 100 mg/kg initial dose, followed by 75 mg/kg every 8 hours.

Infants over 2000 gm— 100 mg/kg initial dose, followed by 75 mg/kg every 4–6 hours.

INFANTS OVER 1 WEEK OF AGE: 100 mg/kg every 4 hours. Reduce dosage in renal insuffi-

line containing gentamicin or other aminoglycosides.

Reconstitute 3- and 6-gm piggyback bottles with 30 and 60 ml of sterile water for injection, respectively.

Dilution for infusion:

3-GRAM BOTTLES

Amount of Diluent	Concentration of Solution
100 ml	1 gm/34 ml
60 ml	1 gm/20 ml
30 ml	1 gm/10 ml

6-GRAM BOTTLES

Amount of Diluent	Concentration of Solution
100 ml	1 gm/17 ml
60 ml	1 gm/10 ml

Do not store reconstituted solutions; discard unused portions.

● TICARCILLIN DISODIUM (Ticar) (Continued)

ACTIONS/ INDICATIONS	DOSAGE	PREPARATION AND STORAGE	DRUG INCOMPAT- IBILITIES	MODES OF IV ADMINISTRATION			CONTRAINDICATIONS; WARNINGS; PRECAUTIONS; ADVERSE REACTIONS
				INJECTION	INTERMITTENT INFUSION	CONTINUOUS INFUSION	
	ciency. No data available for exact dos- age.						

*ADULTS WITH RENAL IMPAIRMENT**

Initial loading dose of 3 gm, followed by:

Creatinine clearance ml/min	Dosage and frequency
>60	3 gm every 4 hours
30–60	2 gm every 4 hours
10–30	2 gm every 8 hours
<10	2 gm every 12 hours
<10 with hepatic dysfunction	2 gm every 24 hours
With peritoneal dialysis	3 gm every 12 hours
With hemodialysis	3 gm after each dialysis

*Manufacturer's dosage suggestion.

NURSING IMPLICATIONS

1. Take anaphylaxis precautions; page 118.
2. Patients with impaired renal function require a reduction in dosage based on creatinine clearance; see Dosage column. Be aware of the patient's BUN and creatinine clearance during therapy. Monitor for signs of bleeding that can be produced by alteration in clotting and prothrombin times in these patients:
   a. Melena, or red blood in stools (guaiac tests can be done periodically to detect occult blood)
   b. Hematuria
   c. Ecchymosis, especially on trunk, inner thighs and inner arms
   d. Nose bleeding
   e. Gum bleeding
   f. Vaginal bleeding
   g. Petechiae
   h. Fall in blood pressure
   i. Hematemesis
   Bleeding could also occur secondary to a reduction in platelet count. Such bleeding usually begins only after the count falls below 100,000/cu.mm. If this occurs, monitor for the signs of bleeding listed above and avoid trau- matic procedures.
3. In patients with pre-existing congestive heart failure, infants and children with cardiac lesions, the elderly, or critically ill, monitor for signs of cardiac decompensation secondary to sodium content of the drug, if dosage is high. Signs and symptoms:
   a. Increasing weight (weigh daily, compare to baseline weight)
   b. Increasing heart rate (take every 4–6 hours or as patient's condition dictates)
   c. Increasing respiratory rate (take with heart rate), dyspnea, orthopnea,

rales
   d. Peripheral edema
   e. Increasing jugular venous distention
   f. Onset of third or fourth heart sounds.
4. Monitor for signs of hypokalemia: weakness, lethargy, irritability, abdominal distention, poor feeding in infants, muscle cramps.
5. Monitor for signs and symptoms of nonsusceptible organism overgrowth in- fection:
   a. Fever (take rectal temperature at least every 4–6 hours)
   b. Increasing malaise
   c. Localized signs and symptoms of a new infection: redness, soreness, pain, swelling, drainage (change in volume or character of pre-existing drainage)
   d. Cough (change in sputum volume or character)
   e. Diarrhea
   f. Perineal or oral rash (*Candida albicans* colonization)
6. In patients with impaired renal function, monitor for signs of neuromuscular irritability, e.g., tremors, spasticity, difficulty moving, convulsions. Report any suspicious sign to the physician.
7. Monitor for signs and symptoms of thrombophlebitis at the injection site, e.g., redness, swelling and pain along the vein tract. If this occurs, discon- tinue the infusion and use another vein. Apply warm compresses to the af- fected area and keep the limb elevated until symptoms subside. Avoid oth- er venipunctures in this extremity until the inflammation resolves.
8. If nausea and vomiting occur and are pronounced, the drug will probably be discontinued. Antiemetic agents can be ordered to control these symp- toms. Monitor intake and output to assist the physician in planning for par- enteral replacement if it is needed to maintain hydration.

● TOBRAMYCIN SULFATE (Nebcin)

ACTIONS/ INDICATIONS	DOSAGE	PREPARATION AND STORAGE	DRUG INCOMPATIBILITIES	MODES OF IV ADMINISTRATION			CONTRAINDICATIONS; WARNINGS; PRECAUTIONS; ADVERSE REACTIONS
				INJECTION	INTERMITTENT INFUSION	CONTINUOUS INFUSION	
				NO	YES	NO	
Aminoglycoside antibiotic, active against: • *Pseudomonas aeruginosa* • *Proteus* • *E. coli* • *Klebsiella-Enterobacter-Serratia* group • *Citrobacter* • *Providencia* • *Staphylococci* • Group D streptococci Used to treat serious infections due to these organisms, of all body systems.	*Normal Renal Function:* ADULTS, CHILDREN AND OLDER INFANTS: *Serious infections*—1 mg/ kg every 8 hours. (3 mg/ kg/24 hrs) *Life-threatening infections* —1.66/kg every 8 hours. Reduce to 1 mg/kg every 8 hrs as soon as possible. NEONATES (ONE WEEK OF AGE OR LESS): Up to 4 mg/ kg/day divided into 2 doses every 12 hrs. Duration 7–10 days. A longer course of treatment may be necessary in severe infections. *Impaired Renal Function:* Follow serum concentration if possible. *Loading dose* — 1 mg/kg. Subsequent doses based on serum levels. Reduce amount of doses or the frequency of administration.	Use D5W, N5, D5/NS, D10W, Normosal-R, RL, Ringer's injection, Sodium Lactate 1/6 M. for infusion. Supplied in 2 ml vials of 10 mg/ml, and disposable prefilled syringes.	Do not mix with any other medication in solution. Do not add to IV tubing containing: Heparin Carbenicillin Penicillin Cephalosporins Calcium Magnesium	NO	Add dose to 50–100 ml of diluent; infuse over 30–60 minutes. *Children*—add dose to 25–50 ml of diluent and infuse over 20–60 min. Do not infuse in less than 20 min.	NO	CONTRAINDICATIONS Hypersensitivity WARNINGS 1. This drug can cause hearing and equilibrium disturbances due to eighth cranial nerve damage. This is more likely to occur in patients with pre-existing impaired renal function or when the drug is given for long periods of time (over 2 weeks) or at higher than recommended doses. The ototoxic effects of this drug are increased by concomitant use of ethacrynic acid, furosemide, and mannitol.[1] 2. Renal damage can also result from administration of tobramycin, and is indicated by casts in the urine, proteinuria, oliguria, rising BUN and creatinine. Renal function should be monitored closely during therapy and the drug discontinued when the above signs of renal damage appear. The possibility of renal damage may be increased by the presence of dehydration, the use of potent diuretics, and certain other antibiotics such as polymyxins, amphotericin B, and vancomycin.[2] 3. Patients with impairment in renal function require a modified dosage schedule because of compromised excretion of the drug (see Dosage column). 4. This drug should be used with caution in premature and full-term neonates (up to 1 week of age) because of the immaturity of their renal function. Follow recommended dosage schedules. 5. Peritoneal and hemodialysis can remove this drug from the serum in the event of overdosage. 6. Avoid serum concentrations greater than 12 mcg/ml. 7. Concurrent or sequential use of other nephrotoxic or ototoxic drugs should be avoided: e.g., streptomycin, neomycin, kanamycin, gentamicin, cephaloridine, paromomycin, viomycin, polymyxin B, colistin, and vancomycin.

● TOBRAMYCIN SULFATE (Nebcin) (Continued)

ACTIONS/ INDICATIONS	PREPARATION AND STORAGE	DOSAGE	DRUG INCOMPAT- IBILITIES	MODES OF IV ADMINISTRATION			CONTRAINDICATIONS; WARNINGS: PRECAUTIONS; ADVERSE REACTIONS
				INJECTION	INTERMITTENT INFUSION	CONTINUOUS INFUSION	
		(Specific dosages related to creatinine clearance are provided by the manufacturer.)					8. Safety for use in pregnancy has not been established. 9. Some groups advocate strict adherence to suggested infusion rate to prevent renal and eighth cranial nerve toxic effects.[3] PRECAUTIONS 1. Neuromuscular blockade and respiratory paralysis may occur, especially in patients with myasthenia gravis, in the presence of severe hypocalcemia, or when neuromuscular blocking agents have been given. This may be reversed by the administration of calcium salts. 2. Cross-allergenicity may occur with other aminoglycoside antibiotics including streptomycin, neomycin, paromomycin, kanamycin, gentamicin, amikacin. 3. Overgrowth of nonsusceptible organisms may occur. ADVERSE REACTIONS 1. Renal damage (see Warning No. 2 above) 2. Neurotoxicity causing eighth cranial nerve damage (see Warning No. 1); symptoms include dizziness, vertigo, tinnitus, roaring in the ears, and hearing loss 3. Increased serum SGOT, SGPT, bilirubin 4. Granulocytopenia, thrombocytopenia 5. Fever 6. Allergic reactions: rash, urticaria, anaphylaxis (1–3%) 7. Gastrointestinal disturbances: nausea, vomiting; these may be secondary to vestibular damage (inner ear) 8. Headache 9. Lethargy

NURSING IMPLICATIONS

1. Monitor for the onset of eighth cranial nerve damage, especially in patients with renal impairment. Signs and symptoms: dizziness, disequilibrium, nystagmus (involuntary movement of the eyes), nausea, and vomiting, tinnitus (ringing in the ears), roaring sound in the ears, hearing loss.

Notify the physician at the onset of any one of these signs and symptoms. Give reassurance to the patient and take precautions to prevent patient injury.

(adults: less than 8–10/minute; children: see chart on page 545), and shallow respirations (muscular weakness inhibits movements of chest muscles and diaphragm).

Notify the physician at the onset of any one of these signs or symptoms, place the patient on bed rest, observe closely and administer respiratory support as indicated (do not leave the patient alone if respirations are less than 8/minute).

5. Monitor for nonsusceptible organism overgrowth infection:

page 546

2. Keep the patient appropriately hydrated to assist in preventing renal toxicity.
3. Monitor for the onset of renal damage, especially in patients who are critically ill and on high doses:
   a. Intake and output recordings at least every 4–8 hours, depending on the patient's condition. Fall in urine output may or may not occur with the onset of renal damage. Notify physician if the average urine output falls below 30 ml/hour for more than 2 consecutive hours (see chart on page 546 for children).
   b. Urinalysis should be done daily to detect the presence of protein and casts in the urine.
   c. Be aware of the patient's serum BUN (normal values: 10–20 mg/100 ml) and serum creatinine (0.7–1.5 mg/100 ml). Renal damage is usually reversible if the drug is discontinued at the first sign of impairment.
4. Monitor for the onset of neuromuscular blockade, especially in patients with myasthenia gravis, hypercalcemia, or in patients who have received a neuromuscular blocking agent (tubocurarine, pancuronium, etc.). Signs and symptoms:
   a. Generalized muscle weakness
   b. Difficulty controlling movements
   c. Respiratory depression as evidenced by a decreased respiratory rate

a. Fever (take rectal temperature at least every 4–6 hours)
b. Increasing malaise
c. Newly appearing localized signs and symptoms of infection: redness, soreness, pain, swelling, drainage (increasing volume, or change in character of pre-existing drainage)
d. Monilial rash (redness and itching) in the perineal area and/or candidal lesions in the mouth (reddened areas with overlying white patches especially on inner cheeks)
e. Cough (change in pre-existing cough and sputum production)
f. Diarrhea
6. Take anaphylaxis precautions, see p. 118.

REFERENCES
1. Barza, Michael, and Scheife, Richard: Drug Therapy Reviews: Antimicrobial Spectrum, Pharmacology and Therapeutic Use of Antibiotics. Part 4: Aminoglycosides. American Journal of Hospital Pharmacy, 34:730, July 1977.
2. Ibid., p. 729.
3. Vanderveen, Timothy W.: Aminoglycoside Antibiotics. American Journal of Intravenous Therapy, July 1977, p. 6.

TOLAZOLINE HYDROCHLORIDE (Priscoline Hydrochloride)

ACTIONS/ INDICATIONS	DOSAGE	PREPARATION AND STORAGE	DRUG INCOMPATIBILITIES	MODES OF IV ADMINISTRATION			CONTRAINDICATIONS; WARNINGS; PRECAUTIONS; ADVERSE REACTIONS
				INJECTION	INTERMITTENT INFUSION	CONTINUOUS INFUSION	
Alpha adrenergic blocking agent, dilates peripheral blood vessels and increases blood flow. Interferes with the vasoconstricting actions of epinephrine and levarterenol. Is classified by FDA as "possibly" effective against spastic peripheral vascular disorders associated with acrocyanosis, acroparesthesia, arteriosclerosis obliterans, Buerger's dis-	ADULTS: Intravenous: individualize according to condition and response seen. Up to 10–50 mg., 4 times a day. Start with low doses and increase until flushing is seen. Keep patient warm. Intra-arterial: only if maximal benefit has been seen in IV route. Give 25 mg as a test dose, then 50–75 mg depending on response.	Supplied in 10-ml multiple-dose vials. Solution concentration is 25 mg/ml.	Do not mix with any other medication in any manner.	YES Slowly undiluted.	NO	NO	CONTRAINDICATIONS 1. Following cerebrovascular accident 2. In known or suspected coronary artery disease 3. Hypersensitivity WARNINGS 1. Stimulates gastric secretion and may activate peptic ulcers. 2. Use with caution in the presence of gastritis. 3. Use with caution in the presence of mitral stenosis (may produce a fall or rise in pulmonary artery pressure). PRECAUTIONS Intra-arterial injections must be done with extreme caution and while the patient is hospitalized. ADVERSE REACTIONS 1. Cardiac arrhythmias 2. Anginal pain 3. Marked hypertension 4. Exacerbation of peptic ulcer 5. Nausea, vomiting, diarrhea

● **TOLAZOLINE HYDROCHLORIDE** (Priscoline Hydrochloride) (*Continued*)

ACTIONS/ INDICATIONS	DOSAGE	PREPARATION AND STORAGE	DRUG INCOMPAT- IBILITIES	MODES OF IV ADMINISTRATION			CONTRAINDICATIONS; WARNINGS; PRECAUTIONS; ADVERSE REACTIONS
				INJECTION	INTERMITTENT INFUSION	CONTINUOUS INFUSION	

ease, diabetic arteriosclerosis, gangrene, endarteritis, frostbite, postthrombotic conditions, Raynaud's disease, and scleroderma.	One to 2 injections daily are usually needed; 2–3/week after response has been obtained; oral form may be used for maintenance. CHILDREN: Not recommended.						6. Flushing (generalized) or chilling 7. With intra-arterial injection, a burning sensation in the affected extremity, transient weakness, postural vertigo, palpitations, apprehension 8. Rarely, a further decrease in already impaired blood supply may occur in a seriously damaged limb with incipient or established gangrene. This may be decreased with a preliminary injection of histamine
							
							MANAGEMENT OF OVERDOSAGE
							1. Manifestations:
							  a. Peripheral vasodilatation, skin flushing
							  b. Hypotension and shock.
							2. Management:
							  a. Place patient in a Trendelenburg position if hypotension produces symptoms such as diaphoresis, dizziness, stupor.
							  b. Administer intravenous fluids.
							  c. If a vasopressor is needed, one having central and peripheral actions such as ephedrine can be used (see page 314 for details on ephedrine). Do *not* use epinephrine or levarterenol since large doses of tolazoline may cause epinephrine reversal, i.e., further reduction in blood pressure followed by an exaggerated rebound.
							  d. Patient should be kept under close observation with frequent monitoring of vital signs until all signs of overdosage have disappeared and vital signs have returned to normal and stabilized.

NURSING IMPLICATIONS
1. Monitor for signs and symptoms of peptic ulcer or worsening gastritis:
   a. Epigastric pain
   b. Flatulance
   c. Melena
   d. Positive guaiac stools
   Antacids may be prophylactically prescribed.
2. Monitor blood pressure and heart rate continuously during injection in patients with mitral stenosis. Notify physician of significant fall or rise in either parameter.
3. Patients with pre-existing cardiac arrhythmias should be monitored electrocardiographically continuously during, and for 4 hours after, each injection.
4. Instruct patients to report chest pain. Notify physician if it occurs. Monitor blood pressure and pulse for abnormalities. Observe until stabilized.
5. Be prepared to manage vomiting to prevent aspiration. If the patient is lethargic or semicomatose, or generally unable to manage secretions, keep suction equipment at the bedside; place patient in a lateral position if possible.
6. Administer supportive care for affected limb to prevent injury:
   a. Monitor circulatory status of the limb, e.g., skin color, temperature, presence or absence of pain.
   b. Monitor neuromuscular status, e.g., ability to move the limb, sensory status and reflexes.
   c. Prevent skin breakdown or other trauma.
   The patient's condition should dictate the frequency of monitoring.
7. Keep the patient warm to increase the effectiveness of the drug.

TRIFLUPROMAZINE HYDROCHLORIDE (Vesprin)

ACTIONS/ INDICATIONS	DOSAGE	PREPARATION AND STORAGE	DRUG INCOMPAT- IBILITIES	MODES OF IV ADMINISTRATION				CONTRAINDICATIONS; WARNINGS; PRECAUTIONS; ADVERSE REACTIONS
				INJECTION	INTERMITTENT INFUSION	CONTINUOUS INFUSION		

Tranquilizer, antiemetic, phenothiazine derivative.
 	
Used in the management of psychotic disorders (except depression) and to control nausea and vomiting.
	ADULTS: 1 mg every 4– 6 hours. Maxi- mum daily dose is 3 mg.
	
	Obstetrics— 8 mg during labor (maxi- mum total dose).
	
	(Maintenance therapy for psychoses is usually given in larger, oral doses.)
	
	CHILDREN: IV route not recommended.
		Color may vary from colorless to light amber. Do not use so- lutions that are darker than light amber or are discolored in any other way.
		
		Supplied in the following forms:
		Multiple-dose vials (20 mg/ ml)
		Multiple-dose vials (10 mg/ ml)
		Prefilled syrin- ges (10 mg/ ml)
			Do not mix with any other medication in any manner.	YES
				
				Slowly, undiluted.
					NO
					
					Do not add to fluids.
						NO
						
						Do not add to fluids.
								CONTRAINDICATIONS
								1. Suspected or established subcortical brain damage; hyperthermia reactions may be induced in such patients
								2. In the presence of large doses of hypnotics
								3. Comatose or severely depressed states
								4. Blood dyscrasias
								5. Liver damage
								6. Renal insufficiency
								7. Hypersensitivity to any phenothiazine
								
								WARNINGS
								Safety for use in pregnancy has not been established.
								
								PRECAUTIONS
								1. Use with caution in patients who have had adverse reactions to other pheno- thiazines.
								2. In the presence of this drug, lower doses of anesthetics and analgesics will be needed.
								3. Do not use prior to spinal anesthesia because of the danger of hypoten- sion.
								4. This drug may potentiate opiates, an- algesics, antihistamines, barbiturates and atropine.
								5. Use with caution if there is a history of seizures.
								6. Patients with mitral valvular insuffi- ciency or pheochromocytoma may have severe hypotensive reactions to this drug.
								7. May cause postural hypotension; keep the patient supine during and for 1 hour after an injection (see Nursing Implications).
								
								ADVERSE REACTIONS SEEN IN SHORT- TERM INTRAVENOUS USE
								1. Neurologic:
								  a. Sedation, drowsiness, and deep sleep
								  b. Blurred vision
								  c. Extrapyramidal reactions such as motor restlessness resembling Par- kinson's disease, drooling, tremors, muscle spasms, shuffling gait, dys-

TRIFLUPROMAZINE HYDROCHLORIDE (Vesprin) (Continued)

ACTIONS/ INDICATIONS	DOSAGE	PREPARATION AND STORAGE	DRUG INCOMPAT- IBILITIES	MODES OF IV ADMINISTRATION			CONTRAINDICATIONS; WARNINGS; PRECAUTIONS; ADVERSE REACTIONS
				INJECTION	INTERMITTENT INFUSION	CONTINUOUS INFUSION	

CONTRAINDICATIONS; WARNINGS; PRECAUTIONS; ADVERSE REACTIONS

tonias (involuntary movements), difficulty swallowing
d. Agitation and nervousness
If these occur, dosage must be reduced or the drug discontinued. Symptoms will subside in 24–48 hours.
2. Rashes usually due to hypersensitivity
3. Hypotension (especially immediately after injection); may be postural type
4. Palpitations, especially immediately after an injection
5. Liver damage producing jaundice (cholestatic hepatitis)
6. Anticholinergic reactions, such as dryness of the mouth, tachycardia, blurred vision, increased salivation, nasal congestion.
7. Exacerbation of seizure disorders.

NURSING IMPLICATIONS
1. Monitor for neurologic disturbances following an injection; see Adverse Reaction No. 1. Report any of these reactions to the physician immediately. If the patient experiences difficulty in swallowing, remain with him until the severity of the reaction is determined. The patient may need parenteral hydration and nutrition until swallowing returns.
2. Examine for rashes; report them to the physician.
3. Keep the patient supine during injection.
4. Monitor blood pressure before, during and after injection. If hypotension occurs continue to take the blood pressure until stabilization occurs. Hypotension can usually be avoided with slow injection. If a patient is to be ambulated after an injection, obtain lying and standing blood pressure. If postural hypotension is significant, report the fact to the physician and keep the patient at rest. As postural effects decrease over time, begin to ambulate the patient if desirable; do so with caution to prevent injury. Warn the patient not to stand up suddenly until the effects of the drug have disappeared. Ambulate the patient with caution if he is experiencing sedation or blurred vision. Initiate safety precautions, such as side rails, to prevent injury.
5. Monitor for jaundice; notify the physician.
6. The patient may experience anticholinergic side effects; see Adverse Reaction No. 6. Inform him of the origin of the symptom and its transient nature.
7. Initiate seizure precautions if not already in effect.
8. This drug can cause the urine to darken or turn orange for 24 hours after administration. Inform the patient of the harmlessness of this effect.

TRIMETHAPHAN CAMSYLATE (Arfonad)

ACTIONS/ INDICATIONS	DOSAGE	PREPARATION AND STORAGE	DRUG INCOMPAT- IBILITIES	MODES OF IV ADMINISTRATION			CONTRAINDICATIONS; WARNINGS; PRECAUTIONS; ADVERSE REACTIONS
				INJECTION	INTERMITTENT INFUSION	CONTINUOUS INFUSION	
Antihypertensive, ganglionic blocking agent, may also have a di-	Titrate with blood pressure response. Initial infusion rate can be 3–	Supplied in ampuls of 50 mg/ ml. Store in refrigerator. Use IV solutions	Do not mix with other medications in IV bottle; drug should	NO	NO	YES
Use a solution of 1 mg/ml (1 gm in 1000 ml	CONTRAINDICATIONS
1. When hypotension may produce a risk, e.g., in severe anemia, hypovolemic shock, asphyxia, uncorrected respiratory insufficiency.

rect peripheral vasodilator effect to lower blood pressure. Used to treat hypertensive crisis. May also be used to control hypertension during surgery and in cases of dissecting aneurysm.

Onset of action is within 1–2 minutes after injection. Maximum effect is seen after 2–5 minutes, and the duration is 10 minutes.

4 mg/min. The range is as low as 0.3 mg/min to 6.0 mg/min.

Dosage recommendations for children are not available.

be titrated alone. Do not add to IV tubing containing:
Aminophylline
Sodium iodide
Sodium bicarbonate

promptly; discard unused portions.

Use infusion pump.

Each infusion should be used for a maximum of 6 hours. Mix a fresh solution after that.

2. When fluids and blood are not available to replace blood volume as needed.

D5W or NS). Titrate with blood pressure response. Use an infusion pump and microdrop tubing.

WARNINGS
1. Use only as infusion.
2. Adequate direct (preferable) or indirect blood-pressure monitoring must be available.
3. Maintain arterial oxygenation.
4. Use with extreme caution in patients with arteriosclerosis, cardiac disease, hepatic, or central nervous system disease, Addison's disease, diabetes mellitus, steroid therapy.
5. Induced hypotension may have adverse effects on the fetus.

PRECAUTIONS
1. Use with caution in patients who have been receiving other antihypertensive agents; in combination with anesthetic agents; during spinal anesthesia; in the elderly or debilitated.
2. This drug liberates histamine; use with caution in patients with any form of allergy, can produce bronchospasm.
3. Diuretics can potentiate this drug.
4. Causes pupil dilation.
5. This drug can decrease renal blood flow and glomerular filtration rate.[1] Use with caution in the presence of renal impairment of any degree.
6. May produce bowel and/or bladder atony, and a meconium ileus in the newborn of a mother who has received this drug during labor.[2]

6. Monitor for the consequences of severe elevation of blood pressure:
a. Encephalopathy: confusion, stupor, nausea, vomiting, visual changes, reflex asymmetries
b. Cerebrovascular accident: muscle weakness, change in mental status
c. Myocardial ischemia and/or infarction: chest pain, ECG changes, arrhythmias
d. Left ventricular failure: shortness of breath, orthopnea, elevated central venous pressure or pulmonary artery (wedge) pressure, tachycardia, rales, third and/or fourth heart sound
e. Renal failure: oliguria, rising BUN and creatinine[3]
Note that a sudden fall in blood pressure below normal levels for the patient can also produce these complications. Be prepared to manage hypotension due to an exaggerated response to the drug. Phenylephrine or metaphentermine can be used. Dopamine should be used if these milder vasopressor agents are ineffective.
7. Monitor for respiratory difficulties produced by bronchospasm, such as tachypnea and wheezing. Notify the physician of this reaction. Keep aminophylline and epinephrine readily available.
8. Monitor for paralytic ileus and urinary retention. Examine for meconium ile-

NURSING IMPLICATIONS
1. Be prepared to accurately monitor arterial blood pressure, preferably by direct arterial cannulation. If this type of monitoring is unavailable, indirect readings using a sphygmomanometer can be used.
2. Patients with a history of cardiac disease including arrhythmias must be monitored electrocardiographically during an infusion of this drug.
3. Keep the patient on bed rest in a supine position during therapy.
4. Be prepared to manage vomiting to prevent aspiration.
5. Keeping in mind the patient's pretreatment blood pressure (indirect and direct), start the infusion at 3–4 mg/minute (using the solution recommended in the Continuous Infusion column, 1 mg/ml, the drip rate or pump rate would be 3–4 ml/minute). Smaller initial doses may be ordered by the physician for patients with renal failure. Observe arterial pressure recordings continuously (indirect readings every 2 minutes). Do not allow the blood pressure to fall too rapidly. The physician should set the blood pressure goal to be reached, and a time limit for when the goal should be reached. If the pressure does not begin to decrease with the initial infusion rate (3–4 mg/minute) within 10 minutes, begin increasing the rate by 0.5 mg (0.5 ml) every 10 minutes until a response is seen.

TRIMETHAPHAN CAMSYLATE (Arfonad) (Continued)

NURSING IMPLICATIONS (No. 8 continued)
9. If the patient will be receiving oral antihypertensive agents on a chronic basis, instruct him on hypertensive self-care.

REFERENCES
1. American Medical Association Committee on Hypertension: The Treatment of Malignant Hypertension and Hypertensive Emergencies. *JAMA,* 228 (13):1675, June 24, 1974.
2. Ibid., p. 1675.
3. Romankiewicz, J. A.: Pharmacology and Clinical Use of Drugs in Hypertensive Emergencies. *American Journal of Hospital Pharmacy,* 34(2):185, February 1977.

SUGGESTED READINGS
American Medical Association Committee on Hypertension: The Treatment of Malignant Hypertension and Hypertensive Emergencies. *JAMA,* 228:1673–1679, June 24, 1974.
Dhar, Sisir K. and Freedman, Philip: Clinical Management of Hypertensive Emergencies. *Heart and Lung,* 5:571–575, January–April, 1976.
Keith, Thomas: Hypertensive Crisis. Recognition and Management, *JAMA,* 237(15):1570–1577, April 11, 1977.
Koch-Weser, Jan: Hypertensive Emergencies. *New England Journal of Medicine,* 290:211–214, January 24, 1974.
Long, M. L. et al.: Hypertension: What Patients Need to Know. *American Journal of Nursing,* 76:765–770, May 1976.
Romankiewicz, J. A.: Pharmacology and Clinical Use of Drugs in Hypertensive Emergencies. *American Journal of Hospital Pharmacy,* 34(2):185–193, February 1977 (references).

TUBOCURARINE CHLORIDE (Curare, d-Tubocurarine)

ACTIONS/ INDICATIONS	DOSAGE	PREPARATION AND STORAGE	DRUG INCOMPATIBILITIES	MODES OF IV ADMINISTRATION			CONTRAINDICATIONS; WARNINGS; PRECAUTIONS; ADVERSE REACTIONS
				INJECTION	INTERMITTENT INFUSION	CONTINUOUS INFUSION	
Neuromuscular blocking agent, nondepolarizing type. Produces flaccid paralysis of skeletal muscles within 2–3 minutes of injection. Effects last 25–90 minutes. There may be prolongation of effects after large or repeated doses.

Used to induce muscle relaxation for tracheal intubation, surgery, electroconvulsive therapy, and mechanical ventilation. Also used to diagnose myasthenia gravis | ADULTS AND CHILDREN: *Anesthesia*— 0.1–0.3 mg/ kg; do not exceed 27 mg. Subsequent doses should be based on patient response; may be ¼–½ of the initial dose every 45–60 minutes. (A test dose 2–3 mg less than the calculated dose may be given to detect hyperactivity.)

Electroconvulsive therapy— 0.1–0.3 mg/ kg with an initial dose 2–3 mg less, then titrate as needed. | Supplied in 3 mg/ml, 5 mg/ ml, and 15 mg/ ml concentrations.

Do not use if more than faintly discolored. | Do not mix with any other drug in syringe; do not inject into IV tubing containing sodium bicarbonate, methohexital, trimethaphan camsylate. | YES

Inject over a 1- to 1½-minute period.

3 mg/ml and 5 mg/ml preparations can be injected undiluted. If 15 mg/ml solution is used, dilute to a concentration of 3 or 5 mg/ml with NS. | YES

But, direct IV injection preferred method because of drug's long duration of action. | YES

But, direct IV injection preferred method because of drug's long duration of action. | CONTRAINDICATIONS
1. Hypersensitivity
2. When histamine release is a hazard

WARNINGS
1. Respiratory support must be immediately available, e.g., positive pressure ventilation, intubation, oxygen.
2. Use with extreme caution in patients with documented myasthenia gravis.
3. Administration of quinidine during postoperative recovery after tubocurarine has been used may result in recurarizing and respiratory paralysis.

PRECAUTIONS
1. The skeletal muscle paralyzing effects (secondary to *normal* dosage) can be reversed with cholinesterase inhibitors (neostigmine, pyridostigmine).
2. Use with caution in patients with respiratory depression, renal or hepatic insufficiency. Respiratory and pulmonary patients will require lower and less frequent doses. Patients with hepatic insufficiency sometimes require a larger dosage to produce adequate paralysis.2
3. Hypotension can result following large doses.
4. Repeated doses may have a cumula- |

when other tests have been inconclusive.

Diagnosis of myasthenia gravis—very small doses of this drug cause an exaggerated response in myasthenia patients. Give 1/15–1/5 of above calculated doses, or 4.1–16.5 mcg/kg.

Lower dosage will be required by patients on aminoglycoside antibiotics, or who have renal impairment; titrate with patient response.

When methoxyflurane or fluroxene anesthetics are used, reduce the initial dose by 33%. If halothane or cyclopropane is used, reduce by 20%.[1]

For controlled respiration—16.5 mcg/kg (average dose: 1 mg) initially; titrate with patient response thereafter.

tive effect.
5. The paralyzing effects of this drug are potentiated and depressed by a variety of factors. See Nursing Implication No. 7.
6. Rapid injection or a large dosage can precipitate the release of histamine which can cause bronchospasm and/or hypotension.
7. Safety for use in pregnancy has not been established. This drug has no direct effect on the uterus or other smooth muscles, and is not thought to cross the placental barrier.[3]

ADVERSE REACTIONS
1. Extension of the drug's pharmacologic actions. Profound and prolonged muscle relaxation may occur, with respiratory depression and possible apnea
2. Hypersensitivity (rare)
3. Histamine release producing bronchospasm
4. Hypotension

NURSING IMPLICATIONS
Postanesthesia Care:
1. Equipment that should be readily available: suction, manual breathing bag, endotracheal tubes and laryngoscope, oxygen.
2. Patients receiving this agent must be intubated to assist in maintaining an adequate airway and ventilation.
3. Be aware of the duration of action of this drug (see Actions/Indications column), and when the patient received the last dose.
4. Be aware of the sequence of progression of the paralytic effects as they will occur after an injection:
   a. Loss of eye movement
   b. Eyelid droop
   c. Stiffness of jaw muscles followed by relaxation
   d. Paralysis of upper trunk muscles spreading to the lower trunk muscles and then to the extremities
   e. Paralysis of pharyngeal muscles (tongue, swallowing, etc.)
   f. Total respiratory paralysis
5. Recovery will be a complete reverse of this sequence.[4]
5. Management of the patient postoperatively is centered around the use of the reversal agent (neostigmine or pyridostigmine) and respiratory support until adequate ventilation has returned. See Nursing Implication No. 10.
6. During recovery, observe for return of the paralytic effects and for incom-

517

TUBOCURARINE CHLORIDE (Curare, d-Tubocurarine) (Continued)

NURSING IMPLICATIONS (No. 6 continued)

plete reversal of the effects by the antagonist agent. Keep reversal (antagonist) agents and atropine readily available. See Precaution No. 1.

7. Be aware of elements which may prolong the paralytic effects of this drug:
   a. Decreased circulation time as seen in congestive heart failure or shock
   b. Low arterial blood pH (less than 7.35)[5]
   c. Decreased hepatic function (the drug is excreted in the bile) and severe renal impairment
   d. Concomitant use of aminoglycoside antibiotics (gentamicin, amikacin, etc.), polymyxin B, or bacitracin
   e. The presence of other drugs such as diazepam (Valium), halothane anesthetic, quinidine, MAO inhibitors
   f. Extremes of age
   g. The presence of myasthenia gravis
   Patients under the influence of any one of these conditions will require prolonged monitoring for recovery from the effects of tubocurarine.
8. The hypotension that can be precipitated by tubocurarine can be treated by withholding additional doses of the drug, fluids, and if necessary, vasopressors. Reversal agents (neostigmine and pyridostigmine) will not reverse the effects that cause hypotension. Monitor blood pressure every 3–5 minutes or as operating room policy or patient condition dictates.
9. Bronchospasm may be serious enough to require treatment with aminophylline or other bronchodilating agents. Monitor for wheezing and decreased lung compliance, cyanosis, etc.
10. Discharge from the recovery room will depend on the following criteria:
   a. Grip strength
   b. Ability to lift the head
   c. Ability to open the eyes
   d. Respiratory status, e.g. vital capacity and tidal volume (it is helpful to have preoperative values for comparison).

Maintenance Care for Ventilatory Control:
1. This drug is usually administered on a p.r.n. basis for control of ventilation. The criteria for when to administer it will be determined by the physician. The criteria will include such situations as:
   a. A respiratory rate greater than ___ per minute (rate prescribed by physician)
   b. When the patient's respiratory effort is out of phase with the respirator
   c. When the patient is struggling against the respirator
   d. When positive end-expiratory pressure (P.E.E.P.) is in use

Monitor for the onset of any of the criteria and administer the drug in the amount ordered. (Be aware of hospital regulations governing the administration of a neuromuscular blocking agent, i.e. storage of the drug, and who may administer it.)

2. Make certain that the endotracheal tube is securely and correctly inserted. Check the connection between the tube and the respirator; it must be tight. KEEP RESPIRATOR ALARM SYSTEMS FUNCTIONING AT ALL TIMES. The patient is totally dependent on the respirator for ventilation.
3. This drug paralyzes skeletal muscles, it does not alter consciousness or relieve pain and anxiety. Therefore, the patient must be adequately sedated and given analgesics appropriate for his condition. He will not be able to make his needs known; the persons caring for him must anticipate those needs. Many institutions assign one or more nurses to stay in constant attendance with these patients.
4. Monitor vital signs before administration and every 5 minutes after until stabilization is seen, then every 15–30 minutes. Repeat the cycle with each dose. Tubocurarine can lower blood pressure initially.
   Monitor for signs of bronchospasm, such as wheezing (by auscultation). Bronchodilator drugs such as aminophylline should be readily available. Notify the physician if bronchospasm is suspected.
   This agent can cause an increase in tracheobronchial secretions. More frequent suctioning may be required, guided by auscultation of the chest.
5. Patients with a history of cardiac arrhythmias should be observed for exacerbation of those arrhythmias via a continuous ECG monitor. Be prepared to treat tachy- and bradyarrhythmias.
6. Because this agent produces muscle paralysis, handle the patient with care to prevent trauma to joints and muscles during turning. Turn and/or position frequently to prevent skin breakdown. Use water mattresses, flotation pads etc., as indicated.
7. When this drug is discontinued, a reversal agent (neostigmine) may be used. Proceed with the nursing management as described under Postanesthesia Care.

REFERENCES
1. Formulary 12:20. American Hospital Formulary Service, American Society of Hospital Pharmacists, Washington, D.C., 1977.
2. Ibid.
3. Wylie, W. D., and Churchill-Davidson, H. C. (editors): *A Practice of Anesthesia* (3rd ed.), Chicago: Year Book Medical Publishers, 1972, p. 877.
4. Ibid., p. 816.
5. Ibid. p. 834.

UREA (Ureaphil)

ACTIONS/ INDICATIONS	DOSAGE	PREPARATION AND STORAGE	DRUG INCOMPATIBILITIES	MODES OF IV ADMINISTRATION			CONTRAINDICATIONS; WARNINGS; PRECAUTIONS; ADVERSE REACTIONS
				INJECTION	INTERMITTENT INFUSION	CONTINUOUS INFUSION	
Osmotic dehydrating agent; can reduce intracranial ede-	Using a 30% solution at a rate of up to 60 gtt/min	Prepare a *30% solution* by adding 105-ml diluent to the 40-	Do not mix with: Aminophylline Sodium bicar-	NO	YES A 30% solution, at a rate	YES A 30% solution, at a rate	CONTRAINDICATIONS 1. Severe renal impairment 2. Active intracranial bleeding 3. Marked dehydration

ma and elevated cerebrospinal fluid pressure. Elevation of blood tonicity causes movement of fluid out of tissues into the blood. Also increases excretion of water in the kidneys.

Used to:
• Reduce intracranial pressure, edema
• Reduce intraocular pressure

(macrodrops), total daily dose should not exceed 120 gm. Titrate with patient's response.

Usual Dosage:
ADULTS: 1.0–1.5 gm/kg.

CHILDREN: 0.5–1.5 gm/kg.

INFANTS UP TO 2 YEARS: 0.1 gm/kg.

gm vial of urea. Use D5W, invert sugar in water for dilution. This produces 135 ml of solution (300 mg/ml).

To make 270 ml of a 30% solution, add 210 ml to the 80-gm vial.

Use immediately; discard unused portions.

Warming diluent to 50°C may shorten reconstitution time. Cool to body temperature before use. Do not infuse in the same IV tubing with blood.

bonate
Do not infuse into a line containing blood.

not greater than 60 gtt/min.
Use an infusion pump.

not greater than 60 gtt/min.
Use an infusion pump.

not greater than 60 gtt/min.
Use an infusion pump.

4. Hepatic failure

WARNINGS
1. Do not infuse into veins of the lower extremities of elderly patients; phlebitis may occur.
2. May produce hyponatremia and hypokalemia.
3. Prevent extravasation; can cause necrosis.
4. If there is liver impairment, administer with caution. This drug may cause a rise in serum ammonia levels.
5. In pregnancy, benefits to the mother must be weighed against possible risks to the fetus.

PRECAUTIONS
1. An indwelling urinary catheter should be used in comatose patients or in the presence of any degree of obstructive uropathy to insure bladder drainage and accurate measurement of urine output.
2. Do not exceed maximum rate of 60 gtt/minute to prevent hemolysis and adverse effects on the vasomotor center of the brain.
3. Reduction of brain edema may result in reactivation of bleeding.
4. Administer with caution in the presence of renal disease. Monitor BUN.
5. If diuresis does not occur within 6–12 hours, discontinue this drug and evaluate renal status.
6. Urea may maintain blood pressure and volume after blood loss, but replacement therapy must be carried out with blood and blood products.
7. Hypothermia therapy, when used with urea, may increase the risk of venous thrombosis and hemoglobinuria.

ADVERSE REACTIONS
1. Headache
2. Nausea and vomiting
3. Syncope
4. Disorientation
5. Reactions are rare if solution is infused slowly and renal status is intact
6. Phlebitis at infusion site

NURSING IMPLICATIONS
1. Use an infusion pump and adhere strictly to suggested infusion rates.
2. Monitor for signs of hypokalemia: unusual weakness, irritability, abdominal distention, poor feeding in infants, muscle cramps.[1]
3. Observe for signs of hyponatremia: confusion, weakness, coma, seizures.[2]
4. Prevent extravasation: see page 118. If this occurs, apply warm compresses until symptoms subside. Avoid trauma to the affected area.
5. Monitor for signs of increasing hepatic coma in susceptible patients: increasing mental depression, increasing disorientation, flapping of hands, slurring of speech.[3]
6. Place urinary catheter in appropriate patients and monitor output (in all patients) hourly during the infusion and every 4 hours after for 24 hours.
7. Weigh patient before and after urea therapy.
8. When appropriate, monitor for signs of increased intracranial bleeding and pressure:[4]
   a. Decreasing level of consciousness

● UREA (Ureaphil) (Continued)

NURSING IMPLICATIONS (No. 8 continued)

b. Change in pupil size and equality
c. Increasing systolic blood pressure
d. Decreasing diastolic blood pressure
e. Decreasing heart rate
f. Irregular and decreasing respiratory rate
Notify the physician at the onset of any of these signs.

REFERENCES

1. Beeson, Paul, and McDermott, Walsh (editors): *Cecil-Loeb Textbook of Medicine* (14th ed.). Philadelphia: W. B. Saunders Company, 1975, p. 1587.
2. Ibid., p. 1582.
3. Ibid., p. 1328.
4. Jimm, Louise R.: Nursing Assessment of Patients for Increased Intracranial Pressure. *Journal of Neurological Nursing.* 6:27, July 1974.

SUGGESTED READINGS

Alexander, Mary M., and Brown, Marie Scott: Neurological Examination. *Nursing '76,* 38–43, June 1976.
Jimm, Louise R.: Nursing Assessment of Patients for Increased Intracranial Pressure. *Journal of Neurosurgical Nursing.* 6:27–38 July 1974.
Mitchell, Pamela, and Mauss, Nancy: Intracranial Pressure: Fact and Fancy. *Nursing '76,* 53–57, June 1976.

● UROKINASE FOR INJECTION (Abbokinase)

ACTIONS/INDICATIONS	DOSAGE	PREPARATION AND STORAGE	DRUG INCOMPATIBILITIES	MODES OF IV ADMINISTRATION			CONTRAINDICATIONS; WARNINGS; PRECAUTIONS; ADVERSE REACTIONS
				INJECTION	INTERMITTENT INFUSION	CONTINUOUS INFUSION	
An enzyme, potent direct activator of the fibrinolytic system. Converts plasminogen to the proteolytic enzyme plasmin. Plasmin degrades fibrin clots from inside and outside the clot. Drug action begins immediately with injection and may last for up to 12 hours after discontinuation. Indicated in the treatment of: • Acute massive pulmonary emboli (obstruction or significant filling	ADULTS: *Loading dose* —4400 IU*/kg infused over 10 minutes, followed by a 12-hour dose of 4400 IU/kg/hr. given as continuous infusion. The volume of infusion fluid should not exceed 200 ml. *Check thrombin time prior to administration. The value should be less than two times the control. See Warning No. 3.* *International Units	To prepare from powder, add 5.2 ml of sterile water for injection. Prepare just prior to use. Discard unused portion. Use NS for infusion. See table below for infusion and dosage preparation.	Do not mix with any other medication in any manner.	NO	NO	YES Use an infusion pump.	CONTRAINDICATIONS This drug, through its effects on the blood coagulation system, increases the risk of bleeding and is contraindicated in: 1. Surgery within the past 10 days, including liver or kidney biopsy, lumbar puncture, thoracentesis or paracentesis, extensive or multiple cutdowns 2. An intra-arterial diagnostic procedure within 10 days 3. Ulcerative wounds 4. Recent trauma with the possibility of internal injuries 5. Visceral or intracranial malignancy 6. Pregnancy, and the first 10 days of the postpartum period 7. Ulcerative colitis, diverticulitis or an actively bleeding lesion or one with a significant potential for bleeding, of the gastrointestinal or genitourinary tract 8. Severe hypertension 9. Acute or chronic hepatic or renal insufficiency 10. Uncontrolled hypocoagulable state, including one that may be caused by a coagulation factor deficiency, thrombocytopenia, spontaneous fibrinolysis, or other purpuric or hemorrhagic disorder 11. Chronic lung disease with cavitation,

defects involving two or more lobar pulmonary arteries or an equivalent amount of emboli in other vessels)

• Pulmonary emboli accompanied by unstable hemodynamics (failure to maintain blood pressure without supportive measures)

In these two clinical situations, urokinase is used for the lysis of these clots.

Diagnoses must be confirmed by objective means, e.g., pulmonary angiogram.

Treatment should be initiated as soon as possible after onset of symptoms and no later than 5 days after onset.

e.g., tuberculosis

12. Subacute bacterial endocarditis or rheumatic valvular disease
13. Recent cerebral embolism, thrombosis or hemorrhage. Treatment with urokinase is contraindicated for 2 months after such events because of the risk of bleeding in the infarcted brain tissue.
14. Any other condition in which bleeding might constitute a significant hazard or be particularly difficult to manage because of its location.

These are not absolute contraindications, but situations in which the risk of hemorrhage must be weighed carefully against the anticipated benefits of using the drug. The risks and benefits of using urokinase must be weighed against those associated with other forms of therapy.

WARNINGS
1. Bleeding
   a. This agent causes a more profound alteration of the hemostatic status than does heparin or coumarin drugs. In its action of stimulating the production of plasmin for lysis of intravascular fibrin deposits, such deposits that provide control of bleeding at needle puncture sites and other trauma will also be subject to lysis, and bleeding may occur. There is a great possibility of bruising or hematoma formation, especially with intramuscular injections. Intramuscular injections must be avoided during urokinase therapy, as should arterial punctures and venipunctures. If an arterial puncture is absolutely necessary, the femoral artery must be avoided in preference to the radial or brachial. Following the procedure, pressure must be applied to the site for at least *15 minutes*, a pressure dressing applied, and the site checked frequently for bleeding.
   b. Spontaneous bleeding from internal sites can occur. The risk is greater in patients with pre-existing hemostatic defects such as abnormalities in platelet count, prothrombin time, partial thromboplastin time, or bleeding time.

*DOSE PREPARATION**

Weight Pounds	*Approx. Equiv. Kilograms*	*Priming Dose Plus 12-Hour Dose*	*Number Vials Abbokinase*	*Volume of Abbokinase After Reconstitution (ml***)* +	*Volume of NaCl 0.9% (ml)* =	*Final Volume (ml)*
81–90	37–41	2,250,000	9	45	150	195
91–100	41–46	2,500,000	10	50	145	195
101–110	46–50	2,750,000	11	55	140	195
111–120	50–55	3,000,000	12	60	135	195
121–130	55–59	3,250,000	13	65	130	195
131–140	59–64	3,500,000	14	70	125	195
141–150	64–68	3,750,000	15	75	120	195
151–160	69–73	4,000,000	16	80	115	195
161–170	73–77	4,250,000	17	85	110	195
171–180	78–82	4,500,000	18	90	105	195
181–190	82–86	4,750,000	19	95	100	195
191–200	87–91	5,000,000	20	100	100	195
201–210	91–95	5,250,000	21	105	95	195
211–220	96–100	5,500,000	22	110	90	195
221–230	100–105	5,750,000	23	115	85	195
231–240	105–109	6,000,000	24	120	80	195
241–250	110–114	6,250,000	25	125	70	195

**After addition of 5.2 ml of Sterile Water for injection, U.S.P., per vial. (See Preparation.)

INFUSION RATE:

Priming Dose	Dose for 12-Hour Period
15 ml/10 min.	15 ml/hr/12 hr

*Courtesy of Abbott Laboratories, North Chicago, Ill. 60064

● UROKINASE FOR INJECTION (Abbokinase) (Continued)

ACTIONS/ INDICATIONS	DOSAGE	PREPARATION AND STORAGE	DRUG INCOMPAT- IBILITIES	MODES OF IV ADMINISTRATION			CONTRAINDICATIONS; WARNINGS; PRECAUTIONS; ADVERSE REACTIONS
				INJECTION	INTERMITTENT INFUSION	CONTINUOUS INFUSION	

CONTRAINDICATIONS; WARNINGS; PRECAUTIONS; ADVERSE REACTIONS

c. Besides its fibrinolytic action, plasmin also degrades fibrinogen Factor V, VII and other proteins. Products of plasmin degradation of fibrinogen and fibrin possess an anticoagulant effect, making any bleeding difficult to control. If serious spontaneous bleeding occurs, the urokinase infusion should be terminated immediately and treatment instituted as described under Adverse Reactions.

2. In patients with a predisposition to cerebral embolism such as in cases of atrial fibrillation, the use of urokinase may be hazardous because of the possibility of bleeding into the infarcted area.

3. Concurrent use of anticoagulants is not recommended and may be hazardous. If the patient has been on heparin, its effects must be allowed to diminish until the thrombin time is less than twice the normal control value before starting urokinase. Also, heparin should not be restarted following urokinase therapy until the thrombin time has returned to less than twice the normal control value. Rethrombosis has occurred after termination of urokinase treatment. To lessen this risk, heparin followed by oral anticoagulants (warfarin) should be part of therapy.

4. Safety and effectiveness of this therapy in children have not been established, and therapy with urokinase is not recommended.

PRECAUTIONS
1. Concurrent use of drugs that may alter platelet function such as aspirin, indomethacin and phenylbutazone should be avoided.

2. Dosage of this drug should not be based on, or altered by, knowledge of the patient's level of fibrinogen, plasinogen, Factor V and Factor VII, fibrinogen degradation products and thrombin time.

ADVERSE REACTIONS

1. Bleeding—The incidence of severe bleeding was between 4 and 6% in clinical trials. Fatalities have occurred due to cerebral hemorrhage during urokinase therapy. Less severe bleeding has occurred at approximately twice the frequency as that occurring with heparin therapy. Oozing of blood from sites of percutaneous trauma is frequent. There may be a moderate fall in hematocrit without detectable bleeding.

   Management of severe bleeding: Discontinue urokinase therapy. If blood loss is large, packed red cell transfusion is indicated. Plasma volume expanders such as fresh plasma and fluids (other than dextran) should be used, along with whole blood. If hemorrhage is unresponsive to blood replacement, aminocaproic acid can be used and may act as an antidote to urokinase effects.

2. Allergic reactions are rare and usually in the form of rash, bronchospasm, and anaphylaxis.

3. Fever can occur and should be symptomatically controlled with acetaminophen rather than aspirin.

NURSING IMPLICATIONS

1. Be aware of contraindications and of clinical situations in which the risk of bleeding is great. Monitor even more cautiously than patients without these risks.

2. Monitor for all signs of bleeding:
   a. Intracerebral bleeding, as indicated by change in mental status, change in neurologic signs (pupil size, hand grip, extremity motion), headache, or change in vision. Check neurologic signs every 2–4 hours.
   b. Gastrointestinal bleeding, as indicated by hematemesis, abdominal pain or tenderness, fall in blood pressure, melena or red blood in the stools.
   c. Respiratory tract bleeding (hemoptysis may already be present secondary to pulmonary embolus) as indicated by hemoptysis, respiratory distress, chest pain.
   d. Bleeding from the urinary tract as indicated by hematuria (micro- and macroscopic) or dark brown urine.
   e. Vaginal bleeding.
   f. Ecchymosis or petechiae.

   Oozing from venipuncture, arterial puncture and intramuscular injections is to be expected. It is advisable to avoid these procedures during urokinase therapy when possible. Pressure should be applied to all venipuncture and arterial puncture sites for 15 minutes followed by the application of a pressure dressing. These sites should be inspected hourly for continued bleeding for the duration of therapy.

3. Avoid other traumatic procedures such as nasogastric intubation and urinary catheterization when possible. When performing endotracheal suctioning, use low vacuum settings (below 110 mm Hg) and keep the frequency and duration of suctioning at a minimum. Watch for increasing blood in the aspirate.

4. Handle the patient carefully to prevent bruising and hematoma formation. Use adequate numbers of personnel when turning to prevent tissue trauma. Use protective devices on the bed (flotation pad, water mattress or air mattress) when possible to lessen trauma to the skin. If a hematoma does occur, notify the physician. Pressure dressings (Ace bandage) and ice packs may be ordered.

5. Monitor blood pressure and pulse indirectly every 1–4 hours depending on the patient's overall condition. If there is an increased risk of bleeding, vital signs should be taken hourly to detect the onset of bleeding.

6. Monitor temperature every 4–6 hours. Fever can occur; acetaminophen will be ordered to control it.

7. The clinician is encouraged to read additional materials on this drug and the conditions for which it is indicated.

SUGGESTED READINGS

Cudkowicz, Leon, and Sherry, Sol: The Venous System and the Lung. *Heart and Lung,* 7(1):91–96, January/February 1978.

———: Current Status of Thrombolytic Therapy. *Heart and Lung,* 7(1):97–100, January/February 1978.

VANCOMYCIN HYDROCHLORIDE (Vancocin)

ACTIONS/ INDICATIONS	DOSAGE	PREPARATION AND STORAGE	DRUG INCOMPAT- IBILITIES	MODES OF IV ADMINISTRATION			CONTRAINDICATIONS; WARNINGS; PRECAUTIONS; ADVERSE REACTIONS
				INJECTION	INTERMITTENT INFUSION	CONTINUOUS INFUSION	
Antibiotic. Useful against gram-positive bacteria such as streptococci and staphylococci. To be used in life-threatening infections that cannot be treated with less toxic drugs or where there has been insufficient response with other drugs. Therapeutic response is usually seen within 48–72 hours.	ADULTS: 2 gm/day in 4 equally divided doses or via continuous infusion. IN THE PRESENCE OF RENAL IMPAIRMENT [1] *Mild impairment*— 1 gm/ day in divided doses *Uremia*— 1 gm every 7 days. (with hemodialysis and peritoneal dialysis, dosage is the same as in uremia), in divided doses. CHILDREN: 40–44 mg/ kg/day (1.2 gm/M²) in 2–4 divided doses or via continuous infusion. NEONATES (PREMATURE AND FULL-TERM) 10 mg/kg/day in 2 divided doses every 12 hrs. Length of therapy is determined by severity of infection and patient response.	Available in 500-mg vials. To reconstitute, add 10 ml sterile water for injection. Refrigerate and discard after 14 days.	Do not mix in solution with any other drug; do not infuse into an IV tubing containing: Chloramphenicol Penicillin G Aminophylline Amobarbital Chlorothiazide Heparin Methicillin Novobiocin Pentobarbital Phenobarbital Secobarbital Sodium bicarbonate Warfarin	NO	YES Dilute dose to *at least* a 5 mg/ml solution (500 mg/100 ml of fluid). Infuse over 20–30 min. PREFERRED MODE OF ADMINISTRATION.	YES Use D5W or NS. Add 12- or 24-hr dose to 1000 ml. D5W or NS and infuse over 12 or 24 hours. (Smaller or larger volumes of fluid may be used depending on patient's fluid needs.)	CONTRAINDICATIONS Hypersensitivity WARNINGS 1. Avoid use in patients with renal insufficiency. This drug may be ototoxic and nephrotoxic in these patients. The risk of toxicity is increased by high serum concentrations for prolonged periods. If this drug must be used, doses of less than 2 gm/day are recommended. 2. Avoid use in patients with pre-existing hearing loss. If it must be used, monitor serum levels. Deafness may be preceded by tinnitus. 3. The elderly are more susceptible to auditory damage. 4. Cessation of therapy may not halt hearing loss. 5. Concurrent or sequential use with other ototoxic-nephrotoxic agents should be avoided (e.g., kanamycin, streptomycin, neomycin, gentamicin, cephaloridine, paromomycin, viomycin, polymyxin B, colistin, tobramycin). 6. This drug is not removed by hemodialysis or peritoneal dialysis.[2] PRECAUTIONS 1. Perform serial auditory function tests and serum drug levels (when possible) in the elderly, in patients with impaired renal function, and in patients on large doses of this drug. 2. Monitor renal, hepatic, and bone marrow function in all patients and discontinue administration if abnormal values develop. Nephrotoxicity in patients with previously normal renal function is rare. If it does occur, it will produce proteinuria, hematuria, and/ or rise in BUN.[3] 3. Prevent extravasation: tissue necrosis and sloughing can result. 4. May cause phlebitis at injection site: this can be prevented with correct dilution of the drug. 5. Overgrowth infections may occur, if so, discontinue vancomycin and initiate appropriate therapy.

ADVERSE REACTIONS
1. Nausea
2. Chills and fever
3. Urticaria and macular rashes
4. Anaphylaxis
5. Rarely, renal impairment
6. Hearing loss secondary to eighth cranial nerve damage

NURSING IMPLICATIONS
1. Monitor for ototoxicity: dizziness, vertigo, tinnitus (most frequent symptom), roaring in the ears, hearing loss. Report onset to the physician.
2. Monitor for nephrotoxicity.
   a. Be aware of the patient's pretreatment BUN.
   b. Measure urine output every 4 hours; report oliguria of 120 ml or less per 4-hour period. (See chart on page 546 for normal urine output in children.
3. Prevent extravasation; see page 96. If it occurs, apply warm compresses continuously for 2 hours and then for 20 minutes every 4 hours. Protect the area from trauma. Observe for tissue breakdown.
4. Change IV site promptly if phlebitis occurs.
5. Monitor for signs and symptoms of nonsusceptible organism overgrowth infection:
   a. Fever (take rectal temperature every four hours)
   b. Increasing malaise
   c. Signs and symptoms of newly developing localized infection—redness, soreness, pain, swelling, drainage (change in volume or character of preexisting drainage).
   d. Cough (change in volume or character of preexisting drainage)
   e. Diarrhea
   f. Oral lesions (thrush) or perineal rash and itching (monilia) secondary to *Candida albicans* infection.
6. Take anaphylaxis precautions; see page 118.

REFERENCES
1. Appel, Gerald B., and Neu, Harold C.: The Nephrotoxicity of Antimicrobial Agents. *New England Journal of Medicine,* 296(12):667, March 24, 1977.
2. ————: The Nephrotoxicity of Antimicrobial Agents. *New England Journal of Medicine,* 296(13):722, March 31, 1977.
3. Ibid.

● VINBLASTINE SULFATE (Velban, VLB)

ACTIONS/INDICATIONS	DOSAGE	PREPARATION AND STORAGE	DRUG INCOMPATIBILITIES	MODES OF IV ADMINISTRATION				CONTRAINDICATIONS; WARNINGS; PRECAUTIONS; ADVERSE REACTIONS
				INJECTION	INTERMITTENT INFUSION	CONTINUOUS INFUSION		
Antineoplastic, mitotic inhibitor (cell-cycle specific).	INITIAL:	Do not mix with any other medication in any manner.	YES	NO	NO		CONTRAINDICATIONS 1. Leukopenia 2. Bacterial infection	
	Adults *Children* First Dose 3.7 mg/M² 2.5 mg/M² Second Dose 5.5 mg/M² 3.75 mg/M² Third Dose 7.4 mg/M² 5.0 mg/M² Fourth Dose 9.25 mg/M² 6.25 mg/M²			Into the tubing of a running IV over 1 minute.	This mode increases the risk of extravasation.		WARNINGS 1. This drug may cause fetal abnormalities. 2. May cause a depression of spermatogenesis.	
Used for palliative treatment of a variety of malignant conditions: • Lymphomas (Hodgkin's, lymphosarcoma, reticulum cell sarcoma, mycosis fungoides); • Neuroblastoma • Letterer-Siwe dis-	These increases are given 7 days apart until the WBC is less than or equal to 3000 cells/cu mm (leukopenia). A maximum dosage	To reconstitute, add 10 ml NS (*with preservative*). This will yield a solution of 1 mg/ml. Refrigerate and discard after 30 days.		Prior to withdrawal of the needle from the vein, rinse the syringe with venous blood. Remove the syringe and flush vein well after injection with 10 ml NS from a separate syringe. Then remove the needle.			PRECAUTIONS 1. Monitor for infection if WBC falls below 2000/cu. mm. 2. There may be a more pronounced leukopenic response in cachectic patients, and in the presence of skin ulcers. The drug should be avoided in both conditions. 3. White cell and platelet counts may fall in the presence of malignant infiltration of the marrow. If this occurs, further use of the drug is inadvisable.	

● VINBLASTINE SULFATE (Velban, VLB) (Continued)

ACTIONS/ INDICATIONS	DOSAGE	PREPARATION AND STORAGE	DRUG INCOMPATIBILITIES	MODES OF IV ADMINISTRATION			CONTRAINDICATIONS; WARNINGS; PRECAUTIONS; ADVERSE REACTIONS
				INJECTION	INTERMITTENT INFUSION	CONTINUOUS INFUSION	
ease May also be effective against: • Choriocarcinomas • Carcinoma of the breast • Embryonal carcinoma of the testis Usually administered concurrently with other antineoplastic agents.	of 18.5 mg/M² should not be exceeded. MAINTENANCE: When the dose which will produce the above degree of leukopenia has been established, a dose one increment *smaller* should be administered at approximately 1-week intervals for maintenance, so that the patient receives the maximum dose that does *not* cause leukopenia. However, subsequent doses should *not* be administered unless the WBC is greater than or equal to 4000 cells/cu mm. Duration of therapy depends on other agents used and the clinical condition of the patient.						4. Do not administer on a daily basis. 5. Do not exceed recommended dosage. 6. Avoid contact with skin and eyes. Rinse well with running water to prevent irritation. 7. Avoid extravasation. ADVERSE REACTIONS 1. Blood: bone marrow suppression, of short duration; leukopenia is usually more severe than thrombocytopenia 2. Skin: hair loss, rashes 3. Gastrointestinal: nausea, vomiting, diarrhea, ulceration of the mouth, pharyngitis, ileus, hemorrhagic colitis, abdominal pain, constipation can also occur in some patients. 4. Neurologic: numbness, paresthesias, peripheral neuritis, mental depression, headache, convulsions (all of these effects are usually seen only with high dose therapy) 5. Miscellaneous: malaise, weakness, dizziness, pain at tumor site

NURSING IMPLICATIONS
1. The patient receiving this medication will be experiencing the emotional and physical effects of the malignancy. Knowledge of the patient's feelings about his disease and its implications will assist in helping him tolerate the chemotherapy. The incidence of uncomfortable side effects and adverse reactions is high. It is within the nurse's role to assist the patient in coping

pain, headaches. Inform the physician at the onset.
  b. If the patient is on high-dose therapy, monitor for seizures.
  c. Monitor for signs and symptoms of mental depression that are related to drug administered. Inform the physician and administer supportive care. Knowing the etiology can relieve the patient of some anxiety.
6. Management of stomatitis:

with the discomforts of the disease and its treatment, and to help him work through depression and anger toward acceptance of the disease at his own pace. Despite the unpleasantness this drug may bring, it can be a source of hope for the patient.

2. Prevent extravasation; see page 96. Follow injection procedure described under Injection column. If it occurs, local injection of hyaluronidase and application of moderate heat will be prescribed by the physician to disperse the drug, help prevent cell damage, and reduce discomfort. Protect the area to prevent further trauma.

3. Management of gastrointestinal disturbances:
   a. Nausea and vomiting are usually mild and of short duration.
   b. Administer an antiemetic, if needed, to correspond to the time when the patient feels his most uncomfortable symptoms occur.
   c. Small frequent meals, timed with periods when the patient feels his best, are advisable. Bland foods are usually tolerated most easily. Carbohydrate and protein content should be high.
   d. If the patient is anorexic, encourage high nutrient liquids and water. Maintain hydration.
   e. Keep an accurate measurement of emesis and stool volumes and total intake and output to guide the physician in ordering parenteral fluids when necessary.
   f. Administer constipating agents as needed for diarrhea. Monitor for signs of hypokalemia (weakness, muscle cramps). Maintain hydration.
   g. Monitor for the onset of obstructive ileus (abdominal pain, distention, obstipation).
   h. Monitor stools for visible and occult blood.
   i. Administer laxatives and stool softeners if constipation occurs.

4. Management of hematologic effects:
   a. Be aware of the patient's white blood cell and platelet count prior to each injection.
   b. If WBC falls to 2000/cu.mm. (rare), take measures to protect the patient from infection such as: protective (reversed) isolation, avoidance of traumatic procedures; maintenance of bodily (especially perineal) cleanliness; carrying out strict urinary catheter care when appropriate, etc. Monitor for infection: temperature every 4 hours, examination for rashes, swellings, drainage and pain. Explain measures to the patient.
   c. If platelet count falls below 100,000/cu.mm., monitor for thrombocytopenic bleeding: petechiae, purpura, hematuria, melena, blood in stools, gum bleeding, vaginal bleeding, epistaxis, hematemesis, etc. Avoid trauma. Transfusions may be ordered.
   d. Instruct patient and/or family on the importance of follow-up blood work and the reporting of the signs and symptoms listed in "b" and "c" above, to the physician if the drug is being administered on an outpatient basis.

5. Management of neurologic side effects:
   a. Instruct the patient and/or family to report numbness, paresthesias,

---

a. Onset of stomatitis may indicate the presence of more serious intestinal ulceration.
b. Administer preventive oral care every 4 hours and/or after meals.
c. For preventive care use a very soft toothbrush (child's) and toothpaste; avoid trauma to tissues.
d. Examine oral membranes at least daily (instruct patient and/or family) to detect the onset of inflammation and erythema.
e. If stomatitis occurs, notify the physician and begin therapeutic oral care:[1]
   (1) *Mild Inflammation:* Remove dentures, use soft toothbrush and a hydrogen peroxide solution (1 part peroxide and 4 parts saline). Do *not* use toothpaste. Rinse with peroxide solution and then water. Replace dentures. This procedure should be carried out every 4 hours and/or after meals.
   (2) *Severe Inflammation:* Remove dentures, use soft gauze pads rather than a toothbrush. Use peroxide solution described above. Rinse with water using an asepto syringe and gentle suction until returns are clear. Do not replace dentures. It may be necessary to carry out this procedure every 2–4 hours.
f. Order a soft, bland diet for patients with inflammation. If stomatitis is severe, the patient may be placed on NPO status by the physician.
g. For patients who can tolerate oral intake, administer Xylocaine viscous or acetaminophen elixir as a mouthwash prior to meals to decrease pain (do not use aspirin rinses), as ordered by the physician.
h. Patients with severe stomatitis may require parenteral analgesia.

7. If rashes occur, administer cool compresses and topical agents as ordered. Keep the patient's environment cool. Turn frequently to prevent skin breakdown.

8. Management of hair loss:
   a. Use scalp tourniquet, if ordered, to help prevent hair loss.
   b. Counsel the patient on the possibility of hair loss to enable him to prepare for this disfigurement.
   c. Reassure him of regrowth of hair following discontinuation of the drug.
   d. Provide privacy and time for the patient to discuss his feelings.

REFERENCE
1. Bruya, Margaret Auld, and Madeira, Nancy Powell: Stomatitis After Chemotherapy. *American Journal of Nursing,* 75(8):1351, August 1975.

SUGGESTED READINGS
   Bruya, Margaret Auld, and Madeira, Nancy Powell: Stomatitis After Chemotherapy. *American Journal of Nursing,* 75(8):1349–1352, August 1975.
   Giadquinta, Barbara: Helping Families Face the Crisis of Cancer. *American Journal of Nursing,* 77:1583–1588, October 1977.
   Gullo, Shirley: Chemotherapy—What to Do About Special Side Effects. *R.N.,* 40:30–32, April 1977.

VINCRISTINE SULFATE (Oncovin)

ACTIONS/ INDICATIONS	DOSAGE	PREPARATION AND STORAGE	DRUG INCOMPATIBILITIES	MODES OF IV ADMINISTRATION			CONTRAINDICATIONS; WARNINGS; PRECAUTIONS; ADVERSE REACTIONS
				INJECTION	INTERMITTENT INFUSION	CONTINUOUS INFUSION	
Antineoplastic agent (cell cycle specific).	ADULTS: 1.4 mg/M² weekly. Other	Reconstitute with solution provided (bacte-	Do not mix with any other medication in	YES Into the tubing	YES In enough NS	NO	CONTRAINDICATIONS None

VINCRISTINE SULFATE (Oncovin) (Continued)

ACTIONS/INDICATIONS	DOSAGE	PREPARATION AND STORAGE	DRUG INCOMPATIBILITIES	MODES OF IV ADMINISTRATION			CONTRAINDICATIONS; WARNINGS; PRECAUTIONS; ADVERSE REACTIONS
				INJECTION	INTERMITTENT INFUSION	CONTINUOUS INFUSION	
Used alone to treat acute leukemias, and in combination with other agents in the treatment of Hodgkin's disease, lymphosarcoma, reticulum-cell sarcoma, rhabdomyosarcoma, neuroblastoma, and Wilms' tumor.	dosage schedules have been used. CHILDREN: 1.5 mg–2.0 mg/M² at weekly intervals.	riostatic sodium chloride solution). Add 10 ml to the 1-mg and 5-mg vials. This results in solution concentrations of 0.1 mg/ml and 0.5 mg/ml respectively. Store in refrigerator, discard after 14 days. Protect stock solutions from light.	any manner.	of a running IV, over 1 minute. Flush vein well after injection.	to make a concentration of at least 1 mg/ml (at least 50 ml). Infuse within 15 minutes.		**WARNINGS** 1. This drug may have adverse effects on the developing fetus. 2. There is insufficient information as to whether this drug may affect fertility in men and women. **PRECAUTIONS** 1. Acute hyperuricemia and uric acid nephropathy may occur. 2. Use with caution in the presence of leukopenia or infection. 3. If CNS leukemia is diagnosed, additional agents and routes of administration may be required, since this drug does not cross the blood-brain barrier. 4. Use caution in determining dosage and in monitoring neurologic side effects, if this drug is used in patients with pre-existing neuromuscular disease or who are on other agents that have neurotoxic effects. 5. Overdosage may cause death. Use extreme caution in determining dose and in administering this drug. **ADVERSE REACTIONS** 1. Blood: bone marrow suppression, producing mild leukopenia beginning on the fourth day of therapy and resolving by the fifth 2. Neurologic: changes are frequently seen and can be dose-limiting, begin with loss of Achilles tendon reflex; parasthesias are common, as are neuritic pain, difficulty walking secondary to muscle weakness; these effects may last through the duration of therapy; seizures have been reported, cranial nerve deficits in the form of ptosis, abducens nerve palsy, seventh cranial nerve dysfunction and vocal cord paralysis 3. Gastrointestinal: constipation secondary to adynamic ileus (occurs more frequently in elderly patients); impaction formation is common; stool softeners should be given prophylactically; nausea and vomiting are rare 4. Hair loss: mild but common, reversible

SUGGESTED READINGS
Bolin, Rose Homan, and Auld, Margaret E.: Hodgkin's Disease. *American Journal of Nursing*, November 1974, pp. 1982–1986.
Bruya, Margaret Auld, and Madeira, Nancy Powell: Stomatitis After Chemotherapy. *American Journal of Nursing*, August 1975, pp. 1349–1352.
Foley, Genevieve, and McCarthy, Ann Marie: The Disease (Hodgkin's) and Its Treatment. *American Journal of Nursing* July 1976, pp. 1109–1114 (references).
_____: The Child With Leukemia In a Special Hematology Clinic. *American Journal of Nursing*, July 1976, pp. 1115–1119.
Giadquinta, Barbara: Helping Families Face the Crisis of Cancer. *American Journal of Nursing*, October 1977, pp. 1583–1588.
Gullo, Shirley: Chemotherapy—What to Do About Special Side Effects. *RN*, April 1977, pp. 30–32.
Hannan, Jeanne Ferguson: Talking Is Treatment, Too. *American Journal of Nursing.* November 1974, pp. 1991–1992.
Martinson, Ida: The Child With Leukemia: Parents Help Each Other. *American Journal of Nursing*, July 1976, pp. 1120–1122.
Showfety, Mary Patricia: The Ordeal of Hodgkin's Disease. *American Journal of Nursing*, November 1974, pp. 1987–1991.
Vietti, Teresa J., and Valeriote, Frederick: Conceptual Basis for the Use of Chemotheraputic Agents and Their Pharmacology. *Pediatric Clinics of North America*, 23:67–92, February 1976, pp. 67–92 (references).

5. Antidiuretic syndrome: high loss of sodium in the urine followed by hyponatremia
6. Stomatitis: rare
7. Prevent extravasation; see p. 96. If it occurs, discontinue injection or infusion promptly. Administer the remainder of the dose in another vein. A local injection of hyaluronidase and the application of moderate heat to the affected area may help to disperse the drug in the tissues to decrease pain and tissue reaction.

NURSING IMPLICATIONS
1. Management of hematologic effects (see Adverse Reaction No. 1):
   a. Bone marrow depression will be minimal and usually does not require special intervention.
   b. Be aware of the patient's white cell and platelet counts.
2. Management of constipation:
   a. Be aware of the patient's previous bowel habits and attempt to maintain them.
   b. Administer stool softeners and laxatives as ordered; keep the patient hydrated.
   c. Monitor stool number.
   d. Observe for abdominal distention and pain.
3. Monitor for signs and symptoms of hyponatremia (see Adverse Reaction No. 5) such as:
   a. Weakness
   b. Changes in mental status such as confusion and drowsiness
4. Stomatitis rarely is a problem with this drug. If the patient develops inflammation of oral mucosa with ulceration, refer to care described under Vinblastine, on page 526 in reference to stomatitis.
5. Management of hair loss:
   a. Use a scalp tourniquet during injection of this drug, if ordered by the physician, to help prevent hair loss.
   b. Counsel the patient on the possibility of hair loss to enable him to prepare for this disfigurement.
   c. Reassure him of regrowth of hair following discontinuation of the drug.
   d. Provide privacy and time for the patient to discuss his feelings.
6. Monitor for neurologic changes (see Adverse Reaction No. 2). Notify physician of onset. Take safety precautions to prevent injury. Reassure him of the reversible nature of these reactions.

● VITAMIN B COMPLEX (Betalin Complex, Solu-B)

ACTIONS/ INDICATIONS	DOSAGE	PREPARATION AND STORAGE	DRUG INCOMPATIBILITIES	MODES OF IV ADMINISTRATION			CONTRAINDICATIONS; WARNINGS; PRECAUTIONS; ADVERSE REACTIONS
				INJECTION	INTERMITTENT INFUSION	CONTINUOUS INFUSION	
Synthetic vitamin B complex factors, essential elements in all metabolic processes. Used to prevent and treat vitamin B deficiencies, when rapid tissue saturation is needed or when oral	ADULTS: 2–5 ml for push injection daily, or 2–10 ml for infusion daily.	Protect infusion bottles from light during infusion. Infusion should last no longer than 8–10 hrs; solution will lose potency after that time. Can be added to solution in plastic IV bags. Refrigerate Betalin	Do not mix in any manner with tetracycline, aminophylline.	YES Undiluted or diluted in NS or sterile water for injection. Slowly, each 1 ml over 2–3 min.	YES Use D5W or D10W.	YES Preferred mode. Use D5W or D10W (and protein hydrolysate). Infusion should last no more than 8 hrs.	CONTRAINDICATIONS Hypersensitivity to thiamine. ADVERSE REACTIONS Allergic reactions to thiamine (see page 499 for detailed information on thiamine).

VITAMIN B COMPLEX (Betalin Complex, Solu-B) (Continued)

ACTIONS/ INDICATIONS	DOSAGE	PREPARATION AND STORAGE	DRUG INCOMPATIBILITIES	MODES OF IV ADMINISTRATION			CONTRAINDICATIONS; WARNINGS; PRECAUTIONS; ADVERSE REACTIONS
				INJECTION	INTERMITTENT INFUSION	CONTINUOUS INFUSION	
route is not available for dependable absorption. Examples: • Prolonged IV therapy • Burns • Extensive surgery or trauma • Malabsorption • Extensive bowel resection		Complex. Do not use if there is a precipitate.					

CONTENTS	SOLU-B per ml.	BETALIN per ml.
Thiamine HCl (V.B₁)	2 mg	5 mg
Riboflavin (V.B₂)	2 mg	5 mg
Pyridoxine HCl (V.B₆)	1 mg	5 mg
Niacinamide	50 mg	75 mg
Calcium Pantothenate	10 mg	—
Pantothenic Acid	—	2.5 mg
Cyanocobalamin (V.B₁₂)	—	2.5 mcgm

NURSING IMPLICATIONS
1. Monitor for allergic reactions; see page 118.
2. See Recommended Daily Dietary Allowances, pages 541–542.

VITAMIN B COMPLEX WITH VITAMIN C (Berocca-C, Berocca-C 500, Betalin Complex F. C., Folbesyn, Solu-B with Ascorbic Acid, Solu-B Forte)

ACTIONS/ INDICATIONS	DOSAGE	PREPARATION AND STORAGE	DRUG INCOMPATIBILITIES	MODES OF IV ADMINISTRATION			CONTRAINDICATIONS; WARNINGS; PRECAUTIONS; ADVERSE REACTIONS
				INJECTION	INTERMITTENT INFUSION	CONTINUOUS INFUSION	
Synthetic vitamin B complex factors, and ascorbic acid, essential elements in all metabolic processes. Used to prevent and treat vitamin B and C deficiencies when rapid tissue saturation is needed or when oral route is not available for dependable	ADULTS: Depending on patient's condition: BEROCCA-C AND BEROCCA-C 500: IV push—2 ml. Infusion—2 –20 ml. daily. BETALIN COMPLEX F.C.:	Dilute in fluids immediately prior to use to prevent loss of potency. Infusion should last no longer than 8–10 hrs, or solution will lose potency. Can be added to fluids in plastic IV bags. See table below for contents of various preparations.	Do not mix in any manner with aminophylline, any antibiotic chlorothiazide, chlorpromazine.	YES. Slowly, diluted or undiluted over 2–3 min into tubing of a running IV. (Infusion modes are preferred.)	YES. Use NS, D5W, D10W, RL, Ringer's injection, sodium lactate, D5/NS, protein hydrolysate.	YES. Use NS, D5W, D10W, RL, Ringer's injection, sodium lactate, D5/NS, protein hydrolysate. Infusion should last no longer than 8 hrs.	CONTRAINDICATIONS Hypersensitivity to thiamine PRECAUTIONS There may be a feeling of warmth or flushing during a rapid injection or infusion. ADVERSE REACTIONS Allergic reactions to thiamine, including anaphylaxis.

absorption. Examples:
• Prolonged IV therapy
• Burns
• Extensive surgery or trauma
• Malabsorption
• Extensive bowel resection

IV push—2 ml.

Infusion—2-10 ml daily.

FOLBESYN:

IV push—2 ml.

Infusion—2 ml daily, or as condition dictates.

SOLU-B WITH C:

IV push—2-10 ml. daily

Infusion—2-10 ml. daily.

CHILDREN: ¼-½ of adult dose depending on body size and clinical situation.

Refrigerate as indicated on individual labels.

Do not use if the solution contains a precipitate.

Protect infusion bottles from light.

COMPARISON OF CONTENTS (mg/ml)

	Berocca-C	Berocca-C-500	Betalin Complex F.C.	Folbesyn	Solu-B with C	Solu-B Forte
Thiamine HCl (B$_1$)	5	5	12.5	5	2	25
Riboflavin (B$_2$)	5	5	3	5	2	5
Niacinamide	40	40	50	37.5	50	125
Pyridoxine (B$_6$)	10	10	5	7.5	1	5
Ascorbic Acid	50	125	75	150	100	100
Sodium Pantothenate	—	—	—	5	10	50
Vitamin B$_{12}$	—	—	—	7.5 mcg	—	—
Folic Acid	—	—	—	0.5	—	—
Pantothenic Acid	—	—	2.5	—	—	—
Dexpanthenol	10	10	—	—	—	—
d-biotin	0.1	0.1	—	—	—	—

NURSING IMPLICATIONS
1. Monitor for allergic reactions; see page 118.

2. See Recommended Daily Dietary Allowances, pages 541-542.

WARFARIN, SODIUM (Coumadin)

ACTIONS/ INDICATIONS	DOSAGE	PREPARATION AND STORAGE	DRUG INCOMPATIBILITIES	MODES OF IV ADMINISTRATION			CONTRAINDICATIONS; WARNINGS; PRECAUTIONS; ADVERSE REACTIONS
				INJECTION	INTERMITTENT INFUSION	CONTINUOUS INFUSION	
Anticoagulant. Works by depressing the formation of prothrombin in the liver. Also interferes with	Must be individualized by frequent prothrombin time determinations.	To constitute from powder, use accompanying diluent. Resultant concentration is 25 mg/ml.	Do not mix in any manner with: Epinephrine Metaraminol Oxytocin Promazine	YES May be injected undiluted over 1 min.	NO	NO	CONTRAINDICATIONS 1. Presence of bleeding or tendency to bleed 2. Blood dyscrasias 3. Purpura 4. Open, ulcerative, traumatic or surgical wounds

WARFARIN, SODIUM (Coumadin) (Continued)

ACTIONS/ INDICATIONS	DOSAGE	PREPARATION AND STORAGE	DRUG INCOMPAT- IBILITIES	MODES OF IV ADMINISTRATION			CONTRAINDICATIONS; WARNINGS; PRECAUTIONS; ADVERSE REACTIONS
				INJECTION	INTERMITTENT INFUSION	CONTINUOUS INFUSION	
the production of vitamin-K dependent factors VII, IX, and X of the clotting system to decrease intravascular clotting. Used for prophylaxis or treatment of pulmonary embolism, venous thrombosis; and the prevention of embolization in atrial fibrillation.	ADULTS: *Initial*—40–60 mg. *Maintenance*—5–10 mg/day. Aim of therapy is to reduce prothrombin activity by 1.5 –2.5 times control (normal). Dosage recommendations for children are not available.	Store reconstituted solution in refrigerator, away from light. Discard after 7 days or sooner if precipitate appears. Exposure to light may cause slight discoloration; solution can still be used. There is some adsorption onto the plastic of intravenous solution bags (11.7% within 24 hours).	Tetracycline Vancomycin Dextrose solutions				5. Ulcerations of the gastrointestinal tract 6. Visceral carcinoma 7. Diverticulitis 8. Colitis 9. Subacute bacterial endocarditis 10. Threatened abortion 11. Recent surgery of the eye, brain or spinal cord 12. During regional or lumbar block anesthesia 13. Vitamin K deficiency 14. Severe hypertension 15. Recent cerebral hemorrhage 16. Severe hepatic or renal disease 17. During continuous tubal drainage of the gastrointestinal and urinary tracts WARNINGS 1. Effects on clotting can be cumulative and prolonged. At the earliest sign of bleeding the drug should be discontinued. 2. Prothrombin times should be done daily to determine stable dose to produce desired anticoagulation. 3. When administered concomitantly with heparin, delay prothrombin time determination for a period of 4 –5 hours after the last dose of heparin. 4. Fetal hemorrhage and death have occurred when used during pregnancy. Fetal abnormalities have also occurred. Risk of withholding the drug should be weighed against possible hazards. 5. This drug is secreted in breast milk; infant should be observed for bleeding, if the drug is used at all. PRECAUTIONS 1. Administer with caution to patients with active TB, moderate hypertension, mild liver or renal dysfunction, severe diabetes, during menstruation and postpartum period, in patients with a history of ulcer disease of the gastrointestinal tract, and in patients in a hazardous occupation.

2. Patients with congestive heart failure usually require lower dosage.
3. If prothrombin time falls below 15% of normal, or if hemorrhage occurs, administer vitamin K (see page 453), whole blood, or fresh frozen plasma, depending on patient needs. Withdrawal of therapy may suffice.
4. Discontinue therapy prior to surgery of the central nervous system or eye.
5. Following surgery of the gastrointestinal tract, stools should be monitored for blood.
6. Any change in dietary fat or vitamin K intake may alter response to warfarin.
7. The newborn infant, with vitamin K deficiency, is sensitive to this drug.
8. An enhanced or prolonged effect of this drug can be seen in renal insufficiency, fever, alcoholism, and scurvy (vitamin C deficiency).

ADVERSE REACTIONS
1. Excess dose (increased prothrombin time beyond therapeutic range) may cause hematuria, bleeding from mucous membranes, hemorrhage from a wound or ulcerative lesion, petechiae, purpuric hemorrhage.
2. Submucosal hemorrhage or intramural hemorrhage of the gastrointestinal tract may cause paralytic ileus and bowel obstruction.
3. Menstrual flow is usually normal, but uterine hemorrhage has occurred.
4. Discontinue the drug with any bleeding.
5. Rare reactions: dermatitis, urticaria, alopecia, priapism (abnormally sustained erection of the penis), fever, nausea, vomiting, diarrhea, hemorrhagic necrosis of the breast.

NURSING IMPLICATIONS
1. Assist in accurate history-taking to detect the presence of contraindications.
2. In the hospital setting, dosage can be easily controlled with daily prothrombin time determinations. However, the early sign of bleeding must be observed for because of the possibility of: (a) patient idiosyncrasy to the drug producing exaggerated depression of prothrombin time; (b) undetected potential bleeding point, e.g., unknown peptic ulcer; or (c) cumulative action of the drug.
The *early signs* of bleeding are:
   a. Micro- and macroscopic hematuria
   b. Occult blood in stool (guaiac)
   c. Gum bleeding
   d. Prolonged bleeding after venipuncture

The latent *overt signs* of excessively prolonged prothrombin time or bleeding are:
   a. Painful swelling in an extremity
   b. Frank hematuria
   c. Melena or bloody stools (be certain that a dark color is not due to a medication such as iron or bismuth)
   d. Epistaxis (nosebleed)
   e. Vaginal bleeding
   f. Fall in blood pressure; unusual rise in pulse
   g. Hematemesis
   h. Ecchymosis (in dark-skinned persons, darker spots on trunk, thighs, inner aspects of upper arms)
   i. Petechiae (may be difficult to see in darker-skinned persons)
3. Instruct the patient who is able to cooperate to report any of the above

● WARFARIN, SODIUM (Coumadin) (Continued)

NURSING IMPLICATIONS (No. 3 continued)

overt signs of bleeding immediately upon detection. Also instruct him/her to report any other unusual pain or symptom. Take care not to frighten the patient with the information. Reassure him/her of the control of the drug with blood tests and an antidote. Those patients who cannot cooperate (comatose or confused) must be observed frequently by the nursing staff. Monitor blood pressure and pulse at least every 4 hours for early signs of hemorrhage.

4. Be aware of the patient's prothrombin time prior to each dose.
5. If the patient must receive intramuscular, subcutaneous, intravenous or intra-arterial injections while on this drug, apply moderate pressure over the injection site for at least 2 full minutes after injection or puncture with a dry sterile gauze pad. Observe the site for external bleeding or hematoma formation hourly for the next 2 to 3 hours. If bleeding occurs, notify the physician. This is a sign of an elevated prothrombin time. Apply a pressure dressing or ice as ordered by the physician.
6. Keep vitamin K (AquaMephyton) on hand.
7. Patients on intravenous warfarin may be placed on chronic oral therapy. If so, instruct the patient and/or family on all self-care information. Such patients and/or families must be reliable and have access to frequent medical follow-up.

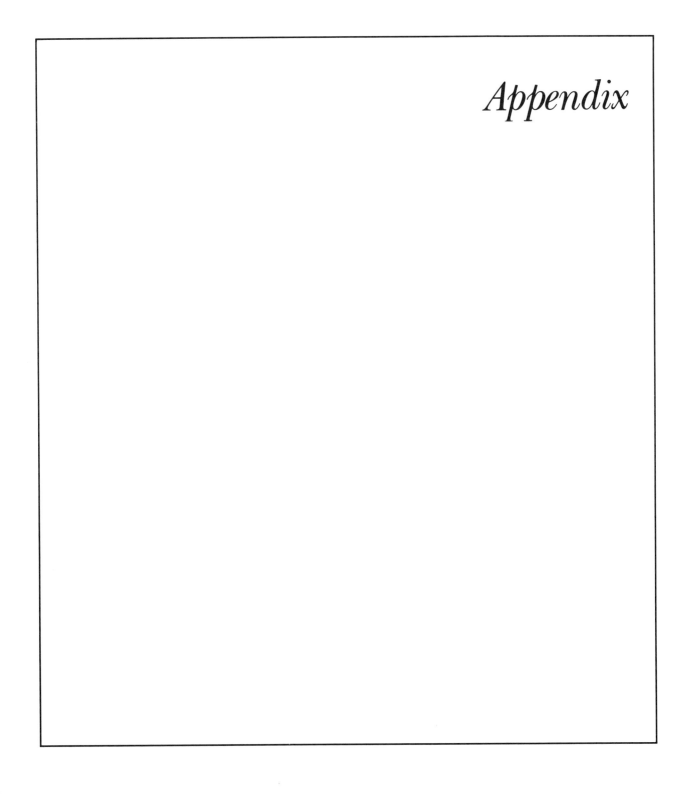

Appendix

Appendix

TABLE 1. METRIC UNITS AND SYMBOLS*

Quantity	Unit	Symbol	Equivalent
Length	millimeter	mm.	1000 mm. = 1 m.
	centimeter	cm.	100 cm. = 1 m.
	decimeter	dm.	10 dm. = 1 m.
	meter	m.	1000 m. = 1 km.
Volume	cubic centimeter	cc. or cm.^{3}	1000 $\begin{cases} \text{cc. or cm.}^3 \\ \text{ml.} \end{cases} = 1 \text{ dm.}^3 \text{ or 1 liter}$
	milliliter	ml.	
	cu. decimeter	dm.^{3}	1000 $\begin{cases} \text{dm.}^3 \\ 1 \end{cases} = 1 \text{ m.}^3$
	liter	L.	
Mass	microgram	μg.	1000 μg. = 1 mg.
	milligram	mg.	1000 mg. = 1 g.
	gram	g.	1000 g. = 1 kg.
	kilogram	kg.	1000 kg. = 1 metric ton (t)

*(From Brunner, L. S., and Suddarth, D. S.: The Lippincott Manual of Nursing Practice (2nd ed.). Philadelphia, J. B. Lippincott, 1978, p. 1827.)

TABLE 2. TABLE OF METRIC AND APOTHECARIES' SYSTEMS*

(Approved *approximate* dose equivalents are enclosed in parentheses. Use *exact* equivalents in calculations.)

Conversion Factors

Metric	*Apothecaries*	*Metric*	*Apothecaries*
1 milligram (mg.)	$\frac{1}{64}$ grain	3.888 cubic centimeters or grams	1 dram (4 cc. or grams)
64.79 milligrams	1 grain (65 mg.)	31.103 cubic centimeters or grams	1 ounce (30 cc. or grams)
1 gram	15.43 grains (15 grains)	473.167 cubic centimeters	1 pint (500 cc.)
1 cubic centimeter (cc.)	16 minims		

WEIGHTS

Metric	*Apothecaries*	*Metric*		*Apothecaries*
0.0001 gram—0.1 mg.—$\frac{1}{640}$ grain ($\frac{1}{600}$ grain)		0.057 gram —57	mg.—$\frac{7}{8}$	grain
0.0002 gram—0.2 mg.—$\frac{1}{320}$ grain ($\frac{1}{300}$ grain)		0.06 gram —60	mg.—$\frac{9}{10}$	grain (1 grain)
0.0003 gram—0.3 mg.—$\frac{1}{210}$ grain ($\frac{1}{200}$ grain)		0.065 gram —65	mg.—1	grain (60 mg.)
0.0004 gram—0.4 mg.—$\frac{1}{150}$ grain		0.07 gram —70	mg.—$1\frac{1}{20}$	grains
0.0005 gram—0.5 mg.—$\frac{1}{120}$ grain		0.08 gram —80	mg.—$1\frac{1}{5}$	grains
0.0006 gram—0.6 mg.—$\frac{1}{100}$ grain		0.09 gram —90	mg.—$1\frac{1}{3}$	grains
0.0007 gram—0.7 mg.—$\frac{1}{90}$ grain		0.097 gram —97	mg.—$1\frac{1}{2}$	grains (0.1 gram)
0.0008 gram—0.8 mg.—$\frac{1}{80}$ grain		0.12 gram —120	mg.—2	grains
0.0009 gram—0.9 mg.—$\frac{1}{75}$ grain		0.2 gram —200	mg.—3	grains
0.001 gram—1 mg.—$\frac{1}{64}$ grain ($\frac{1}{60}$ grain)		0.24 gram —240	mg.—4	grains (0.25 gram)
0.0011 gram—1.1 mg.—$\frac{1}{60}$ grain		0.3 gram —300	mg.—$4\frac{1}{2}$	grains
0.0013 gram—1.3 mg.—$\frac{1}{50}$ grain (1.2 mg.)		0.33 gram —330	mg.—5	grains (0.3 gram)
0.0014 gram—1.4 mg.—$\frac{1}{48}$ grain		0.4 gram —400	mg.—6	grains
0.0016 gram—1.6 mg.—$\frac{1}{40}$ grain (1.5 mg.)		0.45 gram —450	mg.—7	grains
0.0018 gram—1.8 mg.—$\frac{1}{36}$ grain		0.5 gram —500	mg.—$7\frac{1}{2}$	grains
0.0020 gram—2 mg.—$\frac{1}{32}$ grain ($\frac{1}{30}$ grain)		0.53 gram —530	mg.—8	grains
0.0022 gram—2.2 mg.—$\frac{1}{30}$ grain		0.6 gram —600	mg.—9	grains
0.0026 gram—2.6 mg.—$\frac{1}{25}$ grain		0.65 gram —650	mg.—10	grains (0.6 gram)
0.003 gram—3 mg.—$\frac{1}{20}$ grain		0.73 gram —730	mg.—11	grains
0.004 gram—4 mg.—$\frac{1}{16}$ grain ($\frac{1}{15}$ grain)		0.80 gram —800	mg.—12	grains (0.75 gram)
0.005 gram—5 mg.—$\frac{1}{12}$ grain		0.86 gram —860	mg.—13	grains
0.006 gram—6 mg.—$\frac{1}{10}$ grain		0.93 gram —930	mg.—14	grains
0.007 gram—7 mg.—$\frac{1}{9}$ grain		1. gram —1000	mg.—15	grains
0.008 gram—8 mg.—$\frac{1}{8}$ grain		1.06 grams—1060	mg.—16	grains
0.009 gram—9 mg.—$\frac{1}{7}$ grain		1.13 grams—1130	mg.—17	grains
0.01 gram—10 mg.—$\frac{1}{6}$ grain		1.18 grams—1180	mg.—18	grains
0.013 gram—13 mg.—$\frac{1}{5}$ grain (12 mg.)		1.26 grams—1260	mg.—19	grains
0.016 gram—16 mg.—$\frac{1}{4}$ grain (15 mg.)		1.30 grams—1300	mg.—20	grains
0.02 gram—20 mg.—$\frac{1}{3}$ grain		1.50 grams—1500	mg.—22	grains
0.025 gram—25 mg.—$\frac{3}{8}$ grain		2 grams—2000	mg.—30	grains ($\frac{1}{2}$ dram)
0.03 gram—30 mg.—$\frac{2}{5}$ grain ($\frac{1}{2}$ grain)		4 grams	—1	dram (60 grains)
0.032 gram—32 mg.—$\frac{1}{2}$ grain (30 mg.)		5 grams	—75	grains
0.04 gram—40 mg.—$\frac{3}{5}$ grain ($\frac{2}{3}$ grain)		8 grams	—2	drams (7.5 grams)
0.043 gram—43 mg.—$\frac{2}{3}$ grain (40 mg.)		10 grams	—$2\frac{1}{2}$	drams
0.05 gram—50 mg.—$\frac{3}{4}$ grain		15 grams	—4	drams
		30 grams	—1	ounce

LIQUID MEASURES**

Metric	*Apothecaries*	*Metric*	*Apothecaries*
0.03 cubic centimeter	— $\frac{1}{2}$ minim	8 cubic centimeters	—2 fluid drams
0.05 cubic centimeter	— $\frac{3}{4}$ minim	10 cubic centimeters	—$2\frac{1}{2}$ fluid drams
0.06 cubic centimeter	—1 minim	15 cubic centimeters	—4 fluid drams
0.1 cubic centimeter	—$1\frac{1}{2}$ minims	20 cubic centimeters	—$5\frac{1}{2}$ fluid drams
0.2 cubic centimeter	—3 minims	25 cubic centimeters	—$\frac{5}{6}$ fluid ounce
0.25 cubic centimeter	—4 minims	30 cubic centimeters	—1 fluid ounce
0.3 cubic centimeter	—5 minims	50 cubic centimeters	—$1\frac{3}{4}$ fluid ounces
0.5 cubic centimeter	—8 minims	60 cubic centimeters	—2 fluid ounces
0.6 cubic centimeter	—10 minims	100 cubic centimeters	—$3\frac{1}{2}$ fluid ounces
0.75 cubic centimeter	—12 minims	120 cubic centimeters	—4 fluid ounces
1 cubic centimeter	—15 minims	200 cubic centimeters	—7 fluid ounces
2 cubic centimeters	—30 minims	250 cubic centimeters	—8 fluid ounces
3 cubic centimeters	—45 minims	360 cubic centimeters	—12 fluid ounces
4 cubic centimeters	—1 fluid dram	500 cubic centimeters	—1 pint
5 cubic centimeters	—$1\frac{1}{4}$ fluid drams	1000 cubic centimeters	—1 quart

* (From Culver, V. M.: Modern Bedside Nursing. Philadelphia, W. B. Saunders, 1969.)

** Note: A cubic centimeter (cc.) is the approximate equivalent of a milliliter (ml.). The terms are used interchangeably in general medicine.

TABLE 3. CENTIGRADE AND FAHRENHEIT TEMPERATURES*

Celsius (Centigrade)	Fahrenheit
0	32
36.0	96.8
36.5	97.7
37.0	98.6
37.5	99.5
38.0	100.4
38.5	101.3
39.0	102.2
39.5	103.1
40.0	104.0
40.5	104.9
41.0	105.8
41.5	106.7
42.0	107.6

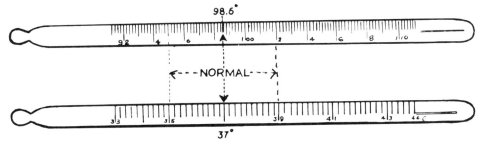

FAHRENHEIT

CELSIUS

To convert degrees F. to degrees C.
Subtract 32, then multiply by 5/9

To convert degrees C. to degrees F.
Multiply by 9/5, then add 32

*(From Brunner, L. S., and Suddarth, D. S.: The Lippincott Manual of Nursing Practice (2nd ed.). Philadelphia, J. B. Lippincott, 1978, p. 1832.)

TABLE 4. COMPARATIVE SCALES OF MEASURES, WEIGHTS AND TEMPERATURES*

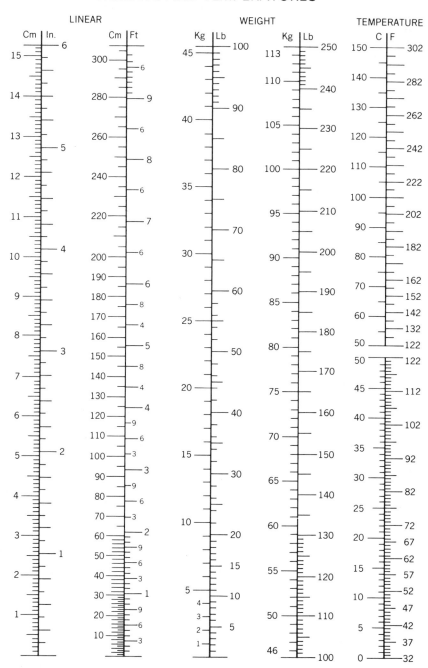

* 2.5 cm = 1 in.   1 kg. = 2.2 lb.

*(From Brunner, L. S., and Suddarth, D. S.: The Lippincott Manual of Nursing Practice (2nd ed.). Philadelphia, J. B. Lippincott, 1978, p. 1833.)

TABLE 5. RECOMMENDED DAILY DIETARY ALLOWANCES

FOOD AND NUTRITION BOARD, NATIONAL ACADEMY OF SCIENCES—
NATIONAL RESEARCH COUNCIL
RECOMMENDED DAILY DIETARY ALLOWANCES,[a] Revised 1974

Designed for the maintenance of good nutrition of practically all healthy people in the U.S.A.

| | AGE | WEIGHT | | HEIGHT | | ENERGY | PROTEIN | FAT-SOLUBLE VITAMINS | | | |
| | | | | | | | | Vita-min A Activity | | Vita-min D | Vita-min E Activity[c] |
	(years)	(kg.)	(lbs.)	(cm.)	(in.)	(kcal.)[b]	(g.)	(RE)[c]	(IU)	(IU)	(IU)
Infants	0.0–0.5	6	14	60	24	kg. × 117	kg. × 2.2	420[d]	1,400	400	4
	0.5–1.0	9	20	71	28	kg. × 108	kg. × 2.0	400	2,000	400	5
Children	1–3	13	28	86	34	1,300	23	400	2,000	400	7
	4–6	20	44	110	44	1,800	30	500	2,500	400	9
	7–10	30	66	135	54	2,400	36	700	3,300	400	10
Males	11–14	44	97	158	63	2,800	44	1,000	5,000	400	12
	15–18	61	134	172	69	3,000	54	1,000	5,000	400	15
	19–22	67	147	172	69	3,000	54	1,000	5,000	400	15
	23–50	70	154	172	69	2,700	56	1,000	5,000		15
	51+	70	154	172	69	2,400	56	1,000	5,000		15
Females	11–14	44	97	155	62	2,400	44	800	4,000	400	12
	15–18	54	119	162	65	2,100	48	800	4,000	400	12
	19–22	58	128	162	65	2,100	46	800	4,000	400	12
	23–50	58	128	162	65	2,000	46	800	4,000		12
	51+	58	128	162	65	1,800	46	800	4,000		12
Pregnant						+300	+30	1,000	5,000	400	15
Lactating						+500	+20	1,200	6,000	400	15

[a] The allowances are intended to provide for individual variations among most normal persons as they live in the United States under usual environmental stresses. Diets should be based on a variety of common foods in order to provide other nutrients for which human requirements have been less well defined. See text for more detailed discussion of allowances and of nutrients not tabulated.

[b] Kilojoules (k J) = 4.2 × kcal.

[c] Retinol equivalents.

[d] Assumed to be all as retinol in milk during the first six months of life. All subsequent intakes are assumed to be half as retinol and half as β-carotene when calculated from international units. As retinol equivalents, ¾ are as retinol and ¼ as β-carotene.

(Reproduced with the permission of the National Academy of Sciences.)

(continued overleaf)

TABLE 5.   RECOMMENDED DAILY DIETARY ALLOWANCES—Continued

FOOD AND NUTRITION BOARD, NATIONAL ACADEMY OF SCIENCES—
NATIONAL RESEARCH COUNCIL
RECOMMENDED DAILY DIETARY ALLOWANCES," Revised 1974

Designed for the maintenance of good nutrition of practically all healthy people in the U.S.A.

WATER-SOLUBLE VITAMINS							MINERALS					
Ascorbic Acid (mg.)	Folacin[f] (μg.)	Niacin[g] (mg.)	Ribo-flavin (mg.)	Thiamin (mg.)	Vita-min B$_6$ (mg.)	Vita-min B$_{12}$ (μg.)	Calcium (mg.)	Phos-phorus (mg.)	Iodine (μg.)	Iron (mg.)	Mag-nesium (mg.)	Zinc (mg.)
35	50	5	0.4	0.3	0.3	0.3	360	240	35	10	60	3
35	50	8	0.6	0.5	0.4	0.3	540	400	45	15	70	5
40	100	9	0.8	0.7	0.6	1.0	800	800	60	15	150	10
40	200	12	1.1	0.9	0.9	1.5	800	800	80	10	200	10
40	300	16	1.2	1.2	1.2	2.0	800	800	110	10	250	10
45	400	18	1.5	1.4	1.6	3.0	1,200	1,200	130	18	350	15
45	400	20	1.8	1.5	2.0	3.0	1,200	1,200	150	18	400	15
45	400	20	1.8	1.5	2.0	3.0	800	800	140	10	350	15
45	400	18	1.6	1.4	2.0	3.0	800	800	130	10	350	15
45	400	16	1.5	1.2	2.0	3.0	800	800	110	10	350	15
45	400	16	1.3	1.2	1.6	3.0	1,200	1,200	115	18	300	15
45	400	14	1.4	1.1	2.0	3.0	1,200	1,200	115	18	300	15
45	400	14	1.4	1.1	2.0	3.0	800	800	100	18	300	15
45	400	13	1.2	1.0	2.0	3.0	800	800	100	18	300	15
45	400	12	1.1	1.0	2.0	3.0	800	800	80	10	300	15
60	800	+2	+0.3	+0.3	2.5	4.0	1,200	1,200	125	18+[h]	450	20
80	600	+4	+0.5	+0.3	2.5	4.0	1,200	1,200	150	18	450	25

' Total vitamin E activity, estimated to be 80 percent as α-tocopherol and 20 percent other tocopherols. See text for variation in allowances.

[f] The folacin allowances refer to dietary sources as determined by *Lactobacillus casei* assay. Pure forms of folacin may be effective in doses less than ¼ of the recommended dietary allowance.

[g] Although allowances are expressed as niacin, it is recognized that on the average 1 mg. of niacin is derived from each 60 mg. of dietary tryptophan.

[h] This increased requirement cannot be met by ordinary diets; therefore, the use of supplemental iron is recommended.

(Reproduced with the permission of the National Academy of Sciences.)

TABLE 6. NOMOGRAM FOR ESTIMATING SURFACE AREA OF INFANTS AND YOUNG CHILDREN

HEIGHT		SURFACE AREA	WEIGHT	
feet	centimeters	in square meters	pounds	kilograms

To determine the surface area of the patient draw a straight line between the point representing his height on the left vertical scale to the point representing his weight on the right vertical scale. The point at which this line intersects the middle vertical scale represents the patient's surface area in square meters. (Courtesy, Abbott Laboratories.)

TABLE 7. NOMOGRAM FOR ESTIMATING SURFACE AREA OF OLDER CHILDREN AND ADULTS

HEIGHT		SURFACE AREA	WEIGHT	
feet	centimeters	in square meters	pounds	kilograms

HEIGHT
feet | centimeters

7' — 220
— 215
10" — 210
8" — 205
6" — 200
4" — 195
2" — 190
6' — 185
10" — 180
8" — 175
6" — 170
4" — 165
2" — 160
5' — 155
10" — 150
8" — 145
6" — 140
4" — 135
2" — 130
4' — 125
10" — 120
8" — 115
6" — 110
4" — 105
2" — 100
3' — 95
10" — 90
8" — 85
6" — 80
— 75

SURFACE AREA
in square meters

3.00
2.90
2.80
2.70
2.60
2.50
2.40
2.30
2.20
2.10
2.00
1.95
1.90
1.85
1.80
1.75
1.70
1.65
1.60
1.55
1.50
1.45
1.40
1.35
1.30
1.25
1.20
1.15
1.10
1.05
1.00
.95
.90
.85
.80
.75
.70
.65
.60

WEIGHT
pounds | kilograms

440 — 200
420 — 190
400 — 180
380 — 170
360 — 160
340 — 150
320 — 140
300 — 130
290
280 — 120
270
260
250 — 110
240
230 — 100
220
210 — 95
200 — 90
190 — 85
180 — 80
170
160 — 75
150 — 70
140 — 65
130 — 60
120 — 55
110 — 50
100 — 45
90 — 40
80 — 35
70 — 30
60 — 25
50 — 20

(Courtesy, Abbott Laboratories.)

TABLE 8. NORMAL VITAL SIGN VALUES IN CHILDREN*

Normal Vital Sign Ranges in Children

Temperature

Oral 36.4–37.4°C. (97.6–99.3°F.)
Rectal 36.2–37.8°C. (97–100°F.)
Axillary 35.9–36.7°C. (96.6–98°F.)

Pulse and Respiratory Rates

Age	Pulse	Respirations
Newborn	70–170	30–50
11 months	80–160	26–40
2 years	80–130	20–30
4 years	80–120	20–30
6 years	75–115	20–26
8 years	70–110	18–24
10 years	70–110	18–24
Adolescence	60–110	12–20

*Blood Pressure**

Age	Mean Systolic	Range in 95% of Normal Children	Mean Diastolic	Range in 95% of Normal Children
6 months–1 year	90	±25	61	±19
2–3 years	95	±24	61	±24
4–5 years	99	±21	65	±15
6 years	100	±15	56	± 8
8 years	105	±16	57	± 9
10 years	109	±16	58	±10
12 years	113	±18	59	±10
15 years	121	±19	61	±10

* Source: The Harriet Lane Handbook, 7th edition, Dennis L. Headings, ed., Copyright © 1975 by Year Book Medical Publishers, Inc., Chicago, 1975, p. 265. Used by permission.

General Considerations for Measuring Vital Signs

1. Vital sign values provide the nurse with only rough estimates of physiological activity. It is important to identify trends, sudden discrepancies and wide deviations from normal.
2. Vital signs should be taken as often as the nurse thinks necessary. They should not be delayed until the next scheduled time if it is suspected that a trend is developing.

Temperature

1. Normal body temperature represents a balance between the body heat produced and body heat lost.
2. The mode for taking the temperature should be kept as constant as possible.
3. Never leave the child alone when taking his temperature.
4. For security, safety, and accuracy keep 1 hand on the thermometer when it is in place.
5. Record the temperature value and method used.
6. Report an elevated or subnormal temperature and initiate whatever nursing measures are indicated by the child's condition.

* (From Johns Hopkins Hospital: The Harriet Lane Handbook, 7th edition. Copyright © 1975 by Year Book Medical Publishers, Inc., Chicago, p. 265. Used by permission.)

Data for ½–5 years from Allen-Williams, G. M.: Pulse-rate and blood pressure in infancy and early childhood. *Arch Dis. Child.*, 20: 125.

Data for 5–15 years from Graham, A. W.; Hines, E. A., Jr.; and Gage, R. P.: Blood pressure in children between the ages of 5 and 16 years. *Amer. J. Dis. Child.*, 69: 203.

*(Reproduced with permission from Johns Hopkins Hospital: The Harriet Lane Handbook, 7th Edition, Dennis L. Headings, Editor. Copyright © 1975 by Year Book Medical Publishers, Inc., Chicago.)

TABLE 9. NORMAL URINALYSIS VALUES IN INFANTS AND CHILDREN*

OSMOLALITY	Premature Infants—100–600 mOsm/L All Other Infants And Children—50–1400 mOsm/L
pH	Newborn—5–7 Thereafter—4.5–8
SPECIFIC GRAVITY	Newborn/Infants—1.001–1.020 Thereafter—1.001–1.030

*Vaughan, Victor C., and McKay, R. James (editors): *Nelson Textbook of Pediatrics* (10th ed.). Philadelphia, W. B. Saunders Company, 1975, p. 1796.

TABLE 10. NORMAL URINE FREQUENCY AND VOLUME IN INFANTS AND CHILDREN*

AGE	AMOUNT
FREQUENCY (VOIDING TIMES/24 HOURS)	
After 72 hours	20
3–6 months	20
6–12 months	16
1–2 years	12
2–3 years	10
3–4 years	9
12 years to adult	4–6
VOLUMES (ml/24 HOURS)	
Newborn	30–300
Neonatal	250–450
Infant	400–600
Child	500–1000
Adolescent	500–1500

*Avery, Gordon B. (editor): *Neonatology: Pathophysiology and Management of the Newborn.* Philadelphia, J. B. Lippincott Company, 1975, p. 489.

TABLE 11. SIGNS AND SYMPTOMS OF INFECTION IN INFANTS AND CHILDREN

1. Subnormal or elevated temperature in the neonate
2. Fever
3. Nausea
4. Vomiting
5. Diarrhea
6. Respiratory distress—tachypnea, nasal flaring, inspiratory chest retractions, expiratory grunting, cyanosis
7. Poor feeding
8. Lethargy
9. Weight loss
10. Mottled skin and jaundice in the infant

TABLE 12. SIGNS AND SYMPTOMS OF ACIDOSIS

INFANTS	CHILDREN
Poor feeding	Drowsiness
Lethargy	Dry skin
Failure to gain weight	Increased respiratory rate
Watery stools	Nausea
Increased respiratory rate	Vomiting
Gray pallor	Abdominal pain
	Lethargy
	Low serum bicarbonate

TABLE 13. SIGNS AND SYMPTOMS OF INCREASED INTRACRANIAL PRESSURE

Restlessness and irritability	Visual abnormalities
High-pitched or shrill cry	Sluggish unequal pupil response to light
Vomiting	Lethargy
Anorexia	Papilledema
Headache	Seizures
Bulging anterior fontanelle (Infants under 18 months)	Stupor
	Increasing temperature
	Coma

CHANGES IN VITAL SIGNS:

Increased blood pressure
Decreased pulse rate
Decreased and irregular respirations

Index

Page numbers in *italics* indicate figures; "t" indicates tabular matter.